Third Edition

Handbook of
Pathology
for Postgraduate Students

Third Edition

Handbook of Pathology for Postgraduate Students

Chief Editor
Sandhya Sundaram MD DNB FICP
Professor and Head
Department of Pathology
Sri Ramachandra Medical College and Research Institute
Chennai, Tamil Nadu

Editorial Board

D Prathiba MD DNB
Former Professor

S Rajendiran MD Dip. RC Path AB (AP & CP) AB (Cyto)
Professor

J Thanka MD DNB FICP
Professor

Febe Renjitha Suman MD
Professor

Assistant Editorial Team

V Pavithra MD
Assistant Professor

Divya D MD
Assistant Professor

Archana B MD
Demonstrator

Gokul Kripesh MD
Demonstrator

Department of Pathology
Sri Ramachandra Medical College and Research Institute
Sri Ramachandra Institute of Higher Education and Research
Chennai, Tamil Nadu

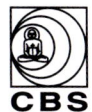

CBS Publishers & Distributors Pvt Ltd

New Delhi • Bengaluru • Chennai • Kochi • Kolkata • Mumbai
Bhopal • Bhubaneswar • Hyderabad • Jharkhand • Nagpur • Patna • Pune Uttarakhand
Dhaka (Bangladesh) • Kathmandu (Nepal)

Disclaimer

Science and technology are constantly changing fields. New research and experience broaden the scope of information and knowledge. The editors have tried their best in giving information available to them while preparing the material for this book. Although all efforts have been made to ensure optimum accuracy of the material, yet it is quite possible some errors might have been left uncorrected. The publisher, the printer and the editors will not be held responsible for any inadvertent errors or inaccuracies.

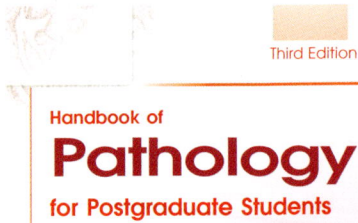

ISBN: 978-93-89688-61-0

Copyright © Editors and Publisher

Third Edition: 2020

First Edition: 2018
Second Edition: 2019

All rights reserved. No part of this book may be reproduced or transmitted in any form or by any means, electronic or mechanical, including photocopying, recording, or any information storage and retrieval system without permission, in writing, from the editors and the publisher.

Published by Satish Kumar Jain and produced by Varun Jain for

CBS Publishers & Distributors Pvt Ltd
4819/XI Prahlad Street, 24 Ansari Road, Daryaganj, New Delhi 110 002, India.
Ph: 23289259, 23266861, 23266867 Fax: 011-23243014 Website: www.cbspd.com
e-mail: delhi@cbspd.com; cbspubs@airtelmail.in.

Corporate Office: 204 FIE, Industrial Area, Patparganj, Delhi 110 092
Ph: 4934 4934 Fax: 4934 4935 e-mail: publishing@cbspd.com; publicity@cbspd.com

Branches

- **Bengaluru:** Seema House 2975, 17th Cross, K.R. Road,
  Banasankari 2nd Stage, Bengaluru 560 070, Karnataka
  Ph: +91-80-26771678/79 Fax: +91-80-26771680 e-mail: bangalore@cbspd.com
- **Chennai:** 7, Subbaraya Street, Shenoy Nagar, Chennai 600 030, Tamil Nadu
  Ph: +91-44-26680620, 26681266 Fax: +91-44-42032115 e-mail: chennai@cbspd.com
- **Kochi:** 68/1534, 35, 36, Power House Road, Opp KSEB, Power House, Ernakulam 682 018, Kochi, Kerala
  Ph: +91-484-4059061-65 Fax: +91-484-4059065 e-mail: kochi@cbspd.com
- **Kolkata:** 6/B, Ground Floor, Rameswar Shaw Road, Kolkata-700 014, West Bengal
  Ph: +91-33-22891126, 22891127, 22891128 e-mail: kolkata@cbspd.com
- **Mumbai:** 83-C, Dr E Moses Road, Worli, Mumbai-400018, Maharashtra
  Ph: +91-22-24902340/41 Fax: +91-22-24902342 e-mail: mumbai@cbspd.com

Representatives

• Bhopal	0-8319310552	• Bhubaneswar	0-9911037372	• Hyderabad	0-9885175004	• Jharkhand	0-9811541605
• Nagpur	0-9421945513	• Patna	0-9334159340	• Pune	0-9623451994	• Uttarakhand	0-9716462459
• Dhaka (Bangladesh)	01912-003485	• Kathmandu (Nepal)	977-9818742655				

Printed at: HT Media Ltd., Greater Noida, UP, India

Contributors

Faculty, Department of Pathology
Sri Ramachandra Medical College and Research Institute

D Prathiba MD DNB
Sandhya Sundaram MD DNB FICP
J Thanka MD DNB FICP
S Rajendiran MD Dip. RC Path AB (AP and CP) AB (Cyto)
Leena Dennis Joseph MD
Febe Renjitha Suman MD
CN Sai Shalini MD
M Susruthan MD
Lawrence D'Cruze MD
N Priyathershini MD

V Pavithra MD
G Barathi MD DCP DNB
S Sri Gayathri MD
Divya D MD
Subalakshmi B MD
GA Vasugi MD DNB
Archana B MD
Arthi M MD
Gokul Kripesh MD
Rithika Rajendran MD

Invited Contributors

Vinod Kumar Panicker MD
Dept. of Transfusion Medicine
SRMC and RI

R Krishnamoorthy MD
Dept. of Transfusion Medicine
SRMC and RI

Malathi N MDS
Oral Pathology
Sri Ramachandra Dental College

Rani Kanthan MS FRCS FRCPSC FCAP MEd
University of Saskatchewan, Canada

Shantha Ravisankar MD
TNGMSSH, Chennai

P Shanthi MD PhD
ALM PGIBMS, Chennai

Marie Therese Manipadam MD
CMC Vellore

N Siddaraju MD
JIPMER, Puducherry

Rajavelu Indira MD
Govt KG Hospital and ISO, Chennai

Shalinee Rao MD
AIIMS, Rishikesh, Uttarakhand

Anila Abraham Kurian MD
Renopath Lab, Chennai

K Swaminathan MD
Tirunelveli Medical College

MP Kanchana MD
Institute of Obstetrics and Gynaecology, Chennai

Foreword

I have great pleasure in congratulating Dr Sandhya Sundaram and the faculty members of Department of Pathology for successfully bringing out the third edition of this book titled *Handbook of Pathology for Postgraduate Students*. It is a sincere and praiseworthy effort by the Department and I am sure that it will prove to be a very useful resource and a ready-reckoner for postgraduate in their exam preparation.

It takes a lot of effort in bringing out the book in terms of content collection, collation, editing, refining and presentation. I am very happy to note that the first edition was very well received and that this edition has further refined the contents.

The effort is greatly commendable. I would like to appreciate Dr Sandhya Sundaram and her team.

I hope that the Department comes out with many such endeavors in future also.

I wish them all the very best.

Dr PV Vijayaraghavan
Vice-Chancellor
Sri Ramachandra Institute of Higher Education and Research
(Deemed to be University)

Foreword

I am delighted to note that Dr Sandhya Sundaram, Professor and Head, Department of Pathology, Sri Ramachandra Medical College and Research Institute, has developed her department's learning resources for postgraduates in pathology into a *Handbook of Pathology for Postgraduate Students*. It is appreciable that the third edition of of the book is being brought out with further updation of information. This Handbook is the collections of key topics in Pathology and the subject matter discussed in the Sri Ramachandra Pathology Annual Rapid Review Course (SPARRC) of the Department of Pathology which is being conducted every year since 2013. The contributors of the chapters include all the faculty members of the department and the invited external experts. It is laudable that the quality of the contents of the chapters are of high order with color photographs of the microscopic pictures of the lesions illustrated. The Handbook also has a chapter on the "Practical tips for the students taking up the MD Pathology Examination" which would be attractive for students.

In view of the current quality requirements of faculty members to write books and volumes on their respective discipline area(s), this effort of Dr Sandhya Sundaram to bring out the edited book as "Sri Ramachandra Medical College and Research Institute publication" is an innovative effort. The efforts of CBS Publishers and Distributors Pvt. Ltd. who have come forward to print and publish this Handbook is appreciated. I am sure that this Handbook would be of immense help to all the Pathology postgraduates across the country. My best wishes for continuation of similar efforts across the institution.

Prof SP Thyagarajan
Former Vice-Chancellor, University of Madras
Professor of Eminence and Dean (Research)
Sri Ramachandra Institute of Higher Education and Research

Messages

I congratulate the Department of Pathology for launching the third edition of the book entitled *Handbook of Pathology for Postgraduate Students*. I am happy that the earlier edition of this book was appreciated by pathology residents and young practising pathologists. It is to the credit of the faculty members of the Department of Pathology and external experts who have contributed to the making of this comprehensive resource material in pathology. I wish the participants all the very best.

Prof KV Somasundaram
Professor of Eminence and Advisor Academic
Sri Ramachandra Institute of Higher
Education and Research
(Deemed to be University)

Modern pathology has become increasingly complex and multifaceted with knowledge that is growing with each passing year. The efforts by the faculty members of Department of Pathology under the leadership of Dr Sandhya Sundaram to compile a concise book entitled *Handbook of Pathology for Postgraduate Students* are laudable. I congratulate the Department for bringing out the third edition of this book which encompasses essential areas of pathology with inclusion of newer entities and updated information of major changes in the old entities. Undoubtedly, the contents of this book will serve as a valuable resource for pathology residents and faculty.

Dr Mahesh Vakamudi
Dean of Faculties
Sri Ramachandra Institute of Higher
Education and Research
(Deemed to be University)

I am happy to note that the Department of Pathology is releasing the third edition of *Handbook of Pathology for Postgraduate Students* as a part of the highly acclaimed rapid revision course conducted by the Department. As in previous years, SPARRC provides an excellent forum for exchanging information and conducting discussions on a wide variety of pathology topics. I congratulate Dr Sandhya Sundaram and her team for compiling this very comprehensive, practical and yet concisely written book in Pathology.

My best wishes.

Dr A Ravikumar
Dean Education
Sri Ramachandra Institute of Higher
Education and Research
(Deemed to be University)

I am delighted that the Department of Pathology has brought out the third edition of the book titled *Handbook of Pathology for Postgraduate Students*. The varied topics highlighted in the book will equip the postgraduates to update their knowledge and excel in their examinations. I congratulate Dr Sandhya Sundaram and the faculty of Department of Pathology for compiling this very useful quick review book for the students.

Dr S Anandan
Dean
Sri Ramachandra Medical College and
Research Institute

Preface to the Third Edition

We are delighted to launch the third edition of the *Handbook of Pathology for Postgraduate Students*. The handbook comprises collection of topics discussed, based on standard reference material and is a combined and earnest effort of the entire faculty of Department of Pathology and invited experts. In this edition, we have added two more chapters based on the feedback by the postgraduate students. Additionally, we have included some more cases for discussion and a detailed list of bibliography and references at the end of the book. While we have taken every effort to screen the contents, some minor errors may have crept while compiling such varied topics and we regret it. We request your honest feedback and suggestions.

Dr Sandhya Sundaram
Chief Editor

Preface to the First Edition

Pathology is the key to the understanding of mechanistic basis of disease and is now being unravelled in a breath taking pace. It is our proud privilege to bring forth this book titled *Handbook of Pathology for Postgraduate Students*, which is a collection of topics from the very popular programme of the Department SPARRC "Sri Ramachandra Pathology Annual Rapid Review Course".

It is a quick review book which is a concise compilation of essential topics for Postgraduates in Pathology. The initial chapters in the book highlight the histologic characterstics of lesions from each organ system, which is a contribution by faculty of Pathology and invited experts. All the photomicrographs are from the case files of Department of Pathology, Sri Ramachandra Medical College and Research Institute and cases shared by our invited experts .We are indebted to our patients for the learning material. Hematology and Cytology cases are also discussed with bulleted learning points. Other essential areas include transfusion medicine, quality control and automation in pathology. Important points from common topics such as immunohistochemistry, autopsy, special stains and pedagogy are presented in a simplified manner. We have also included basics of current topics in pathology such as flow cytometry, molecular pathology, karyotyping, FISH, tissue banking and culture techniques. Some of the "must knows" in pathology has been summarized under the heading, Pearls in Pathology. Simple flow charts showing the approach to lesions are displayed along with useful tips for practical examination. This Handbook comprises collection of topics discussed, based on standard reference material. It is a collective and sincere effort of the entire faculty of Department of Pathology and invited experts. Besides being useful for postgraduates, it will also be useful for young faculty in pathology for easy reference and some of the case based approach maybe useful for undergraduate medical students. We hope that this book will enhance the confidence and knowledge of students of Pathology. Some minor errors may have creeped while compiling such varied topics and is regretted. Feedback and suggestions will be highly appreciated.

Dr Sandhya Sundaram
Chief Editor

Acknowledgments

The information provided in this Handbook for the young budding pathologists would not be possible without the contribution, support and teamwork of a host of dedicated people and Senior Administrative Heads of Sri Ramachandra Institute of Higher Education and Research, Chennai.

We extend our gratitude to our Chancellor Shri VR Venkataachalam, who has given his unstinted support to us in this endeavor. Our special thanks to our Pro-Chancellor Mr RV Sengutuvan for his constant support.

Our sincere thanks to Dr PV Vijayaraghavan, Vice-Chancellor, for giving us the opportunity and encouraging us to bring out this book. Our earnest thanks to Prof SP Thyagarajan, Professor of Eminence and Dean (Research) for his guidance at every stage and Dr S Anandan, Dean, Sri Ramachandra Medical College for his dynamic guidance. We also thank Dr KV Somasundaram, Professor of Eminence and Advisor—academic, Dr TK Parthasarathy, Professor of Eminence and Chief Advisor, Dr JSN Murthy, former Vice-Chancellor, Dr A Ravi Kumar, Dean, Education, Dr Mahesh Vakamudi, Dean of Faculties for their guidance. Our heartfelt thanks to Mr V Swaminathan, Registrar for his valuable suggestions and Mr N Natarajan, Special officer (Admin) for his advice. A word of thanks to Dr D Prathiba, Controller of Examination, for initiating the SPARRC Programme which has culminated in this compilation.

We would also like to thank our invited experts for sharing their wisdom and the faculty of Pathology for the keen enthusiasm. We also acknowledge the technical staff, Department of Pathology, for preparation of excellent glass slides and our energetic postgraduate students who helped with screening of the cases. Thanks to the Departments of Oral Pathology, Transfusion Medicine and Human Genetics, for their help. We thank all our clinical colleagues for their valuable interactions.

Finally, we thank all the pathology postgraduates' students and young faculty for whom this book has been prepared meticulously and we hope you find this helpful for your examinations and practice.

We extend our thanks to Mr SK Jain CMD, Mr YN Arjuna (Senior Vice—President Publishing, Editorial and Publicity), CBS Publishers and Distributors Pvt Ltd. and Mr. Saravanan for taking the effort to perfect the book. In spite of our sincere efforts there may be elements of error and we hope to improve with every edition.

Editors

Contents

Contributors	v
Foreword by Dr PV Vijayaraghavan	vii
Foreword by Prof SP Thyagarajan	viii
Preface to the Third Edition	xi
Preface to the First Edition	xii

1. Lesions of the Head and Neck — 1
2. Oral Lesions — 18
3. CNS Lesions — 23
4. Ophthalmic Lesions — 40
5. Spectrum of Breast Lesions — 46
6. Lesions of the Lung — 67
7. Approach to Gastrointestinal Biopsies — 84
8. Case Files of GIT Lesions — 90
9. Histological Approach to Hepatobiliary Lesions — 98
10. Patterns in Pancreatic and Gallbladder Lesions — 113
11. Medical Renal Disease — 123
12. Pathologic Lesions of Kidneys, Urethra and Urinary Bladder — 134
13. Male Genital Tract Lesions Including Prostate — 153
14. Diseases of the Female Genital Tract — 163
15. Soft Tissue Tumors and Tumor-like Lesions — 179
16. Lesions of the Bone and Joints — 195
17. Skin Lesions — 210
18. Non-neoplastic Lesions of the Lymph Node — 225
19. Diagnostic Approach to Lymphoma — 233
20. Endocrine Pathology — 245
21. Pap Smear—Gynecological Cytology — 261
22. A. Cytology Slide Case Discussion Part I — 272
    B. Cytology Slide Case Discussion Part II — 298
23. Hematology — 313
24. Approach to Bleeding Disorders — 337
25. Automation in Hematology/Clinical Pathology — 340

26. Component Preparation and Therapy	345
27. Blood Bank—Laboratory Procedures	349
28. Immunohistochemistry	352
29. Autopsy Highlights	363
30. Important Histochemical Stains	377
31. Flow Cytometry	387
32. Karyotyping—Basic Essentials	392
33. Fluorescence *in situ* Hybridization (FISH)	396
34. Molecular Pathology: Basics	402
35. Cell Culture and Tissue Banking Techniques	412
36. Quality Control in Histopathology	416
37. Quality Control in Hematology/Clinical Pathology	422
38. Pearls in Pathology	425
39. Criteria Revisited	434
40. Pedagogy in Points	441
41. Current Updates in Pathology	444
42. FAQs in Histotechniques	455

Potpourri of Cases — 464
General Tips for the Examination Going Postgraduates — 468
Glossary — 472
Bibliography — 478

CHAPTER 1

Lesions of the Head and Neck

D Prathiba, Lawrence D'Cruze

Case History: A 20-year-old boy with history of epistaxis.

Diagnosis: Nasopharyngeal angiofibroma

Clinical Features

- Young males (2nd decade).
- Present with nasal obstruction and epistaxis.
- Arise from posterolateral wall-roof of nose.
- Locally aggressive, may extend into sinuses or base of skull.

Gross

Well circumscribed, unencapsulated, polypoid mass.

Microscopy

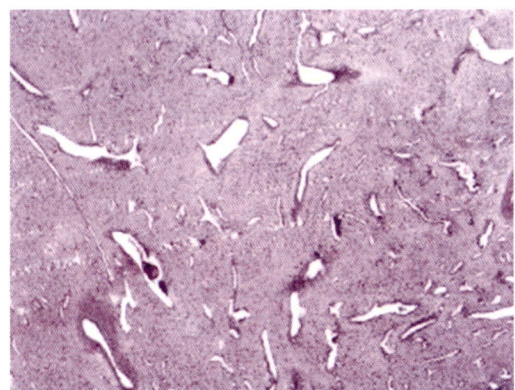

Fig. 1.1

- Fibrocollagenous stromal proliferation, admixed with variable sized staghorn or stellate vascular spaces.
- Vessel wall lack elastic fibers and have a smooth muscle layer (discontinuous) and show marked variation in thickness.
- Stromal cells are spindle-shaped and stellate with plump nuclei, and tend to radiate around blood vessels.

Immunohistochemistry

Stromal cells: Vimentin and c-kit/CD117+; endothelial and stromal cell nuclei AR+ (75%).

Differential Diagnosis

- **Hemangiopericytoma:** All age groups; Females; Cellular tumor, staghorn-shaped irregular vascular spaces, may be hyalinised with spindle (SMA+, CD34–)/round cells: Rare mitosis.
- **Solitary fibrous tumor:** Mixture of hyalinized stroma, ropey collagen, spindle cells, and vessels. Stromal cells CD34+
- **Lobular capillary hemangioma:** Nasal septum (60%), lobular arrangement. Large central vessel surrounded by tightly packed capillaries.
- **Kaposi sarcoma:** Immunocompromised patients/HIV; slit-like vascular spaces with extravasated red blood cells and hyaline globules. HHV-8+
- **Angiosarcoma:** Rare in nasopharynx. Anastomosing, irregularly shaped vascular spaces lined by atypical endothelial cells (CD31+, CD34+). High mitotic rate.

Case History: A 58-year-old lady with right parotid gland enlargement.

Diagnosis: Epithelial–myoepithelial carcinoma

Clinical Features

- Rare tumor
- Frequent local recurrence.
- Painful localized swelling.
- Mean age 60 years; women (60%).

Gross

- Well-delineated and multilobular. Firm, solid, gray-white
- Typically 2–3 cm.

Microscopy

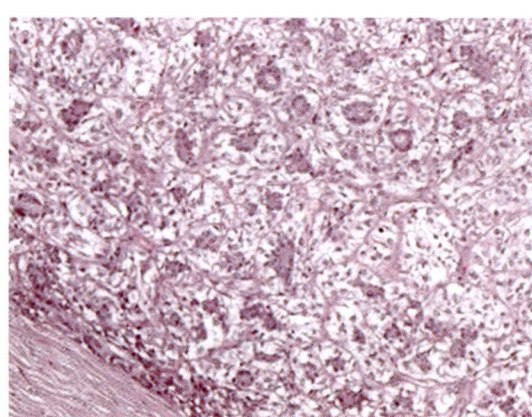

Fig. 1.2

- Biphasic; myoepithelial cells and ductal cells.
- Myoepithelial cells: Relatively large, polygonal to spindle-shaped cells with clear cytoplasm and eccentrically located nuclei.
- Ductal cells: Smaller, uniform cuboidal cells with eosinophilic cytoplasm and round nuclei.
- Cytologic atypia is mild. Variable mitosis.
- Stroma—loose, myxoid to collagenous and hyalinized.
- Infiltration and perineural invasion (occasional).

Immunohistochemistry

- Ductal cells (CK+)
- Myoepithelial cells (p63+, S-100+, SMA+).

Variants

- Apocrine
- Dedifferentiated
- Double clear
- Ex-pleomorphic adenoma
- Oncocytic (senescence phenotype)
- With myoepithelial anaplasia.

Differential Diagnosis

- **Pleomorphic adenoma:** Biphasic epithelial/myoepithelial cells. Myxochondroid matrix merging with epithelial population. Bilayered tubule formation is not prominent, nor is clear cell population.
- **Myoepithelioma:** A spindle cell neoplasm without ductal or tubule formation.
- **Oncocytoma, clear cell type:** Large polygonal cells without biphasic appearance. Clear cell change may predominant but oncocytic granular cytoplasm is still found.
- **Mucoepidermoid carcinoma:** Lack biphasic pattern. Proper sampling will reveal cyst formation, mucocytes and transitional pattern focally in the tumor.
- **Myoepithelial carcinoma:** Unencapsulated, multinodular, invasive. Cytologically bland. Duct formation is not a component of this tumor.
- **Adenoid cystic carcinoma:** Cribriform architecture with ductal cells often inconspicuous and smaller with more hyperchromatic, angulated nuclei. Infiltrative growth/perineural invasion.
- **Clear cell acinic cell carcinoma:** Lacks biphasic appearance. Clear cells are small and nondominant. Basophilic granular cytoplasm predominates. No myoepithelial cell phenotype by immunohistochemistry.
- **Clear cell carcinoma:** Minor salivary glands, unencapsulated, negative for myoepithelial markers.

Prognosis

Recurrence related to margin status, angiolymphatic invasion, necrosis, myoepithelial anaplasia.

Case History: A 58-year-old male, pain in the right maxillary region.

Diagnosis: Mucormycosis

Clinical Features

- Associated with poor glycemic control or immunosuppression.
- Predilection for arterial invasion, extensive emboli and necrosis.

Clinical Forms of the Disease

- Rhinocerebral
- Pulmonary
- Gastrointestinal
- Cutaneous
- Disseminated

Microscopy

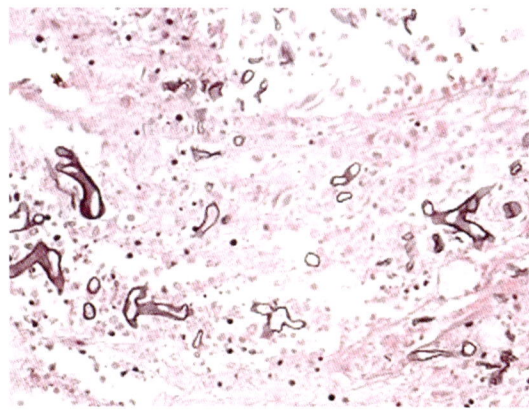

Fig. 1.3

- A septate broad thin-walled hyphae, with irregular nonparallel contours and haphazardly branched.
- Tissue infarction and acute suppurative inflammation (granulomas rare).

Differential Diagnosis

- **Aspergillus:** Septate, narrow, acutely branching hyphae with smooth, parallel walls. Viable hyphae (deeply basophilic); Necrotic hyphae (hyaline). Fruiting bodies may be present.
- **Candida:** Septate, narrow hyphae, with club-shaped pseudohyphae and oval yeast forms present.

Prognosis

Infection once established is difficult to treat and is rapidly fatal.

Case History: A 45-year-old male with swelling of the left parotid region.

Diagnosis: Mucoepidermoid carcinoma

Clinical Features

- Most common malignant salivary gland neoplasm in adults and children.
- Most common radiation induced neoplasm.
- Parotid gland (45%), palate (21%).

Gross

- Ill-defined mass, may be partially encapsulated
- Firm to hard consistency
- Gray-tan cut surface and mucin filled cysts.

Microscopy

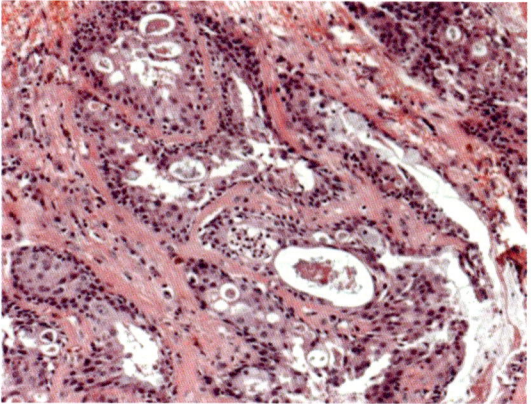

Fig. 1.4

- Irregular invasive borders; tumor nests composed of mucous, squamoid (epidermoid), intermediate cells in variable combinations.
- Stroma is characteristically sclerotic and abundant, with chronic inflammatory cells and occasional extravasated mucin pools.
- No squamous cell carcinoma *in situ*.

Variants of Mucoepidermoid Carcinoma
- Clear cell variant
- Oncocytic variant
- Sclerosing variant
- Sclerosing mucoepidermoid carcinoma with eosinophilia.

Immunohistochemistry
- **MUC1:** Associated with high histologic grade, high recurrence/metastasis rate.
- **MUC4:** It is low histologic grade, low
- **MUC5AC:** Distinguish high-grade mucoepidermoid carcinoma from squamous cell carcinoma.
- **Low grade:** CK 7+ (squamous cell carcinoma usually negative), p63+ in intermediate, epidermoid cells, help distinguish from acinic cell carcinoma and oncocytoma.

AFIP Scoring Point System
- 2 points if <20% intracystic component
- 2 points if necrosis
- 2 points if neural invasion
- 3 points if 4+ mitotic figures/10 HPF
- 4 points if anaplasia

Low grade: Total score is 0–4 points
Intermediate grade: Total score is 5–6 points.
High grade: Total score is >7 points.

Differential Diagnosis
- **Sialometaplasia (from low-grade MEC):** Lobular, lacks cystic growth, no intermediate cells. Squamous metaplasia following FNA. Squamous nests are seen admixed with ductal elements.
- **Mucous extravasation reaction:** Mucous found primarily in macrophages. No intermediate/epithelial cells.
- **Cystadenocarcinoma:** Cystic/papillary architecture. Lacks intermediate cells. Cyst lined by columnar/cuboidal epithelium, monomorphic cells (less variations in cell types).
- **Squamous cell (metastatic) carcinoma:** Known skin/mucosal primary. Well developed keratinization. Lacks intermediate cells and mucocytes.
- **Salivary duct carcinoma:** High grade tumor, high mitosis and comedonecrosis.

Genetic Features
Translocation (11;19) and resultant fusion gene (CRTC1/MAML2).

Poor Prognostic Factors
Histologic grade older male, submandibular gland, extraglandular extension, vascular invasion, necrosis and high mitosis.

Case History: A 38-year-old male with palatal lesion.

Diagnosis: Adenoid cystic carcinoma

Clinical Features
- Parotid gland, submandibular gland, and palate are commonly involved.
- 4th to 6th decades
- Slow growing, indolent, sometimes painful mass.

Gross
Well circumscribed tan, fleshy, firm but it is deceptively infiltrative.

Microscopy

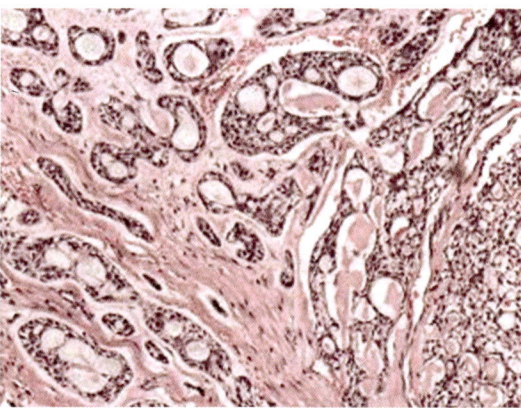

Fig. 1.5

- Cribriform, tubular and solid growth patterns. Stroma is fibrous with variable

amounts of myxohyaline material rather than desmoplastic.
- The cribriform structures are the most characteristic feature. Discrete to coalescent islands comprising small, uniform basaloid cells with angulated nuclei, punctuated by round rigid spaces with PAS+ basement membrane material and mucin, giving rise to a "Swiss cheese" appearance.
- Peripheral–perineural invasion.

Grading
- **Low grade (grade 1):** Tubular and cribriform patterns.
- **Intermediate grade (grade 2):** 30–70% solid.
- **High grade (grade 3):** >70% solid.

Immunohistochemistry
- **Basaloid cells:** CK+, S-100+, p63+
- **Ductal epithelial cells:** CK+, CEA+, CD117+, EMA+

Differential Diagnosis
- **Pleomorphic adenoma:** May show squamous metaplasia and mesenchyme-like areas; plasmacytoid and spindle cells; ducts are present; No invasion.
- **Basal cell adenoma:** In absence of invasive borders the cribriform islands if present appear to be formed by expanded jigsaw puzzle like lobules punctuated by multiple cystic spaces and they merge with the characteristic basaloid lobules of basal cell adenoma. Cells are basaloid with nuclear palisading and round to oval nuclei and nuclear grooving.
- **Basal cell adenocarcinoma:** Discrete jigsaw puzzle like islands; cribriform structures absent or very focal. Lack basophilic mucous substance in stroma which is commonly seen in adenoid cystic carcinoma. Intercellular hyaline droplets are common, it is whereas very rare in ACC.
- **Epithelial-myoepithelial carcinoma:** Dual cell population (ductal and abluminal clear cells). Rare cribriform pattern.

Case History: A 62-year-old male with bilateral parotid enlargement.

Diagnosis: Warthin's tumor (papillary cystadenoma lymphomatosum)

Clinical Features
- Males (usually), smokers, aged 40+ years.
- Parotid gland
- Bilateral
- May occur synchronous with pleomorphic adenoma and salivary duct carcinoma.

Gross
- Well circumscribed, fluctuant mass.
- Cut surface shows brown mucoid and turbid materials in cystic spaces; 10–15% multifocal.
- 2–5 cm in size.

Microscopy

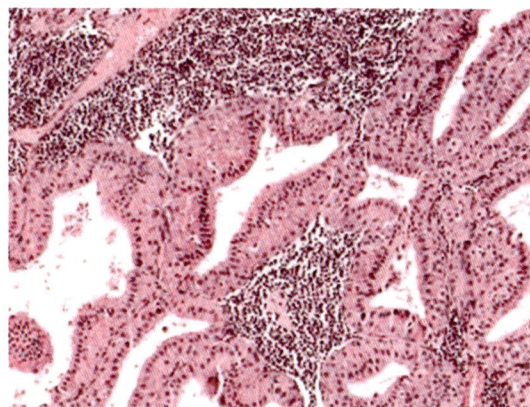

Fig. 1.6

- Double layer of epithelial cells resting on dense lymphoid stroma with variable germinal centers.
- Cystic spaces narrowed by polypoid projections of lymphoepithelial elements.
- Surface palisading of oncocytic columnar cells with underlying discontinuous basal cells.

Differential Diagnosis
- **Oncocytoma:** Lack of prominent lymphoid component, papillae and glands.

- **Squamous cell carcinoma/mucoepidermoid carcinoma (MEC):** Squamous metaplastic Warthin's tumor if infarcted can be mistaken for squamous cell carcinoma/MEC. Warthin tumor lacks keratinization. Compare to low grade MEC Warthin's tumor lack infiltration and tumor cells appear too frankly squamous.

Case History: A 51-year-old male with right submandibular lesion.

Diagnosis: Salivary duct carcinoma (SDC)

Clinical Features
- Rapidly enlarging mass
- Facial palsy (42%)
- Cervical lymphadenopathy.

Gross
- Poorly circumscribed
- Solid, tan, necrosis +, infiltration of adjacent parenchyma (70%).

Microscopy

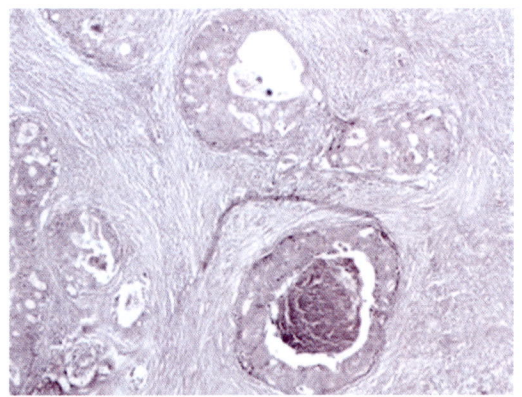

Fig. 1.7

- Glandular/ductal structures with infiltration
- Solid areas, cords, nests, or small cystic spaces.
- Large ducts with "Roman bridges" and comedo necrosis.
- The tumor cells have apocrine appearance, with abundant eosinophilic cytoplasm, large pleomorphic vesicular nuclei, and prominent nucleoli, desmoplasia.
- Perineural and perivascular invasion.
- Numerous mitotic figures.

Variants
- Sarcomatoid variant
- Mucin-rich variant.
- Invasive micropapillary variant.
- Oncocytic variant

Immunohistochemistry
- Androgen receptor expression (>90%)
- CK, EMA, and CEA +++; EGFR (1/2 the cases)
- HER2 positive (17%).

Differential Diagnosis
- **High-grade mucoepidermoid carcinoma:** Resemble SDC particularly in frozen sections. Mixture of cell types such as epidermoid cells and goblet cells is not seen in SDC.
- **Oncocytic carcinoma:** Large tumor cells with granular cytoplasm. Lack comedo necrosis and intraductal like pattern seen in SDC.
- **Cystadenocarcinoma:** Lack comedo necrosis and intraductal like pattern seen in SDC.
- **Intraductal carcinoma:** No invasion. Thorough sampling to rule out invasive component. IHC to demonstrate myoepithelial layer around tumor cells. If invasion is present the alternative interpretation is SDC which is highly aggressive neoplasm.
- **Metastatic breast/prostatic carcinoma:** Clinical history, positive ER/PR and negative AR strongly favor a metastatic breast carcinoma

Case History: A 10-year-old girl with unilateral nasal obstruction.

Diagnosis: Olfactory neuroblastoma (esthesioneuroblastoma)

Clinical Features
- Bimodal (age range: 3 years and 90 years).
- Located at roof of nasal cavity
- Nasal obstruction and hemorrhage.

Gross
- Reddish-gray, vascular
- Polypoid mass with soft consistency.

Microscopy

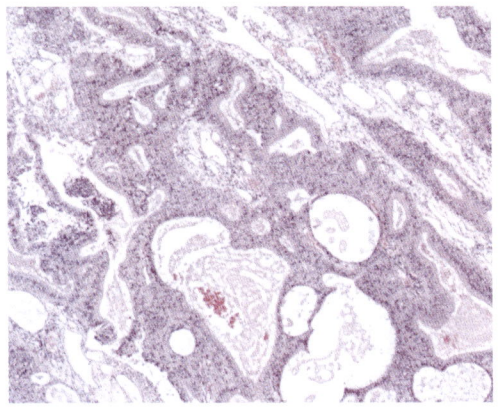

Fig. 1.8

- Lobular nests of uniform, relatively small monomorphic cells with round nuclei, fine and coarse chromatin, scant cytoplasm, and indistinct cell membrane.
- Nests surrounded by fibrovascular cores and sustentacular cells.
- Neoplastic small blue cells infiltrate into the submucosa as single cells and in nests. Neurofibrillary stroma is present.
- Ganglion cells (rare), but when present are diagnostic.
- Homer Wright pseudorosettes or Flexner-type rosettes.

Immunohistochemistry

- Synaptophysin, chromogranin, NSE, NF positive. S-100++ in sustentacular cells surrounding tumor nest.
- CEA and EMA negative.

Differential Diagnosis

- **Non-Hodgkin's lymphoma:** CD45+ and other lymphoid markers.
- **Ewing/PNET:** CD99+, FLI1+, t(11,22)/FLI1-EWSR1 fusion
- **Melanoma:** Positive for S100, SOX10, MelanA, HMB45
- **Small cell undifferentiated neuroendocrine carcinoma:** Diffusely positive for cytokeratin, negative for neurofilament and S100.
- **Rhabdomyosarcoma:** Shows diffuse positivity for desmin and myogenin
- **SNUC:** Tumor cells are negative for synaptophysin and chromogranin.
- **NUT midline carcinoma (NMC):** Positive for NUT (nuclear expression - by IHC); t(15,19) fusion oncogene BRD4-NUT; NMC should be considered in any non-smoking patients with poorly differentiated squamous cell.

Prognosis

Clinical staging for olfactory neuroblastoma, Kadish et al		
Stage	Extent of tumor	5-year survival (%)
A	Tumor confined to nasal cavity	75–91
B	Tumor involves nasal cavity plus one or more paranasal sinuses	68–71
C	Extension of tumor beyond the sinonasal cavities; 20% develop distant metastases, usually to cervical lymph nodes and lung	41–47

Late recurrence (after 10 years) is common.

Hyams (4 grades) histopathological classification for olfactory neuroblastoma							
Grade	Lobular architecture preservation	Mitotic index	Nuclear polymorphism	Fibrillary matrix	Rosettes	Necrosis	Calcification
I	+	Zero	None	Prominent	HW	–	Variable
II	+	Low	Low	Present	HW	–	Variable
III	+/–	Moderate	Moderate	Low	HW	Rare	Absent
IV	+/–	High	High	Absent	+/–	Frequent	Absent

Case History: A 63-year-old lady with a slow-growing right parotid mass.

Diagnosis: Basal cell adenoma (BCA)

Clinical Features
- 6th and 7th decades female
- Solitary, slow-growing mass

Gross
- Well circumscribed
- Solid, occasionally cystic tumor with homogeneous, light tan to brown cut surfaces.
- Cartilage-like or mucoid characteristic of pleomorphic adenoma is lacking.

Microscopy

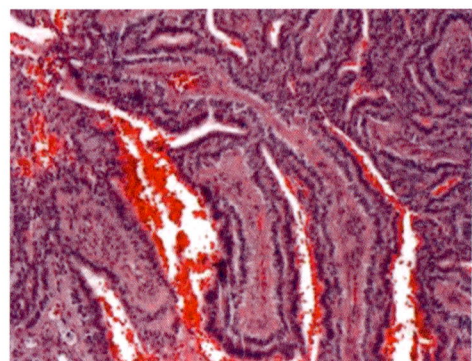

Fig. 1.9

- Tumor surrounded by fibrous capsule. Typical anastomosing jigsaw puzzle-like islands and trabeculae, imparting a plexiform appearance.
- Discrete/anastomosing tubules with lumens containing PAS positive eosinophilic secretion.
- Tumor islands are sharply demarcated from the hyalinized, stroma by basement membrane, differing from the centrifugal or "melting" growth of pleomorphic adenoma.
- *Basal cell adenoma comprises two cell types:* Basaloid cells (with basal cell or myoepithelial phenotype) and luminal cells.
- *Subtypes:* Trabecular type, solid type, tubular type, membranous type.

Differential Diagnosis
- **Pleomorphic adenoma (mixed tumor):** Biphasic population of epithelial and mesenchymal cells in the background of chondromyxoid matrix. Lack jigsaw pattern.
- **Adenoid cystic carcinoma:** Cribriform variant of BCA is mistaken for ACC. Features favoring BCA (Cribriform variant) include tumor encapsulation and expanded jigsaw puzzle-like basaloid islands at least focally.
- **Basal cell adenocarcinoma:** Low grade malignancy similar to basal cell adenoma but infiltrative with perineurial invasion and vascular invasion.

Case History: A 59-year-old male with palatal lesion.

Diagnosis: Clear cell carcinoma: hyalinizing type

Clinical Features
- Adult women
- Slow growing
- Painless submucosal mass
- Minor salivary glands (usually).

Gross
Reddish grey mass

Microscopy

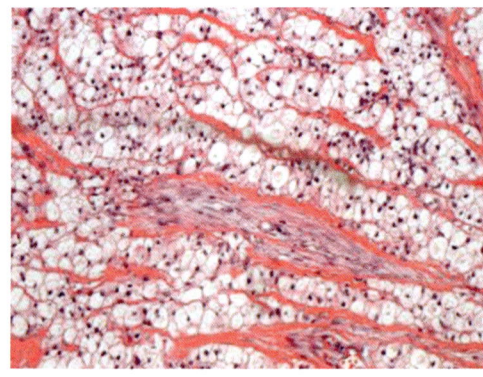

Fig. 1.10

- Infiltrative tumor
- Uniform clear cells forming trabeculae, cords, islands or nests surrounded by abundant hyalinized (PAS+) and focal myxoid stroma.

Immunohistochemistry
Cytokeratin, EMA.

Differential Diagnosis

Differential diagnosis of clear cell tumors of salivary gland

	Clear cell Oncocytoma	CCC	MEC	EMC	Clear cell Myoepithelioma and myoepithelial carcinoma	Acinic cell carcinoma	Metastatic renal cell carcinoma
Nature of the clear cells	Oncocytes	Ductal cells	Intermediate and mucinous cells	Myoepithelial cells	Myoepithelial cells	Acinic cells	Neoplastic renal epithelial cells
Growth pattern	Encapsulated	Infiltrative, solid/trabecular; hyalinized stroma	Infiltrative	Infiltrative; bicellular architecture	Lobules, nest, trabeculae, and fascicles	Infiltration in broad fronts	Prominent sinusoids; hemorrhage and hemosiderin deposition
Cytologic features of clear cells	Round nuclei, centrally located, with peripherally located rim of cytoplasmic granularity	Polygonal cells with water clear cytoplasm; nucleus centrally/eccentrically located	Intermediate cells are large with water clear cytoplasm; mucinous cells have flocculent cytoplasm	Polygonal cells with basally/centrally located nuclei; water-clear cytoplasm	Cells are polygonal or spindly; variable nuclear atypia.	Peripherally located nuclei; sparse basophilic granules in some cells	Water-clear cytoplasm; variable nuclear atypia.
Staining characteristic of clear cells	PTAH+, mitochondrial antibody+	CK+, EMA+ P63−	CK+ p63+	SOX10+, S100+, p63+ (outer layer)	SOX10+ S100+, p63+	SOX10+, PAS-D +	CK+, EMA+, PAX8+, CD10+, myoepithelial markers

Lesions of the Head and Neck

Case History: A 30-year-old female with painful slow-growing right parotid mass.

Diagnosis: Acinic cell carcinoma

Clinical Features

- Slow growing mass, basal malignant tumor (3%).
- Parotid gland (84%)
- Female; mean age 44 years.

Gross

- Circumscribed
- Incomplete capsule
- It can be multinodular or infiltrative.
- Cut surface is solid, firm, cystic areas +/−.

Microscopy

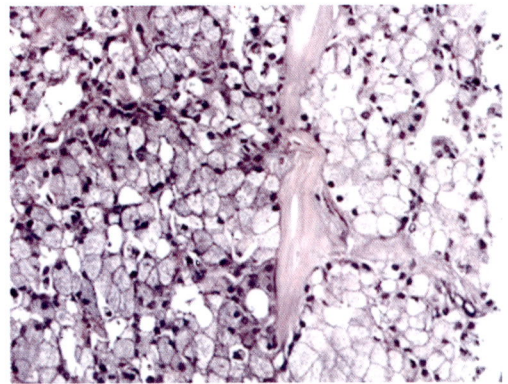

Fig. 1.11

- At scanning power, basophilia and prominent lymphoid infiltrate should raise suspicion of acinic cell carcinoma.
- *Four growth patterns:* Solid, microcystic, papillary, cystic, and follicular; mixed pattern.
- Cells may show acinar, intercalated duct, vacuolated, and clear features.
- Classic acinic cell carcinoma shows sheets of large, polygonal cells with uniform, round, eccentric nuclei and coarsely granular vacuolated cytoplasm.
- Lobular architecture of the normal salivary gland is lacking; normal acinar cells are triangular, whereas tumor cells are polygonal.

Immunohistochemistry

DOG.1

Differential Diagnosis

- **Oncocytoma:** Oncocytes with round nuclei, centrally located, with cytoplasmic granularity. PTAH+
- **Adenoid cystic carcinoma:** Cribriform architecture; CD117+
- **Normal salivary gland tissue:** Especially in biopsies—tumors lack striated and interlobular ducts, lack lobular architecture
- **Metastatic thyroid carcinoma:** IHC for TTF1 and Calcitonin confirms metastatic thyroid (medullary) carcinoma.
- **Granular cell tumor:** Cells with indistinct cell borders and abundant granular cytoplasm with centrally located nuclei. S100+.

Case History: A 20-year-old male with neck swelling.

Diagnosis: Branchial cleft cyst

Microscopy

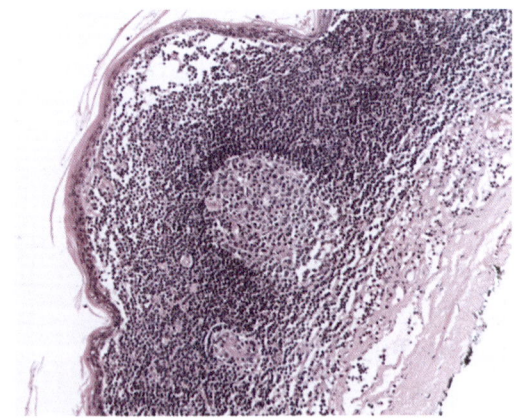

Fig. 1.12

- Cyst and fistulous tract lined by squamous, columnar or ciliated epithelium. Subepithelial stroma contains lymphoid tissue.
- Lining contains mucinous and serous or even sebaceous glands particularly when located in lower neck area.
- Cyst may contain a nucleated squames, histiocytes and cholesterol clefts.

Lesions of the Head and Neck

Differential Diagnosis

- **Squamous cell carcinoma metastatic to lymph nodes with secondary cystic change:** Must be considered in all adult patients with neck mass.
- **Cystic papillary thyroid carcinoma metastatic to lymph node:** TTF-1 and thyroglobulin will be positive.

Case History: A 30-year-old lady presented with lateral nasal wall mass.

Diagnosis: Sinonasal papilloma (schneiderian papilloma)

Clinical Features

Nasal obstruction stuffiness or epistaxis.

Microscopy

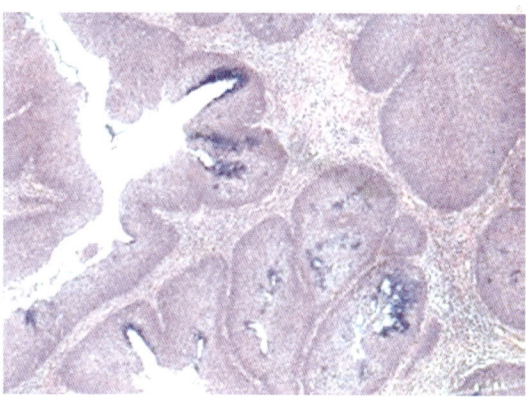

Fig. 1.13

Table 1.1: Types of schneiderian papillomas			
Type	Common location	Pathology	Prognosis
Exophytic/fungiform/septal M > F: Younger age	Nasal septum	**Gross**: Papillary, exophytic, verrucoid; pink-tan appearance, firm to rubbery; attached to mucosa by stalk. **Micro**: Exophytic fronds of bland epithelium—squamous, transitional, or respiratory type; intraepithelial neutrophils and microcysts. Often HPV 6/11+	Local recurrence; No risk of invasive carcinoma
Inverted	Lateral nasal wall; paranasal sinuses	**Gross**: Large, bulky, translucent masses, red-gray, firm to friable. **Micro**: Endophytic or "inverted" growth pattern, thickened squamous epithelial proliferation; epithelium is bland composed of squamous/transitional/columnar cells (all three may be present in a given lesion); admixed mucocytes (goblet cells), intraepithelial mucous cysts, inflammatory cell. Cytologic atypia may be present. Variably positive for HPV and EBV	Local recurrence; ~10% risk of invasive carcinoma
Oncocytic M = F	Lateral nasal wall; paranasal sinuses	**Gross**: Fleshy polypoidal. **Micro**: Exophytic and endophytic pushing nests of columnar, oncocytic cells with abundant, granular eosinophilic cytoplasm; intraepithelial neutrophils and microcysts HPV negative	Local recurrence; ~5–15% risk of invasive carcinoma

Differential Diagnosis

- **Sinonasal inflammatory polyp:** Respiratory lining epithelium lacking hyperplastic changes seen in sinonasal papilloma and also lack microcysts, transmigrating neutrophils as seen in sinonasal papilloma.
- **Nonintestinal type sinonasal adenocarcinoma:** Has oncocytic cytomorphology but shows architectural complexity with marked atypia as compared to the simple exophytic/endophytic growth pattern with bland cells seen in oncocytic papilloma.
- **Nonkeratinizing squamous cell carcinoma:** Infiltrative growth, marked nuclear atypia, frequent mitosis and desmoplastic reaction.
- **Verrucous carcinoma:** Epidermis with hyperkeratosis, papillomatosis, acanthosis and bulbous rete ridges invading deep dermis in a pushing manner which is not encountered in inverted papilloma.

Case History: A 40-year-old female with painless rapidly growing right parotid mass.

Diagnosis: Carcinoma ex-pleomorphic adenoma (CEPA)

Clinical Features
- Parotid gland (>75% of cases)
- Rare <30 years, women
- Long-standing/recurrent parotid mass with recent, rapid growth; typically painless.

Gross
- Poorly circumscribed with infiltrative margins.
- Cut surface is tan-gray with hemorrhage, necrosis, and cystic degeneration.

Microscopy
- Diagnosis requires presence of benign mixed tumor areas (either concomitantly or as recurrence) in addition to malignant carcinomatous component.
- Epithelial component is malignant; most commonly classified as adenocarcinoma NOS.

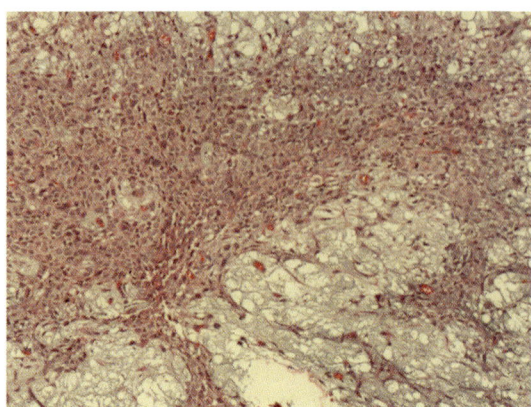

Fig. 1.14

- Infiltrates capsule and adjacent soft tissue; tumor may be localized without capsular involvement (encapsulated, *in situ*, or noninvasive carcinoma ex-mixed tumor) perineural invasion, vascular necrosis and hemorrhage present in high grade tumors.

Differential Diagnosis
- **Salivary duct carcinoma:** The carcinomatous component in a ca-ex-PA may be a high grade (salivary duct carcinoma, SCC, adenosquamous carcinoma) or a low-intermediate grade (PLGA, EMC, ACS, myoepithelial carcinoma). Previous history for evidence of pleomorphic adenoma and/or thorough sampling will identify foci of pleomorphic adenoma (may be chondromyxoid stroma, benign tubular ductular structures/hyalinised nodular stroma with benign epithelial and myoepithelial cells).

Note: Extensive hyalinization in a pleomorphic adenoma is associated with increased risk of malignant transformation. Presence of hyalinised focus/nodule near to a malignancy is evidence of residual pleomorphic adenoma supporting diagnosis of CEPA.

- **Carcinosarcoma:** Epithelial and heterologous mesenchymal malignant components.

Case History: A 51-year-old lady presented with history of blood stained post-nasal drip.

Diagnosis: Nasopharyngeal carcinoma

NPC is a squamous cell carcinoma that originates from nasopharyngeal mucosa showing evidence of squamous differentiation by light microscopy and IHC.

Notes: The designation lymphoepithelioma is a misnomer; this tumor is entirely of epithelial origin with a secondary associated benign lymphoid component.

Regaud and Schmincke are referred to pattern of growth and have no practical significance in diagnosis, treatment or prognosis.

Clinical Features

- Signs and symptoms are often subtle.
- 50% patients presence with asymptomatic cervical neck mass in the posterior cervical triangle/superior jugular nodal chain.
- They also present with nasal discharge, epistaxis and otitis media.

Laboratory Test

- CK positive, highlights malignant cells within lymphoid stroma.
- EBV latent membrane protein-1 (LMP-1) by IHC weak positive (1/3rd)
- ISH demonstrates specific viral mRNA of EBV in tumor cell nuclei (EBER)
- Elevated titres of IgG and IgA in serum (detection rates 93%)
- HLA-A2, HLA-B17 loci, marker of genetical susceptibility to NPC.

Gross

Mucosal bulge to mass lesions in fossa of Rosenmuller. Unidentifiable lesion fortuitously sampled ("blind biopsy").

Microscopy

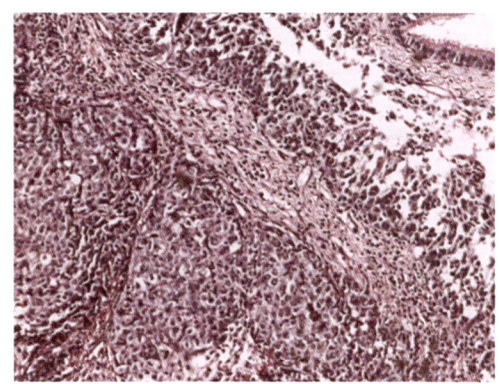

Fig. 1.15

	Keratinizing	Nonkeratinizing	Undifferentiated
Age	Approximately 25	Less common, <15	Most common, >60
Sex, age	M > F; 4th–6th decades	M > F; 4th–6th decades	M > F; 4th–6th decades; may occur in children
H/P	Keratinization, intercellular bridges; conventional squamous carcinoma graded as well, moderately, or poorly differentiated; desmoplastic response to invasion	A little to absent keratinization, growth pattern interconnecting cords (similar to transitional urothelial carcinoma); desmoplastic response to invasion absent	Absence of keratinization, syncytial growth, cohesive or non-cohesive cells with round nucleoli, scant cytoplasm and numerous mitosis; prominent non-neoplastic lymphoid component; typically absence of desmoplastic response to invasion
EBV	Weak association; associated with smoking	Strong association	Strong association
T/t	Radioresponsiveness is not good	Radioresponsive	Radioresponsive
Prognosis	20–40%, 5-year survival	65%, 5-year survival	65%, 5-year survival
Metastasis	Unusual	Cervical LNs unilateral	Often; cervical LNs unilateral

Differential Diagnosis

- **Non-Hodgkin's lymphoma:** IHC: CD45+; CK–
- **Hodgkin's lymphoma:** IHC: Increased eosinophils and plasma cells, CD15+, CD30+.
- **Malignant melanoma:** IHC: HMB45+, S-100+
- **Metastatic carcinoma**
- **Sinonasal undifferentiated carcinoma (SNUC):** Overlapping histology especially with NPC, nonkeratinizing undifferentiated type. Tumor bulk should be located in the sinonasal region but may extend to involve nasopharynx SNUC are EBER negative. No keratinization or lymphocyticin filtrate.

Importance in Differentiating NPC from SNUC

Mark difference in treatment and prognosis between these two types:
- *NPC:* Radio responsive; overall good prognosis.
- *SNUC:* Not radio responsive; poor prognosis and often lethal over relatively short time period.

HPV Associated Head and Neck Squamous Cell Carcinoma (HNSCC)

- Overlapping histology with NPC, nonkeratinizing differentiated and undifferentiated types. EBV-associated HNSCC and HPV-associated NPC can present as neck mass in the face of an occult primary neoplasm. History and IHC (CK/p63) also cannot differentiate these lesions. Presence of EBV support NPC and presence of HPV support oropharyngeal origin.

Rhabdomyosarcoma

Desmin/myogenin positive; CK/EBER negative.

Prognosis of NPC

Better Prognosis

Early clinical stage, younger patient, non-keratinizing histology.

Worst Prognosis

Higher stage, old patient, male gender, HLA Aw33-C3-B58/DR3 haplotype.

Sinonasal Undifferentiated Carcinoma (SNUC)

Tumor bulk should be located in the sinonasal region but may extend to involve nasopharynx. EBV negative. No keratinization or lymphocytic infiltrate.

References

1. Diagnostic histopathology of tumors, christopher D.M. Fletcher, fourth edition.
2. Differential Diagnosis in Surgical Pathology, Gattuso et al, second edition.
3. Pathology outlines.com

Suggested Reading

1. Gland tumors: A clue to the histogenesis for tumor diagnosis.
2. Rie Ohtomo et al; SOX10 is a novel marker of acinus and intercalated duct differentiation in salivary. Modern pathology 2013; 26: 1041–1050.

Lesions of the Head and Neck

APPROACH TO HEAD AND NECK

Nasal cavity and paranasal sinuses

Congenital/Hereditary
Nasal glial heterotopia
Nasal dermoid cyst and sinus

Infectious
- Allergic fungal sinusitis
- Mycetoma
- Rhinoscleroma
- Invasive fungal sinusitis
- Rhinosporidiosis

Inflammatory-immune Dysfunction
Chronic rhinosinusitis
Granulomatosis with Polyangiitis eosinophilic
Angiocentric fibrosis

Reactive
Sinonasal inflammatory polyp
Antrochoanal polyp
Sinonasal hamartoma
Mucocele of paranasal sinus
Extranodal sinus
Histiocytosis with massive lymphadenopathy

Benign Neoplasm
- Sinonasal (schneiderian) Papilloma
- Pleomorphic adenoma
- Ectopic pituitary adenoma
- Meningioma
- Ameloblastoma
- Lobular capillary hemangioma (Pyogenic granuloma)
- Schwannoma/neurofibroma
- Leiomyoma and smooth muscle Tumors of uncertain malignant potential
- Fibromatosis/desmoid-type
- Fibromatosis
- Solitary fibrous tumor
- Myxoma/fibromyxoma

Borderline Neoplasm
Glomangiopericytoma

Malignant Neoplasm
- Squamous cell carcinoma
- Sinonasal undifferentiated carcinoma
- Lymphoepithelial carcinoma
- Sinonasal adenocarcinoma, intestinal type nonintestinal
- Nonsalivary adenocarcinoma
- Olfactory neuroblastoma
- Malignant mucosal melanoma
- Ewing sarcoma, including sinonasal adamantinoma-like teratocarcinosarcoma
- Fibrosarcoma
- Leiomyosarcoma
- Malignant peripheral nerve sheath tumor
- Undifferentiated pleomorphic sarcoma
- Mesenchymal chondrosarcoma
- Angiosarcoma
- Extranodal NK-/T-cell lymphoma
- Biphenotypic sinonasal sarcoma
- NUT midline carcinoma

Pharynx

Congenital/Hereditary
Dermoid cyst, Rathke cleft cyst
Infectious
Infectious mononucleosis

Benign Neoplasm
Nasopharyngeal angiofibroma

Malignant Neoplasm
- Nasopharyngeal carcinoma
- Nonkeratinizing, keratinizing types
- Basaloid squamous cell carcinoma
- Low-grade nasopharyngeal
- Papillary adenocarcinoma
- Diffuse large b-cell lymphoma

APPROACH TO SALIVARY GLAND TUMORS

Why is salivary gland pathology challenging?
1. Rare
2. Broad morphology
3. Complex architecture
4. Overlapping features
5. Pattern matching often does not work
6. Adequate sampling

The approach
1. Look for invasion
2. Cellular composition—one cell or two cell type
3. Architecture
4. Cytology
5. Stroma

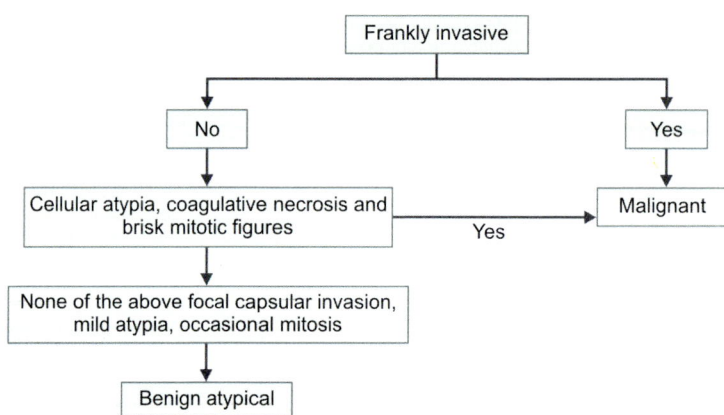

Invasion
Single most important feature
- ✓ benign tumors are circumscribed
- ✓ malignant ones show invasion (exceptions:
  - acinic cell carcinoma
  - Ca Ex PA can be circumscribed = "atypical PA")

Some tumors look benign but have invasion = basal cell adenocarcinoma, oncocytic carcinoma, myoepithelial carcinoma
➢ Be cautious with a poorly sampled salivary gland tumor

Pattern of invasion

Pushing	Irregular
Epithelial-myoepithelial-carcinoma	Everything else
Basal cell adenocarcinoma	
Myoepithelial carcinoma	
Acinic cell carcinoma	

Stroma
➢ Eosinophilic hyaline material—myoepithelial cells
➢ Intraluminal material—ductal cells
➢ Stromal mucin is common; has no value since it can be seen in several tumors
➢ Pleomorphic adenoma—stromal features: Cartilage, mucin in abundance, thick "fluffy" elastic fibers.

Lesions of the Head and Neck

		Tumor Architecture		
Cystic	**Microcystic**	**Cribriform**	**Tubular**	**Papillary**
Warthin's tumor	Acinic cell carcinoma	Adenoid cystic carcinoma	Adenoid cystic carcinoma	Warthin's tumor
Cystadenoma ca	PLGA	SDC	PLGA	Cystadenoma ca
MEC	Myoepithelial ca	PLGA	Epimyoepithalial ca	Papillomas
Acinic cell ca	MEC	PA	PA	Acinic cell ca
Cystic PA	MASC	Cribriform Adenocarcinoma tongue	Cystadenoma ca	PLGA
Lymphoepithelial cyst			SDC	Adenocarcinoma NOS

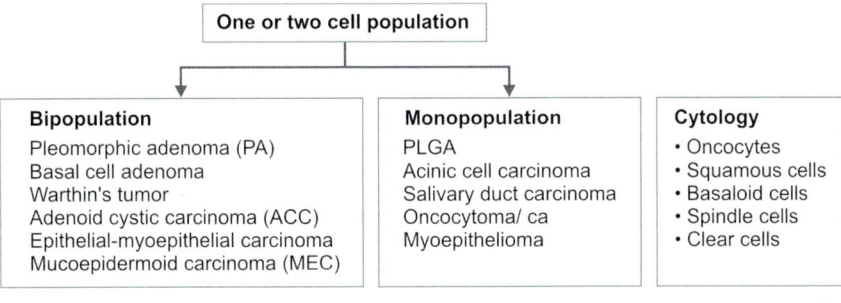

When do we resort to IHC
1. Cell types: One or two cell types
2. Confirm a specific salivary gland tumor type (myoepithelial tumors, MASC, SDC)
3. Ki-67: Adenoma (<5%) vs carcinoma (>10%)*
* Basal cell adenocarcinoma index is low

IHC
1. Luminal cells = epithelial: Low MW keratin+, CD117+, CK7+
2. Abluminal cells = myoepithelial: SMA+, calponin+, p63+, CK14+, mapsin +, CD43
3. High Ki-67 = poor prognosis in MEC, acinic cell carcinoma and adenoid cystic carcinoma
4. Salivary duct carcinoma = AR+
5. Mammary secretory carcinoma – mammaglobin+, S100+, MUC4+
6. CD43: Membranous staining in albuminal cells of adenoid cystic carcinoma (48–100%)

Cytogenetics

Tumor	Cytogenetics	Fusion
Pleomorphic adenoma	Rearranged 8q12 (39%)	PLAG1-CTNNB1
	Rearranged 12q13–15 (8%)	PLAG1-LIFR
	Sporadic non 8q21 or 12q13–15 (23%)	PLAG1-SII
		HMGA2-FHIT
Mucoepidermoid carcinoma	t(11;19)(q21;p13) (70%)	MECT1–MALM2
Adenoid cystic carcinoma	LOH 6q23–25 (76%); t(6;9)(q22–23;p23–24)	MYB-NFIB
Mammary analogue secretory carcinoma	(12;15)(p13;q25)	ETV6-NTRK3
Hyalinizing clear cell carcinoma	t(12;22)(q13;q12)	ESWR1-ATF1

Contributed by Lawrence D'Cruze

CHAPTER 2

Oral Lesions

N Malathi

Case History: A 20-year-old female complaints of pain and swelling in left lower jaw, since 3 months. Impacted 38.

Diagnosis: Odontogenic keratocyst

Clinical Features

- Peak incidence—2nd to 3rd decade of life with male predominance.
- Small odontogenic keratocyst—asymptomatic.
- Large odontogenic keratocyst—pain, swelling, bony expansion, paresthesia of the lower lip or teeth.
- Some extremely large cysts—no symptoms.

Radiographic Features

- Appear as unilocular radiolucencies and these have a smooth periphery, some may have scalloped margins.
- Larger lesions appear as multilocular radiolucencies.

Microscopy

Pindborg and Hansen's Criteria

- The lining epithelium is highly characterized and is composed of parakeratinized surface which is typically corrugated, rippled or wrinkled.
- A remarkable uniformity of thickness of the epithelium usually ranging from 6 to 10 cells thick.
- Prominent palisaded, polarized basal layer of cells often described of having a picket fence or tombstone appearance.

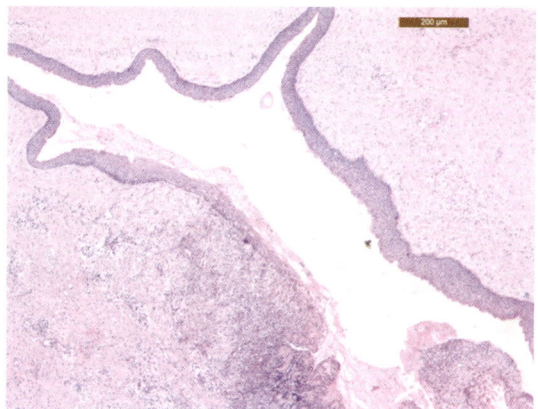

Fig. 2.1

Case History: A 42-year-old female presented with a painful swelling in the left side lower jaw.

Diagnosis: Unicystic ameloblastoma

Clinical Features

- Asymptomatic, sometimes presents as a swelling of the posterior mandible.
- Up to 80% are associated with an unerupted mandibular third molar.

Radiographic Features

Presents as a well-corticated unilocular radiolucency.

Microscopy

Histological Subtypes

- **Luminal variant:** Lined by ameloblastomatous epithelium.

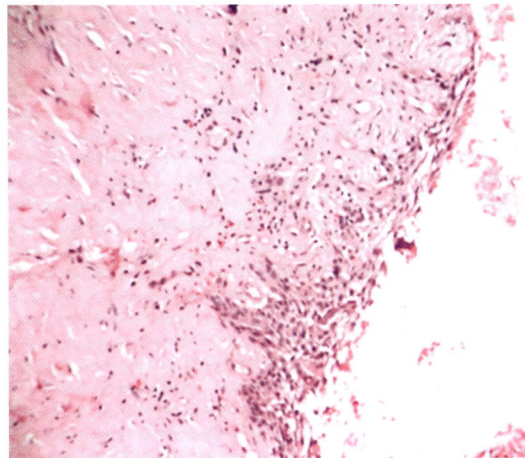

Fig. 2.2

- *Intraluminal variant:* Intralumial extensions may occur. Extensions usually exhibit a plexiform epithelial pattern. No tumor infiltration into the fibrous wall.
- *Mural variant:* The cyst wall is infiltrated by ameloblastomatous epithelium that exhibits either a follicular or plexiform pattern. These epithelial nests, however, do not show the typical histologic features of ameloblastoma: Peripheral palisading and nuclear polarization.

Subgroup	Interpretation
1	Luminal UA
1.2	Luminal and intraluminal UA
1.2.3	Luminal, intraluminal, and intramural UA
1.3	Luminal and intramural UA

Case History: A 23-year-old male with past history of surgical enucleation of radicular cyst presented wih a well-circumscribed swelling present in the body of the left mandible.

Diagnosis Ameloblastoma

Clinical Features
- Average age is 33–39 years with male predominance.
- Slow growing bony expansion. Thinning of the cortical plates, leading to characteristic egg shell crackling.
- When it occurs in the pituitary gland it is termed pituitary ameloblastoma or craniopharyngioma.

Radiography Features
Honeycombed appearance or soap bubble appearance.

Microscopy

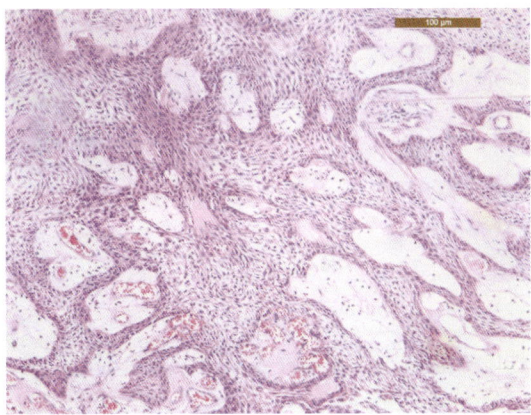

Fig. 2.3

Histological Subtypes
Depends on the pattern of arrangement of odontogenic epithelial islands.
- Follicular ameloblastoma (arranged in follicles).
- Plexiform ameloblastoma (arranged in plexiform strands).
- Acanthomatous ameloblastoma (follicular islands with squamous metaplasia).
- Granular cell ameloblastoma (with granular cells).
- Basal cell ameloblastoma.
- Desmoplastic ameloblastoma.

Case History: A 30-year-old male with ulceroproliferative growth from left retromolar region. Bleeds on touch.

Diagnosis: Ameloblastic carcinoma

Clinical Features
- It is an aggressive neoplasm that is locally invasive.
- Cortical expansion often with perforation.

Radiographic Features
- Ill-defined or irregularly marginated radiolucency is characteristic.

Microscopy

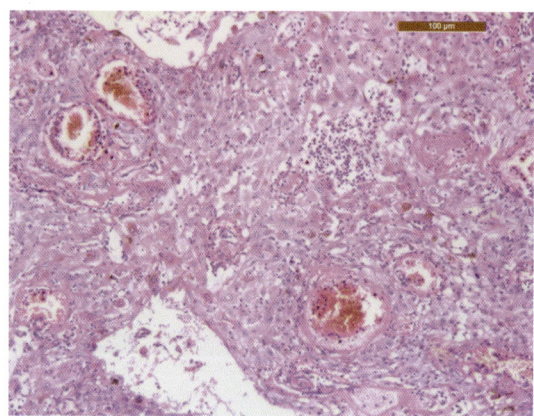

Fig. 2.4

Tall columnar cellular morphology with:
- Pleomorphism
- Mitotic activity
- Focal necrosis
- Perineural invasion
- Nuclear hyperchromatism
- Peripheral palisading
- Reverse or inverted nuclear polarity will be present
- A stellate reticulum structure will usually be seen.
- Cystic spaces may be present that are lined by epithelium.
- Subtle necrosis to comedonecrosis.

Case History: A 43-year-old female swelling over the left retromolar trigone region, soft and non-fluctuant attached to a base.

Diagnosis: Giant cell granuloma

Clinical Features
Mean age: 38 to 42 years. Females affected twice more than males.

Radiographic Features
Pathognomonic: Peripheral "cuffing" of the bone.

Gross
- Pedunculated or sessile lesion.
- Dark red, vascular or hemorrhagic in appearance.

Microscopy

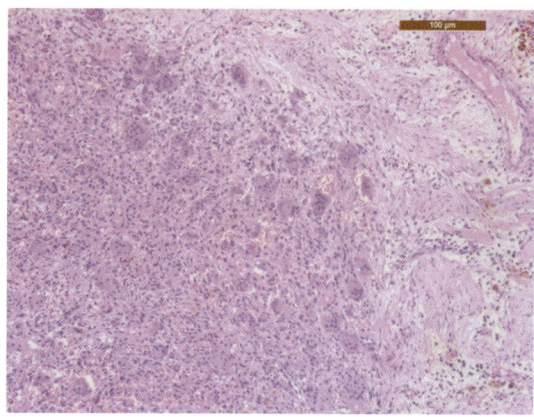

Fig. 2.5

Large number of ovoid or spindle-shaped connective tissue cells with multinucleated giant cells.

Central Giant Cell Granuloma

Types
- *Aggressive:* Quick growing, pain, cortical perforation, and root resorption.
- *Nonaggressive:* Slow growing, no root resorption, or cortical perforation. There is new bone formation.

Radiographic Features
Radiolucent area—smooth or ragged with faint trabeculae and definite loculations.

Microscopy
- Loose fibrillar connective tissue. With proliferating fibroblasts and small capillaries.
- Collagen fibers present a whorled appearance. Multinucleated giant cells prominent.

Case History: An 18-year-old male case of swelling left upper lip causing eversion of lip. Egg shell crackling positive.

Diagnosis: Adenomatoid odontogenic tumor

Clinical Features

- Found in association with unerupted permanent teeth (follicular type).
- Palpable bony-hard swelling with or without slight pain.
- The intraosseous AOTs may cause displacement of neighboring teeth.
- The peripheral variant presents as a fibroma or an epulis-like lesion of the gingiva.

Radiographic Features

Well-defined, unilocular radiolucency.
- *Intraosseous variant:* The radiolucency shows discrete radiopaque foci positive.
- *Peripheral variant:* Erosion of the alveolar bone crest.

Microscopy

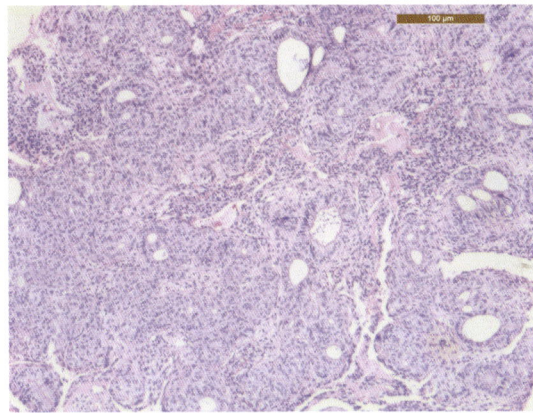

Fig. 2.6

- Solid nodules of cuboidal or columnar cells of odontogenic epithelium forming nests or rosette like structures with minimal stromal connective tissue.
- Between the epithelial cells and in the center of the rosette-like configurations, eosinophilic amorphous material ("tumor droplets") is present.
- Oral analog of 'calcifying epithelioma of Malherbe' (pilomatricoma) and shares histologic features with craniopharyngioma.

Case History: A 35-year-old female with swelling in the right side of face. OPG reveals unilocular radiolucency.

Diagnosis: Calcifying odontogenic cyst (COC)/calcifying cystic odontogenic tumor (CCOT).

COC classified into two types

1. Cystic lesion
2. Solid neoplastic lesion: Dentinogenic ghost cell tumor
   Malignant counterpart: Odontogenic ghost cell carcinoma.

Clinical Features

Swelling, pain and associated with impacted tooth. Two variants:
1. *Intraosseous variant:* Hard bony swelling.
2. *Extraosseous variant:* Painless swelling/nodule mostly seen before molar region.

Microscopy

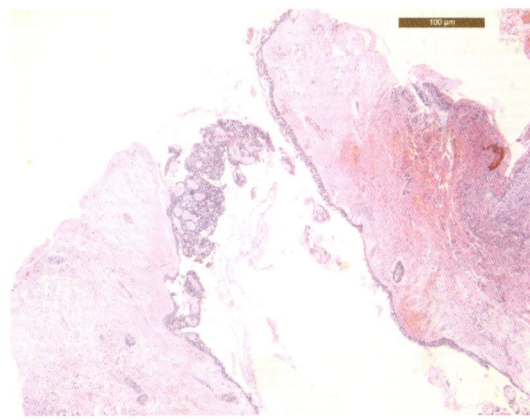

Fig. 2.7

- Cyst lining shows proliferation to the point that it resembles ameloblastoma.
- Within this proliferation epithelial cells undergo characteristic ghost cell keratinization. Dystrophic calcification of ghost cell occurs.
- Solid variant—dentinoid material formed in abundance.

Differential Diagnosis

- Odontoma
- Ameloblastoma
- Ameloblastic fibro-odontoma
- Ameloblastic odontoma

Case History: A 54-year-old female complaints of swelling over the right side of face for the past 2 months.

Diagnosis: Odontome

Odontome classified into two types
1. Compound composite odontome
2. Complex composite odontome

Clinical Features

- Asymptomatic
- Generally consists of unerupted or impacted teeth, retained deciduous teeth, swelling, and infection.
- Occasionally bony expansion with facial asymmetry.

Radiographic Features

Compound

- Radiolucency
- Partial calcification
- Radiopaque with amorphous masses

Complex

- Seen between the roots of teeth and appear as an irregular mass of calcified material surrounded by a narrow radiolucent band with a smooth outer periphery.
- Radiopaque radiolucent lesion.

Microscopy

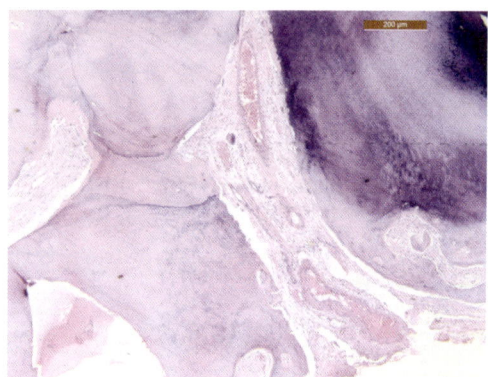

Fig. 2.8

- Haphazard conglomerates of dentin, enamel matrix, cementum and pulp.
- Connective tissue capsule around the odontoma resembles the follicle of tooth.
- Presence of ghost cells.

CHAPTER 3
CNS Lesions

Shantha Ravisankar, Archana B

Case History: A 35-year-old male with temperoparietal SOL.

Diagnosis: Diffuse astrocytoma, WHO grade II

Imaging
CT shows an ill-defined, homogeneous mass of low density, calcification and cystic changes.

Macroscopy
Ill-defined masses with cysts and/or focal calcification.

Microscopy

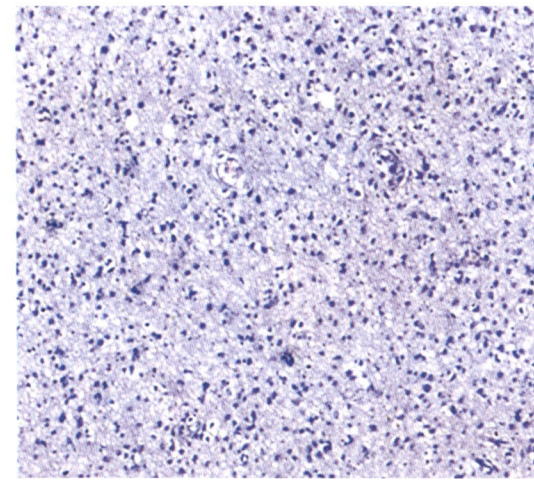

Fig. 3.1

- Scattered gemistocytes characterised by plump, glassy, eosinophilic cell bodies of angular shape.
- Stout, randomly oriented processes, forming a coarse fibrillary network, characterize the tumor cells, and are often useful to discriminate them from the mini gemistocytes found in oligodendroglioma.

Ancillary Tests
- **Immunohistochemistry:** GFAP positive. Ki-67 <4%.
- **Molecular genetics:** Expression of p53 protein and BCL-2 seen.
- **Electron microscopy:** Confirms the presence of abundant, compact glial filaments in the cytoplasm and in cell processes.

Differential Diagnosis
- **Gliosis:** Absence of microcysts, mixed cell population
- **Ganglioglioma:** Admixture of ganglion cells
- **Subependymal giant cell tumor:** Intraventricular, noninfiltrative, larger nuclei.

Case History: A 40-year-old female with parasagittal SOL.

Diagnosis: Rhabdoid meningioma, grade II

Imaging
MRI: Highly vascular dural-based contrast enhancing lesion.

Macroscopy

Irregular firm mass on cut section shows yellowish areas of necrosis.

Microscopy

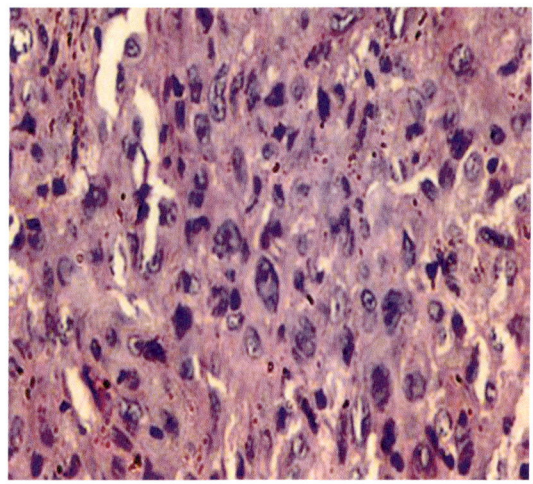

Fig. 3.2

- Groups of rhabdoid cells in the setting of anaplastic features.
- Sometimes cells arranged in zellballen pattern and may resemble paraganglioma.
- Nuclei eccentrically placed with deeply eosinophilic cytoplasm.
- Mitotic figures may be frequent.

Ancillary Tests

- **Immunohistochemistry:** Vimentin positive, EMA variable positive, PR may be positive, Ki67>10% often
- **Molecular genetics:** Increased frequency of allelic losses involving chromosomes 1p, 6q, 10q and 14q.

Differential Diagnosis

- **Metastatic carcinoma:** Cytokeratin positivity
- **Atypical teratoid/Rhabdoid tumor:** Loss of INI1
- **Glioblastoma:** GFAP positive, microvascular proliferation

Case History: A 20-year-old male presented with 4th ventricle SOL.

Diagnosis: Ependymoma, grade II

Clinical Features

- Generally present in young children with a mean age of 4 years.
- Occur infratentorially or supratentorially.

Imaging

- Frequently calcified, intraventricular or paraventricular masses.
- Spinal ependymoma on MRI appears as sausage-shaped enhancing mass.

Macroscopy

Well circumscribed soft grey mass generally related to the ventricle.

Microscopy

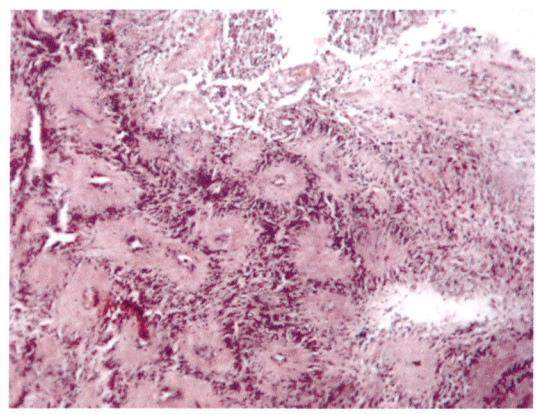

Fig. 3.3:

- Classic ependymoma cells lie close to one another, forming cellular lobules penetrated by areas of diminished cellularity or nuclear free zones. Cells are monomorphic, round to oval bland looking.
- Perivascular pseudorosettes seen. Some ependymomas express epithelial features in the form of round rosettes with central lumina.

Variants

- Papillary ependymoma
- Clear cell ependymoma
- Tanycytic ependymoma
- Cellular ependymoma

Immunohistochemistry

GFAP positive, EMA dot like positivity

Differential Diagnosis

- **Glioma:** No true rosettes, no dot like EMA positivity
- **Central neurocytoma:** Positive for neuronal markers, no EMA positivity

Case History: A 76-year-old male with contrast enhancing SOL lesion in temporo-parietal region.

Diagnosis: Glioblastoma multiforme, grade IV, NOS

Imaging

Pattern of ring-like contrast enhancement that reflects their abnormal vascularization and tendency to spontaneous central necrosis.

Macroscopy

- Relatively circumscribed.
- Appear to be clearly demarcated from neighboring tissue.
- Hemorrhagic discoloration and foci of yellow softening suggest virulent nature.

Microscopy

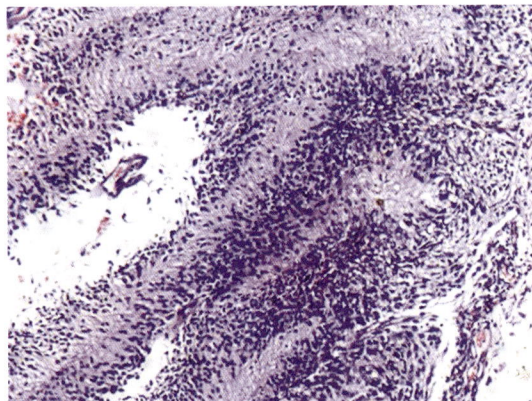

Fig. 3.4

- Highly cellular, mitotically active neoplasm.
- Differentiated elements may be admixed with bizarre giant cells, spindled, epithelioid, rhabdoid, signet ring or small anaplastic forms—devoid of astrocytic features.
- Microvascular proliferation is seen.
- Cellular palisading about foci of necrosis is seen.

Ancillary Tests

- **Immunohistochemistry:** MIB-1 and GFAP-immunoreactive.
- **Molecular genetics:** p53 mutation, loss of heterozygosity on chromosome 17p and EGFR amplification.
- **Electron microscopy:** Intermediate filaments are abundant in astrocytic cells but in undifferentiated tumor cells, intermediate filaments are sparse.

Differential Diagnosis

- **Metastatic tumor:** Displaces rather than infiltrating the glial parenchyma, no fibrillary background, GFAP is negative.
- **Lymphoma:** Angiocentric and angioinvasive, CD45 positive.
- **Meningioma malignant:** EMA positive
- **Other gliomas:** Mitosis, necrosis, endothelial proliferation.

Case History: A 15-year-old boy with suprasellar SOL.

Diagnosis: Craniopharyngioma, WHO grade I

Clinical Features

- Peak age incidence: 5–10 years
- Symptoms and signs due to increased intracranial pressure, compression of the optic pathways.

Macroscopy

- Admixture of cystic and solid components are characteristics.
- Cysts may contain a thick liquid resembling machine oil.

- Papillary variant is more circumscribed and does not contain calcification or oil-like cyst fluid.

Microscopy

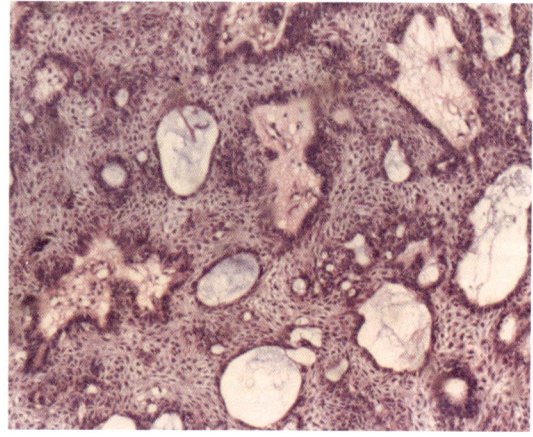

Fig. 3.5:

- Groups of squamous cells, often surrounded by peripheral palisade of columnar cells enclosing stellate reticulum in adamantinomatous type.
- Intercellular accumulations of fluid separates the cells in some parts of the neoplasm.
- Cohesive clusters and sheets of keratinizing a nuclear ghost cells.
- Calcification which may progress to metaplastic bone formation.

Variants

- Adamantinomatous
- Papillary

Differential Diagnosis

- ***Epidermoid cyst:*** Keratohyaline granules seen.
- ***Dermoid cyst:*** Adnexal structures seen.
- ***Pilocytic astrocytoma:*** Microcystic degeneration and loose sheets of astrocytes seen.
- ***Rathke cleft cyst:*** Mostly epithelium will have cilia or goblet cells.

Case History: A 25-year-old female with headache and seizures.

Diagnosis: Meningothelial meningioma, grade I

Clinical Features

- Symptoms by compression of adjacent structures.
- Specific deficits depend upon the location of the tumor.
- Headache and seizures often herald the presence of a meningioma.

Macroscopy

- Most meningiomas are rubbery or firm, well-demarcated, sometimes lobulated, rounded masses that feature broad dural attachment.
- Invasion of underlying dura or of dural sinuses is quite common.

Microscopy

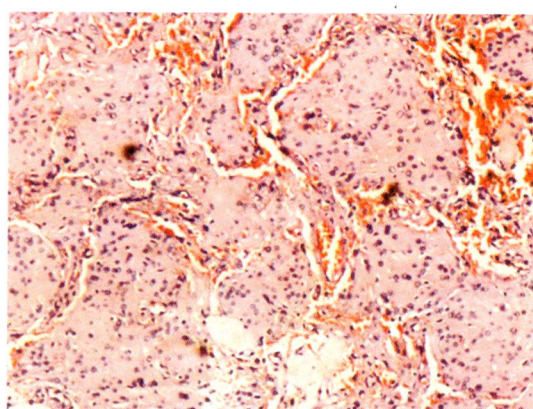

Fig. 3.6

- Tumor cells form lobules, often with whorls and arranged in syncytial arrangement.
- Like normal arachnoidal cap cells, the tumor cells are largely uniform, with oval nuclei with delicate chromatin that on occasion show central clearing, or the formulation of cytoplasmic nuclear inclusions. May contain psammoma bodies.

Ancillary Tests

- **Immunohistochemistry:** EMA and vimentin positive S-100 protein have found varying positivity in meningiomas.
- **Molecular genetics:** Most consistent change being deletion of chromosome 22.
- **Electron microscopy:** Abundance of intermediate filaments complex interdigitating cellular processes and desmosomal intercellular junctions.

Differential Diagnosis

- **Metastatic carcinoma:** Atypia, mitosis, cytokeratin positive
- **Hemangiopericytoma:** Spindle cells with staghorn vessels, storiform pattern, CD34 positive

Case History: A 7-year-old girl presented with posterior fossa cystic SOL.

Diagnosis: Pilocytic astrocytoma, grade I

Clinical Features

- Most common gliomas in children.
- In the visual system it can arise in the optic nerve proper and causes loss of vision.

Imaging

- Well circumscribed and contrast enhancing.
- Cysts may be solitary and massive with the tumor presenting as a mural nodule.
- Bright enhancement on T1-weighted image reflects the proteinaceous content in the tumor and aids in distinction from other forms of astrocytoma.

Macroscopy

- Relatively well circumscribed.
- Often has heterogenous consistency with firm and mucoid areas.
- Focal calcification may be present.

Microscopy

- Typically have a biphasic appearance.
- Compact fascicles of elongated cells with piloid/stellate cells with branching cytoplasmic processes may enclose a fine mesh work of microcysts.

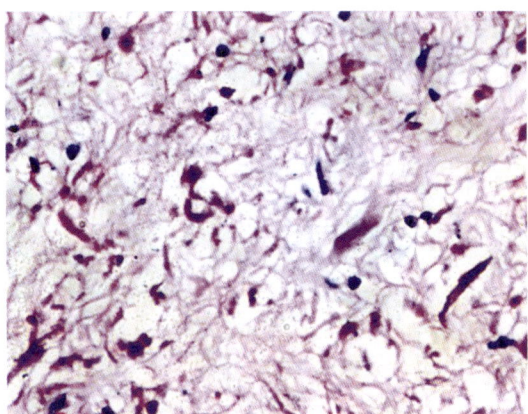

Fig. 3.7

- Nuclear pleomorphism and hyperchromasia may be present.
- Rosenthal fibers and eosinophilic granular bodies are classic features.

Ancillary Tests

- **IHC:** Most cells in PA label with antibodies to GFAP.
- **Molecular genetics:** In patients with NF-1, about 15% develop pilocytic astrocytoma.
- **Electron microscopy:** Reveals abundant cytoplasmic intermediate filaments.

Differential Diagnosis

- **Extensive astrocytic gliosis with Rosenthal fiber formation:** May mimic a PA, either as part of reactive conditions or around neoplasms.
- **Diffuse astrocytomas:** Distinct on neuroimaging. Diffuse astrocytoma do not have the circumscribed nature and biphasic architecture.
- **Glial component of ganglioma:** PA rarely infiltrates the adjacent brain sufficiently to entrap neurons. Neoplastic population of ganglion cells are absent in PA.
- **Glial component of dysembryoplastic neuroepithelial tumor (DNT):** DNT is cortical in location with a nodular architecture. Specific glioneuronal element helps to exclude a diagnosis of PA.

Case History: A 30-year-old female L1–L3 intramedullary SOL.

Diagnosis: Myxopapillary ependymoma, grade I

Important Points

Seen in spinal region. Frequently related to conus or filum terminale. Usually present in patients aged 20–40 years. Associated with type 2 neurofibromatosis. Perivascular and intercellular mucin deposition is a feature.

Microscopy

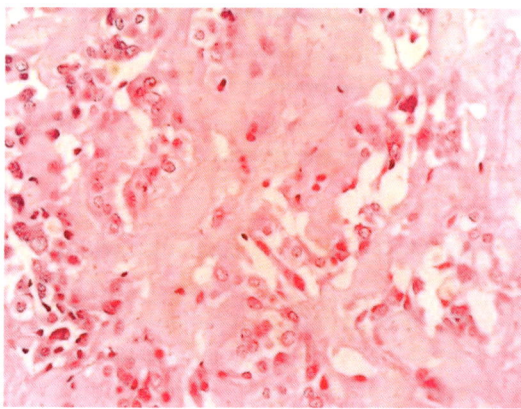

Fig. 3.8

Well-differentiated cuboidal to elongated tumor cells radially oriented around vascularized myxoid cores with a myxopapillary appearance. No atypia, low mitotic count.

Ancillary Tests

- **Immunohistochemistry:** Characterized by immunoreactivity for GFAP, vimentin.
- **Molecular genetics:** Gains in chromosomes 5, 7, 9, 16, 18.
- **Electron microscopy:** Basal bodies and cilia present but difficult to find.

Differential Diagnosis

- **Chordoma:** Presence of physaliphorous cells, keratin positive
- **Myxoid chondrosarcoma:** Lack of GFAP
- **Schwannoma and paraganglioma:** Common intradural tumors in this region.

Case History: A 35-year-old male with temperoparietal SOL

Diagnosis: Oligodendroglioma, grade II

Clinical Features

Majority arise in adults in males. Seizures are the most common presenting symptom.

Imaging

On CT, it appears as hypo/isodense well demarcated and shows little perifocal edema.

Macroscopy

Frontal lobe is involved frequently. It appears well defined, grayish pink, soft with calcifications.

Microscopy

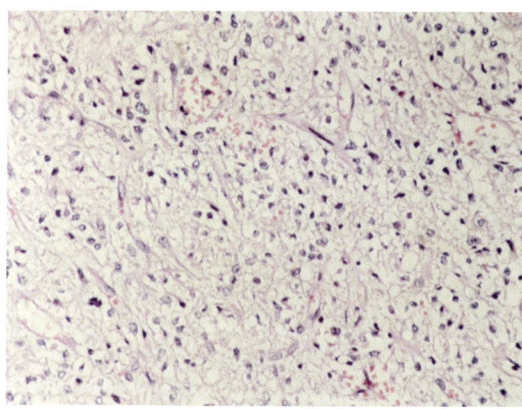

Fig. 3.9

- Monomorphous, moderately cellular, diffusely infiltrating gliomas
- Uniform round to oval nuclei with perinuclear halos giving a honeycomb or fired egg appearance
- Occasional mitotic figures
- Tumor cells are separated by branching chicken wire like capillary network
- Calcospherites noted

Ancillary Tests

- They stain strongly and uniformly with IDH1 R132H as well as IDH2 mutations detected molecularly.
- TP53—lack widespread staining
- GFAP—focally in the gliofibrillary oligodendrocytes and minigemistocytes
- KI67 below 5%
- 1p19q codeletion is the hallmark alteration demonstrated by FISH

Differential Diagnosis

- **Diffuse astrocytoma:** Lack honeycomb pattern, perinuclear halo, diffuse GFAP staining, lack of 1p19q codeletion
- **Pilocytic astrocytoma:** Pediatric, location in cerebellum, brain stem, lack IDH mutations and lack of 1p19q codeletion
- **Clear cell ependymoma:** Perivascular psuedorosettes, dot like EMA positivity
- **Central neurocytoma:** Positive neural markers, intraventricular location, lack of 1p19q codeletion.

Case History: A 40-year-old male with parietal SOL.

Diagnosis: Anaplastic oligodendroglioma, grade III

Clinical Features

Majority arise in adults in males. Seizures are the most common presenting symptom. They develop *de novo* or secondarily from a low grade oligodendroglioma.

Imaging

It appears heterogeneous due to necrosis, hemorrhage, cystic degeneration, calcification. Ring enhancement is uncommon.

Macroscopy

Heterogeneous due to hemorrhage, cyst formations and necrosis.

Microscopy

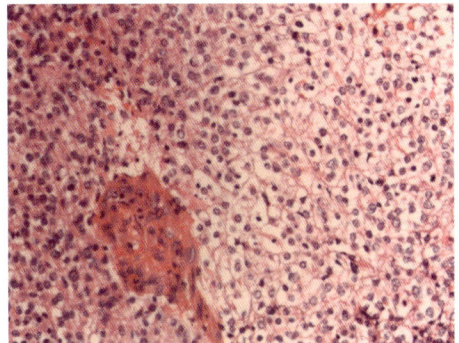

Fig. 3.10

- High cellularity, nuclear pleomorphism, moderate to high mitosis (>6/10 hpf)
- Microvascular proliferation and necrosis
- Infiltration with perineuronal satellitosis

Ancillary Tests

Immunohistochemistry similar to oligodendroglioma except with a high mitosis >5% on MIB labelling index.

Differential Diagnosis

- **Metastatic clear cell carcinomas:** Solid and sharply demarcated, cytokeratin positive
- **Glioblastoma:** 1p19q codeletions absent, presence of EGFR amplification

Case History: An 8-year-old male with IVth ventricle SOL

Diagnosis: Medulloblastoma, grade IV

Clinical Features

They present with raised intracranial pressure. Most common location in children is the cerebellar vermis.

Imaging

- Radiologically they invade the adjacent brain and generally show patchy enhancement with contrast on CT.
- On MRI they appear as solid, contrast enhancing masses.

Macroscopy

- Located in the midline appearing as pink or grey masses that arise in the

region of the vermis to occupy the fourth ventricle.
- Desmoplastic medulloblastoma tends to be more firm and circumscribed.

Microscopy

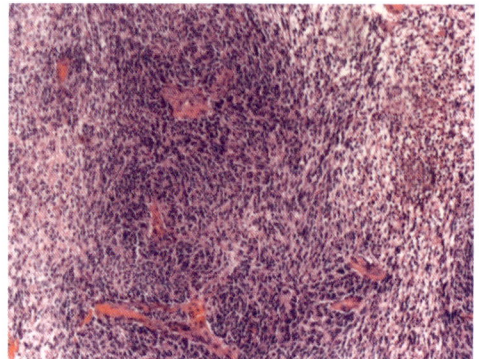

Fig. 3.11

- **Classic medulloblastoma:** It is the most common variant and consists of primitive appearing cells with round to oval hyperchromatic nuclei surrounded by scant cytoplasm. Homer Wright rosettes may be observed. Mitosis and necrosis may also be observed.
- **Large cell/anaplastic medulloblastoma:** Contains cells at least twice the size of those in classic medulloblastoma. Cells are discohesive with uniform round vesicular nuclei, cellular cannibalism and prominent nucleolus. They have higher mitotic counts.
- **Desmoplastic medulloblastoma:** Round to oval islands of low cellularity, reticulin free islands surrounded by highly cellular reticulin forming tumor cells.

Immunohistochemistry
- Synaptophysin positive
- Ki 67%> 30%

Differential Diagnosis
- **Metastatic neuroblastoma, retinoblastoma, lymphoma:** Appropriate IHC
- **High grade gliomas:** Fibrillary matrix with GFAP positivity
- **Germ cell tumor:** Positive for germ cell markers

- **Atypical teratoid rhabdoid tumor (ATRT):** Loss of INI1, vesicular nuclei with prominent nucleoli

Case History: A 22-year-old male lateral ventricle SOL.

Diagnosis: Central neurocytoma, grade II

Incidence and Localization
- Occurs in young-to middle-aged adults.
- Intraventricular in location.

Imaging
- Large, globular, intraventricular mass.
- Many are calcified.
- May be cystic and solid.

Macroscopy

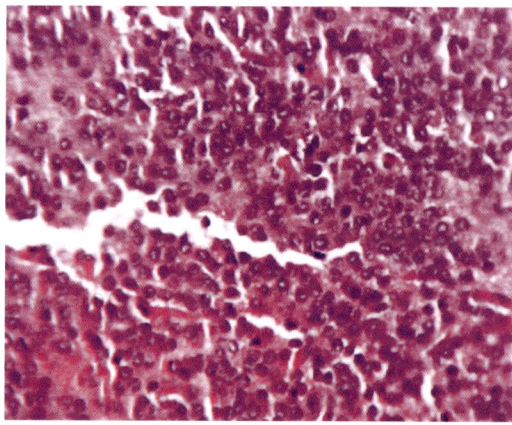

Fig. 3.12

Well circumscribed, grey and gritty.

Microscopy
- Monotonous round to oval cells which have fibrillary cytoplasm and round nuclei with finely granular chromatin.
- Streaming of cells in fine fibrillary background.
- Artifactual perinuclear halo seen.
- Rosettes may be seen.

Ancillary Tests
- **Immunohistochemistry:** Fibrillar zones immunoreactive for both synaptophysin and NSE. Ki-67 index is low.

- **Electron microscopy:** Neuropil produced by neurocytoma cell consists of a dense network of cytoplasmic processes containing microtubules.

Differential Diagnosis

- **Oligodendroglioma:** Chicken wire vasculature with perinuclear halos, molecular studies
- **Cellular ependymoma:** Especially clear cell ependymoma may involve paraventricular region. GFAP will be positive in ependymoma
- **Cerebral neuroblastoma:** Brisk mitosis will be there.

Case History: A 5-year-old male with history of headache and vomiting.

Diagnosis: Choroid plexus papilloma grade I

Clinical Features

Signs and symptoms of increased intracranial pressure. Located supratentorially in the lateral ventricles.

Imaging

Hyperdense contrast enhancing masses within the ventricles.

Macroscopy

- Circumscribed cauliflower-like masses that may adhere to ventricular wall.
- Cysts and hemorrhage may occur.

Microscopy

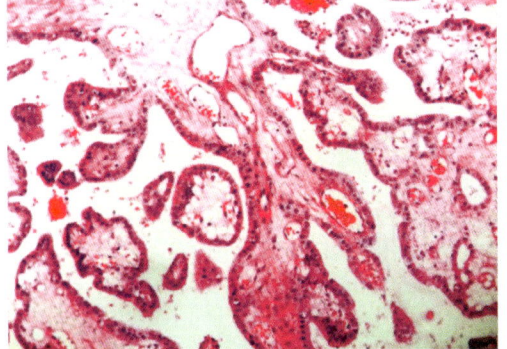

Fig. 3.13

- Benign papilloma is composed of delicate fibrovascular connective tissue fronds covered by a single layer of uniform cuboidal to columnar epithelial cells with round to oval basal nuclei.
- Changes that they can undergo are oncocytic change, mucinous degeneration, melanization and xanthomatous changes with bone or cartilage formation.

Ancillary Tests

- **Immunohistochemistry:** Vimentin and cytokeratin positive.
- **Electron microscopy:** Interdigitating cell membrane junctions, microvilli, occasional apical cilia and a basement membrane at the albuminal pole.

Differential Diagnosis

- **Choroid plexus carcinoma:** Anaplasia, necrosis, mitosis
- **Papillary ependymoma:** Pseudorosettes, GFAP positivity
- **Metastatic papillary carcinoma:** Atypia, mitosis, history and IHC to rule out possible primaries

Case History: A 35-year-old male with lesion in the base of skull.

Diagnosis: Chordoid meningioma, grade II

Incidence and Localization

- Incidence rises with age.
- Common in clivus, sphenoid ridges and other sites common to all meningiomas.
- May be associated with Castleman's syndrome.

Imaging

MRI: Isodense dural masses which may be calcified.

Macroscopy

- Firm irregular masses.
- May be gritty with foci of calcification.

Microscopy

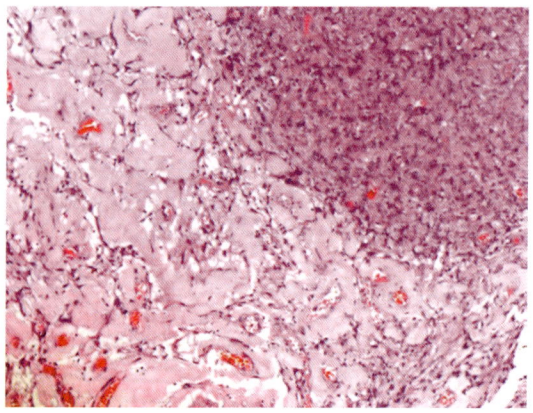

Fig. 3.14

- Cells resembling chordoma cells.
- Cells arranged in trabeculae with eosinophilic, vacuolated cells in a myxoid background.
- Chordoid areas are interspersed by chronic inflammatory cell infiltrate.
- Permeates the bone.

Immunohistochemistry

EMA and S-100 positive.

Differential Diagnosis

Chordoma: Physaliferous cells, S100 and brachury positive.

Case History: A 40-year-old male with cystic SOL in the posterior fossa.

Diagnosis: Hemangioblastoma, grade I

Incidence and Localization

- von Hippel syndrome includes:
  – Intracranial or intraspinal hemangioblastoma.
  – Cystic lesions of liver, kidney, pancreas and epididymis.
  – Benign and malignant renal tumor.
- The age of tumor of adulthood is in between 30 and 65 years.
- Male predominance is noted.
- Cerebellum is the frequent site.

Imaging

- Discrete highly vascular contrast enhancing masses.
- In the cerebellum seen as cystic lesion with mural nodules.

Macroscopy

- Highly vascular nodules abutting the leptomeninges.
- Cut section dark with spongy architecture and extrudes blood on compression.
- Depending on lipid content of stromal cells may appear yellowish.

Microscopy

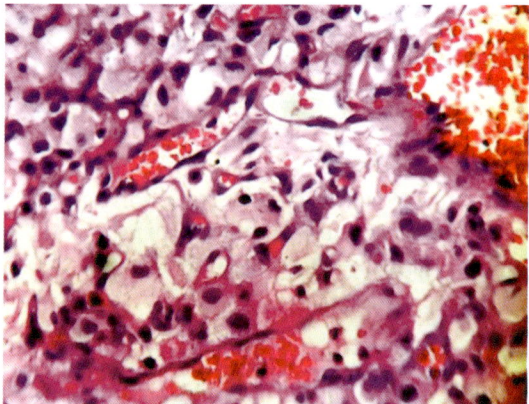

Fig. 3.15

- Cellular variant—cells more in number
- Reticular variant—vasculature is predominant
- Some regions are highly cellular while other consists of pauci-cellular tissue with a network of dilated vessels accompanying cyst-like spaces.
- Stromal cells lie packed between abundant often criss-crossing capillary channels.
- Stromal cells are large and polygonal and variably lipid-rich.
- Mast cells are common features can be demonstrated with toluidine blue.
- Cyst wall of hemangioblastoma consists of a dense non-neoplastic layer of pilocytic gliosis in which Rosenthal fibers are found.

Ancillary Tests

- **Immunohistochemistry:** Stromal cells immunoreactive for NSE, inhibin and GFAP weak positive. Factor VIIIa positive in vacuolated stromal cells.
- **Electron microscopy:** Stromal cells are large and lack specific organelles or cell attachments. Electron dense neurosecretory granules seen in some.

Differential Diagnosis

- **Non-representative biopsy of gliotic cyst wall:** May be mistaken for pilocytic astrocytoma. Unlike hemangioblastomas cerebellar astrocytoma are tumors of young age. Pilocytic astrocytoma has a biphasic histology.
- **Metastatic renal cell carcinoma:** This is entertained when hemangioblastoma lacks cystic areas. RCC shows epithelial characteristics. EMA will be positive in RCC.

Case History: A 60-year-old male with left cerebellar abscess.

Diagnosis: Phaeohyphomycosis

Classification: Clinically phaeohyphomycosis has been classified according to the anatomical site involved, as:
- Cutaneous
- Subcutaneous
- Paranasal sinus
- Cerebral types
- Cerebral phaeohyphomycosis is very rare, but the most serious form of disease, usually caused by *Cladophialophora bantiana*. The portal of entry is not known. Though inhabitation of spores into the lung and colonization and subsequent hematogenous spread has been suggested.

Common Fungal Infections of CNS

- Candidiasis
- Cryptococcosis
- Aspergillosis
- Mucormycosis

Forms of Fungi in CNS Infections

- Yeasts
- Branching hyphae
- Pseudohyphae

Microscopy

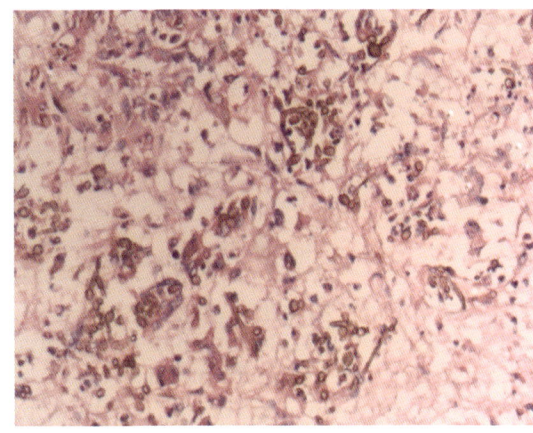

Fig. 3.16

Have a characteristic appearance of irregularly swollen hyphae with yeast-like structures.

Special Stain

Masson-Fontana stain for melanin is used to confirm the presence of dematiaceous hyphae.

Case History: A 2-month-old infant with increase in circumference of head since one month.

Diagnosis: Melanotic progonoma of infancy

Clinical Features

- It is an uncommon, rapidly growing pigmented, osteolytic tumor predominantly involving the maxilla or skull in infants.
- *Histogenesis:* Suggested neural crest origin with biphasic histology of melanin containing cells and neuroblast like cells.
- 98% of them occur in infants less than 1 year.
- Most commonly affects the maxilla and jaw bones of infants.

Microscopy

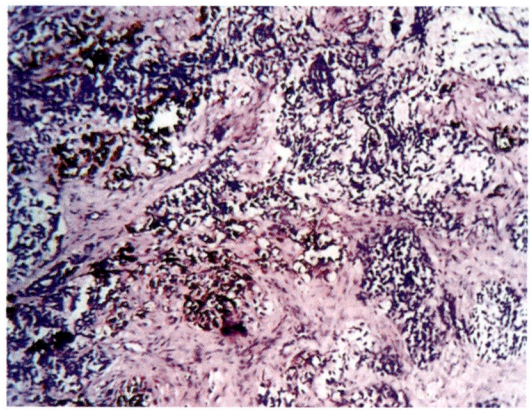

Fig. 3.17

- It is a biphasic tumor
- Composed of nodules of small round blue cell-neuroblast like component
- Larger melanin producing epithelioid cells
- The background consists of dense fibrosis

Ancillary Stains

- Larger cells are positive for keratin and HMB45, masson-fontana, a stain useful to demonstrate melanin pigment.
- Smaller cells are positive for CD57/Leu-7 and NSE.
- Both cell types are usually S-100 negative.
- Electron microscopy: Pigmented cells contain melanosomes, neuroblast-like cells contain neurosecretory granules and cytoplasmic processes.

Differential Diagnosis

- **Neuroblastoma/other small round blue cell tumor:** Typically lack the clinical presentation of a jaw or skull tumor in infants. Biphasic pattern, pigmented cells-rosettes present
- **Melanocytoma:** Well circumscribed lesion, no biphasic pattern
- **Melanoma:** Have prominent necrosis, atypia and mitotic figures.

- **Melanotic medulloblastoma:** Intra parenchymal lesion, rosettes present, hyperchromatic nuclei seen.

Case History: A 48-year-old male with known case of carcinoma lung.

Diagnosis: Metastatic tumor

Clinical Features

- Metastasis to brain affects both cerebrum and cerebellum.
- Most common tumors to metastasize are from lung and breast.

Macroscopy

- 80% located in arterial border zones of cerebral hemispheres.
- Well circumscribed-firm, granular, mucoid or necrotic, varying in color.
- Located at the junction of the gray and white matter.

Microscopy

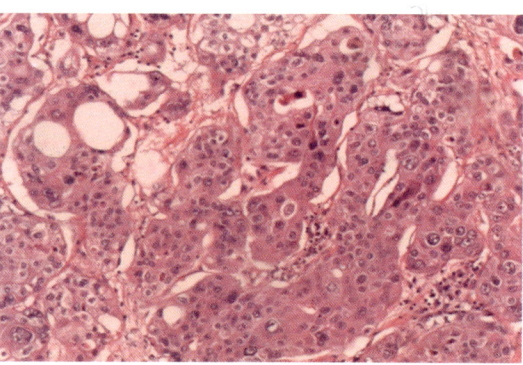

Fig. 3.18

- Discrete parenchymal lesion.
- Vascular proliferation may be seen adjacent to tumor area.
- Necrosis may be present.
- Diffuse leptomeningeal infiltration may be seen.

Ancillary Studies

Immunohistochemistry: Immunoreactivity of the parent neoplasm.

Differential Diagnosis

- **Glioblastoma multiforme:** Endothelial proliferation, GFAP positive and cytokeratin negative.
- **Papillary neoplasms:** Have to be differentiated from choroid plexus carcinoma and other primary papillary tumors of CNS.
- **Primary lymphomas:** Are usually deep seated and angiocentric.

Case History: A 26-year-old male headache and seizures since 3 months, temporal lesion.

Diagnosis: DNET, WHO grade I

Clinical Features

- Uncommon tumor
- Protracted history of partial seizures
- Onset before 20 years of age
- Majority localized to the cerebral cortex

Imaging

- Well demarcated, T1 hypointense
- Internal nodularity
- Thin septations within the tumor
- Pseudocystic appearance due to mucoid accumulation

Macroscopy

Multiple gelatinous nodules

Microscopy

- Mucin rich nodules
- Small oligodendroglia like cells aligned in a columnar fashion along bundled axons and capillaries that are arrayed perpendicular to pial surface
- Myxoid matrix on which mature neurons float.

Ancillary Test

Immunohistochemistry: GFAP positive astroglial cells with entrapped floating neurons positive for neuronal markers and S100.

Differential Diagnosis

- **Oligodendroglioma:** IDH mutation and 1p19q codeletion
- **Ganglioglioma:** Neuronal dysmorphism/inflammatory infiltrates.

Case History: A 15-year-old male with subcortical well circumscribed cystic and solid SOL in the temporal region.

Diagnosis: Papillary glioneuronal tumor

Clinical Features

Arise in the cerebral hemispheres of adults.

Imaging

On MRI they appear as well circumscribed, contrast enhancing lesions with little mass effect or surrounding edema.

Microscopy

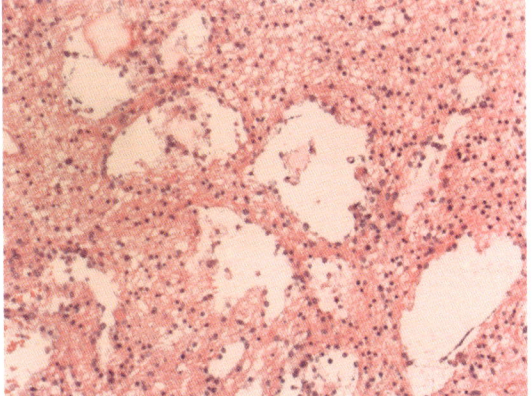

Fig. 3.19

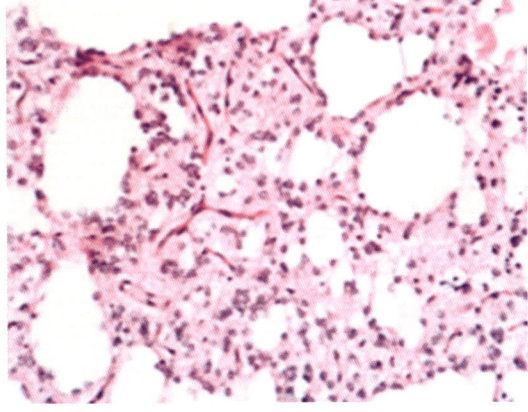

Fig. 3.20

- Circumscribed, noninvasive
- Papillary/pseudopapillary architecture
- Central fibrovascular core surrounded by two distinct cell types
- Inner small cuboidal cells with outer larger clear cells with neurocytic or ganglioid appearance
- Rare to absent mitosis
- IHC: Strong GFAP of the inner layer and strong neuronal markers in the outer layers

Differential Diagnosis

- **Papillary ependymoma:** Rosettes, synaptophysin negative
- **Extraventricular neurocytoma:** No pseudopapillae lined by glial cells
- **Rosette forming glioneuronal tumor:** 4th ventricle, neurocytic rosettes with synaptophysin positive cores.

APPROACH TO CNS LESIONS I

2016 CNS WHO

"ISN-Haarlem" Consensus Guidelines: Diagnostic entities should be defined as narrowly as possible to optimize interobserver reproducibility, clinicopathological predictions and therapeutic planning (avoid waste baskets!)

Diagnoses should be *"layered"* with histologic classification, WHO grade and molecular information as *"integrated diagnosis"*.

COMBINED MORPHOLOGY AND GENETICS

Major changes in 2016 CNS WHO

- Major restructuring and incorporation of genetically defined entities for:
  - Diffuse gliomas
  - Medulloblastomas
  - Embryonal tumors (including removal of the term "primitive neuroectodermal tumor (PNET)"
- Incorporation of a genetically defined ependymoma variant
- Novel approach distinguishing pediatric look-alikes, including new entity of

Diffuse Midline Glioma, H3 K27M

- Addition of other newly recognized entities:
  - Diffuse leptomeningeal glioneuronal tumor
  - Epithelioid glioblastoma
  - Embryonal tumor with multilayered rosettes, C19MC-altered
  - Ependymoma, RELA fusion–positive

Deletion of former entities, variants

  - Gliomatosis cerebri
  - Protoplasmic and fibrillary astrocytoma variants
  - Cellular ependymoma variant
- Addition of brain invasion as a criterion for atypical meningiomas
- Restructuring of solitary fibrous tumor/hemangiopericytoma, including soft tissue type (non-CNS) grading system.

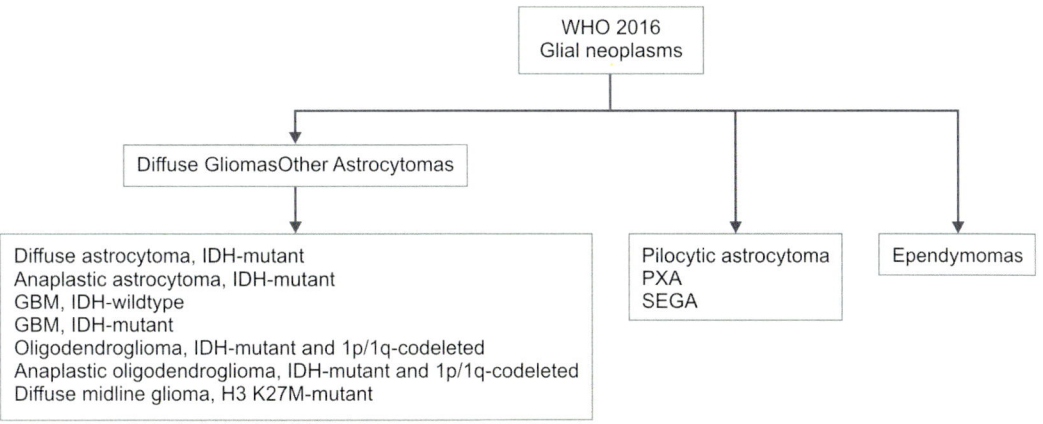

Contributed by Lawrence D'Cruze

APPROACHES TO CNS LESIONS II

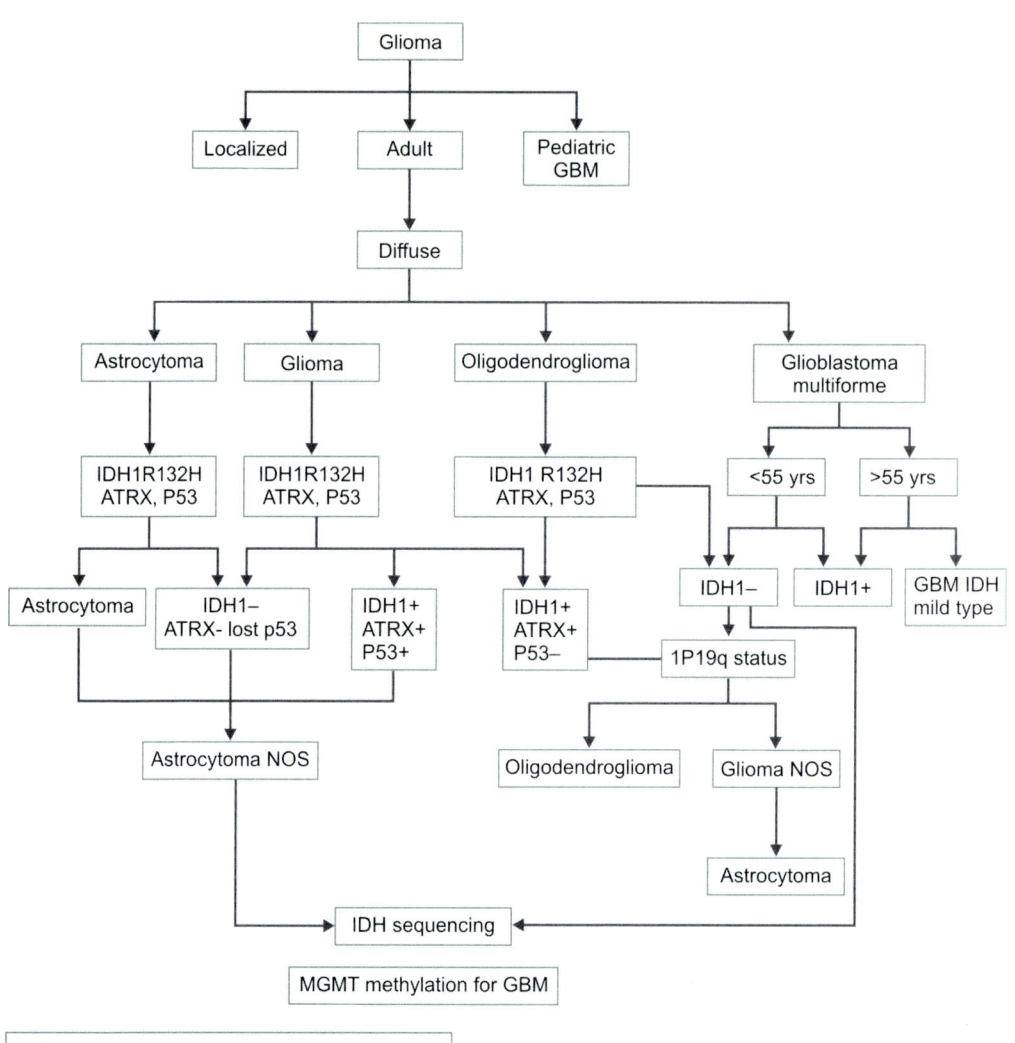

GBM (molecular subgroup)
H3K57M mutation (34%) midline location—very poor prognosis
H3G34R mutation (12%)
IDH mutation (5%)—good prognosis
H3/IDH mild type (29%)
PXA or pilocytic like methylation profiles (20%)
Sublet with BRAF V6000 mutation—good

Contributed by Lawrence D'Cruze

Algorithmic approach for classification of Glioma

Note: See Flowchart

Multilayered Reporting Format

Layer 1: Integrated diagnosis (incorporating all issue-based information)
Layer 2: Histological classification
Layer 3: WHO grade (reflecting natural history)
Layer 4: Molecular information

"Genotype trumps the histological Phenotype"

An NOS designation implies that there is *insufficient information to assign a more specific code*. For a tumor lacking a genetic mutation, the term *wildtype* can be used if the entity exist: If a formal *wildtype* diagnosis is not available, and a tumor lacking a diagnostic mutation is given an NOS designation.

CHAPTER 4

Ophthalmic Lesions

Rajavelu Indira

Case History: A 41-year-old male, blurred vision enucleation done.

Diagnosis: Malignant melanoma of choroid

Clinical Features
- Typically affects adults in sixth decade.
- Sun exposure increases the risk.
- Site—choroid.

Gross
Blackish mass in the vitreous cavity.

Microscopy

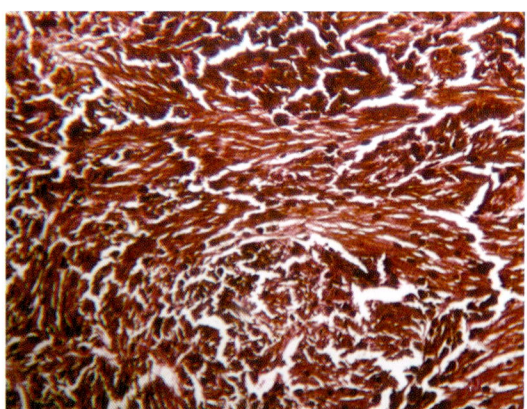

Fig. 4.1

- Corneal and conjunctival mucosa, sclera and ciliary body.
- Nodular infiltrating neoplasm arising from the choroid and composed of spindle shaped cells.
- The cells are arranged in sheets and interlacing fascicles.
- Intracytoplasmic melanin is seen in most of the cells.

Case History: A 50-year-old female fleshy mass with pigmentation in conjunctiva.

Diagnosis: Cancerous acquired melanosis

Clinical Features
- Age group 40 to 50 years.
- Present as an area of brown conjunctival discoloration that can be moved over the sclera.

Gross
Brown black soft tissue.

Microscopy

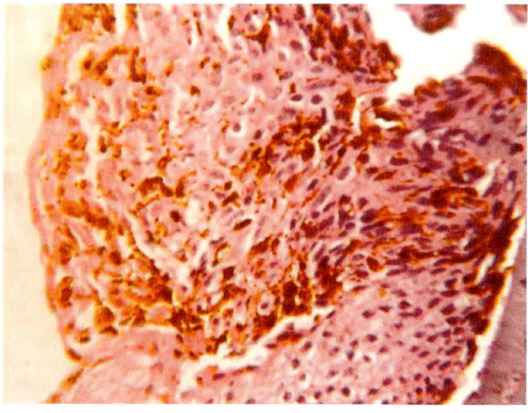

Fig. 4.2

- Hyperplastic stratified squamous epithelium.
- Focal areas show full thickness of the epithelium being infiltrated by atypical melanocytes.
- Subepithelial zone shows dense chronic inflammatory cell infiltration and fibroblasts.

Case History: A 6-month-old girl baby with strabismus and leukokoria ("cat's eye reflex").

Diagnosis: Retinoblastoma

Clinical Features
- Most common intraocular malignancy of childhood.
- Autosomal dominant with 90% penetrance.

Gross
- Creamy white with areas of calcification and necrotic areas
- Endophytic or exophytic (grows outward toward choroid)
- Rarely infiltrative and more often it seeds intraocularly

Microscopy

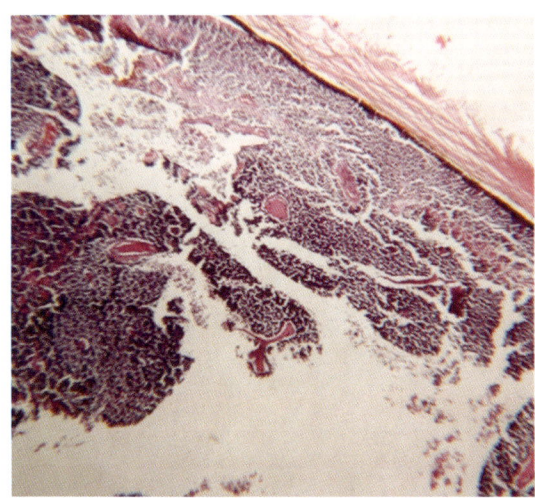

Fig. 4.3

- Cellular neoplasm arising from the retina and extending into the vitreous cavity.
- The tumor cells are small, round to oval having scanty eosinophilic cytoplasm and hyperchromatic nuclei.
- The cells are arranged in sheets and in the form of Flexner Wintersteiner and Homer Wright rosettes.
- Areas of necrosis, hemorrhage and calcification seen.
- Frequent azzopardi phenomena; mitotic figures; variable apoptotic cells
- Differentiated retinoblastoma—bipolar-like cells are present
- Undifferentiated retinoblastoma—large, anaplastic cells without rosette formation.

Immunohistochemistry
- **Positive:** NSE, synaptophysin, S100, Leu7, GFAP, myelin basic protein and p53; high Ki-67
- **Negative:** CD99

Poor Prognostic Factors
Invasion of optic nerve, invasion of uveal tract or sclera, seeding of vitreous, involvement of anterior segment; extensive ocular tissue and tumor necrosis; differentiation does not appear to have prognostic value.

Case History: A 28-year-old female, nodule near the lower eyelid.

Diagnosis: Sebaceous hyperplasia

Clinical Features
- Small, yellowish, slightly umbilicated papules.
- Middle-aged persons.

Microscopy
One or more enlarged, fully mature sebaceous glands with numerous lobules arranged around the central dilated sebaceous duct.

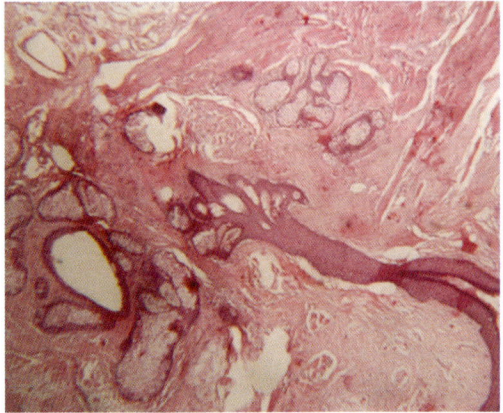

Fig. 4.4

Differential Diagnosis

Basal cell carcinoma

Case History: A 78-year-old female, left upper eyelid mass.

Diagnosis Sebaceous gland carcinoma

Epidemiology

- Middle-aged women are affected.
- Diffuse eyelid thickening/obstructive chalazion/inflammation of conjunctiva, cornea or eyelid.

Gross

- External surface—nodular.
- Cut surface—friable mass with areas of necrosis and hemorrhage.

Microscopy

- Stratified squamous epithelium with an infiltrating neoplasm dispersed as broad papillary fronds, solid sheets and nests.
- The tumor cells are large and polygonal.
- Some cells have eosinophilic cytoplasm and some have foamy vacuolated cytoplasm with hyperchromatic nuclei.
- Nuclear pleomorphism and abnormal mitotic figures seen.
- Well differentiated—better differentiated cells with foamy, finely vacuolated cytoplasm and distinct cell borders.
- Anaplastic—often scant cytoplasm with indistinct vacuoles, central necrosis, pagetoid involvement of overlying skin.

Special Stains

Oil red O on frozen sections—red.

Differential Diagnosis

Basal cell carcinoma: Less pleomorphic, has peripheral palisading.

Case History: A 45-year-old female, lacrimal gland tumor.

Diagnosis: Myoepithelioma of lacrimal gland

Gross

- Well encapsulated nodular mass attached to the lacrimal gland
- Cut surface—grey white, homogeneous.

Microscopy

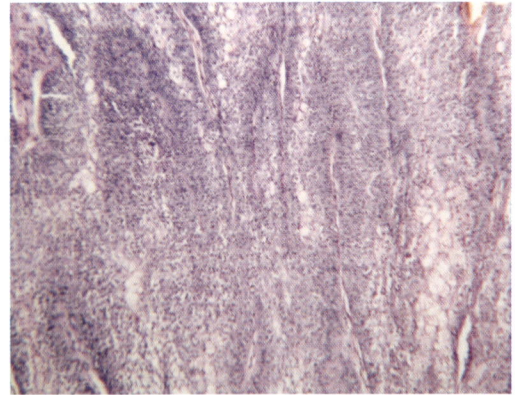

Fig. 4.5

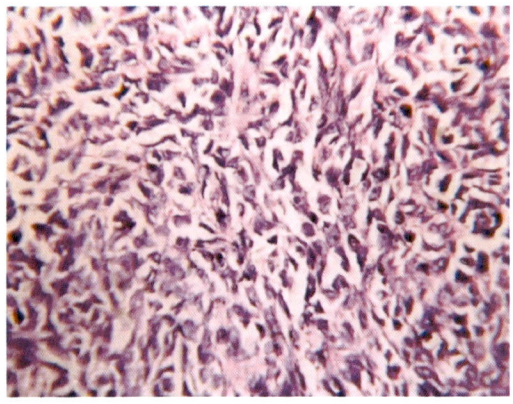

Fig. 4.6

- Partially encapsulated neoplasm composed of round to oval and spindle-shaped cells arranged in nodules and fascicles separated by scanty fibrous stroma.
- Tumor cells have vesicular nuclei and basophilic nucleoli.
- Foci of myxoid stroma and occasional mitotic figures are seen.

Immunohistochemistry
SMA—focal positive.

Differential Diagnosis
- Clear cell variant of oncocytoma
- Mucoepidermoid carcinoma
- Benign fibrous histiocytoma.

Case History: A 4-year-old girl, nodule in lid margin.

Diagnosis: Molluscum contagiosum

Clinical Features
Multiple, small, raised, umbilicated, pearly nodules in young children.

Gross
Small pearly nodule.

Microscopy

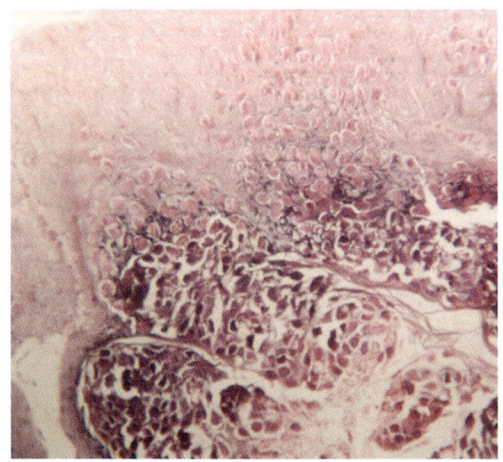

Fig. 4.7

- Acanthotic stratified squamous epithelium with cup-shaped invagination of the epithelium.
- The cells in the deeper layers contain eosinophilic inclusion bodies (Henderson–Patterson corpuscles) in their cytoplasm.

Case History: A 21-year-old male with cystic lesion right lower lid.

Diagnosis: Syringocystadenoma papilliferum.

Clinical Features
- Present at birth or appears in early childhood.
- Solitary or multiple.
- Commonly seen in scalp or face, in association with nevus sebaceous.

Gross
Cyst wall with grey white friable papillary areas.

Microscopy
- Stratified squamous epithelium with cystic invagination extending into the dermis.
- Superficially the invagination is lined with stratified squamous epithelium.
- More deeply the cyst shows broad, branching papillary processes projecting into the lumen.
- These projections are lined by a double-layer of cells—an inner flattened and an outer layer of tall columnar cells with apocrine features.
- Stroma shows numerous lymphocytes and plasma cells.

Immunohistochemistry
Plasma cells are IgA+, IgG+

Case History: A 50-year-old female with circumscribed polypoid, yellowish waxy nodule.

Diagnosis: Conjunctival amyloidosis

Clinical Features
- Occurs in healthy adults who do not have systemic amyloidosis.
- May involve any part of the conjunctiva.

Microscopy

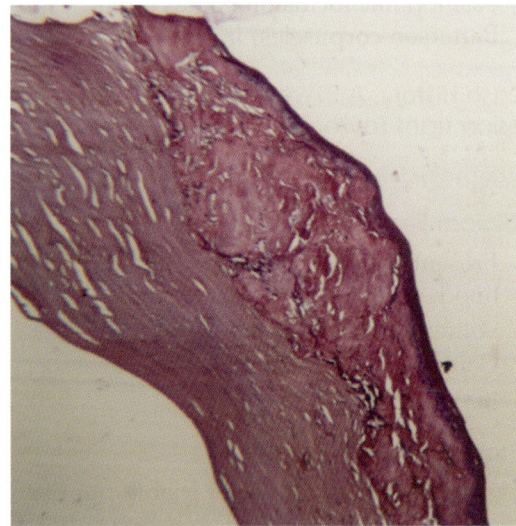

Fig. 4.8

- Stratified squamous epithelium of conjunctiva with goblet cells.
- Subepithelial region shows acellular amorphous deposits of eosinophilic hyaline material.
- A few foreign body type giant cells are seen.

Special Stains

- Congo red—orange.
- Under polarizing microscope—apple green birefringence.

Case History: A 67-year-old male with orbit mass.

Diagnosis: Fibrosarcoma of the orbit

Gross

- Fleshy, hemorrhagic, necrotic, white-tan

Microscopy

- An infiltrating neoplasm dispersed as sheets and interlacing fascicles.
- The tumor cells are spindle-shaped with elongated nuclei.
- Abnormal mitotic figures seen.
- Some cells are round to oval with clear cytoplasm and vesicular nuclei.
- Areas of necrosis seen.

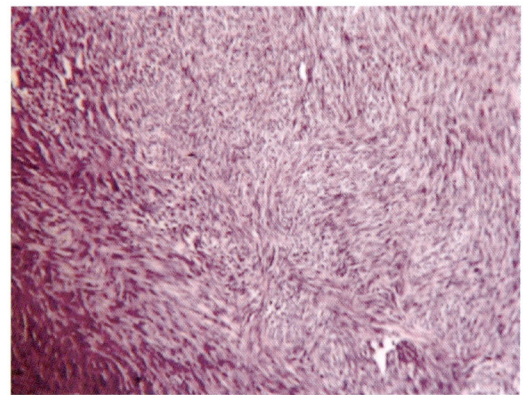

Fig. 4.9

Differential Diagnosis

Malignant peripheral nerves sheath tumor: Monomorphic serpentine cells, palisading, large gaping vascular spaces, perivascular plump tumor cells, geographic necrosis with tumor palisading at edges. Frequent mitotic figures. 5% have metaplastic cartilage, bone, muscle.

Case History: A 50-year-old male with upper lid nodule, infiltration of tarsal plate present.

Diagnosis: Apocrine carcinoma

Microscopy

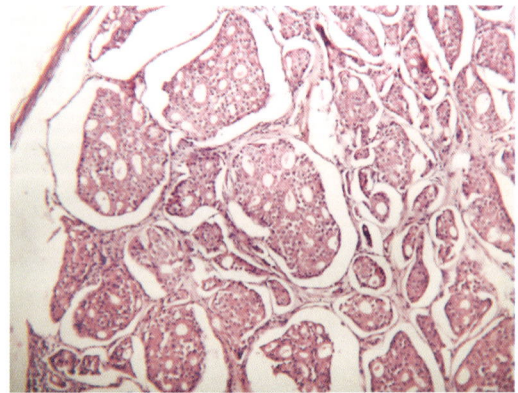

Fig. 4.10

- Thinned out stratified squamous epithelium overlying an infiltrating neoplasm dispersed as tubules, nests, papillary fronds and in a cribriform pattern, separated by thin fibrous stroma.

- The tubules are lined by cuboidal cells having eosinophilic cytoplasm.
- Nuclei are round and exhibit mild variation in size.
- Some have prominent nucleoli.

Case History: A 2-year-old male child with proptosis.

Diagnosis Orbital teratoma.

Radiology

Heterogeneous solid and cystic mass with areas of calcification.

Gross

Solid and cystic, heterogeneous grayish tan and fleshy.

Microscopy

- Tumors with a variety of structures derived from all germ cell layers.
- Squamous epithelium with dermal appendages, choroid plexus, papillary structures, mucinous glands, glial tissues and primitive neuroepithelial tissue with rosettes.

Case History: A 62-year-old female, swelling inferior to medial canthus.

Diagnosis: Filarial lesion

Microscopy

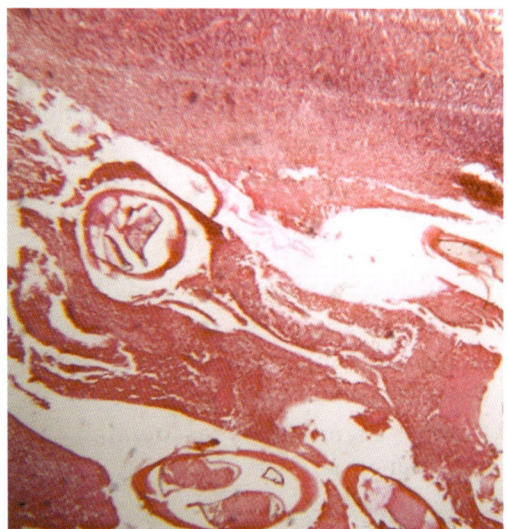

Fig. 4.11

- Fibrous capsule with cut sections of many adult filarial worms.
- The fibrocollagenous capsule is densely infiltrated by acute and chronic inflammatory cells with a predominance of eosinophils.

Case History: A 50-year-old female, with near the lacrimal gland.

Diagnosis: Pleomorphic adenoma of lacrimal gland

Clinical Features

- Most common benign tumor.
- Young adults: M : F 2:1.

Gross

- Lobulated, encapsulated mass.
- Cut surface: Homogenous, firm, myxoid.

Microscopy

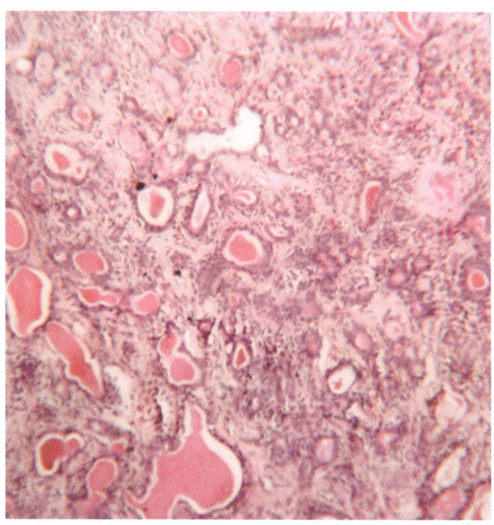

Fig. 4.12

- Encapsulated neoplasm with compressed lacrimal gland tissue outside the capsule.
- The neoplasm is dispersed as ducts, acini and tubules lined by an inner layer of epithelial cells and an outer layer of myoepithelial cells.
- Some of the tubules contain eosinophilic secretions.
- Sheets of spindle-shaped myoepithelial cells are seen in an abundant myxoid stroma.

CHAPTER 5

Spectrum of Breast Lesions

Sandhya Sundaram

Case History: A 6 months post-pregnancy, mass in the upper outer quadrant right breast.

Diagnosis: Granulomatous mastitis with breast abscess

Clinical Features

Rare condition that can either be idiopathic, possibly immune mediated. Unilateral breast mass associated with nipple retraction or skin dimpling reserved for cases in which infection, foreign body exposure, sarcoidosis, and autoimmune disease have been excluded.

Gross

- Discrete, firm mass.
- Foci of necrosis may also be seen.

Microscopy

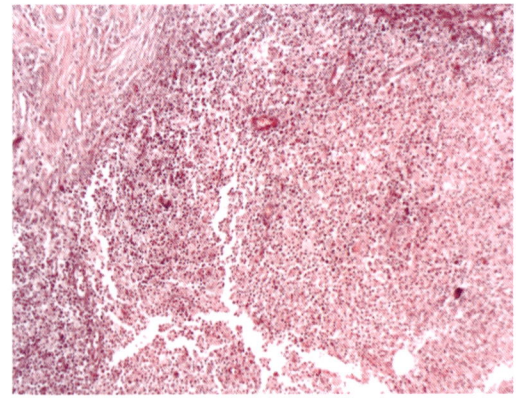

Fig. 5.1

Granulomas are non-necrotizing and centered on the lobules admixed with neutrophils, histiocytes, and multinucleated Langerhans-type and foreign body giant cells. Absence of necrosis but abscess formation may occur.

Ancillary Studies

Because microorganisms are rarely identified using special stains (GMS, PAS, Gram, acid-fast bacilli, Fite) on paraffin-embedded material, fresh tissue should be sent for fungal and mycobacterial cultures to evaluate for infectious agents.

Differential Diagnosis

- **Granulomatous infections:** Tuberculosis, sarcoidosis, actinomycosis, coccidioidomycosis, histoplasmosis, Wegener's granulomatosis, cat-scratch disease.
- **Plasma cell mastitis:** Periductal, plasma cells prominent
- **Fat necrosis and foreign body reaction:** Plastic/silicosis
- **Granulomatous angiopanniculitis:** Involves subcutis and extends into breast
- **Rarely granulomas associated with carcinoma.**

Case History: A 29-year-old female, well-circumscribed mass in the right upper outer quadrant associated with skin discolouration and induration.

Diagnosis: Tubular adenoma

Clinical Features

Seen usually in young women and occasionally in older women

Gross

Well-circumscribed tan yellow, soft to firm mass

Microscopy

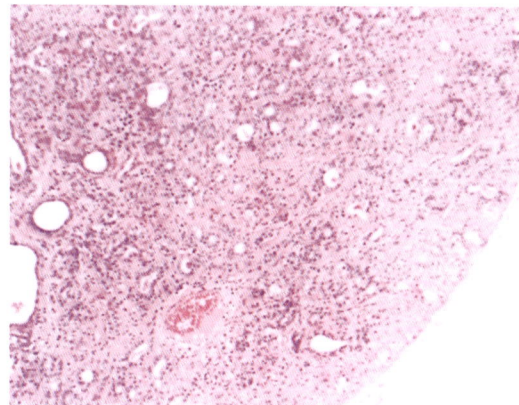

Fig. 5.2

- Closely packed uniform tubules, lined with a single layer of epithelial cells and an attenuated myoepithelial cell layer. No atypia
- Stroma is generally more sparse

Immunohistochemistry

Epithelial cells: EMA+, ER+, PR+
Myoepithelial cells: Vimentin+, SMA+

Differential Diagnosis

- **Fibroadenoma:** More stroma and have less epithelium
- **Adenomyoepithelioma, tubular variant:** Myoepithelial cells appear prominent and not well circumscribed
- **Infiltrating ductal carcinoma:** Atypia with irregular tubules and infiltrative.

Case History: A 32-year-old female, retroareolar mass in the right breast with nipple discharge.

Diagnosis: Intraductal papilloma

Clinical Features

- Occur between age 30 and 50. Present with serous or bloody nipple discharge.
- May be palpable or occult.

Gross

- **Central papilloma:** A few millimeters to >5 cm, well-circumscribed round tumor attached by pedicle to the wall of a dilated duct.
- **Peripheral papilloma:** Grossly occult.

Microscopy

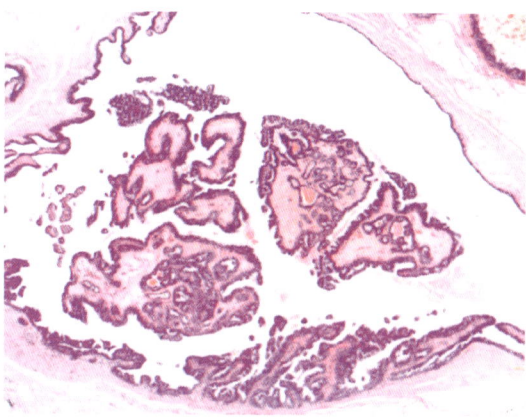

Fig. 5.3

- Cystic space lined by ductal cells filled with branching, dense fibrovascular cores lined by myoepithelial cells and ductal cells.
- Ductal cells are often tall columnar to cuboidal with abundant cytoplasm and oval nuclei and may also show (UDH) usual ductal hyperplasia.
- Can undergo apocrine and squamous metaplasia.
- Sclerosed papillomas have increased collagen in the fibrovascular cores and often calcify.

- Epithelial component—one layer of cuboidal/columnar/may show foci of usual ductal hyperplasia.
- Apocrine metaplasia and squamous metaplasia can occur.

Ancillary Studies
- CK5 and ER can be helpful in distinguishing hyperplasia from atypia in a papilloma, particularly in a core biopsy.
- Hyperplasia is ER positive in a patchy distribution and has high expression of CK5.
- Papilloma with atypia has the reverse immunohistochemical profile, with strong diffuse (>90%) nuclei ER positivity and low CK5 immunoreactivity.

Differential Diagnosis
- **Papillary DCIS:** Delicate or absent fibrovascular core, often atypical nuclei or atypical mitotic figures, pseudo stratification. DCIS may be present.
- **Micropapillary DCIS:** Micropapillae without central fibrovascular core
- **Intraductal papillary carcinoma:** Fine papillae
- **Invasive papillary carcinoma:** Invasion into stroma, no myoepithelial layer.
- **Papilloma with atypia versus papilloma with low-grade ductal carcinoma *in situ***
- **Juvenile papillomatosis.**

Case History: A 62-year-old female, well-circumscribed mass measuring 2 × 2 × 1 cm in left breast.

Diagnosis: Papillary DCIS or intraductal papillary carcinoma

Clinical Features
Clear or blood stained nipple discharge, peripherally located lesions present as mass.

Gross
- Range in size from a few millimeters with mean size of 2 cm.
- Well-circumscribed lesion with cystic and papillary areas.

Microscopy

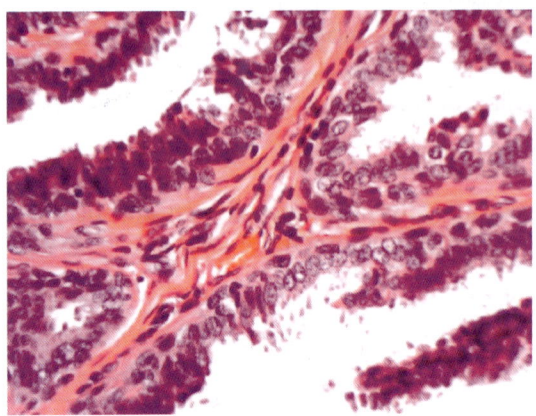

Fig. 5.4

- Ducts or TDLU filled with slender, branching fibrovascular stalks covered by a single cell population of neoplastic epithelial cells. Myoepithelial cell layer is absent within the papillae.
- Cells are polygonal, oval or spindled with abundant granular eosinophilic cytoplasm and bland ovoid nuclei.
- Tumor cells usually show low or intermediate grade nuclear features.
- Tumor cells can form micropapillary, cribriform or solid structures obscuring the spaces between the papillary fronds.
- No benign papilloma areas.

Ancillary Studies
- Myoepithelial cell markers are negative within the papillae but present at the periphery.
- Neoplastic epithelial cells are strongly positive for ER/PR and negative for high molecular weight keratins (CK5/6 and 14).

Differential Diagnosis
- **Apocrine metaplasia**
- **Encapsulated papillary carcinoma:** Myoepithelial cells are absent both within the papillae and at the periphery of duct space.
- **Intraductal papilloma with atypia:** Fibrovascular cores covered by both epithelial and myoepithelial cells.

Case History: A 52-year-old female, well-circumscribed mass in the left breast.

Diagnosis: Adenomyoepithelioma

Clinical Features
- Most commonly occur as mass lesions, which are usually palpable.
- Age ranges from 25 to 82 years, with a mean age of approximately 60 years.

Gross
- Adenomyoepitheliomas range in size from 0.5 to 8 cm.
- Solid and well delineated but with lobulations.
- Cut surface is tan, white, or yellow. Macroscopic cysts of varying size can also occur.

Microscopy

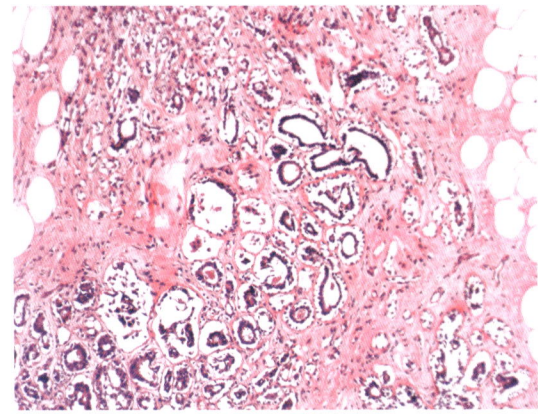

Fig. 5.5

Three main patterns: Tubular, spindled, and lobulated.
- Mixture of epithelial and myoepithelial cells, but the myoepithelial cells are the most prominent component.
- **Tubular type:** Has rounded tubules lined by epithelial cells and surrounded by hyperplastic myoepithelial cells that can expand and obliterate tubular lumens.
- **Spindled type:** Has a predominance of myoepithelial cells with scant epithelial-lined spaces.
- **Lobulated type:** It is characterized by solid nests of myoepithelial cells that compress epithelial-lined spaces.
- Apocrine, squamous, and sebaceous differentiation can be seen in glandular elements. Ancillary studies
- Epithelial component characteristically expresses pan keratins.
- Myoepithelial cells typically show immunoreactivity for smooth muscle actin, calponin, smooth muscle myosin heavy chain, and p63.

Differential Diagnosis
- **Intraductal papilloma:** No prominent myoepithelial component.
- **Invasive carcinoma (on core biopsy):** Unequivocal evidence of invasion.
- **Nipple adenoma:** No prominent myoepithelial component.
- **Tubular adenoma:** Very well- circumscribed (tubular variant is not) myoepithelial cells are inconspicuous or rare.
- **Adenosis tumor:** No prominent myoepithelial component
- **Pleomorphic adenoma (benign mixed tumor) and ductal adenoma.**
- **Metaplastic (spindle cell) carcinoma.**

Case History: A 48-year-old female with malignant breast lump clinically.

Diagnosis: Sclerosing adenosis

Clinical Features
- Most often, sclerosing adenosis has no visible gross findings.
- However, if it has increased fibrosis, it may appear white and vaguely nodular or even as a distinct mass.

Microscopy

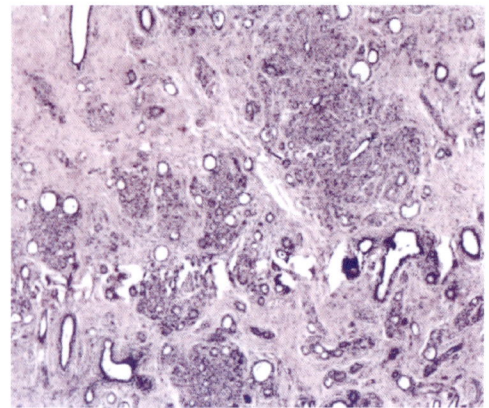

Fig. 5.6

- Characterized by a concomitant marked proliferation and atrophy of the acini.
- When small, the lobular nature is maintained. A terminal duct can be seen and the proliferation of small acini found.
- In sclerotic lesions or in large proliferations, the terminal duct may not be apparent, and the acini may become distorted and look like invasive carcinoma.
- Stroma associated with sclerosing adenosis can be loose or fibrotic.
- Psammomatous type calcification is commonly seen.

Ancillary Diagnostic Studies

Stains for myoepithelial cells such as CD10, p63, calmodulin, SMA positive.

Differential Diagnosis

Invasive ductal carcinoma: Not lobular at low power, marked atypia with no myoepithelial cells.

Case History: A 63-year-old female with bilateral breast mass.

Diagnosis: Mucocele-like lesion

Clinical Features

- Mean age 40 years, range 25–61 years.
- Mucin extravasation or mucocele-like lesions at core biopsy warrant close radiological–pathological correlation and likely excision.
- Often appears malignant radiologically due to microcalcifications.

Microscopy

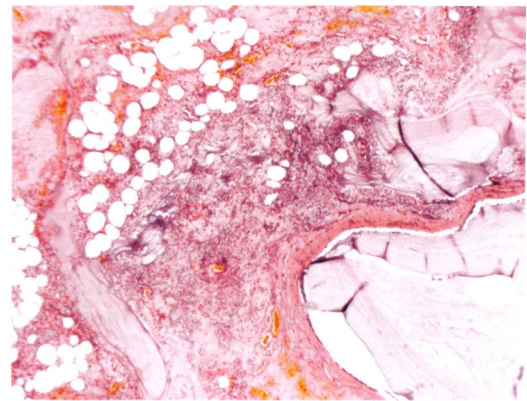

Fig. 5.7

- Mucin containing cysts that often ruptures, with extravasation of mucin into surrounding stroma.
- Epithelium lining the cysts may be benign/flat, hyperplasia, ADH, DCIS or mucinous carcinoma.
- Myoepithelial cells adhere to strips of cells floating in lakes of mucin. Calcifications are often present. Histiocytes and inflammatory cells are seen.

Differential Diagnosis

Mucinous/colloid carcinoma: Low grade tumor cells without adherent myoepithelium floating in a lightly stained amorphous mucin.

Case History: A 25-year-old female, solitary painless firm well-circumscribed mass in upper quadrant—breast.

Diagnosis: Pseudoangiomatous stromal hyperplasia (PASH)

Clinical Features

It is most common in premenopausal women. It represents a myofibroblastic response to endogenous or exogenous hormonal stimuli, predominantly progesterone.

Gross
- Usually unilateral, sharply circumscribed non-encapsulated, firm to rubbery homogenous lobulated nodules.
- Cut surface—tan pink to whitish in color. Range in size from 1 to 12 cm (mean 6 cm)

Microscopy

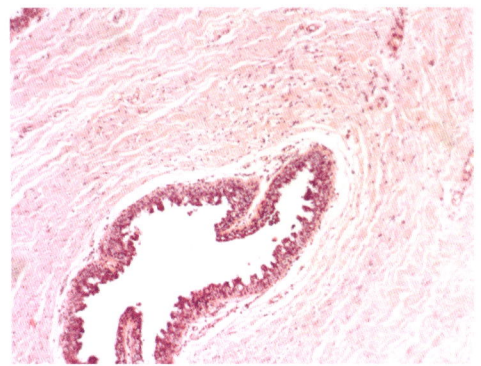

Fig. 5.8

- PASH is characterized by dense fibrous stroma with numerous slit-like spaces devoid of blood.
- A discontinuous layer of bland, mitotically inactive flat, spindle cells, lines the spaces.
- The myofibroblasts rimming the empty spaces resemble endothelial cells.
- Stromal giant cells are rarely present
- No mitotic figures, necrosis, atypia.

Ancillary Studies
- Stromal cells of PASH are usually strongly positive for progesterone receptor and weakly or patchy positive for estrogen receptor.
- Cells lining the spaces are positive for CD34, calponin, desmin and SMA.
- Notably they are negative for CD31, which aids in the differential diagnosis of other vascular lesions.

Differential Diagnosis
- **Low grade angiosarcoma:** The slit like spaces can be deceiving for vascular lesions. Angiosarcoma is very infiltrative with atypical cells and dissects collagen at the edges. Both angiosarcoma and PASH are CD34 positive, but PASH is negative for other vascular markers such as CD31 and von Willebrand factor.
- **Fibroadenoma with prominent stroma.**

Case History: A 42-year-old female, right breast—firm painless mass (m) 9 × 5 × 4 cm.

Diagnosis: Benign phyllodes tumor

Clinical Features
- Middle-aged women, mean 40–50 years.
- Unilateral, firm, painless breast mass. Size >10 cm.

Gross
- Well-circumscribed firm bulging mass.
- Cut surface—tan pink to gray in color. Characteristic whorled pattern with curved clefts resembling leaf buds is seen.

Microscopy

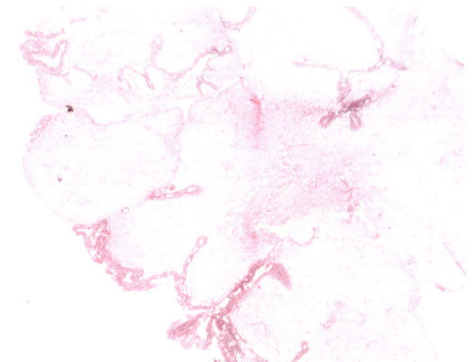

Fig. 5.9

- Circumscribed pushing border, stromal hypercellularity and benign glandular elements with intracanalicular pattern.
- Stroma resembles fibroblasts and myofibroblasts.
- Mitoses are rare, <5/10 HPF.
- Occasional bizarre stromal giant cells may be noted.
- Variable hemorrhage, necrosis, fat, bone, cartilage and skeletal muscle.

Ancillary Diagnostic Studies
- **Epithelial cells:** PR+, GCDFP-15+
- **Stromal cells:** Vimentin, desmin, CD34+

Differential Diagnosis

- **Fibroadenoma:** Stroma less cellular than phyllodes, less stromal overgrowth, no atypia and rare mitosis
- **Leiomyoma:** Smooth muscle morphology and IHC.

Case History: A 48-year-old female, 5 cm firm mass in the left breast.

Diagnosis: High grade Malignant Phyllodes

Clinical Features

- Phyllode tumors tend to occur in older patients, typically 40 to 50 years of age or older.
- Patients usually present with rapidly enlarging breast masses.

Gross

- Phyllode tumors have well-delineated borders but appear more fleshy, with bulging cut surfaces.
- They are typically larger with an average size of 4 to 5 cm. The epithelial component may be grossly conspicuous as cleft-like spaces or cysts.
- In malignant phyllode tumors, Frank necrosis may be seen.

Microscopy

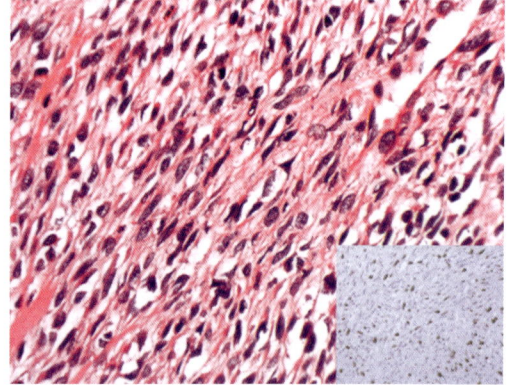

Fig. 5.10: Inset showing high Ki-67 index

- Phyllode tumors are composed of variably cellular stroma admixed with benign glands, which are elongated, slit-like, and often dilated.
- The stromal morphology varies widely, with some cases composed of bland, monomorphic, spindle cells.
- Others show marked nuclear anaplasia similar to pleomorphic undifferentiated sarcomas.
- The epithelial component may show usual ductal hyperplasia or metaplastic changes such as squamous or apocrine.
- The stromal component typically invaginates into dilated glandular lumina, creating the classic "leaflike" pattern.

Ancillary Diagnostic Studies

Ancillary immunohistochemical studies that have been reviewed to aid in distinction of phyllodes tumor from fibroadenoma have not been found useful.

Differential Diagnosis

- Fibroadenoma
- Metaplastic (spindle cell) carcinoma and primary sarcoma

Case History: A 47-year-old female, mammographically detected 5 mm lesion, upper outer quadrant (UOQ).

Diagnosis: Ductal carcinoma *in situ* (DCIS)

Clinical Features

- DCIS accounts for 30 to 40% of all cancers detected mammographically, and it presents as calcifications, soft tissue density, or architectural distortion.
- DCIS has variable risk of progression to invasive disease.
- The risk depends on grade, extent of disease, margin status, and operative and radiation treatment.

LOW-GRADE DUCTAL CARCINOMA *IN SITU*

Gross

Occasionally, DCIS can form a palpable mass, but in the majority of cases, the lesions are microscopic and do not have a typical gross pathology.

Microscopy

- The minimum criteria for low-grade DCIS are a single population of monomorphic cells with distinct cell borders and low-grade but

enlarged nuclei (1.5 times the size of the nucleus of a normal ductal cell nucleus).
- The nuclei stand apart rather than overlap.
- These cytologic and architectural criteria are then coupled with a quantity requirement of at least two ducts or greater than 2 mm.

Ancillary Studies

The usual staining of ERs and PRs in normal and hyperplastic ducts is scattered positivity, whereas low-grade DCIS is usually uniformly positive for the receptors. High-molecular-weight keratin (particularly CK5, CK6, and CK14) is usually positive in hyperplasia but not in low-grade DCIS.

Differential Diagnosis

- High-grade ductal carcinoma *in situ*
- Atypical ductal hyperplasia
- Usual ductal hyperplasia
- Flat epithelial atypia
- Collagenous spherulosis
- Classic lobular carcinoma *in situ*

HIGH-GRADE DUCTAL CARCINOMA *IN SITU*

Clinical Features

High-grade DCIS is the precursor lesion with the highest risk of progression to invasive carcinoma.

Gross

Varies from no findings to mass formation with small streaks of fibrosis.

Microscopy

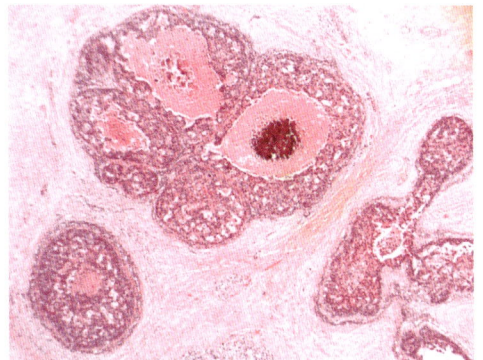

Fig. 5.11

- High-grade DCIS is typified by enlarged cells (nuclei 2.5 times the size of a red blood cell) with coarse chromatin and prominent nucleoli.
- Mitoses are usually present with or without atypical forms. The nuclear membranes are irregular, and there is usually marked anisonucleosis.
- High-grade DCIS is often accompanied by comedonecrosis and calcifications.
- Cribriforming may be present.
- Unlike low-grade DCIS, the 2 mm size requirement is not used when the proliferation has high-grade cytology.
- Usual architectural types: Cribriform, micropapillary, solid, cystic, DCIS associated with mucocele-like lesion, mucinous, papillary and pure micropapillary.

Ancillary Studies

- ER is commonly obtained for DCIS to aid in management and applicability of hormonal treatment.
- E-cadherin may be useful in distinguishing ductal from lobular neoplasia. Myoepithelial stains can be used to assess for invasion. Some may be HER2 amplified.

Differential Diagnosis

- Intermediate-grade ductal carcinoma *in situ*
- Pleomorphic lobular carcinoma *in situ*
- Microinvasive carcinoma
- Invasive cribriform carcinoma.

Case History: A 57-year-old female, excoriation and scaling in the nipple region.

Diagnosis: Paget's disease of the nipple

Clinical Features

- Peak incidence occurs between the sixth and seventh decades. The risk is highest in nulliparous and/or postmenopausal women.
- Patients typically present with an erythematous, eczematous to psoriasiform patch involving or surrounding the nipple.
- Nipple discharge, retraction, pain, burning, and pruritus are common signs and symptoms.

Gross

Grossly, the skin may look irritated with erythema or scale, or architectural distortion may occur such as dimpling of the skin or nipple retraction.

Microscopy

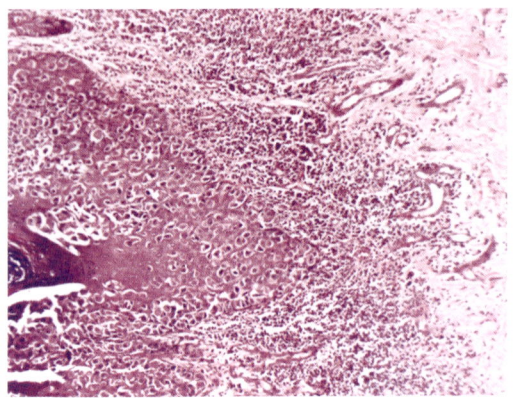

Fig. 5.12

- Large cells with abundant pale cytoplasm and large nuclei with prominent nucleoli termed Paget cells seen within the epidermis.
- Can be present singly or in clusters. Can contain mucin and melanin pigments. 3 variants: Classical, bowenoid, pemphigus-like.

Ancillary Studies

- Almost always positive for keratin 7 and CAM 5.2 and positive for HER2.
- CEA, EMA, GCDFP-15 and p53 may be positive.

Differential Diagnosis

- **Gross hyperpigmentation of the nipple and areola:** Hyperkeratosis, epidermal papillomatosis, and keratotic plugs, but there are no clear cells.
- **Eczema, contact dermatitis, Toker cell hyperplasia, radiation dermatitis, nipple adenoma, and glycogen-rich squamous cells:** Are benign conditions potentially misdiagnosed as PDB.
- **Malignant diseases:** Basal cell carcinoma, malignant melanoma (superficial spreading type, *in situ* or invasive—tumor cells invade dermis, S100+, HMB45+, AE1/3), and epidermotropic metastatic carcinoma.
- **Carcinoma *in situ* of skin:** Has individual cell keratinization and multinucleated giant cells, CK7–, mucin–, HER2–

Case History: A 63-year-old female, firm to hard mass in the left breast close to the nipple and areolar region.

Diagnosis: Squamous cell carcinoma, breast

Clinical Features

Very rare (<0.2% of breast primaries), cutaneous tumors, squamous component of phyllode tumors and squamous-like areas of medullary carcinoma to be excluded.

Gross

- Circumscribed and hemorrhagic tumor.
- May have central cyst with keratin.

Microscopy

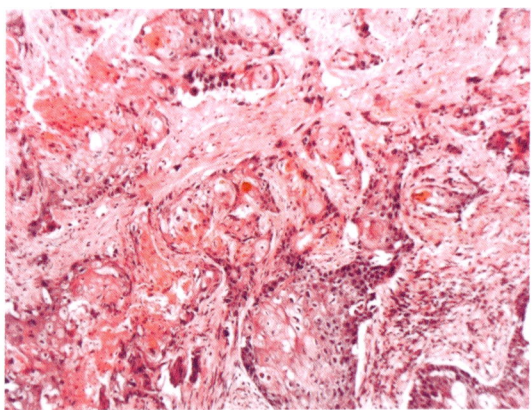

Fig. 5.13

- Tumor composed entirely of malignant squamous cells with variable keratinization and spindle cells.
- Bland squamous cells may line cystic spaces.
- Stroma shows desmoplastic reaction and prominent inflammatory infiltrate.

Ancillary Studies

Triple negative (90%), EGFR (85%), 34 beta E12, CK5/6 (75%), p63 (90%). High Ki-67.

Differential Diagnosis

- Post-traumatic lobular squamous metaplasia.
- Other squamous metaplasia
- Metastasis

Case History: A 66-year-old woman with ill circumscribed firm mass in the left breast

Diagnosis: Metaplastic carcinoma with heterogenous elements

Clinical Features

- Rare (<5% of breast carcinomas)
- More aggressive than invasive ductal NOS due to larger tumor size, higher grade
- Metastases tend to be hematogenous and not nodal
- Represents a type of basal-like carcinoma lacking epidermal growth factor receptor and KIT activating mutations

Gross

- Firm, nodular and well-circumscribed
- Squamous or chondroid areas are pearly white to gray glistening areas on cut surface

Microscopy

- Neoplastic component that is either squamous or non-epithelial should be present
  - May exhibit obviously malignant stroma
  - May resemble pleomorphic MFH or fibrosarcoma
  - May exhibit heterologous differentiation
  - Usually osteosarcoma or chondrosarcoma
  - Less commonly glioma, melanoma, rhabdomyosarcoma, angiosarcoma or liposarcoma
- Stroma may be composed of bland spindle cells (spindle cell carcinoma)
  - p63 positive, often high molecular weight keratin positive
  - May contain fibroblasts and or myofibroblasts
  - May resemble nodular fasciitis or fibromatosis
- Most have a component of ductal carcinoma

Immunohistochemistry

From a diagnostic standpoint the important distinction is from sarcoma

- p63 and CK5/6 appear to be quite specific for this
- It is important to be aware of significant smooth muscle actin and S100 reactivity. Their presence does not rule out carcinoma

Laminin 5	96%
p63	57–86%
CK5/6	50–86%
CD10	85%
Smooth muscle actin	60%
S100	45%

Differential Diagnosis

- **Phyllodes tumor:** Epithelial component is benign. Stromal component negative for high molecular weight keratin and p63. No squamous differentiation.
- **Adenomyoepithelioma:** Epithelial component and stroma is histologically bland with stroma showing myoepithelial differentiation only.

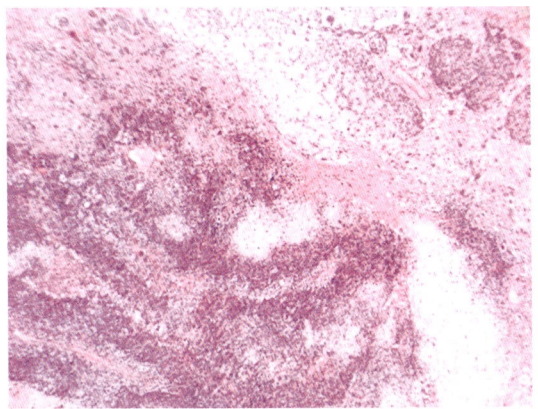

Fig. 5.14

- **Myoepithelial carcinoma:** Ducts with prominent myoepithelial cells at periphery, diffusely S100+
- **Pure sarcoma/nodular fascitis/fibromatosis:** Should be diagnosed only after thorough sectioning and with negative stains for p63, broad spectrum keratin and high molecular weight keratin.

Case History: A 42-year-old female, right axillary lymph node sampling.

Diagnosis: Metastatic carcinoma with apocrine differentiation—lymph node

Clinical Features
- Apocrine carcinoma affects mean age varying from 53 to 62.
- The clinical presentation similar to those of invasive ductal carcinoma NOS.

Gross
Mass of any size and at any site in breast.

Microscopy

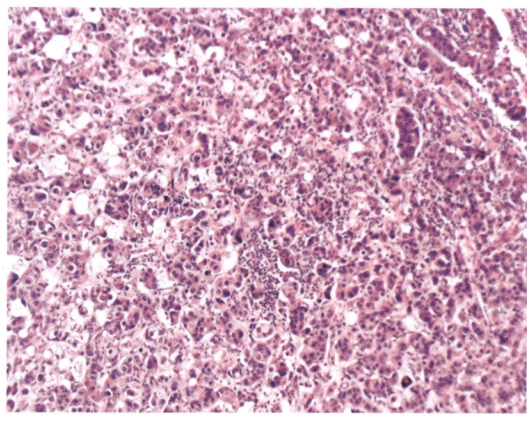

Fig. 5.15

- Apocrine carcinoma is most often arranged in thin cords or trabeculae, or solid nests or as single cells.
- Cytoplasm is usually eosinophilic and granular, it may also appear flocculent or vacuolated.
- The morphologic criteria for apocrine differentiation are defined as:
  - Large cells with abundant granular eosinophilic cytoplasm, usually with a nuclear-to-cytoplasmic ratio of 1:2 or more.
  - Round and/or pleomorphic large vesicular nuclei containing either a single macronucleolus or multiple, smaller nucleoli.
  - Sharply defined cell borders.

Ancillary Studies
- Most apocrine carcinomas show strong reactivity for GCDFP-15.
- The majority of apocrine tumors are negative for ER, PR, and BCL-2 but demonstrate strong expression for androgen receptor.

Differential Diagnosis
- **Apocrine metaplasia**
- **Oncocytic carcinoma:** Indistinguishable on H and E stain; GCDFP15 negative; antimitochondrial antibody stain-strong, diffuse
- **Secretory carcinoma:** Low grade nuclei with inconspicuous nucleoli; cytoplasm granular or clear and vacuolated; PASd shows abundant cytoplasmic mucin
- **Tumors with abundant pale cytoplasm:** Granular cell tumor, xanthogranuloma, and metastatic renal cell carcinoma.

Case History: A 37-year-old female, family history of breast cancer circumscribed lesion, firm to soft in the right breast.

Diagnosis: Carcinoma with medullary features, breast

Clinical Features
Usually occurs age ranging from 45 to 54 years.

Gross
- Well circumscribed and moderately firm.
- Cut surface is fleshy and gray-tan and may appear lobular or nodular. Foci of hemor-

rhage, necrosis, and even cystic degeneration are not unusual.
- Median size of 2 to 3 cm.

Microscopy

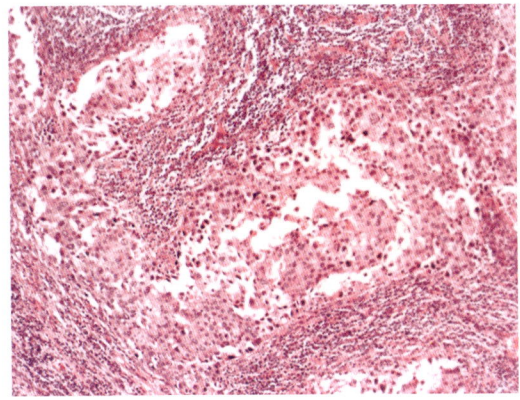

Fig. 5.16

Medullary carcinoma should meet all of the following morphologic criteria as defined by the WHO:
- Syncytial growth pattern in more than 75% of the tumor.
- No glandular or tubular structures, even as a minor component. Lack of tubular differentiation.
- Prominent and diffuse lymphoplasmacytic stromal infiltrate.
- Pleomorphic high-grade vesicular nuclei containing one or several nucleoli.
- Complete histologic circumscription or pushing margins.
- Numerous mitoses.

Ancillary Studies
- Negative for ER, PR, and HER2.
- They have a high Ki-67 proliferation index and often show p53 positivity.

Differential Diagnosis
- **Invasive ductal carcinoma:** Diagnosis of infiltrating ductal carcinoma is suggested only for those carcinomas that lack any of the above required diagnostic criteria. Many of these will be high grade, so the distinction is critical.
- **Lymphoma or melanoma:** Immunohistochemistry can easily resolve this if it is a problem.

Case History: A 57-year-old female, hard mass (m) 4 × 2 × 2 cm irregular with skin puckering in the UOQ—right breast.

Diagnosis: Invasive lobular carcinoma

Clinical Features
Mean age of 63 years. They are often poorly circumscribed and have a higher incidence of multicentric and contralateral disease.

Gross
Slightly larger than invasive ductal carcinomas but these poorly delineated tumors can be difficult to detect on gross.

Microscopy

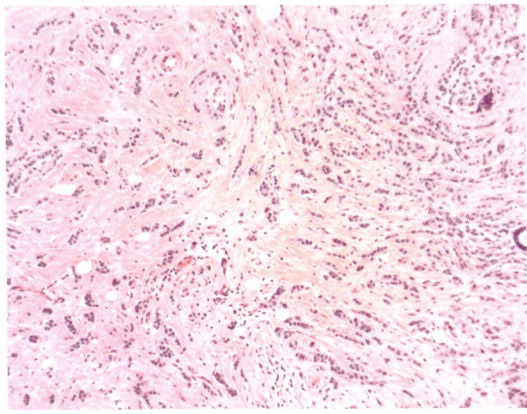

Fig. 5.17

- Classic invasive lobular carcinoma is characterized by small, bland cells that lack cellular cohesion and infiltrate in single lines or thin cords of cells.
- The tumor cells frequently form palisades around normal ductal structures (also termed targetoid distribution).
- No desmoplastic response.
- The cells have bland round-to-oval nuclei that often are eccentrically located and surrounded by a rim of delicate cytoplasm.
- Intracytoplasmic lumens may also be seen and can impart a signet-ring appearance.

- Pleomorphic lobular carcinoma is characterized by tumor cells with grade III nuclei growing in the classic lobular carcinoma pattern of single cell files and lacking E-cadherin expression.
- Variants: Classic type, solid type, alveolar, pleomorphic, tubulolobular and mixed variants.

Ancillary Studies

Immunohistochemical stain for E-cadherin shows lack of membrane reactivity in the majority of invasive lobular carcinomas, reflecting the loss of cellular cohesion characteristic of these tumors.

Differential Diagnosis

- **Invasive ductal carcinoma:** Infiltration in cords of varying thickness; may form ductal structures; E-cadherin positive
- **Lobular carcinoma *in situ* in sclerosing adenosis:** Circumscribed, nodular; Myoepithelial cells present.
- **Gastric carcinoma:** May also display loss of E-cadherin proteins, immunohistochemical stains such as mammaglobin and GATA3 may be of use
- **Lymphoma:** No molding of nuclei; Lymphoid markers positive.

Case History: A 65-year-old female, blood tinged nipple discharge with vague mass in the central portion of the breast for 5 months.

Diagnosis: Invasive micropapillary carcinoma

Clinical Features

Most patients present with a palpable mass. Axillary nodal metastasis is common at the time of presentation.

Gross

The mean size of micropapillary carcinoma is about 4 cm, significantly larger than that of invasive ductal carcinoma NOS.

Microscopy

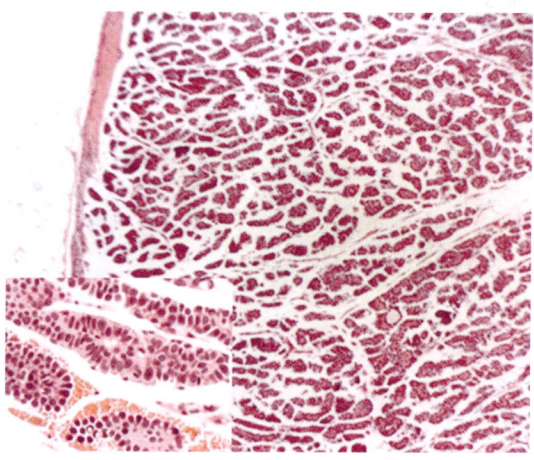

Fig. 5.18

- Hollow or morule-like aggregates of cuboidal to low columnar neoplastic cells devoid of fibrovascular core surrounded by empty stromal spaces.
- Cells display a reverse polarity ("inside out" pattern) where the apical pole of neoplastic cells face the empty stromal spaces which can be demonstrated by MUC1 antibodies.

Ancillary Studies

- Characteristic "inside-out" staining for EMA or MUC1.
- Most tumors are positive for ER and/or PR.
- HER2 gene amplification has been observed in 10 to 45% of cases.

Differential Diagnosis

- **Invasive ductal carcinoma, not otherwise specified**
- **Metastatic micropapillary carcinoma from the other site:** Immunohistochemistry of micropapillary carcinomas of various sites will be helpful.
- **Mucinous carcinoma:** Prominent mucin in spaces; Irregular epithelial clusters; Usually low grade cytology.

Case History: A 43-year-old female, 2 × 2 cm mass right breast with axillary nodes.

Diagnosis: Invasive ductal carcinoma with ductal and lobular features (mixed type carcinoma)

Clinical Features

- Age of onset similar to infiltrating ductal carcinoma.
- May have higher plasma levels of soluble human leukocyte antigens (HLA)-G.

Microscopy

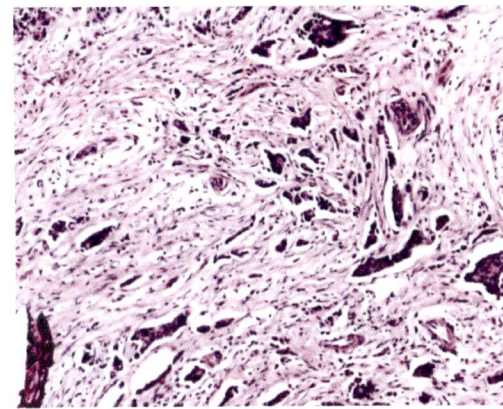

Fig. 5.19

Definite features of invasive ductal carcinoma and invasive lobular carcinoma in same tumor.

Ancillary Studies

E-cadherin patterns include no staining (similar to lobular), full staining (similar to ductal) or staining of ductal areas only.

Differential Diagnosis

Tubulolobular carcinoma: Typical areas of invasive lobular carcinoma with cords of single file cells, which merge with small round to angulated tubules with minute or undetectable lumina.

Case History: A 46-year-old female, radiologically detected one centimeter lesion.

Diagnosis: Invasive tubular carcinoma

Clinical Features

- They are non-palpable and constitute 1–4% of all breast cancers.
- Detected by mammographic screening either as a spiculated lesion or microcalcifications.

Gross

- Tubular carcinomas typically appear as a stellate lesion with a gray-white cut surface and yellow streaks.
- Tumors are usually small in size, ranging from 0.2 to 2 cm.

Microscopy

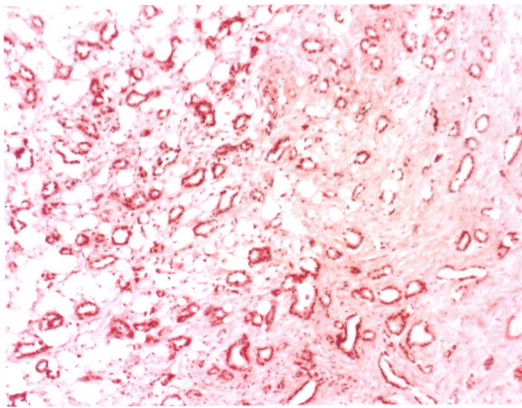

Fig. 5.20

- Tubular carcinoma is composed of well-formed and angulated tubules with open lumens haphazardly arranged in a desmoplastic cellular stroma.
- The tubular structures are lined by a single layer of cuboidal to columnar cells, which often exhibit prominent cytoplasmic apical snouts with stellate infiltrating architecture
- The cytological atypia is mild and shows minimal nuclear pleomorphism with basally located, round to oval nuclei. Nucleoli are inconspicuous and mitotic figures are rare. Intraluminal secretions with microcalcifications are frequently noted.
- Associated with desmoplastic reaction.

Ancillary Studies

Tubular carcinomas invariably express ER, PR, and BCL-2, and they are negative for HER2 and epidermal growth factor receptor (EGFR).

Differential Diagnosis

- **Benign sclerosing lesion:** Circumscribed and nodular; Many ducts have obliterated lumens; Frequent branching; Sometimes more than one layer of cells; Cells smaller, streaming; Myoepithelial cells present.
- **Fibroadenoma:** Biphasic tumor with overgrowth of epithelial and stromal tissue; no true angulated contours of cells, no desmoplastic stroma
- **Microglandular adenosis:** Nodular or diffuse; Uniform small round ducts with small lumens; No apical snouts; Eosinophilic secretion present in at least some lumens; EMA negative
- **Ductal carcinoma, low grade:** Irregular infiltration; May have >10% ribbons or cords; Frequent budding and branching; Frequent budding and branching.
- **Tubulolobular carcinoma:** Mixed tubular and lobular patterns; Linear infiltrative pattern, frequently concentric

Case History: A 70-year-old female, soft circumscribed mass in the UOQ left breast.

Diagnosis: Mucinous carcinoma breast

Clinical Features

- Accounts for approximately 2% of all breast carcinomas.
- Occurs in patients >55 years of age
- MRI: Stimulates a benign process.

Gross

- Gelatinous lesion with pushing margins and a soft consistency.
- Size ranges from <1 to >20 cm.

Microscopy

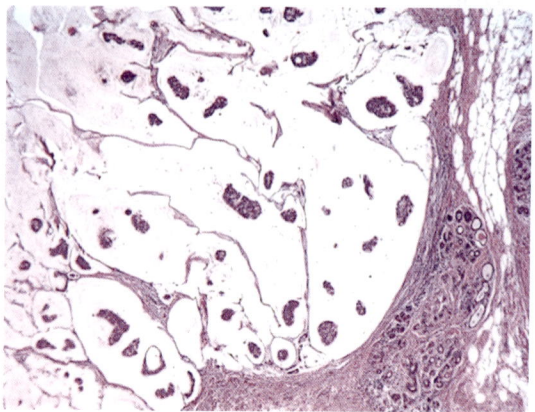

Fig. 5.21a

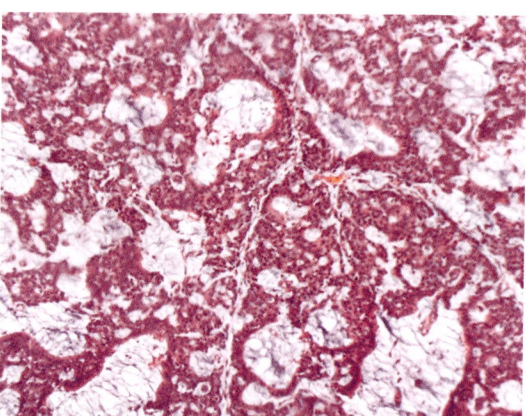

Fig. 5.21b

- Nests of cells floating in lakes of mucin partitioned by delicate fibrous septa containing capillary blood vessels.
- Cell clusters are variable in shape and size with low nuclear atypia.
- Type A: Mucinous carcinoma classical non-endocrine type with large quantities of extracellular mucin.
- Type B: Mucinous carcinoma with large cell clusters showing frequent neuroendocrine differentiation.
- Pure tumor is composed of >90% mucinous carcinoma.

Ancillary Studies

- More than 90% are positive for ER and 70% for PR. The vast majority of the tumors lack HER2 overexpression.
- Type B is positive for chromogranin, synaptophysin, or neuron-specific enolase by immunohistochemistry.
- Mucinous carcinoma displays a CK7 positive and CK20 negative keratin profile. These tumors consistently lack CDX2.
- Recent studies have demonstrated WT1 nuclear expression.

Differential Diagnosis

- **Mucocele-like lesion:** Seen in premenopausal women with an average age of 40 years. Identifying the presence of benign ducts distended by mucinous material adjacent to a mucocele like lesion can be a helpful clue in pointing toward a benign process with a myoepithelial cell layer.
- **Fibroadenoma with myxoid stroma:** Has compressed spaces lined by 2 layers
- **Matrix-producing metaplastic carcinoma**
- **Invasive micropapillary carcinoma:** Less extracellular mucin than mucinous carcinoma; cells have abundant eosinophilic cytoplasm, round vesicular nuclei and prominent nucleoli; extensive true angiolymphatic invasion; often psammoma bodies
- **Signet ring carcinoma:** Characterized by cells with intracellular mucin that indents the nucleus.

Case History: A 63-year-old female, form mobile mass (M) 3 x 2 x 2 cm, freely mobile in left lower outer quadrant

Diagnosis: Rosai-Dorfman disease of breast

Clinical Features

- Rosai-Dorfman disease limited to the breast is an extremely rare entity.
- Painless palpable breast masses
- These lesions in the breast commonly have an appearance that is indistinguishable from breast carcinoma on mammogram and ultrasound.

Microscopy

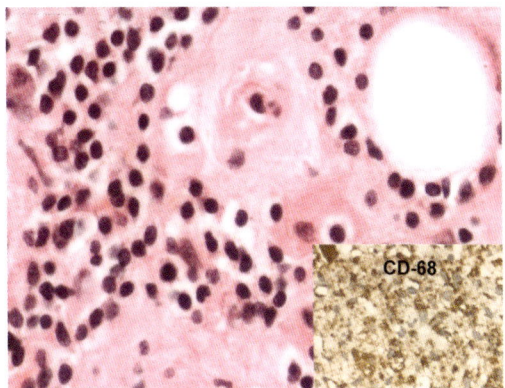

Fig. 5.22

- Marked lymphoplasmacytic and histiocytic (large with abundant cytoplasm) inflammation
- Emperipolesis (phagocytosis of lymphocytes by histiocytes)

Ancillary Studies

- Strong staining of histiocytes with S-100 or CD68 or CD163
- Lymphocytes and plasma cells polyclonal

Case History: A 57-year-old female, postmenopausal 2 months history of left breast mass. 2 x 1 cm, ill-defined.

Diagnosis: Adenosquamous carcinoma, breast

Microscopy

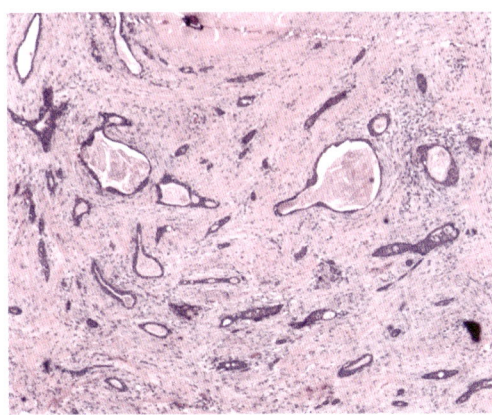

Fig. 5.23

- While focal squamous differentiation has been observed in 3.7% of infiltrating duct carcinomas, a prominent admixture of invasive ductal and squamous cell carcinoma is rarely observed.
- The squamous component is often keratinizing, but ranges from very well-differentiated keratinizing areas to poorly differentiated non-keratinizing foci.

Ancillary Studies

The squamous component is negative for both ER and PR, while the positivity of the ductal carcinoma component for ER and PR depends on its degree of differentiation.

Prognosis: Relatively good prognosis with rare lymph node metastasis.

Case History: A 36-year-old female, grayish red mass in the left breast, no calcification on imaging.

Diagnosis: Angiosarcoma, breast

Clinical Features

- Clinically diffuse breast enlargement is present. Skin involvement is associated with discoloration of skin:
  1. *Primary:* Arises in breast parenchyma.
  2. *Secondary:* Skin, chest wall, breast parenchyma secondary to surgery and postoperative radiation for breast carcinoma.
- Incidence: 0.5% of breast carcinoma.

Gross

Usually 1–25 cm with spongy hemorrhagic appearance with ill-defined borders. Poorly differentiated tumors have a solid fibrous appearing areas.

Microscopy

- In well-differentiated forms, ectatic and often angulated or branching vascular spaces dissect through and infiltrate adipose tissue or pre-existing tissue such as breast epithelium or cutaneous adnexal structures.

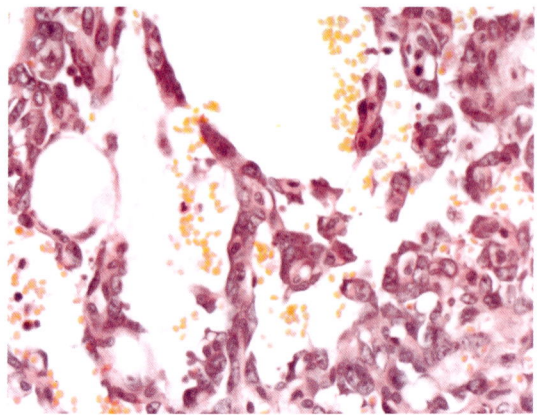

Fig. 5.24

- The endothelial lining cells may be flattened with no significant nuclear atypia, but areas with more significant nuclear pleomorphism, cellular stratification, and/or cellular tufting are commonly seen at least focally.
- In more poorly differentiated tumors, there may be confluent spindling of the neoplastic endothelial cells and fascicle formation.
- In these poorly differentiated angiosarcomas, extravasated red blood cells, blood lakes, and necrosis are often seen, whereas areas with obvious vasoformation are typically identified around the periphery.
- Finally, epithelioid angiosarcomas are composed of plump, round neoplastic cells with amphophilic cytoplasm and round nuclei, often with prominent nucleoli. These epithelioid angiosarcomas may grow in a sheet-like fashion.

Ancillary Studies

CD31 is the most utilized adjunctive immunohistochemical marker of endothelial differentiation.

Differential Diagnosis

- **PASH:** No endothelial lining of spaces; No red blood cells in spaces; No infiltration of fat; Lining is CD31 negative

- **Angiolipoma**
- **Benign vascular lesion:** Hemangiomas, vascular malformations and angiomatosis.
- **Atypical vascular lesion:** Almost all have received radiation; Usually in the skin of the breast; Small non-hemorrhagic lesion
- **Invasive carcinoma and melanoma:** Positive for other specific lineage markers

Case History: A 70-year-old female, presented with right breast nodule. USG showed well-demarcated lobulated mass of 5.1 × 4.5 cm.

Diagnosis: Pleomorphic sarcoma, breast

Clinical Features
- Undifferentiated pleomorphic sarcomas often grow rapidly and may be painful.
- Incidence: 1% of all breast carcinomas.

Gross
- Well-circumscribed masses with heterogeneous composition.
- They have been identified as pale, fibrous and fleshy areas admixed with zones of (cystic) necrosis, hemorrhage, or myxoid features.

Microscopy

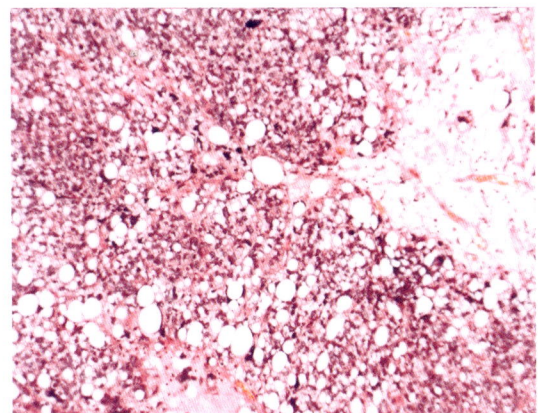

Fig. 5.25

- Lesion exhibits cells showing marked pleomorphism admixed with bizarre giant cells, spindle cells, and variable foamy cells.
- A storiform growth pattern and variable chronic inflammatory cells are also common.
- Numerous atypical mioses seen.
- Rarely metaplastic bone or cartilage seen.

Ancillary Studies
Desmin, vimentin, smooth muscle antigen, CK, leukocyte common antigen, CD34, HMB-45, SMA, EMA, and S-100 protein should all be analyzed in sarcoma patients.

Differential Diagnosis
- **Metaplastic (spindle cell) carcinoma:** Should show at least some keratin or myoepithelial marker expression
- **Malignant phyllodes tumor.**
- **Inflammatory myofibroblastic tumor (IMT):** Neoplasm of myofibroblastic origin, often admixed with prominent inflammatory infiltrate consisting of lymphocytes, plasma cells, macrophages, eosinophils and histiocytes. Immunohistochemistry of IMT shows strong SMA reactivity within the spindle cells frequently and occasional immunoreactivity for ALK.
- **Myofibrosarcomas:** Electron microscopy examination has been considered a gold standard for diagnosis of myofibrosarcoma, Most myofibrosarcomas are immunoreactive for SMA and expression of CK, EMA, CD34, desmin or S100 protein is seen sporadically.
- **Pleomorphic liposarcoma:** MDM2 amplified
- **Pleomorphic leiomyosarcoma**
- **Pleomorphic rhabdomyosarcoma**
- **Breast sarcoma:** May be misdiagnosed as benign spindle cell lesions such as myofibroblastoma, nodular fasciitis and fibromatosis.

Case History: A 55-year-old female, hard mass (m) 2 × 2 × 1 cm irregular in the upper inner quadrant—left breast.

Diagnosis: Granular cell tumor of breast

Clinical Features
- Uncommon
- <1 per 1000 malignancies.
- Usually in inner quadrants of breast.

Gross

- Usually small, sometimes can reach up to 5 cm in diameter.
- They have a hard consistency and ill-defined margins resembling invasive carcinoma clinically.
- Cut surface is firm, homogenous, gray-white-yellow having ill-defined/infiltrative margins.

Microscopy

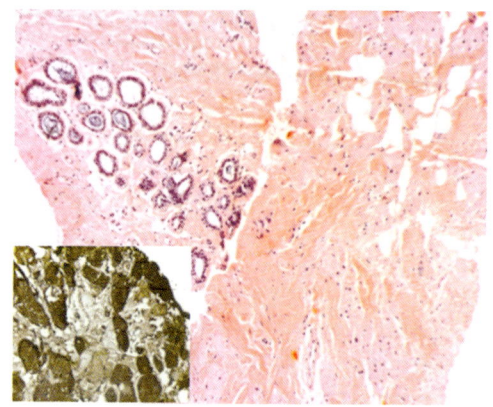

Fig. 5.26: Inset shows inhibin positivity

- Infiltrating sheets/cords of polygonal bland cells with well-defined cell borders and abundant eosinophilic granular cytoplasm.
- Round/oval nuclei with prominent nucleoli.
- The stroma is collagenous. May be close to small nerve bundles and have infiltrative margins.
- Overlying epithelium may show pseudo-epitheliomatous hyperplasia.

Ancillary Studies

PAS, S-100, inhibin positivity.

Differential Diagnosis

- **Alveolar soft part sarcoma**—cells are divided into packets by thin-walled vessels.
- **Apocrine carcinoma**—usually ductal carcinoma also present, keratin+, mucin+, S-100–
- **Histiocytic tumors**
- **Renal cell carcinoma.**

Case History: A 28-year-old female, primi presented with rapidly enlarging breast mass.

Diagnosis: Lactating adenoma

Gross

- Well circumscribed, lobulated, solitary or multiple.
- Cut surface—gray tan. Necrosis or infarction common.

Microscopy

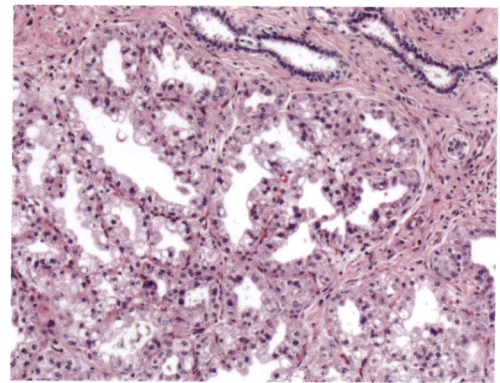

Fig. 5.27

- Cuboidal cells with actively secreting closely packed glands.
- Cells have a foamy to finely vacuolated cytoplasm, uniform nuclei, fine chromatin and prominent nucleoli.
- Background shows abundant foamy material.

Differential Diagnosis

Delayed involution of lacatation.

Case History: A 65-year-old female, left breast irregular mass (m) 5 × 3 × 3 cm.

Diagnosis (a) Encapsulated papillary carcinoma
Diagnosis (b) Invasive solid papillary carcinoma

Clinical Features

- Postmenopausal women, mean age 63–67 years.
- Palpable circumscribed mass, bloody nipple discharge.

- Uncommon histological pattern <1% of breast carcinomas.

Gross
- Nodular, circumscribed mass.
- Whitish grey or yellowish brown, fleshy firm or soft.
- Range from a few millimeters to several centimeters.

Microscopy

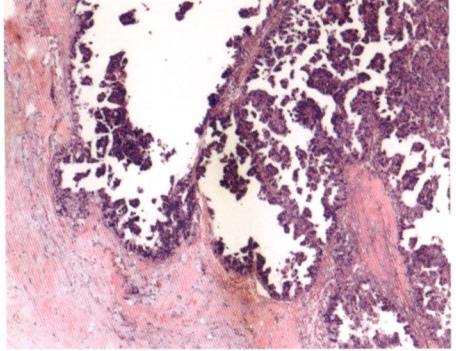

Fig. 5.28a

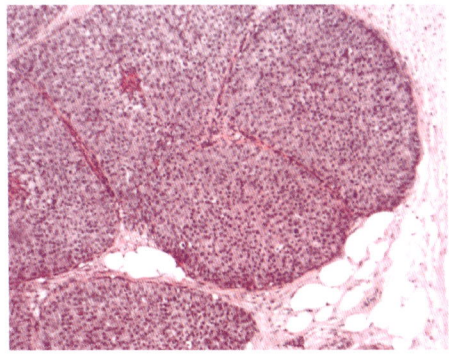

Fig. 5.28b

- Multiple circumscribed cellular mass comprised of closely apposed solidified rounded duct-like structures arranged in contiguous or geographic patterns.
- Cells have moderate to abundant cytoplasm, hyperchromatic nucleus, moderate or marked mucin, often papillary DCIS, microcalcifications.
- The cellular nests frequently lack peripheral myoepithelium.
- The presence of geographic jigsaw pattern with irregular margin coupled with absence of myoepithelial cells marks the distinction *in situ* and invasive disease.
- May have neuroendocrine features.

Ancillary Studies
- Mucin—mucicarmine, alcian blue and PAS+. ER+, HER2/neu−.
- Variable positivity for chromogranin and synaptophysin.

Differential Diagnosis
Intraductal papilloma and metastatic papillary carcinoma.

Suggested Reading
Theory topics:
- Role of tumor microenvironment in carcinoma breast
- Molecular dynamics in breast cancer.
- Sub-classification of triple negative breast carcinoma.

APPROACH TO BREAST LESIONS

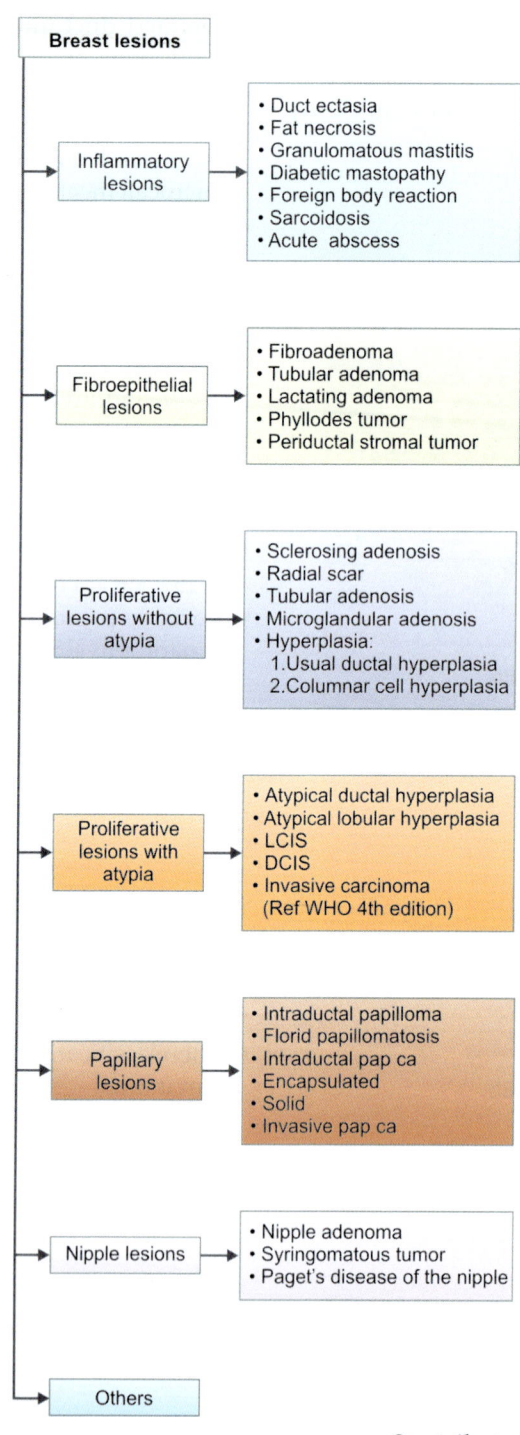

Contributed by Sandhya Sundaram

CHAPTER 6

Lesions of the Lung

Rani Kanthan

Case History: A 50-year-old man presenting with acute respiratory failure.

Diagnosis: Acute respiratory distress syndrome with hyaline membranes

Conditions Associated with Development of ARDS

- Infection
- Sepsis
- Diffuse pulmonary infections
- Viral
- Mycoplasma
- *Pneumocystis pneumonia*
- Miliary tuberculosis
- Gastric aspiration

Morphology

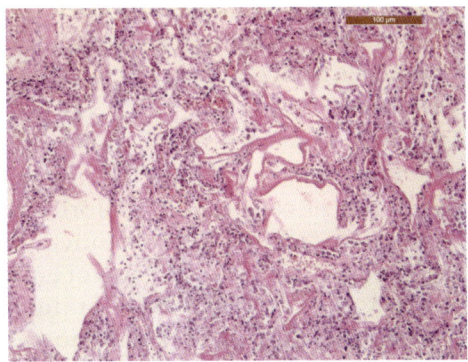

Fig. 6.1

Acute Stage
- Lungs—heavy, firm, red, and boggy.
- Congestion, interstitial and intra-alveolar edema, inflammation, fibrin deposition, and diffuse alveolar damage.
- Alveolar walls—waxy hyaline membranes.

Organizing Stage
- Type II pneumocytes proliferate, and granulation tissue forms in the alveolar walls and spaces.

Case History: A 50-year-old woman presenting with past history of breast cancer.

Diagnosis: Metastatic lymphangitis carcinomatosis

Clinical Features
- 6–8% of patients with pulmonary metastases.
- Breathlessness and a non-productive cough.

Morphology

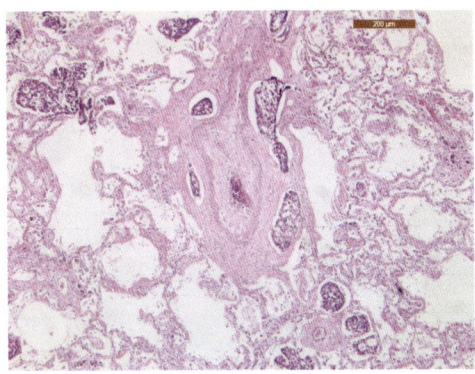

Fig. 6.2

- The spread of tumor cells to the pulmonary lymphatic system or the adjacent interstitial tissue results in thickening of the bronchovascular bundles and septa.
- Desmoplastic reaction—proliferation of neoplastic cells, and lymphatic dilation by edema fluid or tumor secretion contribute to this interstitial thickening.

Imaging
Nodular thickening and ground-glass attenuation.

Transbronchial Biopsy
Required for a definitive diagnosis.

Differential Diagnosis
Sarcoidosis: Nodules in sarcoidosis mainly central regions of the middle and upper. Pulmonary lymphangitic carcinomatosis—usually lower lobes.

Case History: A 50-year-old female with recurrent pneumonia.

Diagnosis: Bronchiectasis

Clinical Features
Cough, fever and copious amounts of foul-smelling, purulent sputum.

Gross
- Markedly distended peripheral bronchi, usually in lower lobes, can trace up to pleural surface.
- Bronchial walls are irregularly thickened.

Microscopy

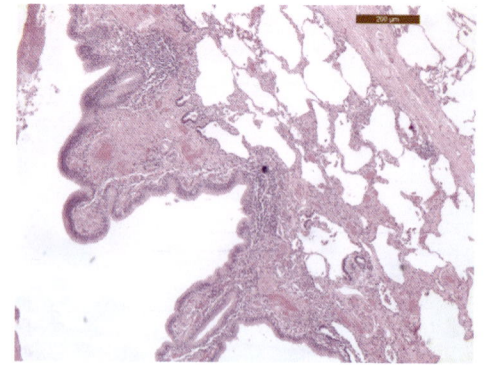

Fig. 6.3

- Chronic inflammation, ulceration of bronchial wall, ossification of bronchial cartilage.
- Thickened pleura with variable inflammation and fibrosis of alveoli.

Case History: A 74-year-old man with past history of tuberculosis with a dry persistent cough.

Diagnosis: Metastatic chordoma of the lung

Clinical Features
- 55–65 years.
- Spheno-occipital—children.
- Over 60% cases occur in men.
- Chondroid chordomas are more common in women.

Gross
Soft, gelatinous, hemorrhagic, gray tumor.

Microscopy

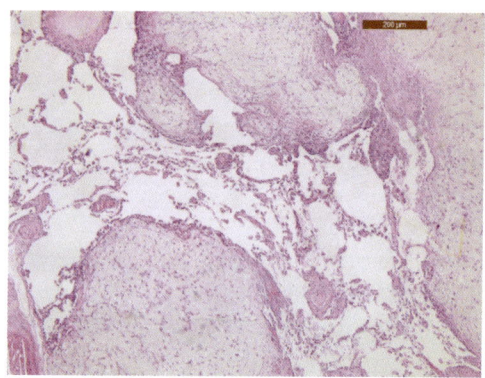

Fig. 6.4

- Lobules separated by fibrous tissue with the tumor cells arranged in cords, columns or trabeculae.
- Basophilic to metachromatic mucinous or myxoid stroma.
- Two types of cell—small, uniform, non-vacuolated cells with ovoid nuclei and larger cells with multivacuolated or bubble-like cytoplasm and vesicular nuclei: "Physaliphorous cells"—diagnostic of chordomas.

Ancillary Tests
- **PAS:** The physaliphorous cells are positive.

- **Alcian blue and mucicarmine:** The matrix is positive.
- **Immunohistochemistry:** S-100, keratin (CK8/18, CK19, AE1–AE3), EMA, 5′-nucleotidase, glycogen, neural-type cadherin, brachyury.
- **Molecular genetics:** Aneuploid.
- **Electron microscopy:** Mitochondria—endoplasmic reticulum complexes, parallel bundles of criss-crossing tubules, desmosomes.

Differential Diagnosis

- **Chondrosarcoma:** Not midline, no fibrous septa, EMA and keratin negative
- **Metastatic renal cell carcinoma:** Prominent vascularity, not lobulated, S100 negative
- **Myxopapillary ependymoma:** Negative for epithelial markers
- **Parachordoma:** Soft tissue tumor composed of epithelioid cells, smaller "glomoid" cells and spindle cells, negative for CK7, CK19, CK20, CEA

Case History: A 50-year-old woman presenting with an enlarged uterus.

Diagnosis: Metastatic endometrial stromal sarcoma

Clinical Features

- Metastases to lung—rare
- Occur a mean 10 years after diagnosis of uterine tumor.

Microscopy

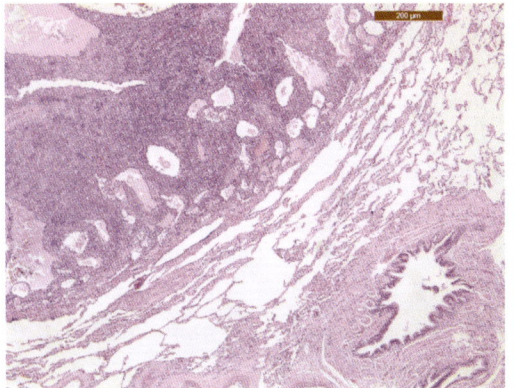

Fig. 6.5

- Well circumscribed
- Solid tumor composed of plump spindle cells in short fascicles, often with hyalinized areas.
- May have cystic or sex cord-like areas

Ancillary Tests

Immunohistochemistry: Vimentin, ER, PR, CD10 positive.

Differential Diagnosis

- Endometriosis
- Hemangiopericytoma
- Lymphangioleiomyomatosis
- Benign metastasizing leiomyoma
- Sclerosing hemangioma
- Solitary fibrous tumor

Case History: A 48-year-old man presenting with an endobronchial lesion.

Diagnosis: Neuroendocrine tumor—carcinoid

Clinical Features

- 1–2% of all lung malignancies in adults and roughly 20–30% of all carcinoid tumors.
- Locally invasive, rarely metastasizes
- Usually age <40 years. Occasionally as part of MEN syndrome.

Gross

Usually well defined, smooth, ivory to pink, cut surface, no necrosis.

Microscopy

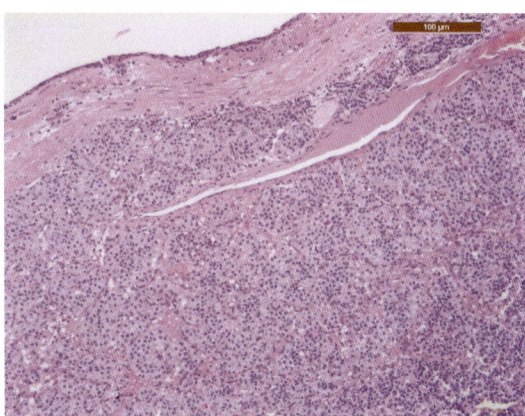

Fig. 6.6

- Nests or trabeculae of medium-sized polygonal cells with lightly eosinophilic cytoplasm, low nuclear grade, round to oval finely granular nuclei; may have rosettes or small acinar structures with variable mucin.
- Scanty vascular stroma, occasionally amyloid stroma with bone.
- No/minimal mitotic activity (<2/10 HPF), no necrosis.

Ancillary Tests
- **Positive stains in central carcinoid:** Keratin, serotonin, neuron-specific enolase, chromogranin A and B, synaptophysin, CD57/Leu 7, pancreatic polypeptide, N-CAM
- **Positive stains in peripheral carcinoid:** Congo red (amyloid), TTF1 (usually), calcitonin (often)
- **Electron microscopy:** Dense core neurosecretory granules.

Case History: A 44-year-old male with hypogammaglobulinemia and pneumonia.

Diagnosis: Aspergillus with pneumocystis pneumonia

Clinical Features
- **HIV patients:** More indolent course.
- **Others:** More acute and severe illness.

Imaging
- Usually atypical interstitial pneumonia
- Lung biopsy is rarely required for diagnosis.

Gross
- Invasive disease—targetoid lesions with peripheral consolidation and central thrombosed vessels due to angioinvasive fungi.
- Variable bronchopneumonia or lobar pneumonia.

Microscopy

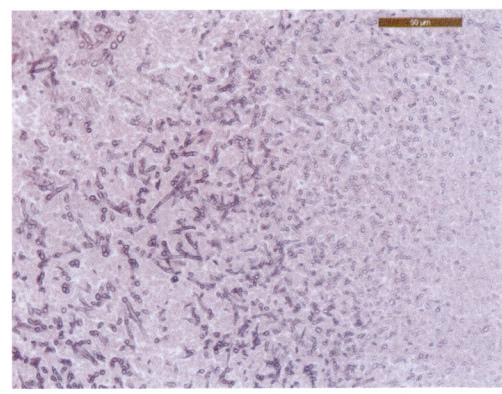

Fig. 6.7

- Alveolar spaces filled with pink, foamy amorphous material (proliferating fungi), cell debris.
- Mild inflammatory reaction with fibrin exudate, hyaline membranes.
- Solitary necrotizing granulomas and miliary disease are also described.
- *P. jiroveci* 4–6 microns, cup/boat-shaped cysts.
- *Aspergillus dichotomous* (into two nearly equal branches, or 45 degrees) branching, hyphae with frequent septation, diameter ranges from 2.5 to 4.5 μm.
- May see Aspergillus fruiting body (pathognomonic), and often invades vessels.

Special Stains
GMS, Warthin-Starry, other silver stains and Gram-Weigert.

Differential Diagnosis
- **Alveolar proteinosis:** Diffuse pulmonary opacification and intra-alveolar PAS-positive material.
- **BOOP:** Bronchiolar and alveolar plugs of loose fibrous tissue

Case History: A 77-year-old woman with a solitary nodule in the upper lobe of the right lung.

Diagnosis: Pulmonary hamartoma/chondroma

Clinical Features
May present as intrabronchial polypoid mass causing obstruction.

Imaging
Commonly, presents as incidental coin lesion (rounded abnormality) with popcorn pattern of calcification.

Gross
- 4 cm or less, sharply delineated and lobulated.
- Glistening cut surface (cartilage) with ill-defined clefts.

Microscopy

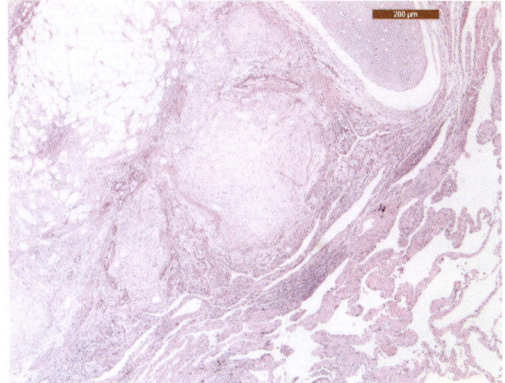

Fig. 6.8

- Islands of mature hyaline cartilage, fat, smooth muscle and clefts lined by respiratory epithelium.
- Periphery of cartilage—immature myxomatous tissue. Resembles breast fibroadenoma if no cartilage present.
- 15% have papillary projections resembling immature placental villi with stromal macrophages and lymphocytes and abundant mast cells.

Differential Diagnosis
- Benign metastasizing leiomyoma
- Leiomyosarcoma
- Lymphangioleiomyomatosis
- Native pulmonary muscle proliferation

Case History: A 45-year-old with lesion left lung.

Diagnosis: Aspergillus with poorly differentiated squamous cell carcinoma

Clinical Features
- Bronchial obstruction (pneumonitis, atelectasis).
- May spread to thoracic wall, diaphragm, mediastinum.

Gross
- Usually central portion of lung affecting larger bronchi but may be peripheral.
- Invades peribronchial soft tissue, lung parenchyma and nearby lymph nodes.
- May compress pulmonary artery and vein.

Microscopy

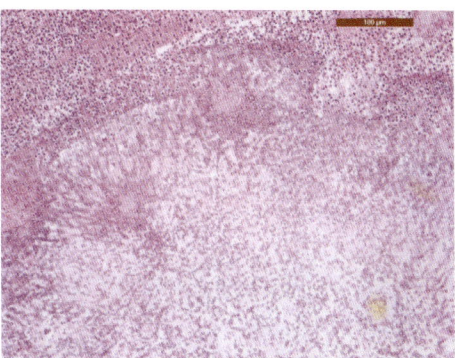

Fig. 6.9a

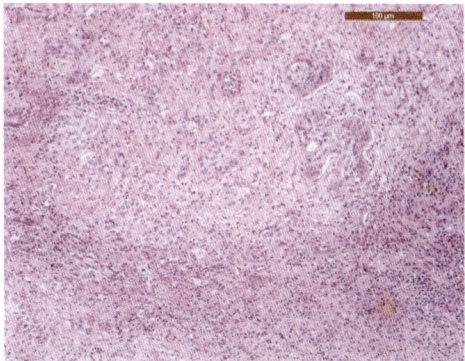

Fig. 6.9b

- Sheets or islands of large polygonal malignant cells containing keratin (individual cells or keratin pearls) and intercellular bridges.

- Adjacent bronchial dysplasia or carcinoma *in situ* is common.
- May have focal areas of intracytoplasmic mucin.

Ancillary Tests

Immunohistochemistry: p63, CK5/6 (87–100%), EMA, thrombomodulin (87–100%) shows positivity. Variable CD15, CEA, HPV, mesothelin (16–31%), p53, p40, S-100. Negative vimentin (usually), TTF1 (usually), Napsin A.

Case History: A 20-year-old woman with a cystic lesion, right middle lobe of the lung.

Diagnosis: Pulmonary—hydatid cyst. Hydatidosis (echinococcosis)

Introduction

- Infestation by *Echinococcus granulosus* (which is usually cystic)
- Rarely by *Echinococcus multilocularis* (which causes alveolar echinococcosis).

Microscopy

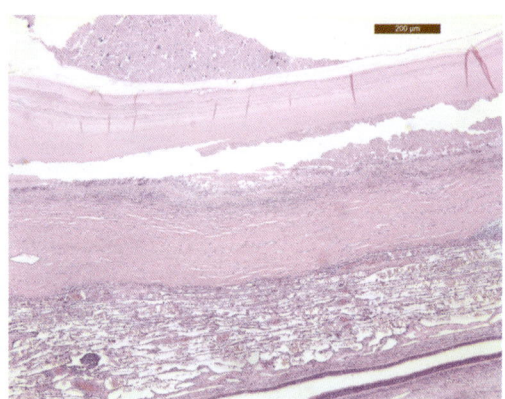

Fig. 6.10

- Outer chitinous (or fibrous laminar) layer, inner germinal layer.
- Cyst wall surrounded by granulation tissue or a fibrous capsule (so-called 'pericyst layer').
- Calcification suggests the cyst is dead. The viable cyst—colorless fluid, which contains daughter cysts and brood capsules with scolices.

Case History: A 75-year-old woman with a mass in periphery of the right lower lobe.

Diagnosis: Adenocarcinoma—acinar and papillary types

Gross

- Poorly circumscribed gray-yellow lesions, single or multiple, may be mucoid.
- 77% involve visceral pleura producing puckering/pleural retraction, 65% are peripheral.
- Usually not cavitary and often associated with a peripheral scar or honeycombing.

Microscopy

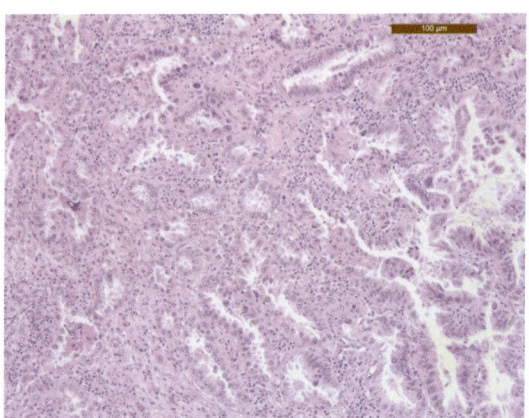

Fig. 6.11

- Glandular differentiation with tubules or papillae and mucin secretion.
- Either *in situ*, minimally invasive or invasive (mucinous or serous).
- Tumors 1.5 cm or less—usually one cell type, larger tumors are often mixed.
- Vascular invasion common.

Ancillary Tests

- **Immunohistochemistry:** Positive-mucin, low molecular weight keratin (CK7), EMA, CEA, TTF1. Negative-CK20, keratin 5 (usually), P504S, p63 (cytoplasmic expression associated with bad prognosis). Mucinous bronchoalveolar: CK20+, TTF1– but CDX2+.

- **Molecular studies:** EGFR mutation, K-ras mutation (with mucinous adenoma) and ALK-1 mutation (extensive signet ring morphology).

Differential Diagnosis
Metastatic adenocarcinoma: (TTF1 negative).

Case History: A 68-year-old woman—wedge biopsy lesion lung carcinoma.

Diagnosis: Cryptococcal mucoid pneumonia

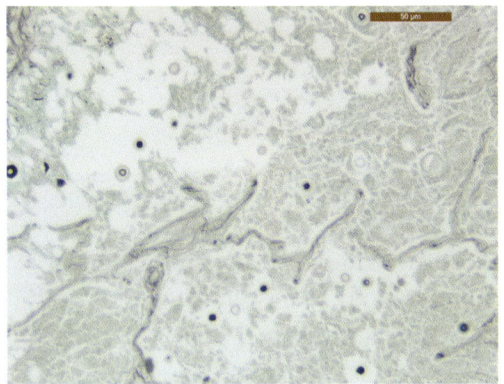

Fig. 6.12

Case History: A 64-year-old woman with prior breast cancer with a pulmonary nodule.

Diagnosis: Cryptococcal granulomatous nodule

Clinical Features
- Affects immunocompromised hosts predominantly and is the commonest cause of fungal meningitis.
- AIDS associated cryptococcosis the CD4+ lymphocyte count is below $200/mm^3$.
- Symptoms—cough, low-grade fever and pleuritic pain.

Laboratory Diagnosis
Clinical material: Bronchial washings, blood
- *Direct microscopy*
  a. *For exudates and body fluids*—thin wet film under a coverslip using India ink to demonstrate encapsulated yeast cells. Sputum and pus may need to be digested with 10% KOH prior to India ink staining.

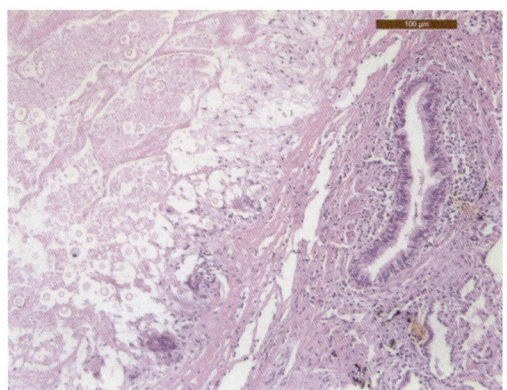

Fig. 6.13

  b. *For tissue sections*—PAS digest, GMS and H&E, mucicarmine stains and polysaccharide capsule. Globose to ovoid, budding yeast cells surrounded by wide gelatinous capsules.
- *Culture:* Primary isolation media, like Sabouraud's dextrose agar. Translucent, smooth gelatinous colonies, later becoming very mucoid and cream in color.
- *Serology:* Detection of cryptococcal capsular polysaccharide antigen.

Interpretation
- Demonstration of encapsulated yeast cells in CSF, biopsy tissue, blood or urine—significant, even in the absence of clinical symptoms.
- Positive sputum specimens—considered potentially significant.

Case History: A 69-year-old man with a mass in the right lung.

Diagnosis: Carcinosarcoma lung

Clinical Features
- Usually men, heavy smokers, 5th–6th decade.
- Central endobronchial type: Slow growing and locally invasive.
- Peripheral invasive type: Also called parenchymal carcinosarcoma—metastasize early and widely.

Imaging

- Solitary huge mass or extensive opacity due to associated obstructive pneumonitis and atelectasis.
- Intratumorous calcifications on CT scans—ossification in the osteosarcomatous component.

Microscopy

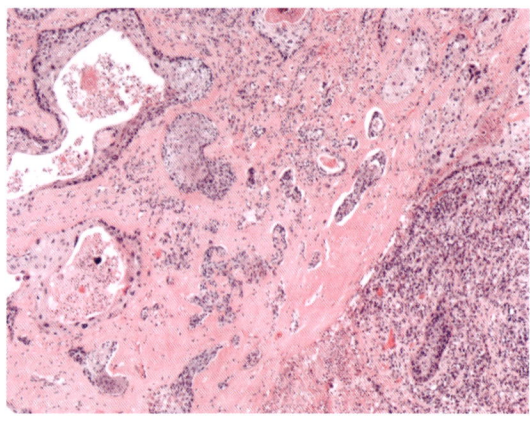

Fig. 6.14

- Carcinomatous component—squamous cell carcinoma (69%), adenocarcinoma (20%), large cell carcinoma (11%).
- Sarcoma elements—cartilage or skeletal muscle.

Ancillary Test

Immunohistochemistry: CEA, S-100 protein, cytokeratin and vimentin.

Case History: A 16-month-old baby—lungs at autopsy, cause of death.

Diagnosis: Aspiration pneumonia

Clinical Features

- Fever or hypothermia
- Tachypnea, tachycardia, hypotension, decrease breath sounds, altered mental status.
- 5–15% of 4.5 million cases of community acquired pneumonia result from aspiration pneumonia.

Imaging

Infiltrates in lung field. Bilateral or unilateral.

Microscopy

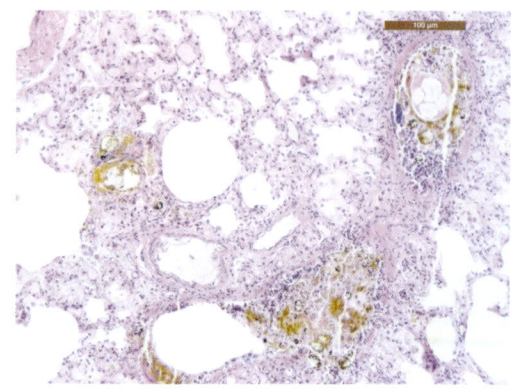

Fig. 6.15

- Neutrophilic infiltration.
- Foreign materials, e.g. plant matter.
- Foreign body giant cell reaction.

Differential Diagnosis

All infectious pneumonias.

Case History: A 74-year-old man with mass left upper lobe, cancer.

Diagnosis: Blastomycosis—necrotizing granuloma

Clinical Features

- Most individuals—asymptomatic, not detected until the infection has spread to other organs.
- Other symptoms develop after an incubation period of 3–15 weeks continued suppuration, necrosis and cavitation.
- A few acute onset of infection—high fever, chills, productive cough, myalgia, arthralgia and pleuritic chest pain—recover after 2–12 weeks of symptoms, some return months later with lesions at other sites. Others will fail to recover—chronic chest infection or disseminated infection.

Laboratory Diagnosis

- **Clinical material:** Bronchial washings and tissue biopsies.

- **Direct microscopy:** Exudates and body fluids—centrifuged, 10% KOH and Parker ink or calcofluor white mounts. Tissue sections: PAS digest, GMS or Gram stain

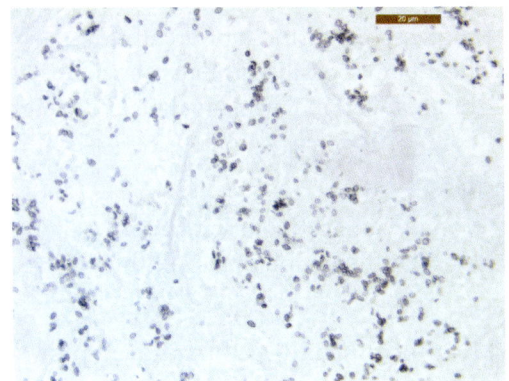

Fig. 6.16

- **Histopathology:** Large, broad-base, unipolar budding yeast-like cells, 8–15 m in diameter.
- **Culture:** Clinical specimens primary isolation media: Sabouraud's dextrose agar, brain–heart infusion agar supplemented with 5% sheep blood.

Case History: A 54-year-old female with a mass in left upper lobe, cancer.

Diagnosis: Coccidioidomycosis—necrotizing granuloma

Clinical Features

- 60%—benign, transient chest infection that does not require medical attention.
- 40%—acute febrile "flu-like" illness starting 7–28 days (average 10–16 days) recover completely usually.

Laboratory Diagnosis

- **Clinical material:** Bronchial washings and tissue biopsies.
- **Direct microscopy**
  a. *Skin scrapings:* 10% KOH and Parker ink or calcofluor white mounts.
  b. *Exudates and body fluids centrifuged:* Sediment examined 10% KOH and Parker ink or calcofluor white mounts,
  c. *Tissue sections:* PAS digest, GMS or Gram stain.
- **Direct microscopy of skin scrapings:** 10% KOH and Parker ink solution—characteristic endosporulating spherules (sporangia) of *Coccidioides immitis*. Presence of spherules with endospores is diagnostic.

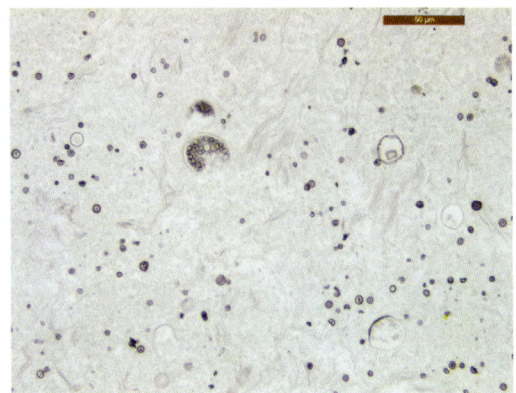

Fig. 6.17

- **Tissue section:** Typical endosporulating spherules of *Coccidioides immitis*.
- **Culture:** Clinical specimens: Primary isolation media, like Sabouraud's dextrose agar and brain–heart infusion agar supplemented with 5% sheep blood. Culture—suede-like to downy, greyish white colony with a tan to brown reverse.
- **Serology:** Immunodiffusion and/or complement fixation tests for detection of antibody.

Case History: A 21-year-old with recurrent pneumothorax.

Diagnosis: Eosinophilic granuloma

Clinical Features

- 20–39 years, often associated with smokers
- Asymptomatic.
- Sometimes cough and dyspnea.
- Associated with pneumothorax, *Pneumocystis carinii* pneumonia.

Imaging

Chest X-ray, CT: Honeycombing pattern.

Gross

Lesion of upper lobes, local or diffuse, with nodules and cavitary lesions and late honey-combing.

Microscopy

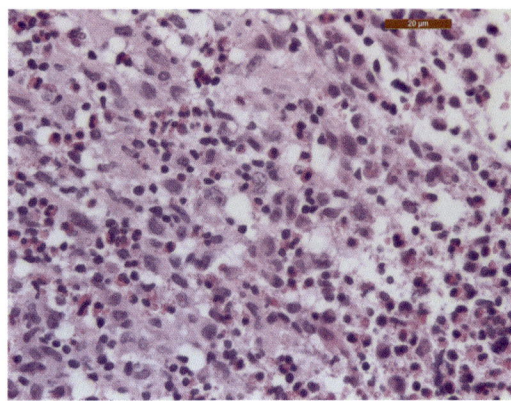

Fig. 6.18

- Interstitial scarring with nodular aggregates of Langerhans cells with a bronchiolocentric distribution.
- Langerhans cells have abundant eosinophilic cytoplasm and grooved nuclei with indented nuclear membranes, prominent eosinophils and mesothelial cells.
- Frequent hemosiderin, necrosis, alveolar lining cell hyperplasia, pigmented alveolar macrophages.
- Variable vasculitis.

Ancillary Test

- **Immunohistochemistry:** Positive: CD1a, S-100, HLA-DR
- **Electron microscopy:** Birbeck's granules (pentilaminar intracytoplasmic structures, tennis racket shaped).

Differential Diagnosis

- **Eosinophilic pleuritis:** No Langerhans cell, although mesothelial cells may appear similar
- **Reactive Langerhans cells in inflammatory conditions:** No sheets or groups of Langerhans cells.
- **Desquamative interstitial pneumonitis.**

Case History: A 68-year-old woman with recurrent right-sided pleural effusion.

Diagnosis: Malignant mesothelioma

Clinical Features

- Progressive shortness of breath.
- Chest pain, possibly unilateral.
- Cough, fever, malaise, myalgia and weight loss.

Imaging

- Strongly suggestive of malignancy.
- Pleural effusion, pleural wall thickening.

Gross

- Multifocal studding of lung or pleural surfaces.
- Circumferential or nodular pleural thickening.

Microscopy

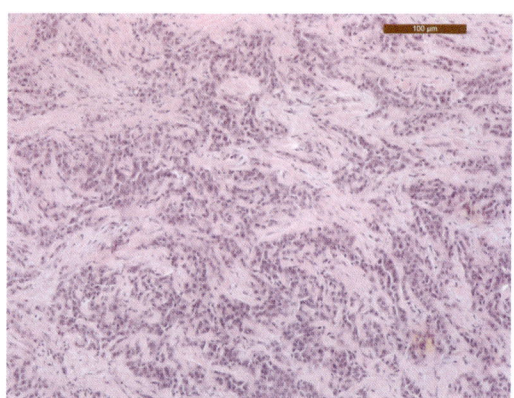

Fig. 6.19

Stromal or fat invasion is helpful in diagnosis. Three broad histopathological types:

- Epithelioid: Includes tubulopapillary, deciduoid, clear cell, and small cell types.
- Sarcomatoid: Desmoplastic and lymphohistiocytoid types.
- Biphasic/mixed

Ancillary Test

- Vacuoles contain hyaluronic acid which is positive for alcian blue and digestible by hyaluronidase and negative for PAS-D.

- Mucicarmine should not be used to distinguish mesothelioma and adenocarcinoma because it may stain hyaluronic acid as well as mucin in adenocarcinoma.
- **Immunohistochemistry:** Calretinin, cytokeratin and WT1, D2-40
- **Electron microscopy:** Long, slender microvilli (length >15 × diameter) with tonofilaments but without glycocalyx.
- **Molecular genetics**
  - BAP1 (BRCA associated protein 1)
  - Homozygous deletions of p16/CDKN2A at 9p21.

Differential Diagnosis

- **Adenocarcinoma:** Negative for calretinin, D240, CK5/6, and WT1.

  Special stain: Alcian blue with hyaluronidase and PAS-D will be positive.

  Electron microscopy: Apical microvilli—shorter and has glycocalyx. Perinuclear tonofilament bundles, basal lamina and long desmosomes are absent.
- **Atypical mesothelial hyperplasia**
- **Fibrous pleurisy:** Thickened pleura is composed of fibrous tissue without elastic fibers
- **Synovial sarcoma:** Shows IHC positivity for CK7, vimentin, BCL2, CD99 (focal), variable EMA; SYT-SSX1 or SYT-SSX2 fusion transcript due to t(X;18) (p11.2;q11.2)

Case History: A 56-year-old woman with a pleural-based mass.

Diagnosis: Solitary fibrous tumor of the pleura

Clinical Features

Associated with pulmonary osteoarthropathy, digital clubbing and hypoglycemia, which regress after tumor resection.

Gross

- Arises from pleural surface by a pedicle.
- Solitary, well circumscribed, may be encapsulated and composed of dense, gray-white fibrous tissue with firm, whorled cut surface (like uterine leiomyoma), large tumors may be cystic and hemorrhagic.

Microscopy

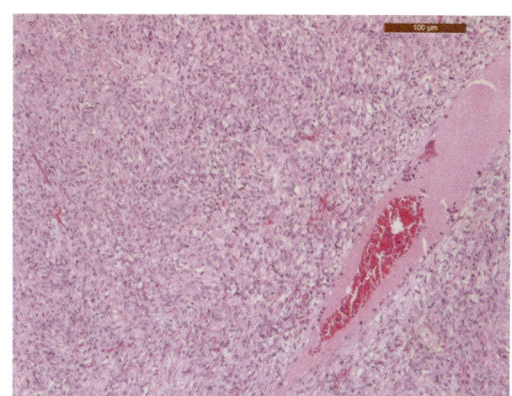

Fig. 6.20

- Fibroblast-like cells with variable cellularity in collagenous, keloid-like stroma, reticulin fibers, hemangiopericytoma-like vessels.
- No/rare mitotic activity, no atypia. May entrap mesothelium or epithelium at periphery.
- Differentiate from malignant by: Fascicles or patternless pattern of spindled or plump cells in dense collagenous stroma. Increased cellularity, marked nuclear atypia, prominent necrosis, high mitotic activity.

Ancillary Test

Immunohistochemistry

Positive: CD34 (strong), CD99, vimentin.
Negative: Cytokeratin, EMA, S-100, smooth muscle actin, desmin.

Differential Diagnosis

- **Fibrosarcoma:** Highly cellular fibroblastic proliferation in herringbone pattern (cells in columns of short parallel lines with all the lines in one column sloping one way and lines in adjacent columns sloping the other way). Cells have scant cytoplasm, tapering elongated dark nuclei with increased granular chromatin, variable nucleoli. Mitotic activity **present**, often with abnormal forms. Variable collagen.

- **Malignant peripheral sheath tumor:** Immunohistochemistry—CD99/O13 (86%), S100 (62%), CD57 (55%), collagen IV, p53 are positive.
- **Sarcomatoid/desmoplastic mesothelioma:** Diffuse on X-ray, infiltrative, often atypia or mitotic figures.
- **Spindle cell carcinoma:** Carcinoma composed exclusively of spindle-shaped tumor cells. Tumor cells often obliterate vessels.

Case History: A 64-year-old man with a right upper lobe mass.

Diagnosis: Small cell carcinoma lung

Clinical Features

When associated with paraneoplastic syndromes due to production of ACTH (Cushing's syndrome), ADH (hyponatremia), calcitonin (hypocalcemia), gonadotropins (gynecomastia), parathyroid hormone (hyperparathyroidism), serotonin (carcinoid syndrome); also encephalomyelitis, Lambert-Eaton syndrome, sensory neuropathy, the patient will present with abovementioned symptoms.

Gross

- Usually central/hilar, white-tan, soft, friable, extensive necrosis.
- Peripheral nodules have fairly well-defined border and fleshy cut surface.

Microscopy

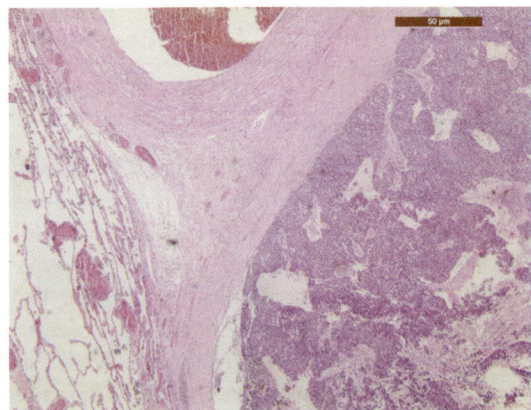

Fig. 6.21

- Sheets, ribbons, clusters, rosettes or peripheral palisading of small to medium sized (2–4 × neutrophils) round/oval cells with minimal cytoplasm, salt and pepper chromatin without prominent clumps, hyperchromatic, indistinct nucleoli, nuclear molding, smudging, frequent mitotic figures.
- Azzopardi phenomena (basophilic nuclear chromatin spreading to wall of blood vessels), indistinct cell borders. Stroma is scanty, vascular, delicate. Necrosis and apoptotic debris-common.

Ancillary Test

- **Immunohistochemistry:** Positive-pan-keratin TTF1; neuron-specific enolase, CD117, chromogranin, synaptophysin, calretinin, thrombomodulin, keratin 5.
- **Electron microscopy:** Occasional round, membrane bound, dense core neurosecretory granules, 100–200 nm in diameter.

Differential Diagnosis

- **Atypical carcinoid tumor:** Less nuclear atypia, <20 mitotic figures per 10 HPF, no extensive necrosis, more intense neuroendocrine staining.
- **Metastatic small cell carcinoma.**

Case History: A 77-year-old man with a right middle lobe mass.

Diagnosis: Extranodal marginal zone B cell lymphoma of mucosa—associated lymphoid tissue (malt lymphoma)

Clinical Features

- Indolent, when it spreads, tends to involve other mucosal sites such as Waldeyer's ring.
- May transform to diffuse large B cell lymphoma.
- Develops in background of *H. pylori* infection or rarely post-transplant.

Microscopy

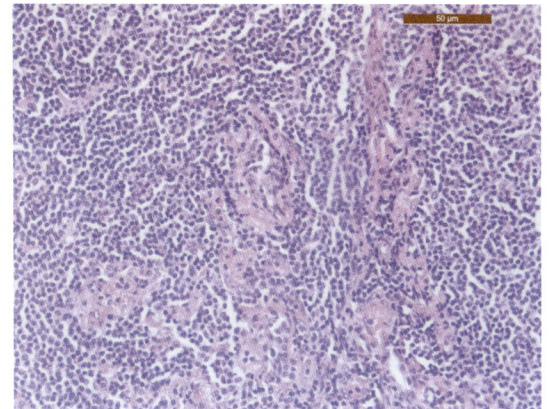

Fig. 6.22

- Dense, monotonous population of centrocyte-like cells, often with residual germinal centers and lymphoepithelial lesions.
- Commonly lymphoepithelial lesions or follicular colonization. Adjacent mucosa has epithelial erosion, intestinal metaplasia, *H. pylori,* lymphoid follicles, atrophy, atypical regenerative changes, and dysplasia.

Ancillary Test

Immunohistochemistry: Positive stains: B cell markers (CD19, CD20, CD79a), CD43.

Differential Diagnosis

Lymphoid hyperplasia or other benign process.

Case History: (a) A 77-year-old man with a right middle lobe mass.

Diagnosis: Adenocarcinoma with bronchoalveolar features, non-mucinous variety with Clara cell differentiation

(b) A 50-year-old woman with a right upper lobectomy.

Diagnosis: Adenocarcinoma with bronchoalveolar features, mucinous type

Clinical Features

Multifocal/lobal/bilateral involvement is frequent in invasive mucinous, rare in nonmucinous (AIS/MIA/LPA).

Microscopy

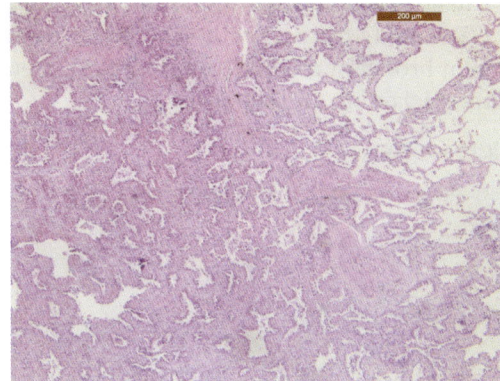

Fig. 6.23a

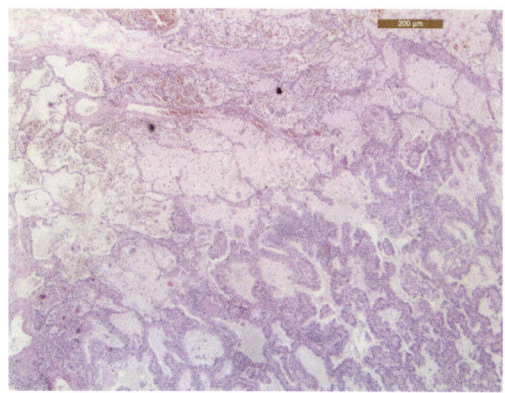

Fig. 6.23b

- *Invasive mucinous:* Composed primarily of mucin filled columnar or goblet cells.
- *Non-mucinous tumors:* Composed primarily of type II pneumocytes or Clara cells.

Genetic Abnormalities

- KRAS ENL4-ACK transinvasive mucinous adenocarcinoma.
- They present at higher stage and have multifocal invasive.

Case History: (a) A 73-year-old woman with effusion and nodular airspace disease.

Diagnosis: Alveolar septal pulmonary amyloidosis

(b) A 83-year-old woman with a solitary nodule left lung.

Diagnosis: Nodular pulmonary amyloidosis

Imaging

- **Chest X-ray:** Diffuse interstitial infiltrate.
- **CT lung:** Diffuse septal thickening. Prominent bronchovascular core structure, pleural thickening and pleural effusion.

Microscopy

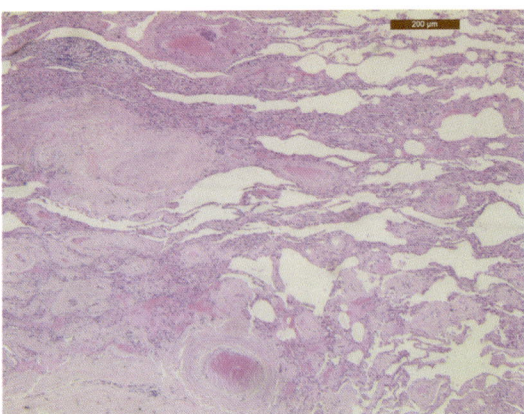

Fig. 6.24a

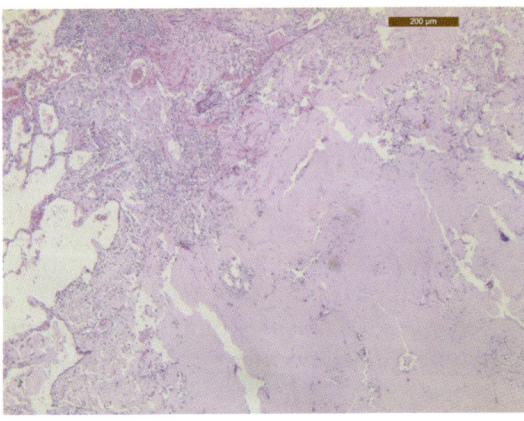

Fig. 6.24b

Diffuse hyaline thickening of the alveolar septum and pulmonary vasculature.

Ancillary Test

Apple green birefringence by Congo red on a polarizing microscope.

Differential Diagnosis

- Advanced UIP or other diffuse fibrosing lung diseases.
- Light chain deposition disease.

Case History: A 49-year-old man with lesion left lung cancer.

Diagnosis: CMV pneumonitis

Clinical Features

Commonly found in immunocompromised.

Imaging

Chest X-ray: B/L interstitial infiltrates.

Lab Investigations

Culture, serology and PCR for CMV.

Gross

Lung is firm. Hemorrhagic lung nodules may be present.

Microscopy

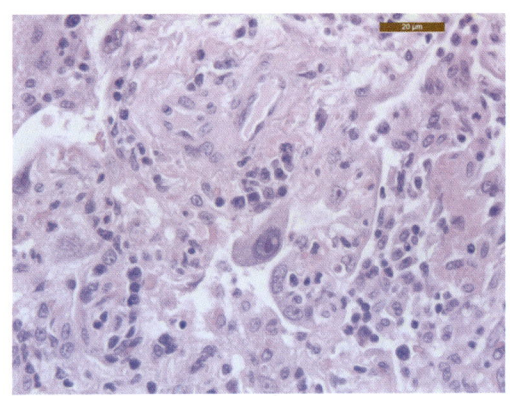

Fig. 6.25

- Hemorrhagic necrosis. Mononuclear infiltrate, mild edema and pneumocyte hyperplasia.
- Within the cells, prominent basophilic intranuclear inclusions with a central halo and smaller basophilic intracytoplasmic inclusions.
- Fibrin-rich eosinophilic hyaline membrane around the alveoli.
- Fibrosis of the collapsed alveoli. Squamous metaplasia due to terminal bronchial injury.

Ancillary Tests

- PAS and GMS positive.
- **Immunohistochemistry:** CMV is confirmatory.

- **Electron microscopy:** 150–200 nm particle with a round core and double membrane.

Differential Diagnosis
- Drug-induced lung injury particularly in bone marrow transplant recipients.
- Herpes simplex virus.
- Herpes varicella zoster viral infection of the lung.

Case History: A 68-year-old man with lesion left lung cancer.

Diagnosis: Busulphan pneumonitis

General Pathologic Findings
- Most of the inflammatory changes in lung related to drug toxicity is non-specific.
- In chronic drug toxicity, lung fibrosis may occur, sometimes with honeycomb remodeling such cases UIP may be stimulated.
- Tissue eosinophilia can occur.

Microscopy

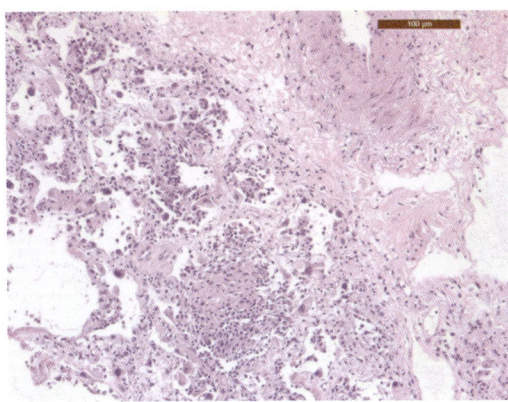

Fig. 6.27

- Nonspecific lung injury with hyaline membranes.
- Atypical type 2 pneumocytes with markedly enlarged pleomorphic nuclei and prominent nucleoli.

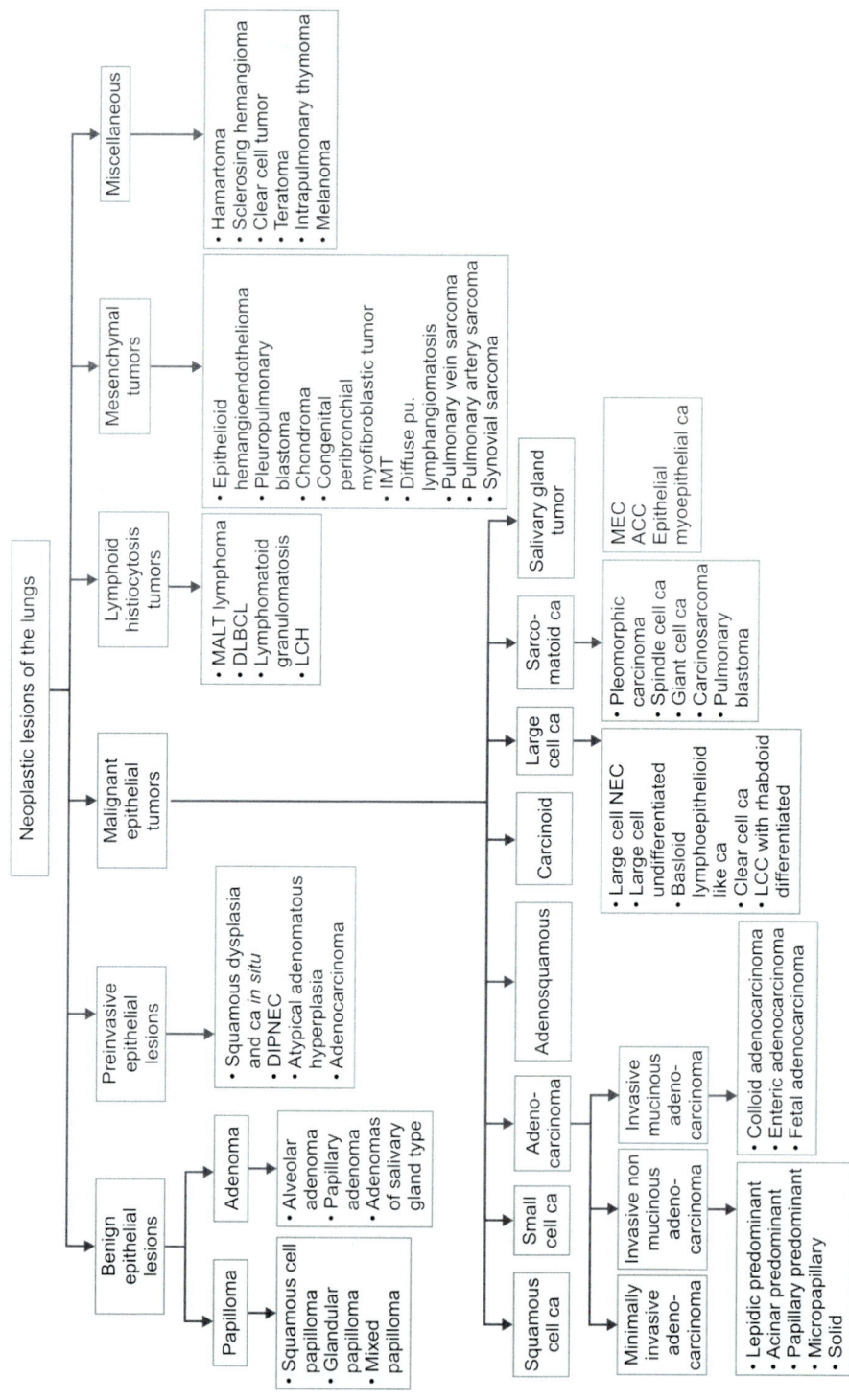

Lesions of the Lung

APPROACHES TO NONNEOPLASTIC LESIONS OF THE LUNGS

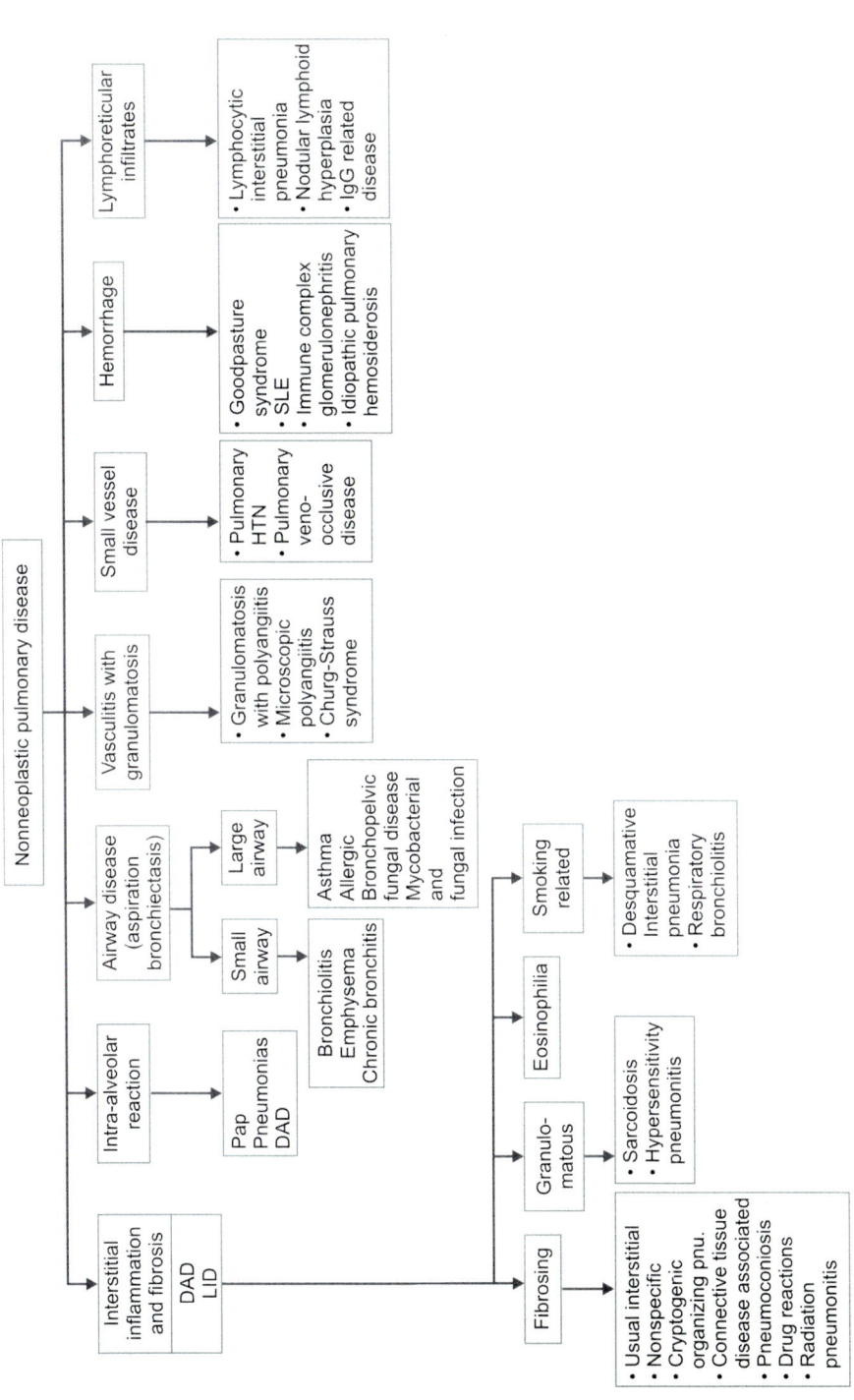

Contributed by Archana B

CHAPTER 7

Approach to Gastrointestinal Biopsies

S Rajendiran

SYSTEMATIC APPROACH

It is very essential for identifying the pathologic lesions in GI biopsies. It starts with clinical features, endoscopic appearance and ends with… not a pathologic diagnosis but with a final diagnosis… correlating with clinical and pathologic features… and… last but not the least… response to the treatment. Please remember the "Patient" is our boss and getting his well being should be the aim of all the physicians involved in his/her care including the clinicians, radiologists and pathologists. The components as are follows:

Patient	Complaints
Clinician	Clinical history, physical examination, lab investigations, provisional diagnosis, endoscopy, appearance, biopsy
Radiologist	Radiological investigations
Pathologist	Biopsy interpretation
	Gross appearance (proper orientation for embedding), microscopy
	Low power—architecture
	Medium and high power—cytologic features
	Final pathological diagnosis
	Clinical, radiological and pathological correlation, final diagnosis
	Treatment
	Response to the treatment follow up
	Happy patient (clinician, radiologist and pathologist)

The pathologists, especially, the one in the training should be aware of this holistic approach and should be knowing that a "live patient" is there behind every "specimen". It is our duty to help them to get rid of their disease and make them happy as they are our "Boss"….

With this in our mind, let us now see… how we can do our job in a systematic way in the interpretation of the GI biopsies. Knowing the normal histology is very essential and it should not be ignored.

A few general concepts should be stressed

1. GI tract is made up of:
   a. *Mucosa:*
      i. Lining epithelium
      ii. Subepithelial glands
      iii. Lamina propria
      iv. Muscularis mucosa
   (it is a miniature of muscularis propria and has 2 layers, inner circular and outer longitudinal)
   b. *Submucosa:* Blood vessels, nerve plexus (Meissner), connective tissue
   c. *Muscularis propria*
      i. Inner circular
      ii. Outer longitudinal
      iii. Inter-Auerbach plexus
   d. *Serosa or adventitia:* Depending upon the mesothelial lining, if present, it is serosa.

2. In the mucosal biopsies we should be predominantly getting mucosa and a portion of submucosa. This is very important in 2 aspects:
   a. Mucosal biopsies may not be representative of submucosal lesions like lipoma or GIST.
   b. When you see muscularis propria or possible serosa/adventitia or a lot of adipose tissue, immediately call the clinician and rule out perforation. (Histopathological "panic/critical value".)
3. Lamina propria can have lymphocytes, plasma cells (for IgA secretion) and scattered eosinophils and neutrophils as a normal component. You have to understand that a high number of capillaries are there in the lamina propria and these cells can be seen within them and should not be interpreted as ... "Inflammatory cells"... (in that case we all have 4,000 to 11,000 inflammatory cells in our blood .... Hope you catch the point ... hahaha ...).
   When and how should we be calling inflammation ... and differentiate it from normal component ...?
   a. **Acute inflammation**
      i. You should be seeing the neutrophils entering the glandular epithelium (cryptitis) and/or pass into the intraglandular lumen (crypt abscess).
      ii. Collection of 5 or more inflammatory cells in one focus in lamina propria (microabscesses).
      iii. Ulceration of the surface epithelium with fibrino-purulent exudation.
      Scattered neutrophils in the lamina propria does not qualify for acute inflammation
   b. **Chronic inflammation**
      i. *Architectural disarray:* Normally the surface epithelium gives rise to non-branching glands with uniform size, shape and distribution (SSD). On longitudinal sections they look like test tubes in a rack and on tangential sections they look like round donuts. Any disturbance in the uniform size, shape and distribution should be considered as chronic inflammation.
      ii. *Basal plasmacytosis:* Presence of plasma cells in between the crypt and muscularis mucosa.
      iii. Granulomas in the lamina propria.
      iv. Lymphoid aggregates in stomach (*H. pylori* associated).
      Scattered plasma cells in the superficial lamina propria does not qualify for chronic inflammation.
   c. **Specific entities**
      i. Lymphocytic colitis/enteritis/gastritis (microscopic colitis)—25 lymphocytes per 100 epithelial cells. Should not be counting in the areas above lymphoid aggregates as there will be more in those areas (to confuse you more ... You can see more police in front of the police station but ... not in the other areas ... normally ...).
      ii. Eosinophilic colitis/enteritis/gastritis —15 eosinophils per one HPF (X40).
4. For dysplasia, the following criteria should be followed:

	Criteria	Normal	LG dysplasia*	HG dysplasia*
1.	Cells	Single layer	Stratified	Stratified
2.	Polarity	Maintained	Maintained	Lost
3.	Cribriform, micropapillary	Absent	Absent	Present
4.	Nuclei position	Basal	Up to middle 1/3rd	Upper 1/3rd, at apex
5.	Mucin	Present	Less	Absent
6.	Macro-nucleoli	Absent	Absent	Present
7.	Mitosis	Absent	Present	Present
8.	Apoptosis	Absent	Present	Present

* Dysplastic changes should be seen involving the surface epithelium.

5. The microscopic changes to be seen broadly in each component of the GI biopsy as follows (changes involving muscularis propria and serosa/adventitia not included as they won't be present in an endoscopic biopsy):
   a. **Surface epithelium**
      Architectural changes
      i. Loss of normal structure (e.g. loss of villi, variation in SSD)
      ii. Ulceration
      iii. Loss of mucin
      iv. Hyperplasia
      v. Others
      Cytological changes
      i. Intraluminal organisms
      ii. Inflammation
      iii. Regenerative changes
      iv. Metaplasia
      v. Dysplasia (low and high)
   b. **Glands**
      Architectural changes
      i. Variation in SSD
      ii. Cryptitis
      iii. Crypt abscess
      Cytological changes
      i. Organisms
      ii. Atrophy
      iii. Metaplasia
      iv. Dysplasia (low and high)
   c. **Lamina propria**
      i. Edema
      ii. Muscularization
      iii. Inflammation: Acute—microabscesses, chronic—granulomas
      iv. Organisms (CMV, TB)
      v. Fibrosis
      vi. Atypical/foreign cells (inflammation, radiation, benign, malignant)
   d. **Muscularis mucosa**
      i. Hyperplasia with extension into lamina propria.
      ii. Atypical/foreign cells (inflammation, radiation, benign, malignant)
   e. **Submucosa**
      i. Vascular changes (portal gastropathy)
      ii. Neural hypertrophy (Crohn disease)
      iii. Atypical/foreign cells (inflammation, radiation, benign, malignant)
6. Previously diseases are classified into congenital, acquired, inflammatory and neoplastic lesions. Now they are approached as follows:
   a. Non-proliferative lesions (e.g. diverticulosis)
   b. Proliferative lesions without atypia (e.g. hyperplastic polyps)
   c. Proliferative lesions with atypia
      i. Non-invasive (low and high grade dysplasias)
      ii. Invasive (carcinoma)
         1. Microinvasive, widely invasive
         2. With lymph node mets
         3. With systemic mets

In case of invasive malignancy, look for the background metaplastic/dysplastic changes ...what we call as "Field effect" and its presence confirms the primary origin from that particular site. Otherwise, we have to think of secondary from other organs.

We have seen the general approach to GI biopsies in detail. Let us now see the organ specific entities starting from esophagus. The major classification of lesions is:
1. Normal
2. Inflammatory
3. Neoplastic

One thing, as a pathologist, we should not hesitate to say... "Normal" when the microscopic findings are devoid of findings. This helps the clinicians to form a reasonable differential diagnosis or it will help them to focus other causes for a particular clinical symptom. Reporting... "non-specific gastritis" is neither helping the clinician nor the patient. Avoid the terminology... "non-specific inflammation"... as much as possible... it should be.... specific inflammation ..."

We are not going to deal with neoplastic lesions in this discussion and hence will mainly concentrate in the inflammatory lesion.

Esophagus
a. **Neutrophilic**
   1. Infection—HSV, CMV, Candida
   2. GERD
   3. Pill/medication
b. **Lymphocytic**
   1. GERD
   2. Infection
   3. Dysmotility
   4. HIV/CVID
   5. Crohn
c. **Eosinophilic**
   1. GERD
   2. Eosinophilic esophagitis
   3. Parasitic infection
d. **Granuloma**
   1. Crohn
   2. Sarcoidosis
   3. Infection
   4. Medication
e. **Pauci-inflammatory**
   1. Corrosive injury
   2. GVHD (apoptosis)
   3. Collagen vascular disease
   4. Amyloidosis
f. **Others**
   1. Lichen planus
   2. Pemphigus

Stomach
a. **Neutrophilic**
   1. Phlegmonous gastritis
   2. Helicobacter gastritis
   3. CMV
b. **Lymphocytic**
   1. Autoimmune gastritis
   2. Lymphocytic gastritis
   3. Collagenous gastritis
c. **Eosinophilic**
   1. Parasitic infection
   2. Eosinophilic gastritis
d. **Pauci-inflammatory**
   1. Reactive gastropathy
   2. GAVE/PHG
   3. GVHD (apoptosis)
   4. Medication effect
   5. Amyloidosis
e. **Lamina propria infiltrate**
   1. Granuloma
   2. Xanthoma
   3. Siderosis
   4. Calcinosis

Small Intestine
a. **Flat mucosa (classic celiac pattern)**
   1. Celiac disease
   2. Autoimmune enteropathy (AIE)
   3. Tropical sprue
   4. Refractory sprue
   5. IBD
   6. Others
      i. Microvillous inclusion disease
      ii. Tufting enteropathy
      iii. CVID
b. **Partial/complete preservation of villi**
   1. Lymphocytic
      i. Celiac disease
      ii. AIE
      iii. Peptic duodenitis
      iv. IBD
      v. Immunodeficiency
   2. Eosinophilic
      i. Parasitic infection—Giardia
      ii. Eosinophilic enteritis
   3. Pauci-inflammatory
      i. Infections
      ii. GVHD (apoptosis)
      iii. Immunodeficiency
   4. Lamina propria infiltrates
      i. Whipple
      ii. MAI
      iii. Siderosis
      iv. Melanosis
      v. Granuloma

c. **Normal villi with minimal lamina propria inflammation**
   1. Luminal parasites (Giardia, cryptosporidium, strongyloidiasis)
   2. Erosion/hemorrhage (NSAID)
   3. Foveolar metaplasia (peptic injury, gastric heterotopia, NSAID)
   4. Cytoplasmic vacuoles (abetalipoproteinemia)
   5. Intraepithelial lymphocytes (latent celiac disease)
   6. Increased apoptosis (GVHD, CMV, AIE, CVID, mycophenolate)
   7. Absent plasma cells (agammaglobulinemia)
   8. Pigment (melanosis, calcium, iron)
   9. Vascular ectasia (lymphangiectasia)
   10. Perivascular deposits (amyloid).

Colon

- Normal
- Inflammatory
- LP infiltrate
- Neoplasia

Inflammatory	
Acute	
Ischemic/hemorrhagic	*Non-ischemic/hemorrhagic*
1. Ischemia	1. Infection
2. Infection	2. Medications
3. Radiation	3. Early or fulminant IBD
4. Medications	
Chronic	
Preserved architecture	*Disturbed architecture*
1. Microscopic colitis	1. IBD
2. Early IBD	2. Diverticular disease
3. Medications	3. Chronic ischemia
4. Diverticulosis	4. Radiation
5. Infection	5. Prolapse
	6. Medications
	7. Diversion colitis
	8. Infections
Eosinophilic	
1. Eosinophilic colitis	
2. Mastocytosis	
3. Infections (parasitic)	
4. IBD (treated)	

Pauci-inflammatory	
With increased apoptosis	*Without apoptosis*
1. GVHD	1. Infection in immunocompromised hosts
2. Mycophenolate-induced colitis	i. Sporochetosis
3. Infections (CMV, HIV)	ii. CMV
4. CVID	iii. Cryptosporidium
5. Cord colitis syndrome	2. Mucosal prolapse injury
6. Bowel preparation effect	3. Amyloidosis

LP infiltrate	
Non-pigmented	*Pigmented*
1. Histiocytic 　i. Xanthoma/muciphages 　ii. MAI 　iii. Granuloma/CGD 2. Neoplastic 　i. Signet cell carcinoma 　ii. Granular cell/mast cell/Langerhans cell	1. Melanosis coli 2. Brown bowel syndrome

Conclusion

Systematic approach is very important in the interpretation of the endoscopic biopsies of the GI tract. Pathologic findings should correlate with the clinical and endoscopic features.

In any discrepant/difficult cases, please call the clinician and discuss about the difficulties you are facing, explain the differential diagnosis and ask his permission to carry on appropriate additional histochemical, immunohistochemical or molecular ancillary studies.

Give her/him a call with the results of the additional studies and your final diagnosis. Close communication is a must and ... please believe me ... the more you call your clinicians the more respect and affection the clinicians will develop on you.

References

1. www.pathologyoutlines.com
2. Amitabh Srivastava, MD, Department of Pathology Brigham and Women's Hospital and Massachusetts General Hospital, Boston, MA Algorithmic Approach to Interpretation of Tubal Gut Biopsies.

   (General approach to GI lesions are discussed and this will help the readers to diagnose the lesions in a systematic way. For the individual cases, the diagnosis has been provided and the readers are requested to refer to www.pathologyoutlines.com)

CHAPTER 8

Case Files of GIT Lesions

S Rajendiran

UPPER GIT LESIONS: CASE LIST

- Candidiasis: Esophagitis
- Cytomegalovirus: Esophagitis
- Herpes simplex virus: Esophagitis
- Barrett esophagus
- Moderately differentiated squamous cell carcinoma
- Adenocarcinoma with focal papillary pattern
- Poorly differentiated carcinoma
- Basaloid squamous cell carcinoma
- Granulomatous gastritis
- Gastric fundic gland polyp
- Peutz-Jeghers polyp
- Hyperplastic polyp with xanthoma
- Poorly differentiated carcinoma with focal signet cells
- Signet cell carcinoma
- Mucinous carcinoma of stomach
- Moderately differentiated adenocarcinoma—intestinal type
- Lymphangiectasia
- GIST: Stomach

LOWER GIT LESIONS: CASE LIST

- *Stongyloides stercoralis* with focal pyloric metaplasia
- Whipple disease
- Peutz-Jeghers polyp
- HG dysplasia, lymphangitis carcinomatosa
- Eosinophilic appendicitis
- *E. vermicularis*
- Neuroendocrine carcinoma grade I (carcinoid)
- Hirschsprung disease
- CMV colitis
- Ulcerative colitis
- Ischemic colitis and sigmoid volvulus
- Radiation colitis
- Tubular adenoma
- Moderately differentiation adenocarcinoma and tubular adenomas
- Mucinous adenocarcinoma: Rectosigmoid
- NHL—diffuse large B cell type: Rectal
- NHL—diffuse large B cell type: Illeocaecal
- Malignant GIST: Mesocolon
- Fibroepithelial polyp: Anal canal
- Benign granular cell tumor: Anal region
- Malignant melanoma: Anal canal

GIT LESIONS

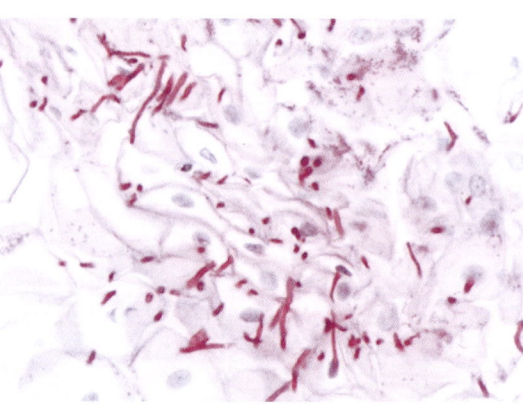

Candidial esophagitis

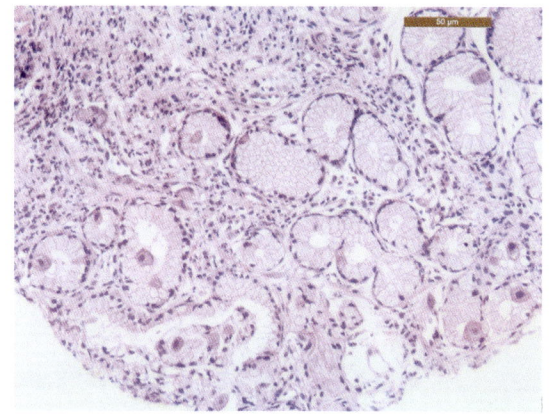
Cytomegalovirus esophagitis

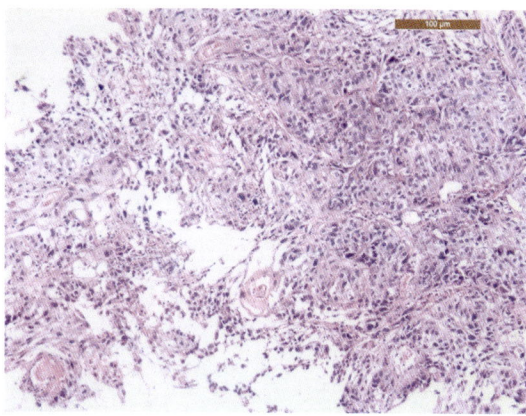
Moderately differentiated squamous cell carcinoma

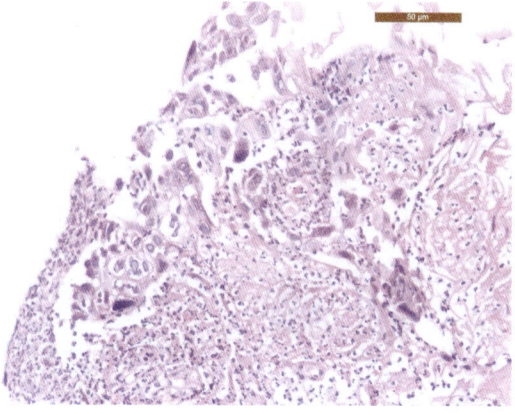
Herpes simplex virus—esophagitis

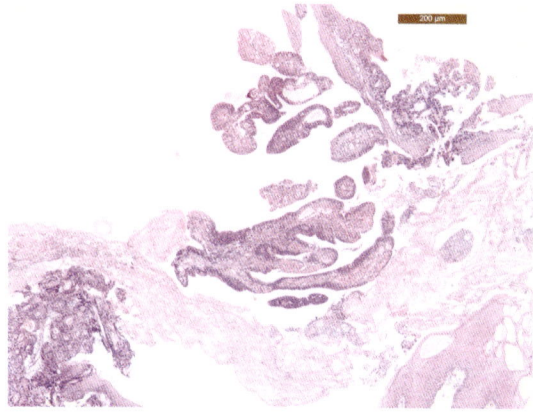
Adenocarcinoma with focal papillary pattern

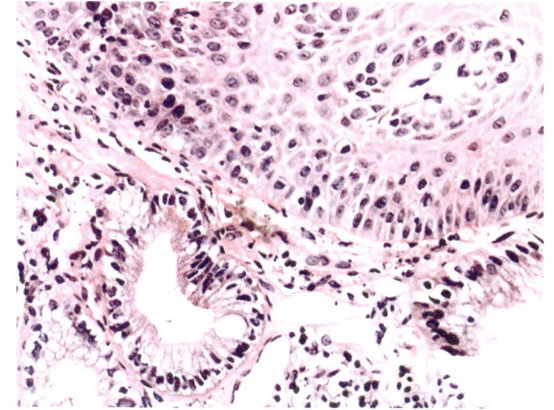
Barrett esophagus

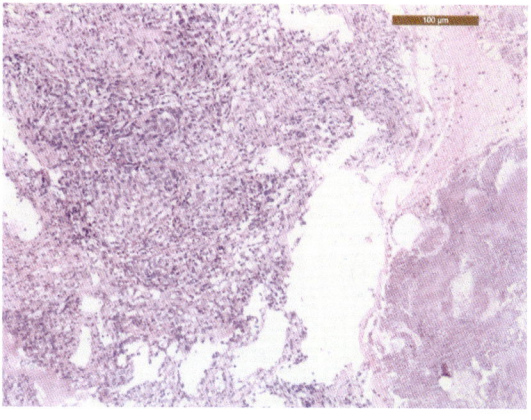
Poorly differentiated carcinoma

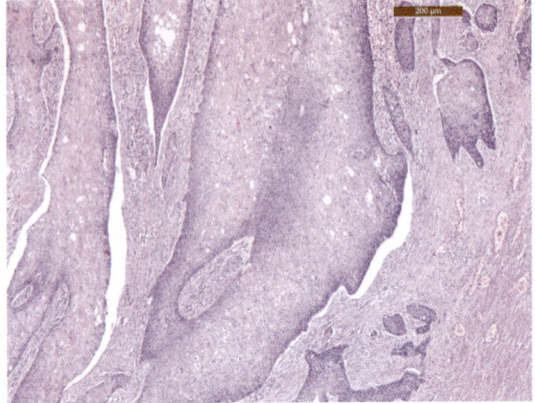
Moderately differentiated squamous cell carcinoma

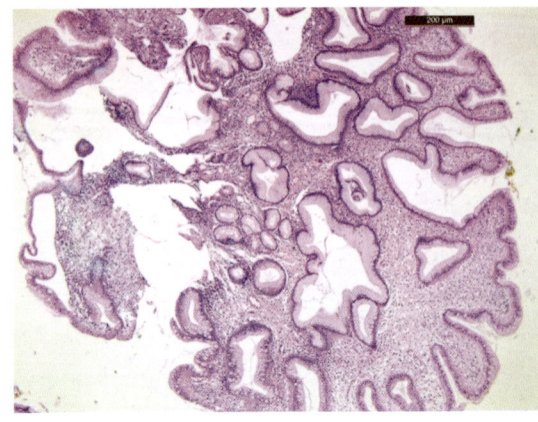
Gastric fundic gland polyp

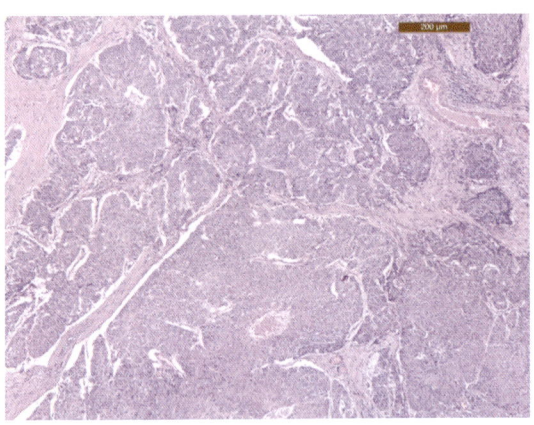
Basaloid squamous cell carcinoma

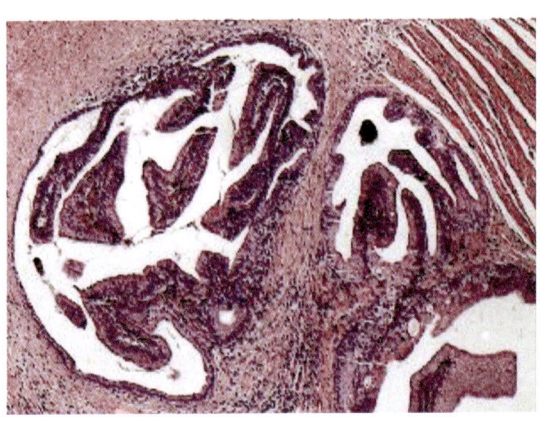
Peutz-Jeghers polyp

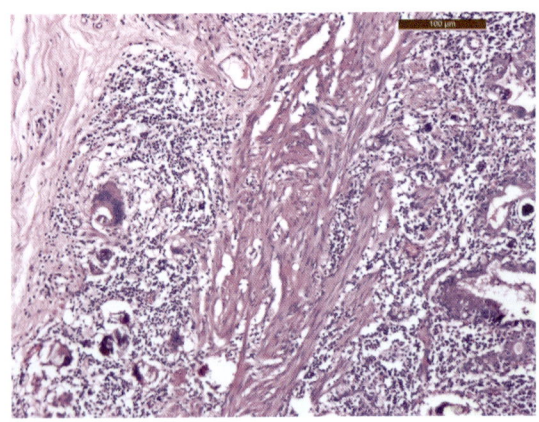
Granulomatous gastritis

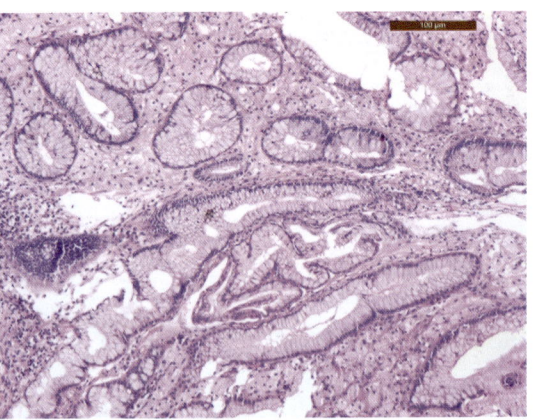
Hyperplastic polyp with xanthoma

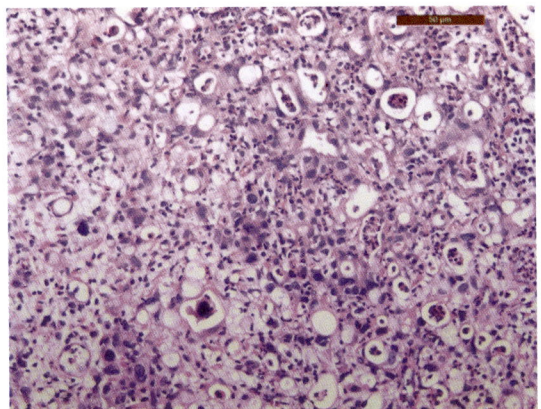

Poorly differentiated carcinoma with focal signet cells

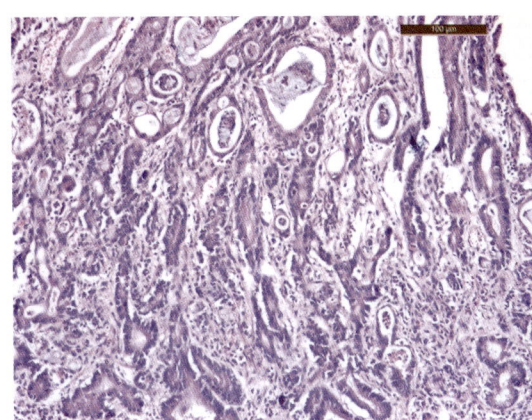

Moderately differentiated adenocarcinoma of the stomach—intestinal type

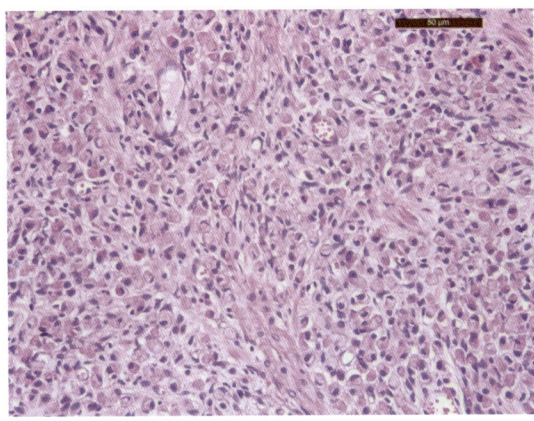

Signet cell carcinoma

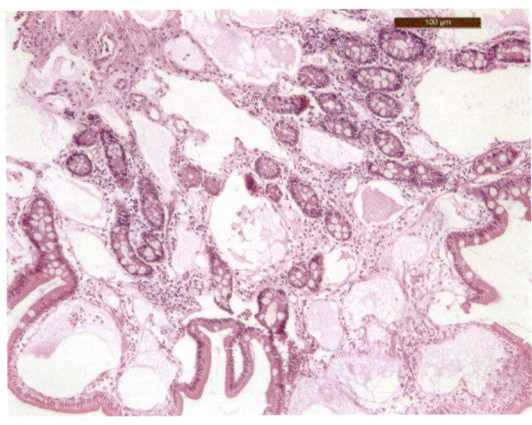

Lymphangiectasia

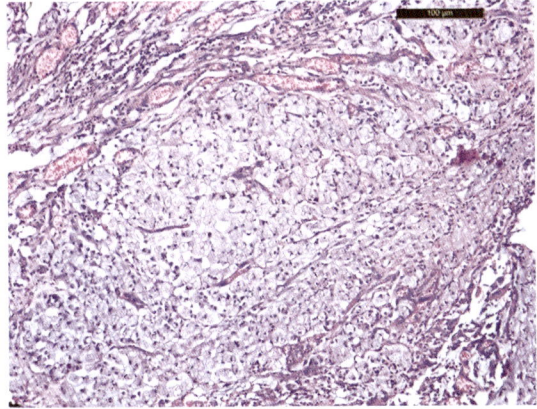

Mucinous carcinoma of the stomach

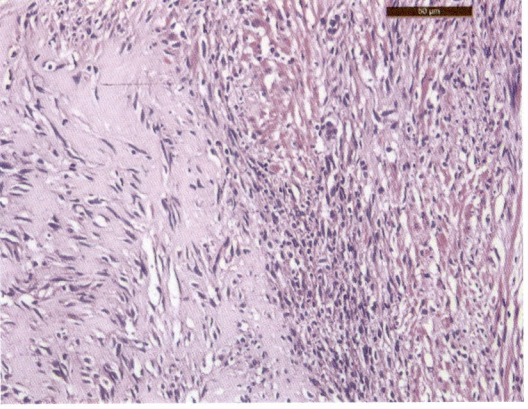

GIST— stomach

GIT 2

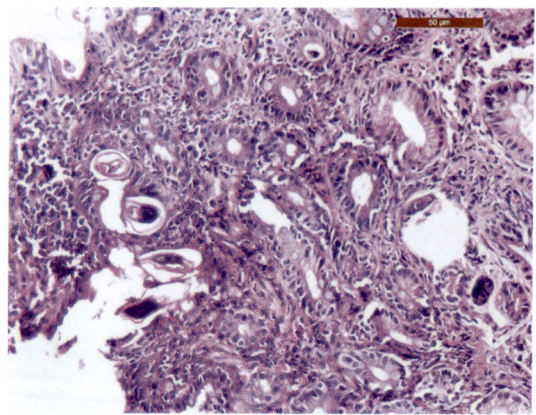

Strongyloides stercoralis with focal pyloric metaplasia

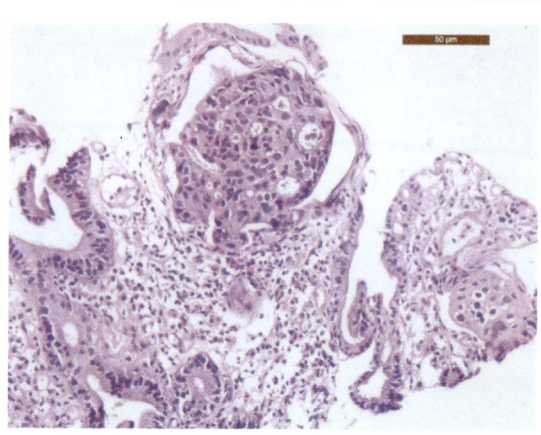

Lymphangitis carcinomatosa

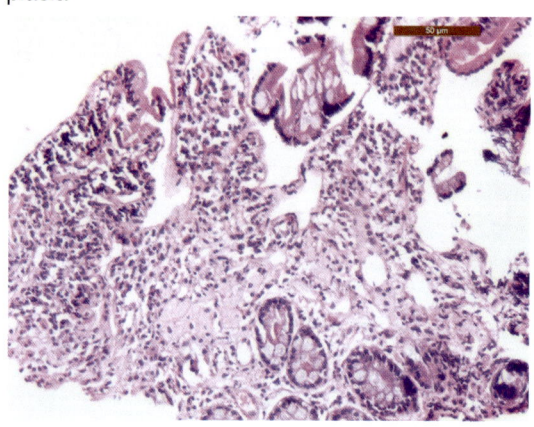

Whipple disease

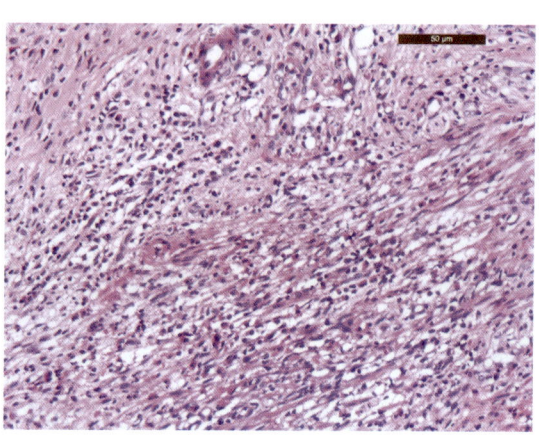

Eosinophilic appendicitis

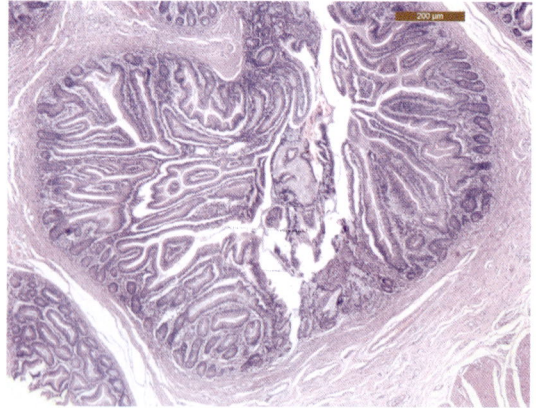

Diverticulosis

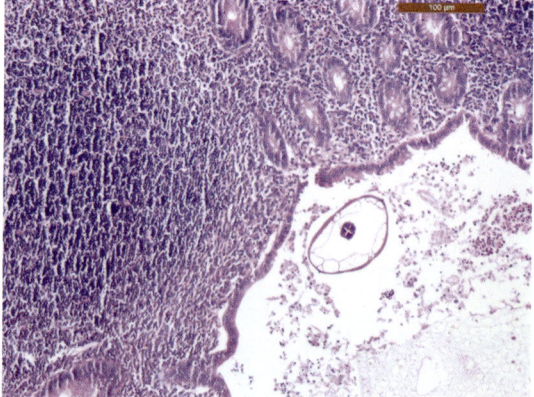

E. vermicularis

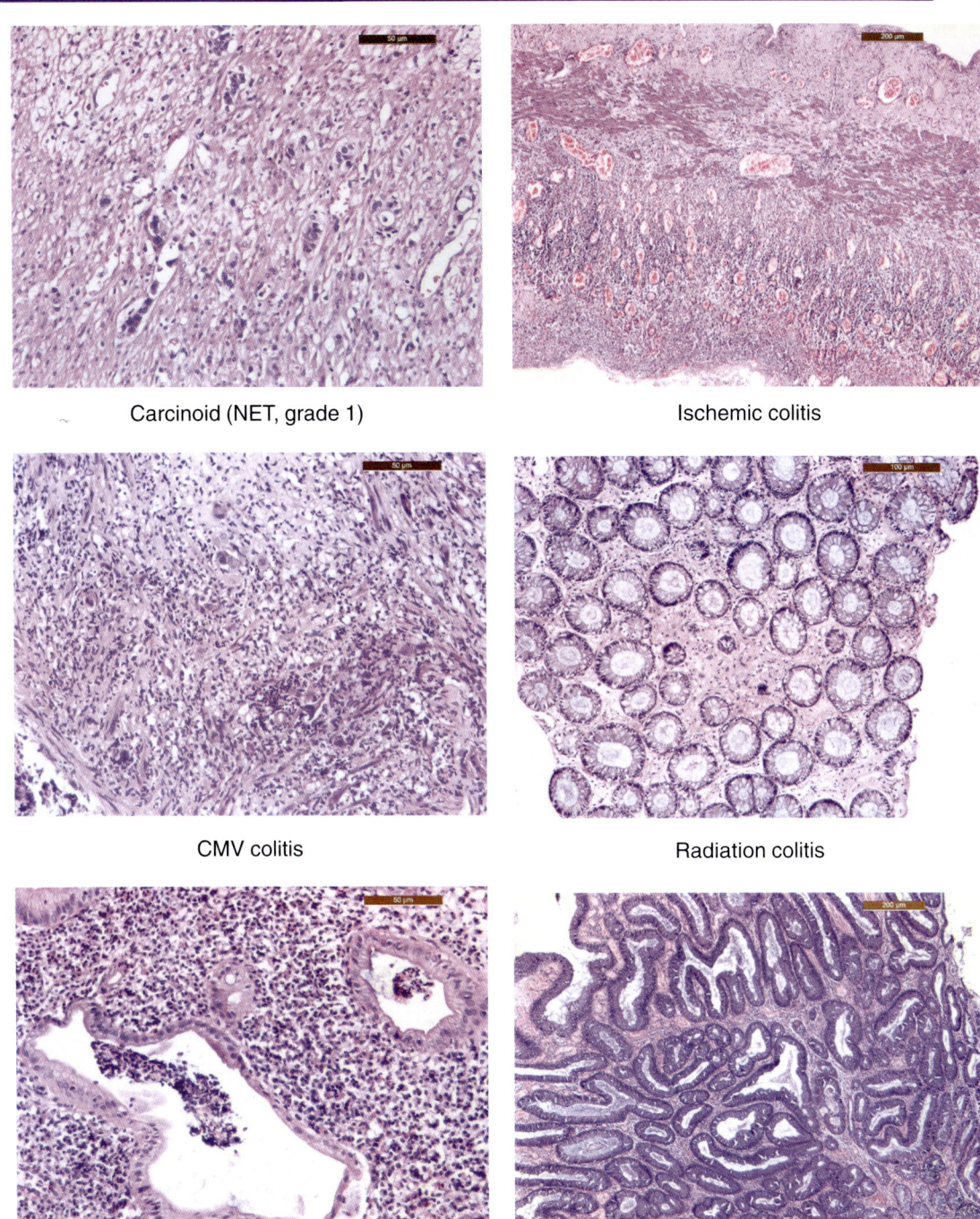

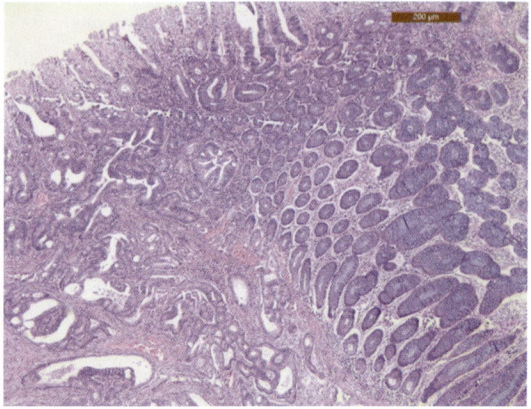

Moderately differentiated adenocarcinoma and tubular adenoma

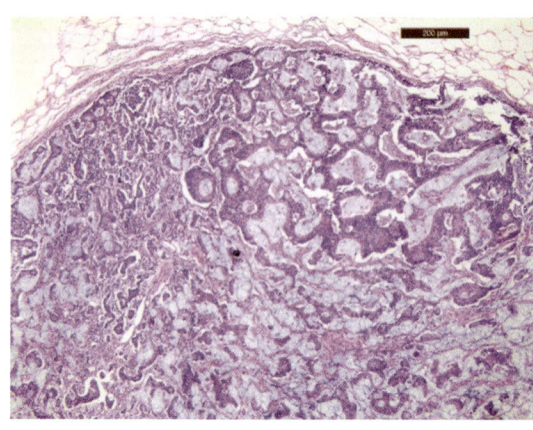

Mucinous carcinoma metastasis to lymph node

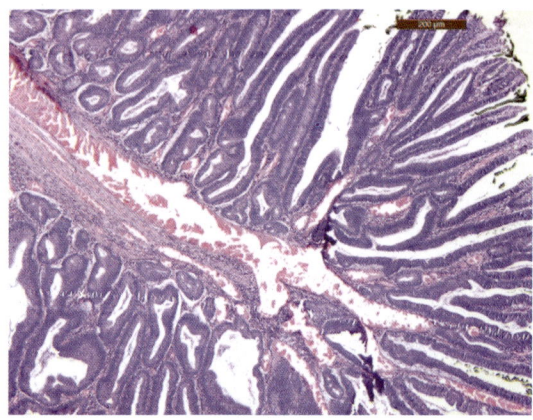

Tubulovillous adenoma

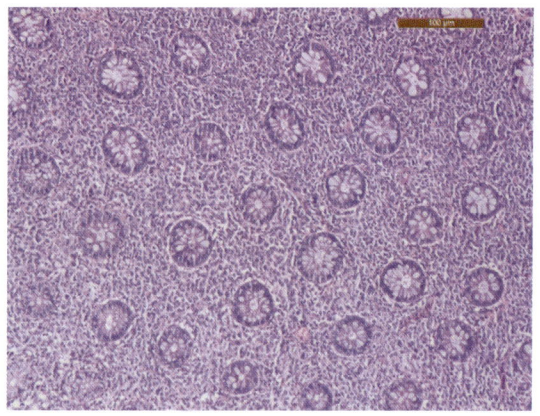

NHL diffuse large B cell—rectal

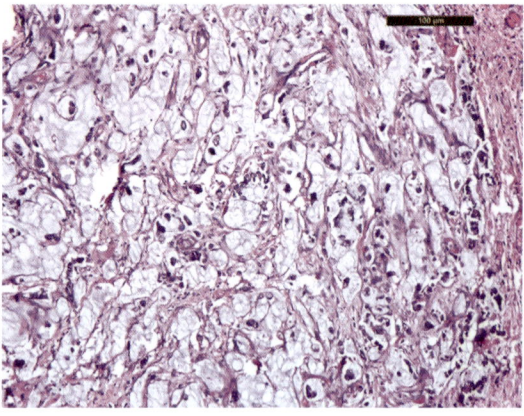

Mucinous adenocarcinoma

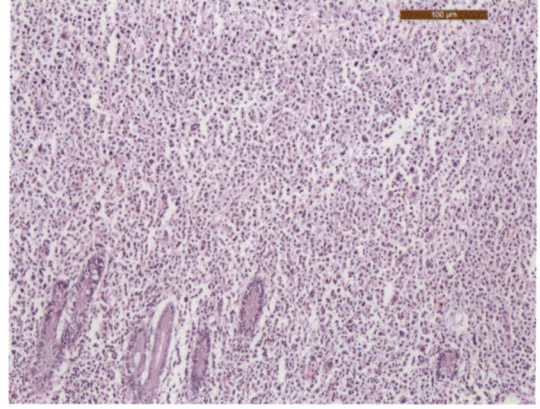

NHL diffuse large B cell—ileocaecal region

Case Files of GIT Lesions

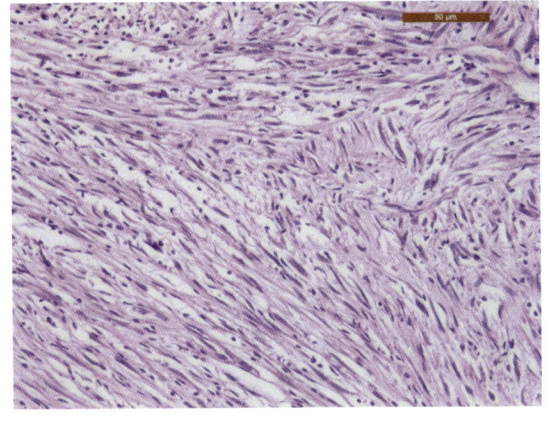

GIST

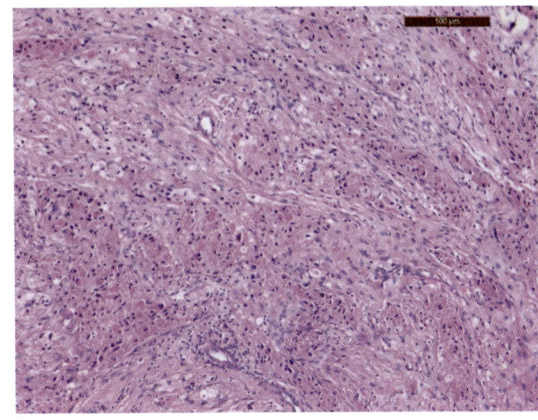

Benign granular cell tumor: Anal region

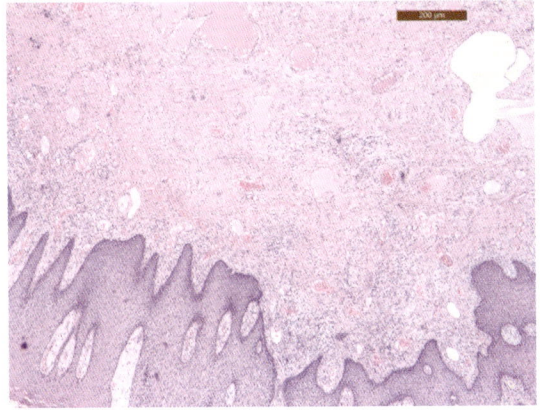

Fibroepithelial polyp

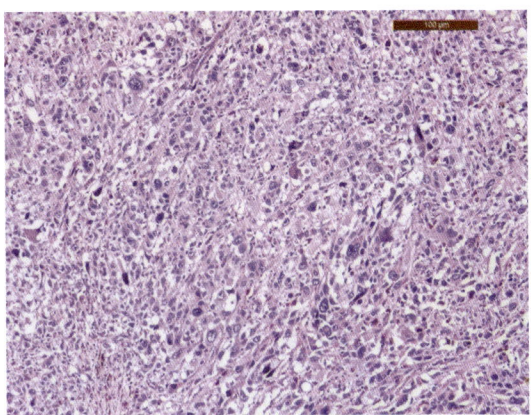

Malignant melanoma—anal canal

CHAPTER 9

Histological Approach to Hepatobiliary Lesions

J Thanka

Case History (a): A 14-year-old girl with jaundice.

Diagnosis: Chronic active hepatitis

(b): A 60-year-old female with nodular lesion liver.

Diagnosis: Chronic active hepatitis with cirrhotic changes

Clinical Features

- Wide spectrum of clinical manifestations.
- Hepatomegaly or other stigmata of chronic liver disease, such as palmar erythema.
- Patients with advanced cirrhosis may develop ascites or esophageal varices.
- Serum enzyme levels usually fluctuate, but may be elevated 2X to 10X.

Microscopy

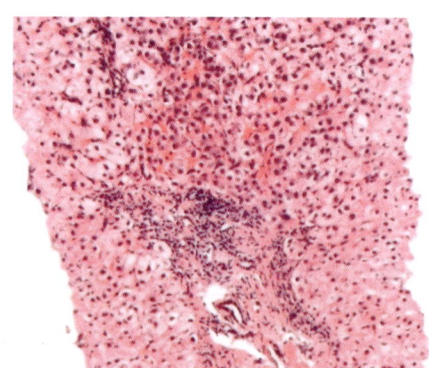

Fig. 9.1a

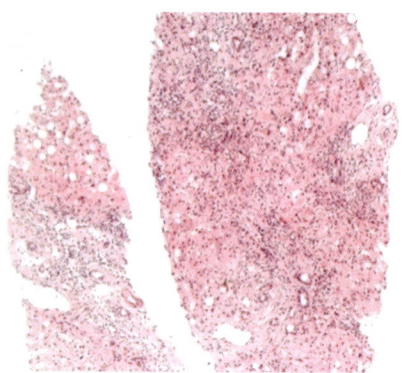

Fig. 9.1b

- Portal inflammation
- Interface hepatitis: Also known as piecemeal necrosis.
- Parenchymal inflammation and necrosis.
- Cirrhosis

Ancillary Studies

- **Immunohistochemistry:** Hepatitis B core antigen (HBcAg), HBsAg, and hepatitis B early antigen (HBeAg).
- **Electron microscopy:** HBsAg in hepatocyte cytoplasm. (22 nm spheres and rods)

Differential Diagnosis

- **Cases without interface hepatitis, differential diagnosis include:**
  1. Acute hepatitis
  2. Non-specific inflammation

3. Primary biliary cirrhosis
4. Lymphoma
- **Chronic hepatitis with lobular lesions, differential diagnosis include:** Acute hepatitis.
- Serologic markers of viral infection are virtually essential to establish or exclude the diagnosis
- **Cases with interface hepatitis:**
  1. Primary biliary cirrhosis.
  2. Primary sclerosing cholangitis.
  3. Wilson disease.
  4. α_1-antitrypsin deficiency
  5. Lymphoma.

Case History: A 57-year-old female with deviated liver enzymes.

Diagnosis: NASH—Non-alcoholic Steato Hepatitis

Clinical Feature

A manifestation of the metabolic (insulin resistance) syndrome.

Gross

- Early: Large, soft, greasy, yellow liver.
- Late: Shrunken, mottled red brown liver with bile staining.
- End stage: Cirrhosis.

Microscopy

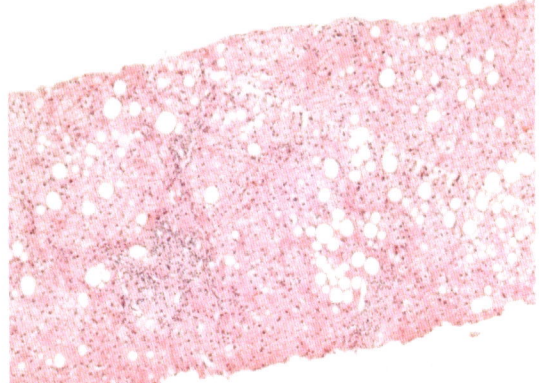

Fig. 9.2

Essential Features

Steatosis, predominantly macrovesicular. Mild mixed acinar inflammation hepatocellular injury in the form of:
- Hepatocellular ballooning, often most prominent in zone 3
- Pericellular fibrosis

Other Features

- Glycogenated nuclei in zone 1
- Lipogranulomas in the lobular parenchyma or portal tracts
- Occasional acidophil bodies
- Mallory hyaline in zone 3, typically inconspicuous
- Mild iron deposits in hepatocytes or sinusoidal cells
- Megamitochondria
- Unusual features
- Predominantly microvesicular steatosis
- Prominent portal and/or acinar inflammation, numerous plasma cells
- Prominent bile ductular reaction, cholestasis
- Perivenular fibrosis, hyaline sclerosis
- Marked lobular inflammation.

Differential Diagnosis

- Alcoholic liver disease
- Fatty liver of pregnancy.

Case History: A 1-month-old girl baby with increased liver enzymes.

Diagnosis: Neonatal hepatitis

Causes

- Alpha-1antitrypsin deficiency
- Cystic fibrosis
- Hypopituitarism
- Alagille syndrome
- Progressive familial intrahepatic cholestasis,
- Congenital infections such as cytomegalovirus, hepatitis-B, herpes simplex, human herpesvirus-6, rubella, syphilis, toxoplasmosis and varicella
- Down syndrome
- Trisomy 18
- Idiopathic

Clinical Feature
Prolonged jaundice beyond 2 weeks of age.

Microscopy

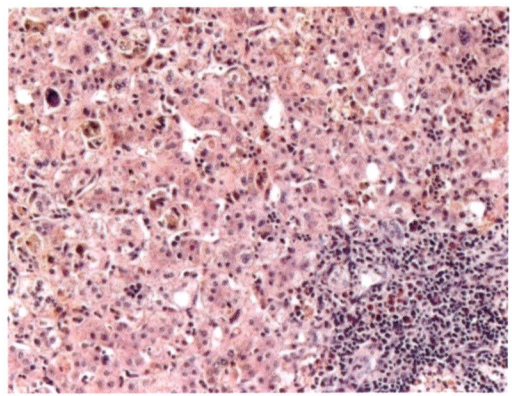

Fig. 9.3

- Cholestasis with variable, spotty or confluent to bridging necrosis.
- Giant cell transformation (4–10 nuclei).
- Portal and lobular lymphocytic inflammation.
- Regenerative changes.
- Extramedullary hematopoiesis.
- Canalicular and hepatocellular bilirubinostasis.
- Portal tract changes: Mononuclear inflammatory cell infiltrate.

Differential Diagnosis
Extrahepatic biliary atresia: Ductular reaction and portal fibrosis are essential discriminatory histological features suggestive of extra hepatic biliary atresia.

Case History: A 43-year-old male liver with gallbladder.

Diagnosis: Cirrhosis

Clinical Features
- Anorexia
- Weight loss, weakness
- Signs and symptoms of hepatic failure, signs and symptoms of portal hypertension.

Gross
- *Early:* Enlarged with or without greasy surface.
- *Late:* Shrunken with diffuse nodularity. Micronodular <3 mm and macronodular >3 mm.

Microscopy

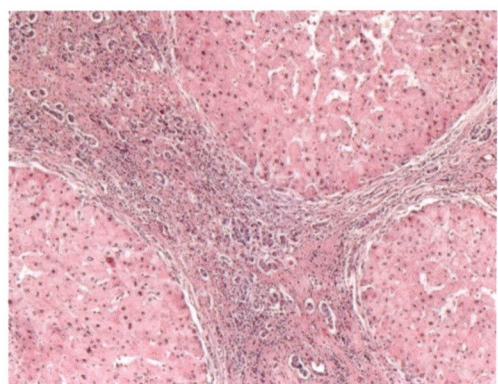

Fig. 9.4

- Diffuse nodules of regenerating hepatocytes surrounded by fibrous bands.
- Arteries, bile ductules, and inflammatory infiltrate within fibrous septa.
- Garland shaped nodules in biliary type cirrhosis.

Grading: Modified histological activity index (HAI grading): Necroinflammatory scores (Table 9.1).

Table 9.1	
A. Periportal or periseptal interface hepatitis (piecemeal necrosis)	
Absent	0
Mild (focal, a few portal areas)	1
Mild/moderate (focal, most portal areas)	2
Moderate (continuous around <50% of tracts or septa)	3
Severe (continuous around >50% of tracts or septa)	4
B. Confluent necrosis	
Absent	0
Focal confluent necrosis	1
Centrolobular necrosis in some areas	2
Centrolobular necrosis in areas	3
Centrolobular necrosis + occasional portal-central (P-C) bridging	4
Centrolobular necrosis + multiple P-C bridging	5
Panlobular or multilobular necrosis	6

Contd.

C. Focal (spotty) lytic necrosis, apoptosis, and focal inflammation
  - Absent — 0
  - One focus or less per 10X objective — 1
  - One to four foci per 10X objective — 2
  - Five to 10 foci per 10X objective — 3
  - More than 10 foci per 10X objective — 4

D. Portal inflammation
  - None — 0
  - Mild, some or all portal areas — 1
  - Moderate, some or all portal areas — 2
  - Moderate/marked, all portal areas — 3
  - Marked, all portal areas — 4
  - **Maximum possible score for grading** — 18

Staging: Modified HAI staging—architectural changes, fibrosis and cirrhosis (Table 9.2).

Table 9.2: Modified histological activity index—staging: Architectural changes, fibrosis and cirrhosis*

Change	Score
No fibrosis	0
Fibrous expansion of some portal areas, with or without fibrous septa	1
Fibrous expansion of most portal areas, with or without short fibrous septa	2
Fibrous expansion of most portal areas with occasional portal-portal (P-P) bridging	3
Fibrous expansion of portal areas with marked bridging (portal-portal) (P-P) as well as portal-central (P-C)	4
Marked bridging (P-P and/or P-C) with occasional nodules (incomplete cirrhosis)	5
Cirrhosis, probable or definite	6
Maximum possible score in staging	**6**

Additional features which should be noted but not scored:
Intralobular fibrosis, perivenular (chicken-wire fibrosis)
Phacosclerosis of terminal hepatic venules (central veins)
*Data (adapted to new terminologies) from Ishak et al, with permission from authors and publisher.

Special Stains
- **Trichrome:** Useful for determining the extent and pattern of fibrosis.
- **Reticulin:** Useful for identifying thickened hepatic plates within regenerative nodules.

Differential Diagnosis

Table 9.3: Differential diagnosis of cirrhosis

Disease	Diffuse involvement of the liver	Septa	Nodules
Cirrhosis	+	+	+
Nodular regenerative hyperplasia	+	–	+
Focal nodular hyperplasia	–	+	+

Case History: A 45-day-old child with liver biopsy.

Diagnosis: Hemophagocytic syndrome

Types
- Genetic—rare, infants/young children, rapidly fatal, autosomal recessive or parental consanguinity.
- Acquired—EBV infection in immunocompromised patients.

Diagnostic Criteria
Repeated sampling of bone marrow, CSF, lymph node, liver and spleen.

Table 9.4: Diagnostic guidelines for HLH

The diagnosis of HLH requires a molecular diagnosis consistent with HLH or 5 of 8 of the below criteria

1. Fever
2. Splenomegaly
3. Cytopenias affecting 2 lineages
   a. Hemoglobin <9 gm/dl
   b. Platelets <100 × 10^9/L
   c. Neutrophils <1.0 × 10^9/L
4. Hypertriglyceridemia and/or hypofibrinogenemia
   a. Triglycerides 265 mg/dl
   b. Fibrinogen 150 mg/dl
5. Hemophagocytosis in marrow, spleen, or lymph nodes
6. Low or absent NK cell activity
7. Ferritin 500 μg/L
8. sCD25 (i.e. sIL2R) ≥2400 U/ml

Clinical Features
- Fever
- Jaundice
- Hepatosplenomegaly.

Microscopy

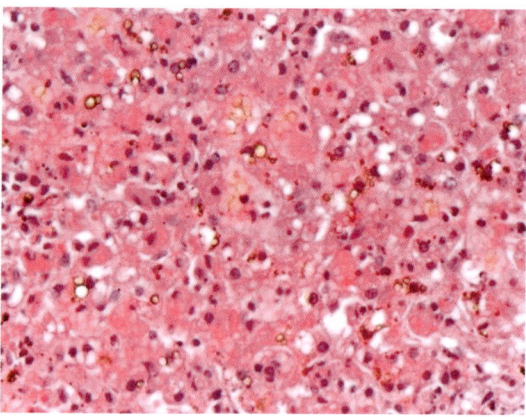

Fig. 9.5

- **Liver:** Increase number of histiocytes showing evidence of phagocytosis of erythroid cells, platelets and granulocytes.
- **Spleen:** A rarefaction of the white pulp with hemophagocytic histiocytes with erythrophagocytosis present in lymph node, bone marrow and spleen with abundant lymphocytes, plasma cells and plasma cell precursors in the cords.

Differential Diagnosis
- **Malignant histiocytosis:** Where atypical architectural effacement will be pronounced.
- **Peripheral T-cell lymphoma:** Where atypical cells will be seen.

Case History: A 55-year-old male with hepatomegaly.

Diagnosis: Extramedullary hematopoiesis

Common sites: Fetal yolk sac, liver, spleen, lymph node.
Other sites: Pleura, lungs, GIT, breast, skin, brain, kidney and adrenal glands.

Microscopy

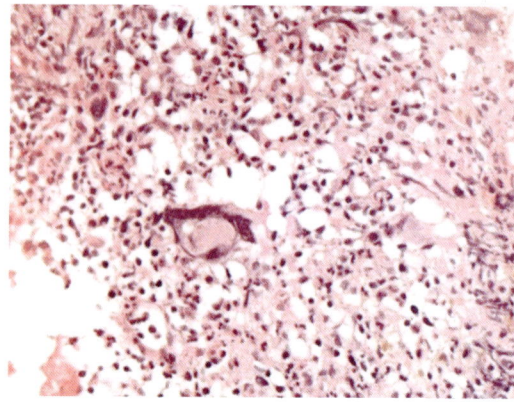

Fig. 9.6

- Erythroid precursors in sinusoids
- Myeloid precursors in portal tracts
- Also megakaryocytes within sinuses.

Differential Diagnosis
- Abscess/infections
- Lymphoproliferative disorder
- Prominent megakaryocytic component: May suggest atypical or malignant diagnosis.

Case History: A 32-year-old female with excision biopsy liver.

Diagnosis: Hydatid cyst

Sites
- 60–70% in liver, also brain, lungs.
- Frequently communicates with biliary tract.

Gross
- 75% solitary
- Unilocular white cyst with fluid filled.

Microscopy
Three layers in cyst wall:

Innermost (germinal layer)
- 10–25 microns, contains nuclei, gives rise to brood capsules attached by short stalk in infectious cysts.
- Also protoscolices with double row of refractile, birefringent, acid-fast hooklets 22–40 microns and 4 round suckers that comprise "hydatid sand".

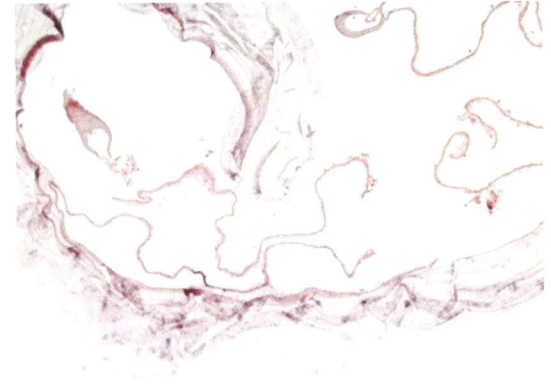
Fig. 9.7

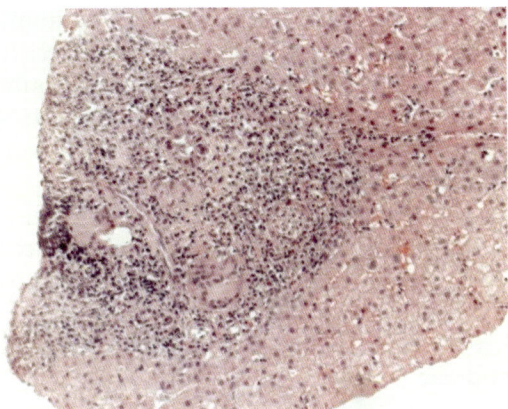
Fig. 9.8

Laminated membrane
Beneath germinal layer is 1 mm thick, vascular, eosinophilic, refractile and chitinous; strongly PAS+, GMS+.

Outer layer
Dense fibrovascular tissue with chronic inflammatory cells, variable calcification develops after 5+ years.

Case History: A 38-year-old female with liver biopsy.

Diagnosis: Overlap syndrome

Introduction
The term overlap syndrome describes variant forms of the major hepatobiliary autoimmune diseases, autoimmune hepatitis (AIH), primary biliary cirrhosis (PBC) and primary sclerosing cholangitis (PSC).

Autoimmune Hepatitis
Types
- **Type 1:** AIH (bimodal, 10–25 years, 45–70 years)—ANA, SMA positive
- **Type 2:** AIH (<15 years)—anti-LKM antibody, anti-LC antibody positive.
- **Type 3:** AIH (severe disease, relapse after drug withdrawal requires transplantation)—soluble liver antigen (SLA), LP antigen positive, p-ANCA positive.

Diagnosis
- Elevated serum liver tests (ALT).
- Presence of elevated serum immunoglobulin (IgG >1.5 times the normal) or gamma-globulins and of serum antibodies [anti-nuclear antibodies (ANA), anti-smooth muscle antibody (ASMA), and anti-liver kidney microsomal antibody (ALKM)].
- Absence of AMAs and viral markers.
- Lack of evidence of alcohol/drug-induced liver disease.
- IgG is also a marker for monitoring treatment response.

Histopathology
- Chronic hepatitis pattern of injury, with portal and periportal—lymphoplasmacytic infiltrates and interface hepatitis.
- The severity of necro-inflammatory activity is quite variable, ranging from mildly active hepatitis to bridging necrosis to massive hepatic necrosis.
- Emperipolesis
- Hepatocyte regeneration may be prominent, with regenerating rosette-like structures.

Primary Biliary Cirrhosis
Diagnosis
- Cholestatic serum enzyme pattern
- Elevated serum IgM

- The presence of AMAs detected by immunofluorescence (positive in 95% of cases) or PBC-specific AMA-M2 directed against E2 subunit of pyruvate dehydrogenase complex and detected by ELISA or immunoblotting.
- A florid bile duct lesion of mid-sized intrahepatic bile ducts and bile duct paucity.

Gross

Liver turns green, granular, then micronodular.

Microscopy

- Florid duct lesion sometimes also called chronic non-suppurative destructive cholangitis.
- The three components of florid duct lesion are inflammation, injury to bile duct epithelial cells and disruption of the bile duct basement membrane.
- The inflammatory infiltrate is composed of lymphocytes, scattered eosinophils, macrophages and a variable number of plasma cells and is intimately associated with the bile duct.
- The basement membrane becomes disrupted and fragmented best visualized on PAS stain.
- The cirrhosis has a typical biliary pattern, in which the nodules have an irregularly shaped 'jigsaw puzzle piece' profile.

Criteria for Diagnosis

- 2/3rds of the following typical features of AIH and PBC are required for diagnosis of overlap syndrome:

AIH	PBC
1. ALT more than 5 times	1. ALP more than 2 times
2. IgG or SMA more than 2 times	2. GGT more than 5 times
3. Moderate to severe interphase/lobular activity	3. AMA positive or florid duct lesion

Histologic Staging of PBC

- **Stage 1:** Damage to interlobular bile ducts is seen in the form of florid duct lesion.
- **Stage 2:** Expansion of portal tracts with piecemeal necrosis and ductular proliferation but no bridging.
- **Stage 3:** Scarring or pre-cirrhotic stage, with bridging fibrosis.
- **Stage 4:** Cirrhosis.

Case History: An 8-month-old boy baby, abdominal distension, ultrasound—cystic lesion.

Diagnosis: Mesenchymal hamartoma

Clinical Features

- Child presenting with abdominal distension or upper abdominal mass.
- Older children/adult presents with abdominal pain/jaundice.
- Serum AFP levels may be elevated.

Gross

- Solitary, unencapsulated, well circumscribed with satellite lesions. 75% in right lobe.
- Cut surface—multiple cysts—a few mm to 14 cm solid in infants.
- Fibrotic/multiloculated in older patients.
- Cysts have clear/mucoid, solid pink white areas.

Microscopy

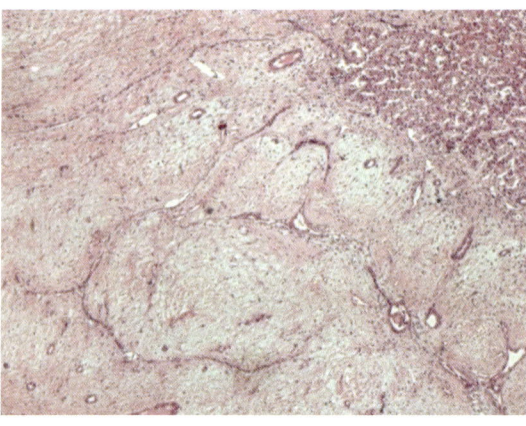

Fig. 9.9

- Epithelial and mesenchymal components are seen.
- Stroma consists of primitive mesenchymal tissue composed of bland stellate and spindle cells with myofibroblasts in an edematous/myxoid matrix with variable collagen.
- Fluid in degenerated mesenchyma leads to alveolar pattern, simulating lymphangioma.
- Some area may resemble hemangioendothelioma due to vascular proliferation.

Ancillary Tests
- **Electron microscopy:** Myofibroblastic features
- **Immunohistochemistry:** Positive—vimentin, CK7, SMA, desmin, actin, glypican 3. Negative—CK20

Differential Diagnosis
- **Mixed epithelial mesenchymal hepatoblastoma:** Epithelial component has embryonal and fetal hepatocytes; mesenchymal component has spindle cells, osteoid, cartilage
- **Infantile hemangioma:** Females more common, vascular channels of variable size
- **Infantile hemangioendothelioma:** More vascular
- **Bile duct adenoma**
- **Bile duct hamartoma:** Usually multiple with fibrous background
- **Embryonal sarcoma:** Marked cellularity and atypical cells, eosinophilic PASD globules

Case History: A 66-year-old male with end-stage liver disease, total hepatectomy specimen.

Diagnosis: Intraductal papillary biliary neoplasm

Clinical Features
- Patients usually present with obstructive jaundice.
- Males are more affected, with a mean age of 58 years.

Gross
- Extrahepatic intraductal papillary neoplasms of the bile duct presented as solid intraluminal tumors 0.8–5 cm in size or papillary mucosal lesions measuring 1–3 cm and dilating the bile duct.
- Intrahepatic intraductal papillary neoplasms of the bile duct present mostly as a cystic lesion 0.5–14 cm than as clearly visible intraluminal 2.1–6.5 cm or intrahepatic tumors 4.5–8.5 cm.
- The cystic lesion appears well defined with the cyst containing mucoid and haemorrhagic contents.
- The wall of the cyst is lined by friable papillary tumor mass.

Classification
Based on the cellular phenotype they are classified as:
- Intestinal type (most common)
- Pancreatic biliary
- Gastric
- Oncocytic

Microscopy

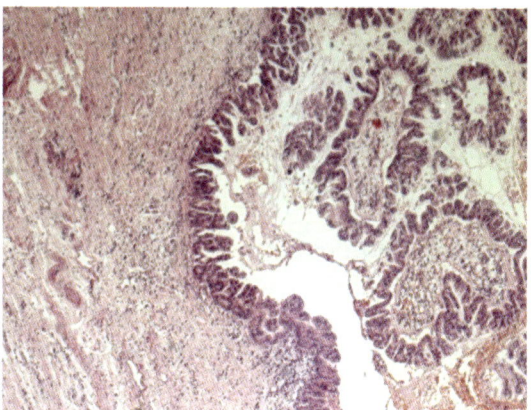

Fig. 9.10

Pancreaticobiliary Variant
- Complex arborizing papillae lined by cuboidal cells, often with round nuclei containing a single prominent eccentric nucleolus.

- The bile duct is packed with fine papillary tumor, which was composed of aborizing complex branch and abundant micropapillae, lined by pseudostratified, biliary type cells with frequent cytoplasmic mucinous vacuoles and prominent nucleoli.

Cystic (Intestinal Variant)

- Long finger-like projections and lined by columnar cells with cigar-shaped nuclei were classified as intestinal type.
- These were morphologically indistinguishable from colonic villous adenomas.
- The cells contained variable amounts of mucin in the apical cytoplasm.
- Nuclei were pseudostratified with varying degrees of atypia.

The other two variant gastric and oncocytic types are lined by the respective type of epithelium.

Histological grading was done into three classes (adenoma, carcinoma or borderline). Based on:
- Degree of cytologic and structural atypia
- Increased nuclear/cytoplasmic ratio
- Loss of polarity
- Pleomorphism and hyperchromatism
- Prominent nucleoli and abnormal mitosis (1–3/10 HPF)
- Cribriform pattern and multilayering, and presence of invasion.

Immunohistochemistry

- Pancreaticobiliary type is positive for MUC 1 and negative for MUC 2.
- Intestinal type is positive for MUC 2 and negative for MUC 1.
- Gastric and oncocytic types are positive for MUC 5AC and negative for MUC 1 and 2.

Case History: A 58-year-old female with decompensated liver disease.

Diagnosis: Hepatocellular carcinoma

Clinical Features
- Abdominal pain
- Ascites
- Hepatomegaly
- Obstructive jaundice

Laboratory Investigation
Elevated serum AFP (70% sensitive).

Gross
- Unifocal, multifocal or diffusely infiltrative soft tumor, paler than normal tissue, may be green due to bile.
- Extensive intrahepatic metastases are common.
- Snake-like masses of tumor may involve the portal vein, hepatic vein or inferior vena cava.
- Hemorrhage and necrosis are common.

Microscopy

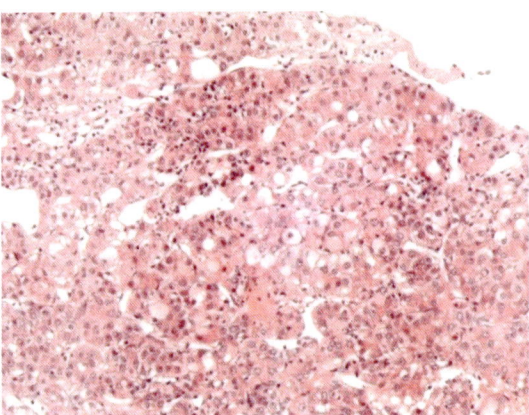

Fig. 9.11

- Trabecular pattern with 4+ cells surrounded by layer of flattened endothelial cells; also clear cell, giant cell, pelioid, pseudoglandular, sarcomatoid, and solid.
- Presence of sinusoidal vessels surrounding tumor cells.
- Scanty stroma.
- Cells are polygonal with distinct cell membranes, abundant granular eosinophilic cytoplasm, higher NC ratio than

normal, round nuclei with coarse chromatin and thickened nuclear membrane; may have prominent nucleoli.

Common Features
- Portal vein thrombosis
- Vascular invasion
- Mitotic figures.

Immunohistochemistry
- Hep Par-1
- Glypican 3
- Polyclonal CEA in canalicular pattern (50–90%, in better differentiated tumors)
- AFP (15–70%, not in small tumors)

Differential Diagnosis
- **Adenoma/macroregenerative nodule:** (Difficult if small sample): No cirrhosis in adenoma, not trabecular, no extensive pseudoglandular growth pattern, different clinical history, reticulin framework slightly maintained, minimal atypia, no mitotic figures; no thick fibrous pseudocapsule; negative for GPC3 and AFP.
- **Focal nodular hyperplasia:** No cytologic atypia, no ductular reaction, arteries are abnormally structured; note that "focal nodular hyperplasia-like nodules" may be present in cirrhotic livers and mimic HCC on imaging.
- **Angiomyolipoma, epithelioid:** spindle cell component, thick-walled vessels, HMB45+, actin+, CK–
- **Metastatic tumors**

Case History: A 50-year-old male with mass right lobe of liver.

Diagnosis: Fibrolamellar variant of hepatocellular carcinoma

Clinical Features
- <10% of HCC, but 35% of patients <50 years old; no gender preference.
- Similar symptoms to classic HCC.
- Not associated with hepatitis B virus, cirrhosis or metabolic abnormalities.

X-ray
- Central scar
- Often calcified

Laboratory Investigation
Serum -fetoprotein elevated.

Gross
- Single, large, hard, scirrhous, well-circumscribed, bulging, white-brown tumor with fibrous bands throughout and central stellate scar.
- Only liver tumor that is more common in left lobe, but may involve both lobes.
- Variable bile staining, hemorrhage and necrosis.

Microscopy

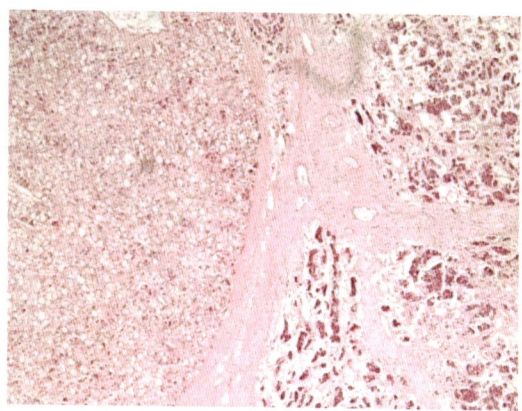

Fig. 9.12

- Nests, sheets or cords of well-differentiated oncocytic cells in background of dense, acellular collagen bundles arranged in parallel lamellae that may contain small, thick-walled vessels.
- Cells are large and polygonal with well-defined cell borders, abundant granular and eosinophilic cytoplasm due to abundant mitochondria, often pale bodies (ground glass cells) or PAS+ hyaline globules, vesicular nuclei and prominent nucleoli.
- Vascular invasion and necrosis common; fibrotic tissue coalesces into central scar; remaining liver is unremarkable.

- Radiologic calcification corresponds to necrosis with foreign body type reaction.
- Variable: Focal nuclear pleomorphism, conventional hepatocellular carcinoma, trabecular, adenoid or pelioid patterns.

Ancillary Tests

- **Immunohistochemistry:** Hep Par and CK7. Others: Also fibrinogen (pale bodies), copper, copper-binding protein, bile, α_1-antitrypsin, polyclonal CEA and CAM 5.2 (CK8/18).
- **Electron microscopy:** Numerous mitochondria

Differential Diagnosis

- **Focal nodular hyperplasia:** Ductular reaction around central scar, lesional cells are not characteristically oncocytic, does not have the nuclear features of fibrolamellar carcinoma
- **Neuroendocrine tumors:** Positive for neuroendocrine markers
- **Paraganglioma:** May have abundant oncocytic cytoplasm; round nuclei without the typical features of fibrolamellar carcinoma, vascular stroma without dense fibrosis; positive for neuroendocrine markers and negative for cytokeratin
- **Cholangiocarcinoma:** Truly glandular, often conspicuous pleomorphism
- **Metastatic carcinoma with sclerotic stroma:** Conspicuous pleomorphism

Case History: A 1-year-old boy with liver tumor.

Diagnosis: Hepatoblastoma

Clinical Features

- About one-third are associated with a variety of congenital anomalies, syndromes, or other childhood tumors.
- Beckwith-Wiedemann syndrome and familial adenomatous polyposis.
- Patients may present with virilization; result of ectopic sex hormone production.

Laboratory Investigation

Serum AFP is often elevated.

Gross

Solitary, unencapsulated, often large mass measuring up to 25 cm in diameter. Variegated cut surface with areas of necrosis, cystic changes, and hemorrhage. Normal surrounding liver can be seen.

Microscopy

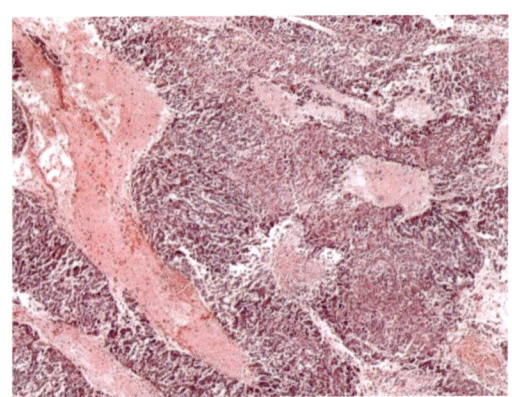

Fig. 9.13

Two types: Epithelial (75%). Mixed (epithelial and mesenchymal) (25%).

Epithelial Type

Fetal component

- Fetal-type cells are polygonal and large with round to oval nuclei and with single nucleoli and clear or granular cytoplasm.
- Cells are organized into irregular plates with bile canaliculi and sinusoids. Commonly associated with extramedullary hematopoiesis.

Embryonal component

- Embryonal-type cells are smaller and elongated with hyperchromatic nuclei and scant cytoplasm.
- Predominantly solid pattern with rosette-like clusters, cords, ribbons, and rarely tubules.

Variants of Epithelial

- Anaplastic
- Macrotrabecular

Mixed epithelial and mesenchymal type
- Fetal and embryonal epithelium component admixed with mesenchymal elements.
- Mesenchymal component is usually osteoid, cartilage, or undifferentiated spindled cells.

Immunohistochemistry
- Keratin low molecular weight (keratins 8 and 18) and pan-keratin, and EMA are typically positive.
- Hep Par-1, neuron-specific enolase (NSE), S-100 protein, chromogranin and CEA are often positive.
- AFP positive in fetal and embryonal cells
- BCL-2 variably positive.

Electron Microscopy
Immature hepatocytes in epithelial areas.

Molecular Genetics
- Complex karyotype with gain of chromosome 2 and X.
- 11p15LOH in Beckwith-Wiedemann syndrome
- Trisomy 2q and 20q
- Wnt signaling pathway abnormality.

Differential Diagnosis
- **Metastatic primitive tumor of infancy:** (Nephroblastoma and neuroblastoma)
- **Hepatocellular carcinoma of childhood:** Resembles macrotrabecular variant of hepatoblastoma, uncommon in children, larger more pleomorphic tumor cells, no extramedullary hematopoiesis.

Case History (a): A 43-year-old female with liver tumor

Case History (b): A 27-year-old male with liver secondaries

Case History (c): A 77-year-old female with biopsy from right lobe liver.

Diagnosis: Metastasis liver

Clinical Features
- Hepatomegaly
- Right upper quadrant abdominal pain.
- Anorexia
- Weight loss.
- Biliary obstruction, acute hepatic failure leading to jaundice.
- Metastasis from carcinoid tumor results in classical carcinoid syndrome including flushing, diarrhea and palpitation.
- Metastatic NETs from GI tract can be asymptomatic.
- Abnormal liver function test.

Radiology
- May show single or multiple nodules on ultrasound scan or CT scan.
- Areas of necrosis within the tumor appears as cystic lesion.

Gross
- Hepatic metastases are usually discrete and well-demarcated from adjacent liver parenchyma often with a hyperemic rim.
- May be single or multiple, occasionally with infiltrative growth; may mimic either intrahepatic cholangiocarcinoma or HCC.
- Diffusely infiltrative patterns may resemble primary liver tumors.
- Occasionally metastases from the breast, prostate, or stomach can spread through the liver as small punctate lesions simulating cirrhosis.
- Colonic metastases are usually multiple large nodules with marked central umbilication on the surface of the liver.
- Extensive necrosis seen following chemotherapy.
- Metastatic sarcoma shows characteristic "Fish flesh" appearance.
- Hemorrhage is seen in metastatic angiosarcoma, choriocarcinoma or thyroid carcinoma.
- Squamous cell carcinoma firm/white and granular.
- Mucinous carcinoma shows soft, glistening cut surface.
- Melanomas are brown to black.
- Metastatic adenocarcinoma has been reported to grow within bile duct stimulating primary hepatocellular carcinoma.

Microscopy

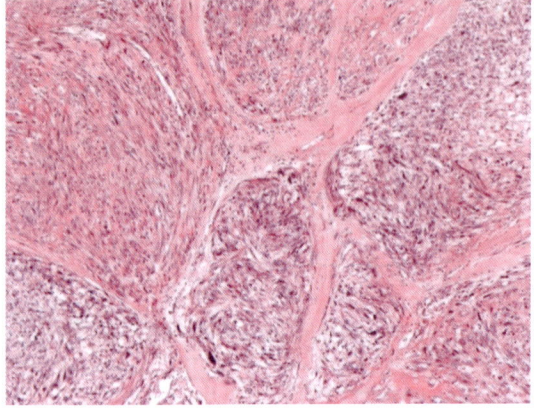

(a)

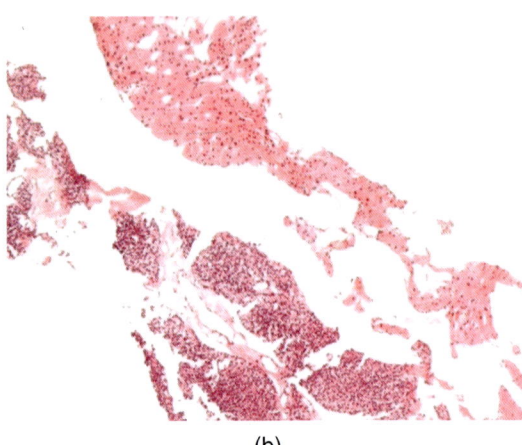

(b)

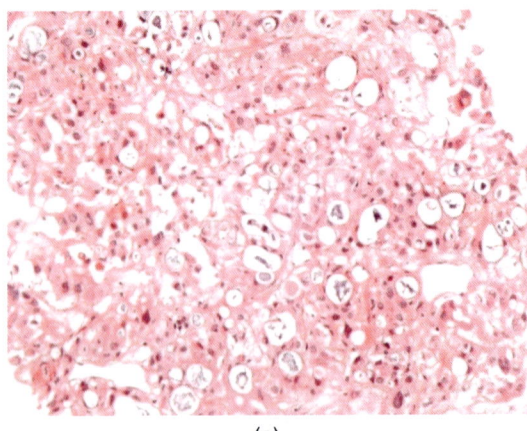

(c)

Fig. 9.14a to c

- *Colon:* Prominent central dirty necrosis in metastatic glandular lumens; mucin production can be abundant and may undergo calcification.
- *Squamous cell carcinoma:* Polygonal cells with abundant eosinophilic cytoplasm with keratin pearls. If basaloid cells predominate think upper aerodigestive tract or anal origin.
- *Lung and breast:* Often medium-sized nodules without necrosis or hemorrhage and with early central umbilication; may be histologically indistinguishable if poorly differentiated.
- *Gallbladder:* Tumor clusters around gallbladder bed and diminish in size with infiltration of hepatic parenchyma.
- *Malignant melanoma:* Large epithelioid or spindled cells with prominent nucleoli with or without pigment.
- *Prostate:* Epithelial cells with prominent nucleoli acinar differentiation may not be conspicuous in some cases.

Immunohistochemistry

Primary	IHC markers
Thyroid	
Papillary/follicular carcinoma	Thyroglobulin + TTF-1+
Thyroid medullary carcinoma	Calcitonin +
Mammary cancer	ER PR HER2/neu (similar to molecular subtype)
Pulmonary	
Small cell carcinoma	TTF 1+ p63 – Synaptophysin + Chromogranin +
Non-small cell carcinoma	TTF 1+ EGFR+ CK7+ CK20– p63 + (squamous)

Upper GI		**Tumors of germ cell and**	
GIST	DOG 1+	**sex cord stromal tumor**	
	CD117+	Seminoma and	PLAP+
	CD34 +	intratubular germ	OCT 4+
	Negative: S-100, actin,	cell neoplasia	NANOG+
	desmin		CD117+
Primary	IHC markers	Embryonal carcinoma	AE1/3+
Lower GI	CK7−		CAM 5.2+
	CK20+		OCT 4+
	CDX2+		NANOG+
	CEA+		SOX 2+
	MUC 2+	Yolk sac tumor	AE 1/3+
	MUC 5 AC −		CAM 5.2+
Pancreaticobiliary	CK7+		NSE+
Pancreatic	CK20+		AFP+
adenocarcinoma	CEA+		CD10+
	CEA 19-9+	Choriocarcinoma	AE 1/3+
	MUC 5AC +		CAM 5.2 +, hCG +
	MUC 2+, CDX2 variable		Inhibin +
Cholangiocarcinoma	CK7+, CK20+	**Prostate**	PSA +
	CEA+		PRAP+
	CK19+	**Melanoma**	HMB45
Urothelial carcinoma	CK7+		Melan A/Mart 1+
	CK20+	**In children**	
	Uroplakin+	Rhabdomyosarcoma	MSA +
	Thrombomodulin +		Desmin +
	p63+		Myogenin + (most
	CK5/6 variable		specific)
	HMW keratin +		Myo D1+
	WT1−, MUC 2−	Wilms' tumor	**Positive stains**
Renal cell carcinoma			1. Blastema—WT 1
Clear cell RCC	Pan CK+		2. Epithelium—WT1, EMA
	CAM 5.2+		3. Stroma—weak WT 1+
	MUC 1 (EMA)+		Negative stains
	CD10+		CK7
	CK 7−		CD57
	CK20−		p53
	AE 1/3+	Neuroblastoma	**Positive stains**
Papillary RCC	AE 1/3+		NSE
	Pan CK+		Synaptophysin
	AMACR+		Chromogranin
	CD10+		CD57
Chromophobe	Pan K+		CD56
	MUC 1+		Alk 1
	CD10−		GFAP
Oncoytoma	Pan K+		**Negative stains**
	CD10 low+		EMA, HMB45, CD99
			CD45, S-100

112 Handbook of Pathology

APPROACH TO HEPATOBILIARY PATHOLOGY

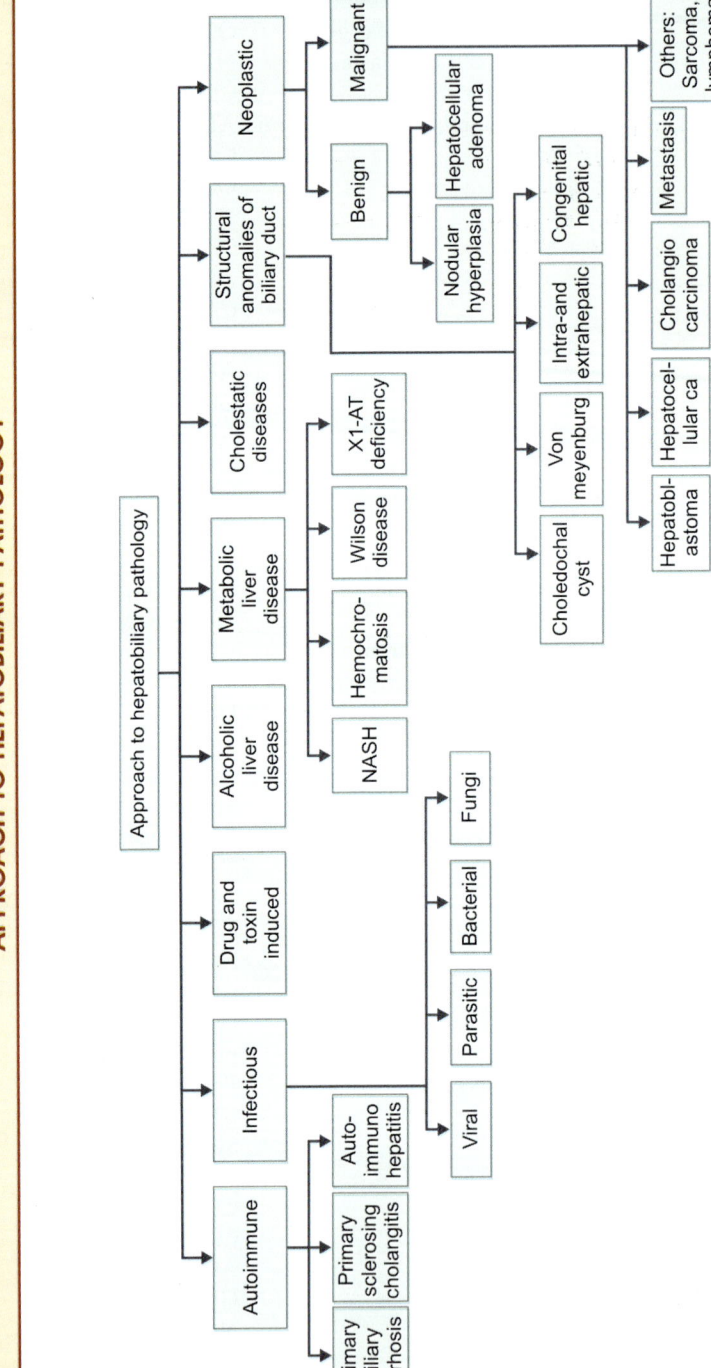

Contributed by Arthi M

CHAPTER

10 Patterns in Pancreatic and Gallbladder Lesions

J Thanka

Case History: A 30-year-old female with gallbladder polyp.

Diagnosis: Adenoma of the gallbladder

Clinical Features
- More common in adults/women.
- Associated with Peutz-Jeghers and Gardner's syndrome.

Gross
- 90% single and well-demarcated.
- Typically 3–25 mm polypoidal, mostly sessile.

Microscopy

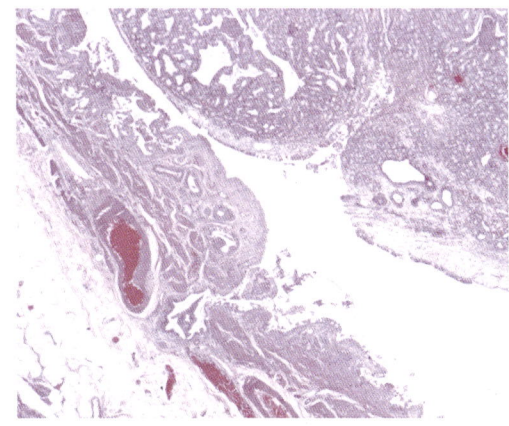

Fig. 10.1

Types based on:
Architecture
a. Tubular b. Papillary c. Tubulopapillary

Cytology
a. Pyloric b. Intestinal c. Biliary

Pyloric type (most common)
Tightly packed tubular glands pyloric or Brunner's gland appearance. Squamoid morule formation is seen.

Intestinal type
Tubular and papillary or both lined by pseudostratified, mucin depleted cells with cigar-shaped nuclei. Associated with high grade dysplasia. Frequency of carcinoma *in situ* is higher.

Biliary type
Complex branching papillae. Lined by cuboidal epithelium.

Immunohistochemistry
- Pyloric type: MUC5AC, MUC6, ER (+)
- Intestinal type: CDX2 (+)

Differential Diagnosis
Invasive adenocarcinoma: Pagetoid Spread of the dysplastic cells into the Rokitansky Aschoff sinus

Case History: A 70-year-old male with calculous cholecystitis.

Diagnosis: Adenocarcinoma gallbladder

Clinical Features
- Age peak—seventh decade, uncommon in patients younger than 50 years.
- More common in females than males. Upper abdominal pain.

- Increased serum alkaline phosphatase levels are the most common findings at presentation.

Gross
- Most common in fundus followed by body and neck.
- Two growth patterns
  1. Diffuse growth.
  2. Polypoidal or papillary mass.

Microscopy

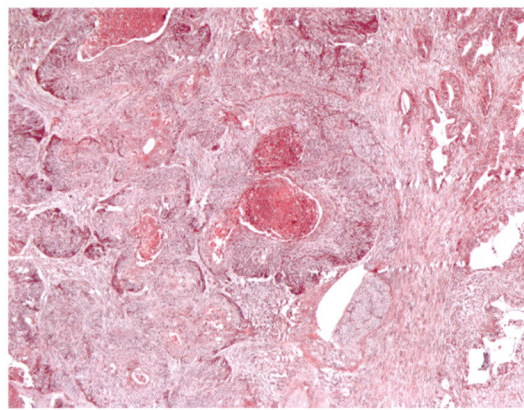

Fig. 10.2

- Infiltrative or exophytic
- Well formed glands in papillary architecture with wide lumina, atypical cuboidal cells, high-grade nuclei.
- May extend to Rokitansky-Aschoff sinuses (but this does not signify deep invasion).
- Superficial portion is often better differentiated than deeper portion.
- May have foci of intestinal differentiation.

Variants
- Intestinal type
- Signet ring cell type
- Mucinous
- Adenosquamous
- Squamous
- Small cell
- Undifferentiated
- Medullary
- Hepatoid
- Clear cell

Immunohistochemistry
- Cytokeratin (+): CK7 most commonly expressed.
- CA19-9, CEA, MUC 1 and epidermal growth factor receptor.

Differential Diagnosis
- Rokitansky-Aschoff sinuses.
- Luschka ducts.

Case History: A 50-year-old male with obstructive jaundice.

Diagnosis: CMV cholangitis

Modes of Transmission
1. Transplacental
2. Blood transfusion
3. Transplant
4. Venereal

Clinical Features
- Abdominal pain
- Cholestasis.

Gross
Diffuse thickening of the wall with luminal narrowing.

Microscopy

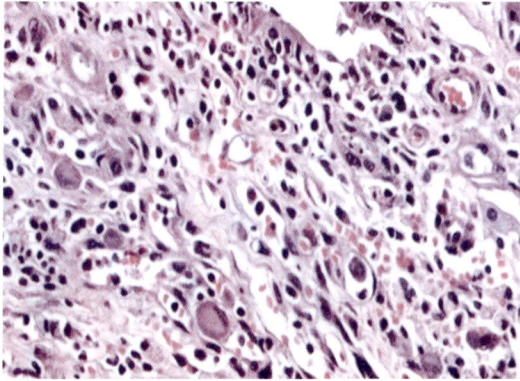

Fig. 10.3

- Diffuse fibrosis and inflammatory infiltrate. Individual cells are large (>2–4 times a normal cell). Intranuclear and intracytoplasmic inclusions.

- Round to oval basophilic intranuclear inclusions with a peripheral halo and marginated chromatin.

Immunohistochemistry
Anti-CMV antibody (+).

Differential Diagnosis
- IgG-4 related disease
- Hodgkin's lymphoma
- Transplant rejection.

Case History: A 47-year-old male with CBD stricture, cholangiocarcinoma.

Diagnosis: Granular cell tumor

Clinical Features
- Age—young to middle age.
- Sex—women (91%)

Gross
- Usually single (83%) but may be multicentric.
- Non-encapsulated. <3 cm, yellow-tan-white.

Microscopy

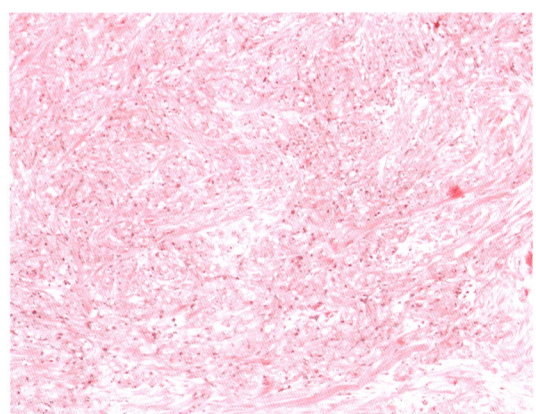

Fig. 10.4

- Large polygonal cells with abundant, eosinophilic, granular cytoplasm.
- Central, small, dark, and uniform nuclei.

Ancillary Tests
- **Histochemistry:** PAS (+) granules.
- **Immunohistochemistry:** S-100 (+), CD68 (+), inhibin alpha (+).
- **Electron microscopy:** Numerous lysosomes/phagosomes and granules.

Case History: A 63-year-old female with pancreatic lesion.

Diagnosis: Mucinous cystic neoplasm

Clinical Features
Common in middle-aged women.

Imaging
Appears as a multilocular cyst on CT images.

Gross
- **Location:** Body and tail.
- **Size:** Can measure up to 36 cm. Irregular lesion with a smooth glistening capsule.
- **C/S:** Shows a multilocular cyst with papillary excrescences. Cyst exudes thick mucoid fluid.

Microscopy

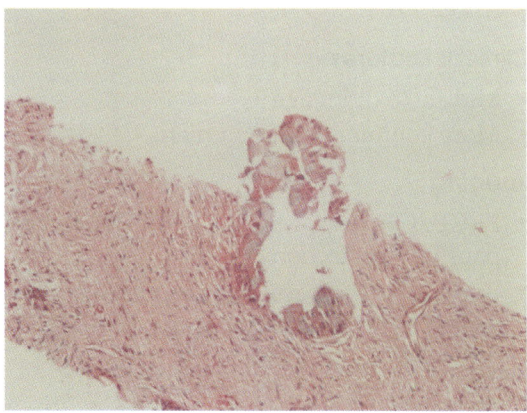

Fig. 10.5

- Cyst lined by non-ciliated silomucin producing columnar cells, goblet cells, absorptive type cells and cuboidal cells.
- There can be focal loss of epithelium and atypia can also be seen.

- Abrupt transitions to papillary formations are common.
- The surrounding stroma is plump and spindled.

Immunohistochemistry

- **Epithelium:** CEA/CA19/MUC5AC/MUC 1/EMA (+)
- **Stroma:** Vimentin/SMA/ER, PR/CD10/ inhibin/calponin (+).

Differential Diagnosis

- **Intraductal pancreatic mucinous neoplasm:** Usually located in the head and communicates with a duct
- **Pancreatic pseudocyst:** No lining epithelium. High amylase, elastase and low CEA levels in the cyst fluid
- **Pancreatic ductal adenocarcinoma:** No lining epithelium. High amylase, elastase and low CEA levels in the cyst fluid
- **Ovarian mucinous tumors.**

Case History: A 54-year-old male with pancreatic head mass.

Diagnosis: Intraductal pancreatic neoplasm with high-grade dysplasia

Clinical Features

- Middle to older age
- More commonly seen in men.

Imaging

- ERCP/CT: It appears as a cystic lesion with papillary projections.
- Bulging of the papillae into the duodenal lumen is a characteristic sign.

Gross

- Dilated principal pancreatic duct, filled with mucus is noted in the head and body of pancreas.
- Irregular, nodular or fungating soft to firm papillary projections are seen on the surface of the lesion.
- Surrounding pancreas is pale and firm due to chronic obstructive pancreatitis.
- Multicystic grape-like clusters ranging from 1–10 cm is seen in the uncinate process if branch ducts are involved.
- Cyst wall is thin and flat or has a papillary lining.
- *Note:* Extensive sampling is required to rule out invasion.

Microscopy

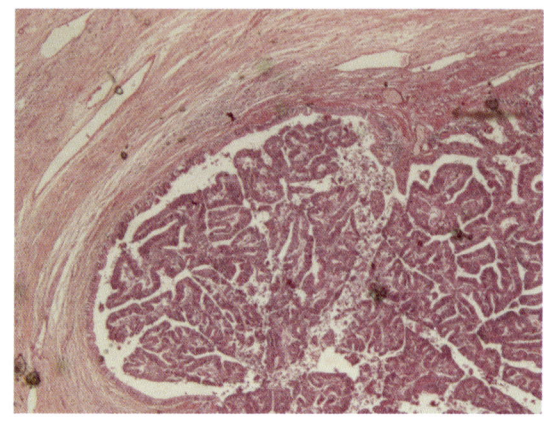

Fig. 10.6

- Complex papillary architecture.
- The papillae are lined by tall columnar cells with clear to eosinophilic cytoplasm/gastric/intestinal/oncocytic/tubulopapillary type of epithelium.
- Adjacent parenchyma shows features of chronic pancreatitis and atrophy.

Immunohistochemistry

- **Pancreaticobiliary type:** MUC 1, 6 (+)/ MUC 2 (–)
- **Gastric type:** MUC 5AC/MUC 6 (+), MUC 2 (–)
- **Intestinal type:** MUC 1 (–), MUC 2 (+), CDX2 (+)
- **Oncocytic type:** MUC 1/MUC 2/MUC 6 (+)

Differential Diagnosis

- Cystic mucinous neoplasm of the pancreas
- Invasive ductal adenocarcinoma
- Chronic pancreatitis

Table 10.1

	Mucinous cystic neoplasm	IPMN
Sex	F > M	M > F
Age	40–50 years	60–70 years
Location	Tail—not in the ducts	Head and body—in the ducts
Gross	Cystic	Cystic with papillae >1 cm
Microscopy	Ovarian stroma (+)	No ovarian stroma

Case History: A 70-year-old female with mass in tail of pancreas.

Diagnosis: Pancreatic microcystic adenoma (synonym—serous cystadenoma)

Imaging

CT shows a honeycombed appearance with a central scar. Incidental finding.

Gross

- Can be found anywhere in the pancreas.
- Size: Around 11 cm
- Partly encapsulated, lobulated lesion.
- C/S: Sponge-like, soft
- Irregular, central calcified scar. Exudes clear watery fluid.

Microscopy

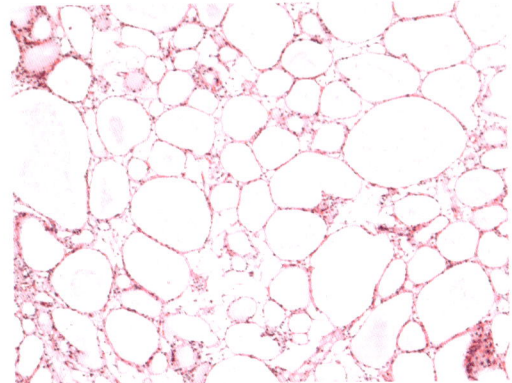

Fig. 10.7

- Small cysts arranged in an honeycomb pattern.
- Large irregular cysts can also be seen.
- Lined by cuboidal cells and surrounded by myoepithelial cells with central round hyperchromatic nuclei.

Ancillary Tests

- **Histochemistry:** PAS (+)
- **IHC:** Keratin/CA19-9/CA15-3/EMA/inhibin/MUC 1, 6 (+)
- **Electron microscopy:** Microvilli seen on the apical surface. Glycogen granules present.

Differential Diagnosis

- **Lymphangioma:** Lymphocytes present. Factor VIII (+)
- **Mucinous cystic neoplasm:** Larger cystic spaces, Mucin (+) CEA (+)
- **Pancreatic pseudocyst**
- **Solid pseudopapillary tumor.**

Case History (a): A 27-year-old female with pancreatic tumor

Case History (b): A 26-year-old female cystic pancreatic tumor.

Diagnosis: Solid pseudopapillary neoplasm

Clinical Features

Exclusively in adolescent girls, young women.

Imaging

- Shows a heterogenous lesion with a little vascularity. No duct dilation.
- Degenerated with blood and cyst formation.

Gross

- Location: Body and tail
- Size: More than 10 cm
- Encapsulated solid and cystic lesion
- C/S: It is soft with hemorrhage and necrosis.

Microscopy

- Predominantly pseudopapillary.
- Others include trabecular, solid, cystic, pseudomicrocystic. Branching pseudopapillae lined by bland fragile epithelium; cells with clear to eosinophilic cytoplasm, oval grooved nuclei, finely stippled chromatin and inconspicuous nuclei.

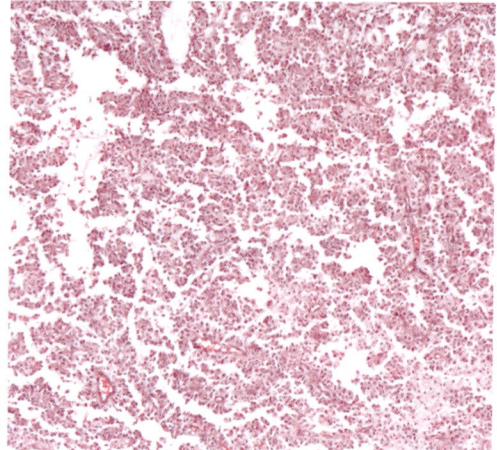

Fig. 10.8

- Foam cells, clusters of lipid or cholesterol crystals surrounded by foreign body giant cells. Intra and extracellular eosinophilic globules are seen. Mitoses are a few in number.

Histochemistry
PAS (+) eosinophilic globules.

Immunohistochemistry
Vimentin/NSE/CD10/PR (+)

Case History (a): A 49-year-old male
Case History (b): A 70-year-old female
Case History (c): A 68-year-old female with pancreatic mass.

Diagnosis: Adenocarcinoma of the pancreas

Clinical Features
- 60–80 years of age.
- Carcinoma of the head presents with painless obstructive jaundice.
- Carcinoma of the body and tail are asymptomatic and present with distant metastasis.
- Thromboembolism is more common.

Gross
- Location: 2/3rds occur in the head and cause duct dilation.
- Size: 2.5–3.5 cm.
- Single or multicentric due to cancerization of the ducts. Rarely mutifocal. Poorly defined pale hard mass.

Microscopy

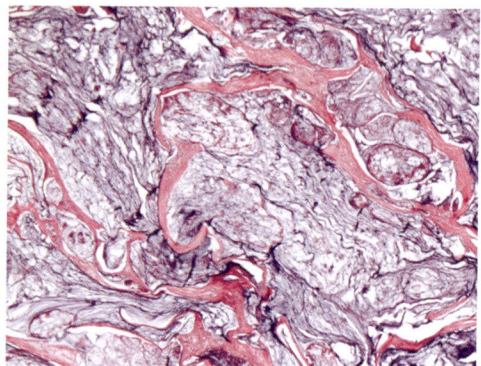

(a) Pancreatic mucinous adenocarcinoma

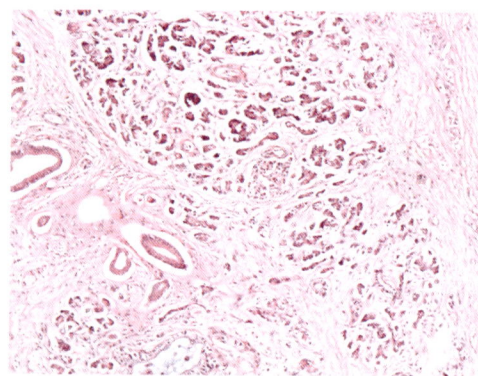

(b) Pancreatic ductal adenocarcinoma

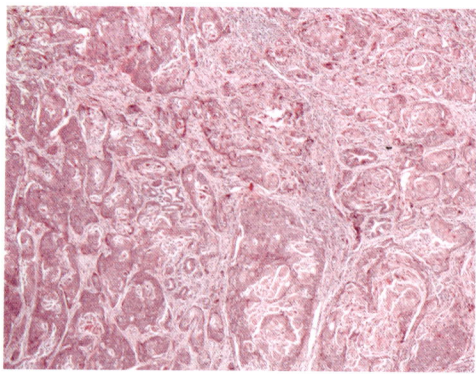

(c) Pancreatic adenosquamous carcinoma

Fig. 10.9a to c

- Individual tubular glands surrounded by stroma.
- Typically good architectural differentiation with marked atypia and extensive desmoplasia.
- Mucin production is specific for ductal origin.
- Normal pancreas may show atrophic changes, chronic inflammatory infiltrate, fibrosis, ductal dilation beyond tumor mass.
- Angiolymphatic invasion in 50%.
- High-grade PanIN in 20%, distal to the main tumor mass or at the margin, low-grade PanIN in 30%.

Variants

Adenosquamous, mucinous, papillary, microglandular, oncocytic, clear cell

- Adenosquamous: Older men. Risk factor: Ionizing radiation K-ras mutation. Carcinoma of head of pancreas. Poor prognosis. IHC-AE1: AE3 (+).
- Mucinous/non-cystic colloid: Older age group. >50–80% is extracellular mucin.
- Better prognosis than usual type IHC-MUC 2/ MUC 5AC (+)

Ancillary Tests

- **Serum tests:** Span 1, CA19-9.
- **Immunohistochemistry:** Mapsin/S-100P/IMP3/MUC 1, 4, 5, 6/CA19.9/CA125/DUPAN2/CK7, 8, 17, 18, 19, HER2/neu (+)

Case History: A 29-year-old female with mass in the tail of pancreas.

Diagnosis: Neuroendocrine tumor of pancreas

Clinical Features

- F > M
- 30–60 years of age
- Associated with MEN.

Two types

1. *Functional:* Symptoms are due to production of hormones.
2. *Non-functional:* Symptoms are due to pressure of the mass.

Types

1. Pancreatic neuroendocrine microadenoma
2. Neuroendocrine tumor (NET)
   - NETG1
   - NETG2
   - Non-functional pancreatic NET G1, G2

Table 10.2

Feature	Well differentiated	Moderately differentiated	Poorly differentiated
Architecture	Haphazard	Haphazard	Haphazard
Desmoplasia	+	++	+++
Glandular formation	+++	+	Cells arranged in solid sheets
Mitosis/10 HPF	<5	6–10	>10

Table 10.3: Differential diagnosis

Features	Chronic pancreatitis	Ductal adenocarcinoma
Gross	Focal segmental or diffuse hard mass with irregular scar	Solitary, hard, poorly demarcated lesion
Architecture	Preserved Fibrosis with chronic inflammatory infiltrate	Infiltrating atypical glands
Cytology	No pleomorphism	Pleomorphism and mitosis
Perineural invasion	–	+
Adjacent mucosa	Atrophy/hyperplasia/metaplasia	Intraepithelial lesion

Table 10.4

Type	Sex	Number	Location	Symptoms	Incidence	Malignancy	IHC
Insulinoma	F	Solitary	Head and tail	Whipple's triad	Common	Males, >2 cm, >2% MIB	Amyloid polypeptide
Gastrinoma	M	Multiple in MEN 1	Head	Zollinger-Ellison syndrome	1/5	+	Gastrin
Glucogonoma	F	Solitary	Tail	Necrotizing migratory erythema DM	10%	+	Pancreatic polypeptide
Somatostatinoma	F	Solitary	Head	Non-specific	Rare	+	Synaptophysin

3. Neuroendocrine carcinoma (NEC)
   - Large cell NEC
   - Small cell NEC
4. EC cell and serotonin producing NET (carcinoid)
5. Gastrinoma
6. Glucagonoma
7. Insulinoma
8. Somatostatinoma
9. VIPoma

Gross

- Size: 1–15 cm (<0.5 cm microadenoma, >2 cm is nonfunctional).
- Solitary, discrete, completely or partially encapsulated.

Microscopy

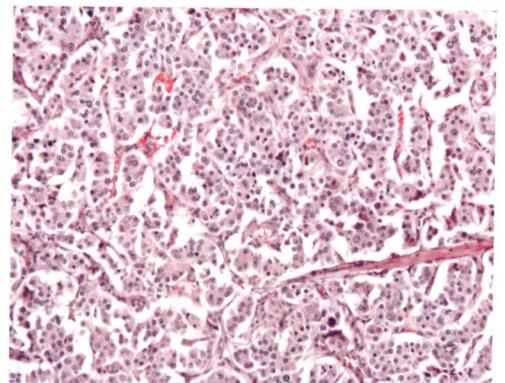

Fig. 10.10

- Patterns: Ribbon/trabercular/festooned/gyriform
- Acinar/duct-like
- Solid/medullary
- Classic features—insulinoma: Ribbon-like arrangement of cells, amyloid deposits
- Somatostatinoma: Psammoma bodies
- Others: VIP/serotonin and ACTH producing tumors.

Ancillary Tests

- **Histochemistry:** PAS (+) extracellular material (α_1-antitrypsin), amyloid and silver staining.
- **Immunohistochemistry:** CEA/NSE/CD56, 57, 8, 18, 19 (+)
- **Electron microscopy:** Dense—core neurosecretory granules.

Grading

Table 10.5

Grading of GEP-NETs	Mitotic index	Ki-67 Li
Grade 1 (G1)	Mitotic count <2 per 10 HPF	≤2
Grade 2 (G2)	Mitotic count 2–20 per HPF	3–20%
Grade 3 (G3)	Mitotic count >20 HPF	>20%

Differential Diagnosis

- **Solid ductal adenocarcinoma**
- **Chronic pancreatitis:** Cases with islet cell hyperplasia resemble pancreatic endocrine neoplasms

- **IPMN:** Small, incidentally identified pancreatic endocrine tumors compress main pancreatic duct and present clinically, radiologically, and grossly as intraductal papillary mucinous neoplasm
- **Pseudoneoplastic islet cell lesions:** Islets aggregate while rest of pancreas atrophies; islets at tail are compact, islets in head are diffuse and may appear infiltrative, usually have trabecular pattern and are pancreatic polypeptide positive; usually no perineurial invasion
- **Solid pseudopapillary neoplasm:** Clear cytoplasmic vacuoles on cytology, alpha1-antitrypsin+, vimentin+, CD10+, PR+, nuclear staining for beta-catenin

Case History: A 5-month-old baby with repeated hypoglycemic attacks.

Diagnosis: Nesidioblastosis congenital hyperinsulinism of infancy

Types
- Focal
- Diffuse

Clinical Presentation
- Repeated attacks of hypoglycemia in the neonatal period, drowsy, sometimes leading to seizures.
- Rarely present in adult hyperglycemia associated with Zollinger-Ellison syndrome.

Gross
Gross of the pancreas appears normal.

Microscopy

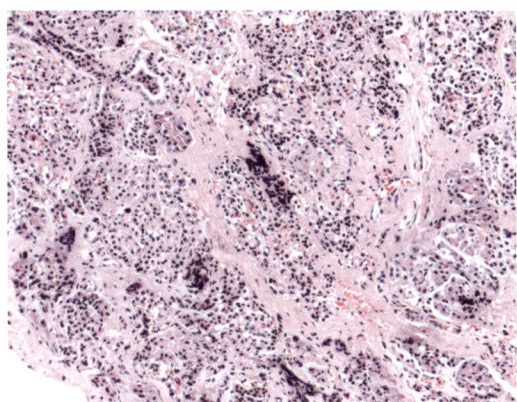

Fig. 10.11

- Ductoendocrine proliferation, numerous small and large endocrine areas.
- Islands of islet cells interspersed among exocrine glands.
- Hypertrophied islet cells show nuclear enlargement with presence of giant bizarre nuclei.

Criteria for Diagnosis
- Exclusion of insulinoma by macroscopic, microscopic and immunohistochemical examination.
- Multiple β cells with an enlarged and hyperchromatic nucleus and abundant clear cytoplasm.
- Islets with normal spatial distribution of the various cell types.
- No proliferative activity of endocrine cells.

Immunohistochemistry
Positive for synaptophysin and chromogranin.

APPROACH TO PANCREATIC PATHOLOGY

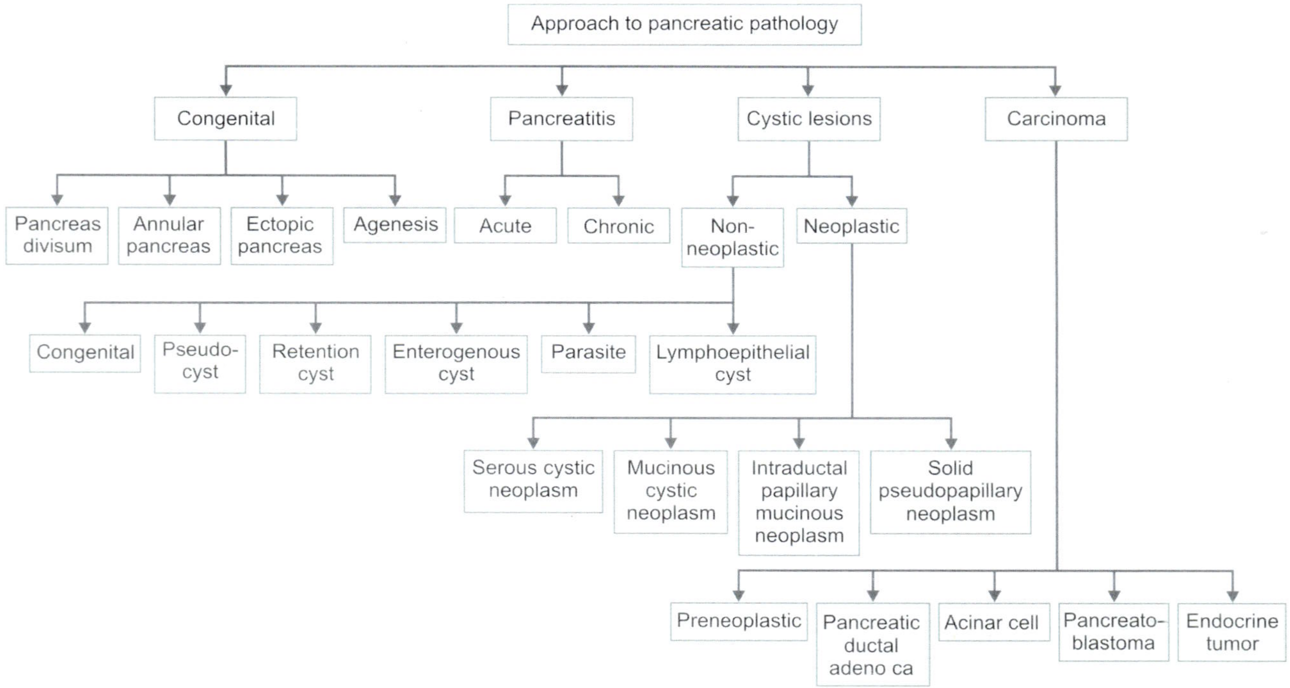

Contributed by Arthi M

Approach to pancreatic pathology

- Congenital
  - Pancreas divisum
  - Annular pancreas
  - Ectopic pancreas
  - Agenesis
- Pancreatitis
  - Acute
  - Chronic
- Cystic lesions
  - Non-neoplastic
    - Congenital
    - Pseudo-cyst
    - Retention cyst
    - Enterogenous cyst
    - Parasite
    - Lymphoepithelial cyst
  - Neoplastic
    - Serous cystic neoplasm
    - Mucinous cystic neoplasm
    - Intraductal papillary mucinous neoplasm
    - Solid pseudopapillary neoplasm
- Carcinoma
  - Preneoplastic
  - Pancreatic ductal adeno ca
  - Acinar cell
  - Pancreato-blastoma
  - Endocrine tumor

CHAPTER 11

Medical Renal Disease

Anila Abraham Kurian, Barathi G

Case History: A 47-year-old male.

Indication for biopsy: Renal failure:
- S. electrophoresis—distinct band in gamma region
- S. creatinine—5.5 mg/dl
- Proteinuria—1+

Diagnosis: Cast nephropathy

Definition
- Disorder in which monoclonal urinary immunoglobulin light chains (Bence Jones proteins) lead to acute or chronic renal failure.
- Cast nephropathy can occur as the first manifestation of multiple myeloma or can develop later during the course of myeloma.

Clinical Features
Renal failure

Gross
No specific gross features.

Microscopy
- Glomerular and vascular compartments—normal.
- Tubular casts are usually seen in distal nephron, mainly collecting ducts.
- May be seen in proximal tubule as a result of retrograde filling.

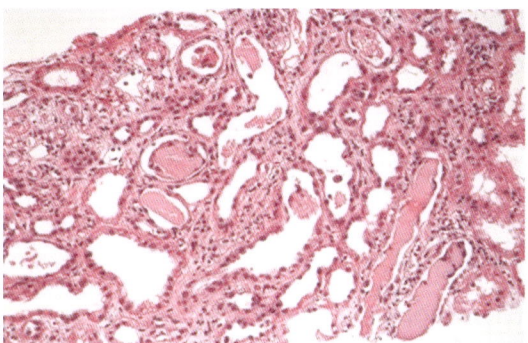

Fig. 11.1

- Casts are variably eosinophilic with irregular, angulated, geometric shapes and fracture planes.
- Multinucleated giant cells may be seen surrounding the casts.

Ancillary Tests
- **Special stains:** Some casts are congophilic.
- **Immunofluorescence microscopy:** Only when the casts are acutely formed, monotypic light chain staining is seen.
- **Electron microscopy:** Fibrillary material admixed with cellular debris. Granular electron dense material and occasionally crystalline structures may be seen.

Differential Diagnosis
Rifampicin-induced light chain proteinuria.

Case History: A 58-year-old male known hypertensive, not a diabetic.

Indication for biopsy: Nephrotic syndrome
- S. creatinine—0.8 mg/dl
- Proteinuria—4+
- Urine PCR—4.5

Diagnosis: Primary membranous nephropathy

Definition
Membranous nephropathy is a pathologic diagnosis defined by the presence of subepithelial immune deposits that induce a spectrum of changes in the glomerular basement membrane.

Clinical Features
- Nephrotic syndrome. Have normal renal function and normal BP.
- Microscopic hematuria occurs in 50%.

Gross
No specific gross features.

Microscopy

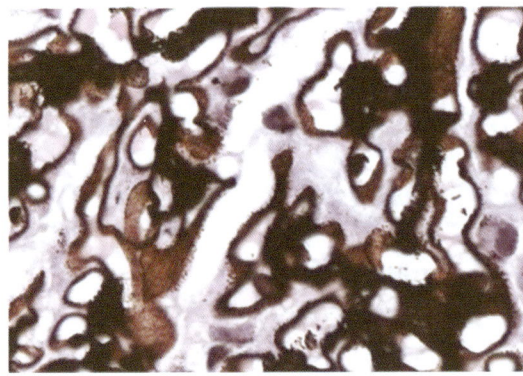

Fig. 11.2

- The pathology of primary and secondary forms is often similar or even identical. Glomeruli: Normocellular. Glomerular capillary wall thickening.
Proximal tubule: Lipid and protein resorption droplets.
Degree of interstitial fibrosis and tubular atrophy are important prognostic markers.

Ancillary Tests
- **Special stains:** PAS and silver stains: Glomerular basement membrane spikes, internal vacuolizations. Trichrome—subepithelial fuchsinophilic deposits.
- **Immunofluorescence microscopy:** Granular global subepithelial deposits that stain strong for IgG. C3 staining present but less intense.
- **Electron microscopy:** Hallmark—subepithelial electron dense deposits.

Differential Diagnosis
Secondary forms of membranous nephropathy.

Case History: A 45-year-old female with BP 140/90 mmHg, not a diabetic.

Indication for biopsy: Rapidly progressive renal failure:
- S. creatinine—6 mg/dl
- Proteinuria—3+
- Urine RBC—20–25/HPF

Diagnosis: Crescentic glomerulonephritis: Antiglomerular basement membrane disease

Classification of Crescentic Glomerulonephritis
- Pauci-immune crescentic glomerulonephritis
- Immune complex associated crescentic glomerulonephritis.
- Anti-GBM associated crescentic glomerulonephritis.

Clinical Features
Present with rapidly progressive glomerulonephritis, hematuria and proteinuria in the non-nephrotic range.

Gross
Numerous petechial spots.

Microscopy
- Presence of glomerular crescents. Earliest glomerular lesion is focal and segmental necrotizing glomerulonephritis. Neutrophilic infiltrate is seen at the site of necrosis.

Medical Renal Disease

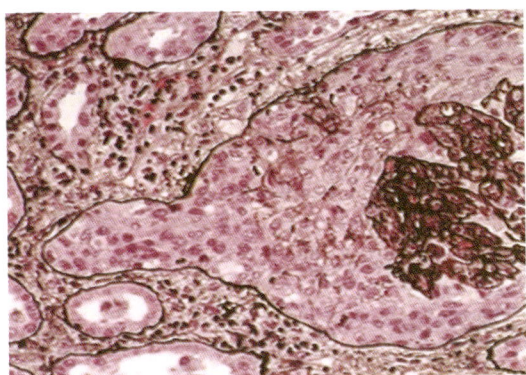

Fig. 11.3

- Glomerular capillaries and mesangium are normocellular. With time, the cellular crescents evolve from cellular to fibrocellular then into fibrous crescents.
- Tubules: Red cells, red cell casts and pigment casts. Epithelial cell injury.
- No significant vascular pathology.

Ancillary Tests

- **Special stains:** PAS and methenamine silver: Highlights the areas of segmental necrosis and the breaks in GBM and Bowman's capsule.
- **Immunofluorescence microscopy:** The diagnostic feature—marked diffuse, global, linear staining for IgG and C3 less intense granular or discontinuous linear staining.
- **Electron microscopy:** No ultrastructural diagnostic features.

Differential Diagnosis

ANCA-associated glomerulonephritis.

Case History: A 35-year-old female with H/O fever 2 weeks back and hematuria.

Indication for biopsy: Renal failure/proteinuria
- S. creatinine—2.6 mg/dl
- Proteinuria—3+
- Urine PCR—0.6
- Urine RBC—30–40/HPF

Diagnosis: Infection related glomerulonephritis

Clinical Features

Acute renal failure with microscopic hematuria and proteinuria.

Gross

Kidney is enlarged and may have flea-bitten appearance.

Microscopy

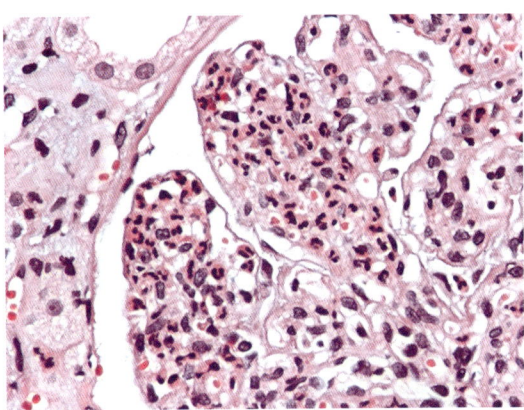

Fig. 11.4

- Diffuse and global enlargement of glomeruli.
- Glomerular tufts: Hypercellular.
- Hypercellularity: Increased number of mesangial cells and proliferation of the capillary endothelial cells and filling of the capillary lumen by leukocytes.
- Capillary lumen is obscured. Late microscopic finding; mesangial hypercellularity, some degree of mesangial matrix expansion.

Ancillary Tests

- **Special stains:** PAS or methenamine silver stain, 'endocapillary' hypercellularity—best appreciated.
- **Trichrome stain:** Subepithelial fuchsinophilic (red) deposits.

- **Immunofluorescence microscopy:** IgG and C3—coarse granular, 'lumpy bumpy' staining of glomerular capillary loops.
- **Electron microscopy:** Subepithelial, variably electron dense 'hump-like' deposits along the peripheral and paramesangial regions of glomerular capillary loops.

Differential Diagnosis

- MPGN
- Dense deposit disease
- Cryoglobulinemic glomerulonephritis
- Lupus nephritis.

Case History: A 51-year-old male with hypertension for 2 years, diabetes for 6 years.

Indication for biopsy: Nephrotic syndrome.
- S. creatinine—1.5 mg/dl
- Proteinuria—4+
- Urine PCR—2.5

Diagnosis: Diabetic nephropathy

Clinical Features

Proteinuria, nephrotic syndrome and progressive renal failure.

Gross

Early stage kidneys are enlarged. As the disease progresses, size decreases and surface becomes finely granular.

Microscopy

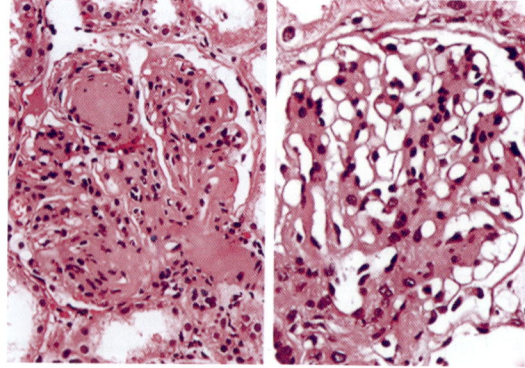

Fig. 11.5

- Affects all 4 compartments
- It has 2 forms: Diffuse and nodular
- Thickening of glomerular basement membrane.
- Mesangial matrix accumulation may show diffuse or nodular pattern mesangial nodules (Kimmelstiel-Wilson nodules).
- Capsular drop
- Fibrin cap
- Tubular basement membrane thickening
- Tubular atrophy and interstitial fibrosis
- Armanni-Ebstein change (very rare)
- Afferent and efferent arteriolar hyalinosis
- Arteriosclerosis

Mesangial Nodules—Kimmelstiel-Wilson Nodules

- Variation in the size of nodules—typical
- Eosinophilic, strongly PAS positive and dark-blue with Masson's trichrome. Congo red negative.

Ancillary Tests

- Immunofluorescence microscopy
- Linear positivity along the glomerular capillary walls and tubular basement membranes is common with IgG and albumin.
- Electron microscopy—earliest change: Increase in thickness of glomerular basement membrane.

Differential Diagnosis

For nodular diabetic glomerulosclerosis:

- Light chain deposition disease (LCCD)/ heavy chain deposition disease (HCDD)/ light and heavy chain deposition disease (LHCDD)
- Amyloidosis
- Membranoproliferative glomerulonephritis
- Fibrillary glomerulonephritis
- Immunotactoid glomerulonephritis
- Collagenofibrotic glomerulopathy
- Fibronectin glomerulopathy
- Idiopathic nodular glomerulosclerosis

Case History: A 65-year-old female, not a diabetic or hypertensive.

Indication for biopsy:
- S. creatinine—0.8 mg/dl
- Proteinuria—3+; PCR: 6

Diagnosis: Amyloidosis

Clinical Features
Proteinuria, nephrotic syndrome and progressive renal failure.

Gross
Kidneys are enlarged.

Microscopy
Amorphous eosinophilic material in the glomeruli, interstitium and vessel wall. Amyloid—first noted in the mesangium and then extends to peripheral capillary walls.

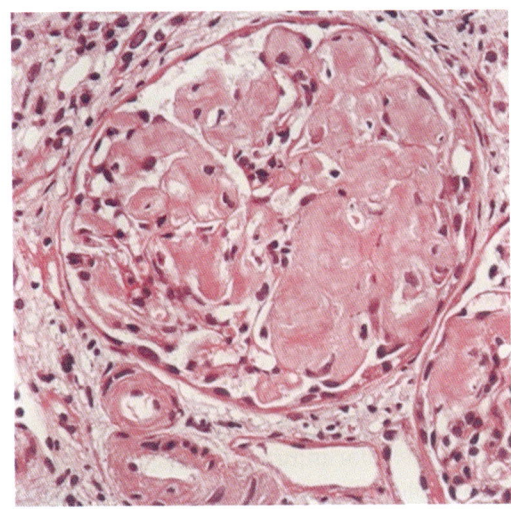

Fig. 11.6

Ancillary Tests
- **Special stains:** Weakly PAS positive, blue with trichrome and negative for silver stain.
- **Congo red stain:** Salmon pink on bright field and apple green birefringence on polarization using immunofluorescence microscopy.
- **Immunohistochemistry:** To identify precursor protein and characterize the type of amyloid present.
- **Electron microscopy:** Randomly dispersed non-branching fibrils of 8–10 nm diameter.

Differential Diagnosis
- Early amyloidosis *vs* minimal change glomerulopathy.
- Other glomerulopathies with mesangial nodularity (*see* DDs for diabetic nephropathy).

Case History: A 40-year-old female, not a diabetic or hypertensive, history of backache for 10 days, on NSAIDs.

Indication for biopsy: Unexplained renal failure
- S. creatinine—1.8 mg/dl
- Proteinuria—nil

Diagnosis: Acute tubular injury

Definition
Acute deterioration of renal function associated with tubular epithelial cell injury.

Clinical Feature
Oliguria, elevated serum creatinine, blood urea nitrogen and serum potassium levels.

Gross
Kidneys—enlarged. Cut surface: Pale, turgid cortex and congested medulla.

Microscopy

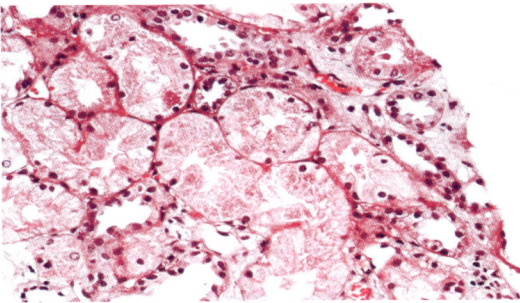

Fig. 11.7

- Tubules: Single epithelial cell necrosis, apoptosis and segmental coagulative necrosis of tubules.

- Injured epithelial cells loose adhesion for the tubular basement membranes, accumulate in lumen as necrotic cellular casts.
- Tubules may have dystrophic calcium deposits.
- Evidence of epithelial regeneration present.
- Interstitium—mild edema with sparse mononuclear cells and neutrophilic infiltrates.

Ancillary Tests
- **Special stains:** PAS—diminished or absent brush border.
- **Immunofluorescence and electron microscopy:** Non-specific.

Differential Diagnosis
Tubular autolysis

Case History: A 43-year-old male, hypertensive—3 years, on irregular treatment, not a diabetic.

Indication for biopsy
- S. creatinine—3.2 mg/dl
- Proteinuria—2+

Diagnosis: Hypertensive arterionephrosclerosis

Clinical Features
Asymptomatic: Advanced stages may present with progressive renal failure.

Gross
Cortex thinned out, has a granular subcapsular surface.

Microscopy

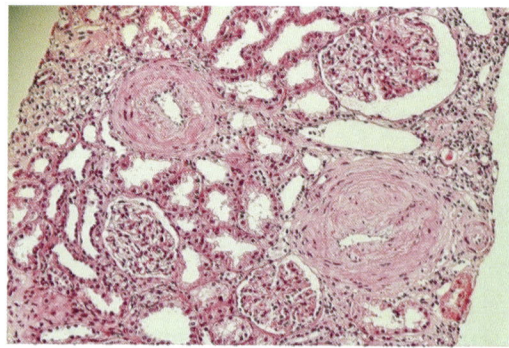

Fig. 11.8

- Glomeruli: May be normal or may show ischemic changes with retracted capillary loops and wrinkled basement membranes.
- Tubules: Atropic and contain hyaline casts.
- Interstitium: It is widened in areas of atrophic tubules.
- Blood vessels: Changes vary with the size of the vessel involved.
- Hyalinosis: Hyaline glassy eosinophilic staining, slightly PAS positive, blue with Masson's trichrome and unstained with silver.
- Arcuate and interlobular arteries: Intimal fibrosis. Internal elastic lamina is reduplicated. Mild intimal fibrosis—media thickened. Advanced intimal fibrosis—media focally has reduced number of smooth muscle cells that are replaced by fibrous tissue.

Ancillary Tests
- **Immunofluorescence microscopy:** IgM, C3 may show non-specific changes.
- **Electron microscopy:** Non-contributory.

Changes seen in Malignant Hypertension
- Segmental fibrinoid necrosis of the glomerular capillary tuft.
- Thrombotic microangiopathy: Dilated capillaries filled with fibrin thrombi in acute form and subendothelial widening and double contours in chronic form.
- Acute tubular injury.
- Fibrinoid necrosis of afferent arterioles.
- 'Onion skin' thickening of small arterioles (thickening of intima with mucoid matrix and widely spaced concentrically arranged cells).

Case History: A 22-year-old female; fever for 1 month, on NSAIDs, acute renal failure.

Indication for biopsy:
- S. creatinine—2.3 mg/dl
- Proteinuria—1+

Diagnosis: Granulomatous tubulointerstitial nephritis

Definition
Presence of clustered epithelioid macrophages in the interstitium.

Clinical Features
Progressive renal failure

Gross
Diffuse enlargement of the kidney. Cut surface—visible nodules.

Microscopy

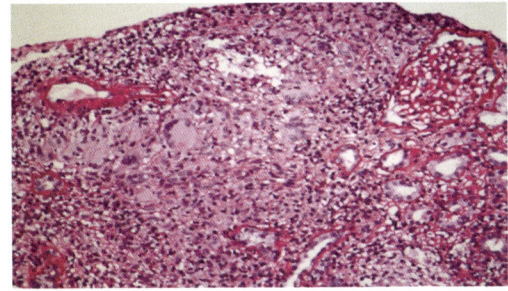

Fig. 11.9

- A few focal clusters (variable) of epithelioid macrophages and large confluent masses.
- Tubular epithelial injury, tubulitis. Glomeruli and blood vessel—unremarkable.

Ancillary Tests
- **Immunofluorescence microscopy:** Non-specific
- **Electron microscopy:** May help to identify the infectious microorganism.

Differential Diagnosis
- **Infections:** Tuberculosis, fungal
- **Sarcoidosis:** Well-formed, discrete and non-necrotizing granuloma with numerous giant cells.
- **Drug-induced granulomas:** Poorly formed.
- **Malakoplakia:** Michaelis-Gutmann bodies (PAS).

Case History: A 30-year-old female; indication for biopsy: SLE, developed hypertension and proteinuria. Urine RBC: Plenty.

Indication for biopsy:
- S. creatinine—1.8 mg/dl
- Proteinuria—3+
- Serology—ANA+, anti-dsDNA +, C3, C4 – low.

Diagnosis: Diffuse lupus nephritis (lupus nephritis, class IV)

Definition
Active/chronic endocapillary and extracapillary glomerulonephritis involving >50% of all glomeruli sampled, typically with subendothelial immune deposits, and usually with mesangial alterations.

Clinical Features
Hypertension, proteinuria and renal insufficiency in >50% of cases.

Microscopy

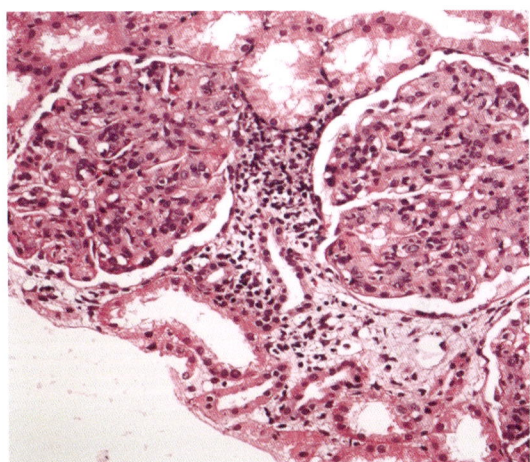

Fig. 11.10

- Diffuse proliferative lupus nephritis—endocapillary and mesangial proliferation with leukocytic infiltration, wireloops and hyaline thrombi, necrotizing lesions and crescents in varying combinations. Chronic proliferative lesions progress to segmental or global glomerulosclerosis.
- IV (A)—purely active lesions
- IV (C)—purely chronic lesions
- IV (A/C)—mixed features
- Lupus related vascular disease is more common in class IV than in other classes.

Ancillary Tests

- **Immunofluorescence microscopy:** Immune deposits can be detected in all renal compartments, glomeruli, tubules, interstitium and blood vessels. Staining pattern is usually 'full-house' when deposits containing all 3 immunoglobulin classes (IgG, IgM, IgA), both complement components (C3, C1q), and both light chains (kappa, lambda) are present. Location of the immune deposits varies with the class of the disease. In lupus nephritic class IV, deposits are identified as subendothelial peripheral capillary wall and mesangial in location.
- **Electron microscopy:** Diffuse segmental or global subendothelial peripheral capillary wall and mesangial electron dense deposits.

Differential Diagnosis

- MPGN
- Infection related glomerulonephritis.

Case History: A 22-year-old male with nephrotic syndrome.

Indication for biopsy: Facial puffiness and pedal edema:
- Proteinuria—3+
- Urine RBC—2–3/HPF

Diagnosis: Focal segmental glomerulosclerosis (FSGS)

Definition

- Refers to a pattern of glomerular scarring that affects a subset of glomerular (i.e. focal), and involves only a portion of the glomerular tuft (i.e. segmental).
- It can be primary or secondary.
- Secondary's FSGS may be genetic, virus associated, drug-induced or adaptive.

Gross

- Kidneys are enlarged and swollen.
- In cases where FSGS has progressed to ESRD, the kidneys show bilateral symmetric shrinkage.

Light Microscopy

- Segmental solidification of the glomerular capillary tuft by an acellular matrix that is eosinophilic, PAS reactive and argyrophilic.
- May be accompanied by hyalinosis and adhesion to Bowman's capsule.
- Juxtamedullary glomeruli are more vulnerable due to greater single nephron GFR and higher glomerular capillary pressures and flow rates.
- Visceral epithelial cell hyperplasia leads onto the formation of a single-layered cobble stone appearance overlying the segmental sclerosis lesion.

Ancillary Tests

- **Immunofluorescence study:** There is often segmental glomerular staining for IgM and C3 (consistent with non-specific trapping in areas of sclerosis)
- **Electron microscopy:** Podocyte foot process effacement overlying areas of segmental sclerosis and in more than 50% of the capillary surface area in the non-sclerotic glomeruli. The mean foot process effacement is significantly greater in primary FSGS compared to MCD and secondary FSGS.

Morphologic Variants of FSGS

1. Collapsing variant
2. Tip variant
3. Cellular variant
4. Perihilar
5. NOS

Differential Diagnosis

Post-inflammatory scarring from immune complex-mediated glomerulonephritis and pauci-immune glomerulonephritis.

Case History: A 2-year-old male child with nephrotic syndrome.

Indication for biopsy: Facial puffiness and pedal edema
- Proteinuria—4+

Diagnosis: Minimal change disease (MCD)

Definition
It is characterized clinically by nephrotic syndrome and pathologically by minimal or no glomerular alternations by light microscopy, absence of glomerular immune deposits by IF and the presence of foot process effacement by EM.

Laboratory Findings
Highly selective proteinuria.

Gross
- Both the kidneys are enlarged
- C/s swollen, edematous

Light Microscopy
- Minimal or no glomerular abnormality
- Tubular epithelial cells may show clear vacuoles.

Ancillary Tests
- **Immunofluorescence:** No immunoglobulins or complement staining seen.
- **Electron microscopy:** Extensive foot process effacement seen.

Differential Diagnosis
Unsampled FSGS.

ACUTE TUBULOINTERSTITIAL NEPHRITIS (TIN)
Gross Pathology
- External surface is smooth
- Kidneys are pale, edematous and enlarged with the degree of enlargement proportional to the extent of involvement.

Light Microscopy
- The cellular infiltration and edema in the interstitium are multifocal and vary in intensity.
- Although neutrophils are common in acute TIN, mononuclear cells, including lymphocytes and macrophages, are also seen and are usually the predominant cell types.
- Drug reactions are frequently, though not always, associated with eosinophilic infiltration.
- Tubular injury includes tubulitis, tubular basement membrane breaks, necrosis of tubular cells and later atrophy and loss of tubules, depending on the stage of the disease.

Ancillary Tests
- **Immunofluorescence study:** Helps in the determination of underlying etiology (in cases of secondary TIN).
- **Electron microscopy:** Limited value.

IgA NEPHROPATHY
Introduction
It is the most common form of primary glomerulonephritis in the world.

Clinical Features
Most common presentation in children is macroscopic hematuria and in adults asymptomatic urinary abnormalities.

Gross Pathology
In most patients, kidneys appear normal grossly.

Light Microscopy
- Mesangial hypercellularity may be mild, moderate or marked, more often segmental.
- Endocapillary proliferation—usually focal and segmental.
- Crescents usually focal and non-circumferential.
- Tubulointerstitial scarring can be seen at any stage of IgA nephropathy.

Ancillary Tests
- **Immunofluorescence:** Dominant or co-dominant IgA staining in the mesangium.
- **Electron microscopy:** Granular electron dense immune deposits in the mesangium.

Differential Diagnosis
- Extrarenal and renal hematuric disease.
- Prodigious amounts of IgA may deposit in *Staphylococcus* associated IRGN. These cases

are characterized by positive culture, hypocomplimentemia and subepithelial humps.

The Oxford Classification and its Clinical Applicability (MEST SCORE)

- M0 or M1, indicating mesangial hypercellularity in <50% versus >50% of glomeruli.
- E0 or E1, indicating endocapillary hypercellularity in zero versus one or more glomeruli.
- S0 or S1, indicating segmental sclerosis in zero versus one or more glomeruli.
- T0, T1 or T2 indicating IFTA in <25%, 26 to 55% or >50% of renal cortex, respectively.
- C0, C1 or C2 indicating no crescents, crescents in less than one-fourth of the glomeruli and crescents in more than one-fourth of the glomeruli.

ATHEROEMBOLIC RENAL DISEASE (AERD)

Definition

AERD is defined as renal failure occurring secondary to renal artery, arterioles or glomerular capillary occlusion by atheromatous plaque dislodged from major arteries. It may occur spontaneously or after invasive vascular procedures.

Clinical Features

The classic triad of a precipitating factor, skin lesions and renal failure is highly suggestive of AERD.

Laboratory Findings

C3 hypocomplementemia, eosinophilia, increased C-reactive protein and elevated ESR.

Light Microscopy

- Needle shapes, biconvex clefts are seen in the arcuate and interlobular arteries, as the lipids are dissolved during fixation.
- Surrounding the cleft-like spaces, foreign body type giant cells may be seen.
- Cholesterol emboli rarely lodge in the afferent arteriole and in the glomeruli.
- Eosinophilic and neutrophilic infiltration is seen initially. This is followed by mononuclear cell accumulation in the interstitium.

Ancillary Tests

Immunofluorescence study and electron microscopy: Noncontributory.

International Society of Nephrology/Renal Pathology Society (ISN/RPS) 2003 and Classification of Lupus Nephritis

Class I: Minimal mesangial lupus nephritis—normal glomeruli by light microscopy, but mesangial immune deposits by immunofluorescence.

Class II: Mesangial proliferative lupus nephritis—purely mesangial hypercellularity of any degree or mesangial matrix expansion by light microscope, with mesangial immune deposits.

A few isolated subepithelial or subendothelial deposits may be visible by immunofluorescence or electron microscopy, but not by light microscopy.

Class III: Focal lupus nephritis—active or inactive focal, segmental or global endo- or extracapillary glomerulonephritis involving <50% of all glomeruli, typically with focal subendothelial immune deposits with or without mesangial alterations.

Class III (A): Active lesions; focal proliferative lupus nephritis.

Class III (A/C): Active and chronic lesions; focal proliferative and sclerosing lupus nephritis.

Class III (C): Chronic inactive lesions with glomerular scars: Focal sclerosing lupus nephritis.

Class IV: Diffuse lupus nephritis—active or inactive diffuse, segmental or global endo- or extracapillary glomerulonephiritis involving ≥50% of all glomeruli, typically with diffuse subendothelial immune deposits, with or without mesangial alterations. This class is divided into diffuse segmental (IV-G) lupus nephritis when 50% of the involved glomeruli have global lesions. Segmental is defined as a glomerular lesion that involves less than half of the glomerular tuft. This class includes cases with diffuse wireloop deposits but with a little or no glomerular proliferation.

Class IV-S (A): Active lesions; diffuse segmental proliferative lupus nephritis.

Class IV-G (A): Active lesions; diffuse global proliferative lupus nephritis.

Class IV-S (A/C): Active and chronic lesions; diffuse segmental proliferative and sclerosing lupus nephritis.

Class IV-G (A/C): Active and chronic lesions; diffuse global proliferative and sclerosing lupus nephritis.

Class IV-S (C): Chronic inactive lesions with scars; diffuse segmental sclerosing lupus nephritis.

Class IV-G (C): Chronic inactive lesions with scars; diffuse global sclerosing lupus nephritis.

Class V: Membranous lupus nephritis: Global or segmental subepithelial immune deposits or their morphologic sequelae by light microscopy and by immunofluorescence or electron microscopy; with or without mesangial alterations class V lupus nephritis may occur in combination with class III or IV in which case both will be diagnosed class V lupus nephritis may show advanced sclerosis.

Class VI: Advanced sclerosing lupus nephritis—≥90% of glomeruli globally sclerosed without residual activity.

Indicate and grade (mild 25%, moderate 25 to 50%, severe >50%) tubular atrophy, interstitial inflammation and fibrosis, severity of arteriosclerosis or other vascular lesions.

a. Indicate the proportion of glomeruli with active and with sclerotic lesions.

b. Indicate the proportion of glomeruli with fibrinoid necrosis and/or cellular crescents.

References

1. Heptinstall's Pathology of the Kidney, seventh edition.
2. Silva's Diagnostic Renal Pathology, second edition.

Activity and chronicity index	
	Score
Index of activity	**(0–24)**
Endocapillary hypercellularity	(0–3+)
Neutrophil infiltration/karyorrhexis	(0–3+)
Subendothelial hyaline deposits	(0–3+)
Fibrinoid necrosis	(0–3+) × 2
Cellular crescents	(0–3+) × 2
Interstitial inflammation	(0–3+)
Index of chronicity	**(0–12)**
Glomerular sclerosis	(0–3+)
Fibrous crescents	(0–3+)
Tubular atrophy	(0–3+)
Interstitial fibrosis	(0–3+)

CHAPTER 12

Pathologic Lesions of Kidneys, Urethra and Urinary Bladder

Sandhya Sundaram

Case History: A 7-year-old boy with mass abdomen.

Diagnosis: Wilms' tumor

Clinical Features

- Abdominal mass and abdominal pain
- Hematuria, hypertension
- Acute abdominal crisis (secondary to traumatic rupture)

Gross

- Solitary, rounded, multinodular masses sharply demarcated from the adjacent renal parenchyma by a peritumoral fibrous pseudocapsule.
- Pretreated cases: Areas of necrosis seen

Microscopy

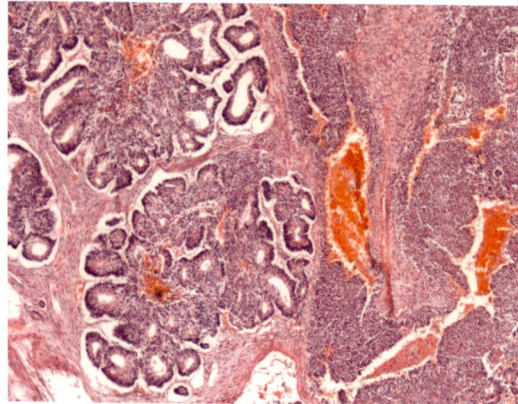

Fig. 12.1

Triphasic/biphasic/monophasic lesions

- *Blastemal cells:* Small, closely packed, mitotically active, rounded or oval cells with scant cytoplasm. Nuclei are overlapping, evenly distributed, slightly coarse chromatin and small nucleoli.
- *Epithelial component:* Tubular/glomerular differentiation.
- Heterologous epithelial elements—mucinous, squamous and neuroepithelial.
- *Stromal component:* Fibroblast like stroma, skeletal muscle, adipose tissue, cartilage, bone, ganglion cells and neuroglial tissue. Any one component >2/3rds categorised accordingly, e.g. epithelial predominant.
- Prognosis depends on presence/absence of anaplasia whether diffuse/focal (refer criteria)

Immunohistochemistry

Blastema: WT1, desmin, focal vimentin
Epithelium: WT1, keratin and EMA
Stroma: Weak WT1, according to histology

Genetics

- WT1 gene on chromosome 11p13. WT2 (11p15.5)
- TP53 related with anaplasia

Staging

- Children Oncology Group (COG)
- International Society of Paediatric Oncology (SIOP)

Anaplasia
Focal or diffuse

Differential Diagnosis
- **Mesoblastic nephroma**—congenital, mesenchyme predominant
- **Multicystic nephroma**—older, predominantly cystic, with hobnailing of cells, benign? Diff Wilms
- **Pediatric RCC**
- **Nephroblastomatosis**—diffuse process if blastema predominates. DD includes: Intrarenal neuroblastoma and EWS/PNET
- **If cystic**—polycystic kidney and renal dysplasia.

Case History: A 5-year-old boy with abdominal mass.

Diagnosis: (a) Neuroblastoma poorly differentiated type (b) Ganglioneuroblastoma (c) Ganglioneuroma

Anatomic sites are related to distribution of neural crest cells.
- Paravertebral region from neck to pelvis
- Adrenal medulla
- Extra-adrenal retroperitoneum
- Posterior mediastinum
- Hereditary NB gene (HNB1)—distal short-arm of chromosome 16p.

Laboratory Findings
- Elevated levels of catecholamines and their metabolites (VMA, HVA, MHPG).
- VMA/HVA ratio >1.5 or more is associated with improved prognosis.
- Increased serum neuropeptide Y is seen in neuroblastoma as compared to ganglioneuroblastoma or ganglioneuroma.
- Increased serum ferritin is associated with poor prognosis.
- LDH: Elevated levels indicate high tumor load.

Gross
- Lobulated masses with diameter between 6–8 cm with delicate membranous capsules
- Soft, fleshy, grey, partially hemorrhagic tumor
- Tumors with large expanses of differentiated ganglioneuroma associated with neuroblastoma foci have grey hemorrhagic nodules set in a firm white grey tumor mass.

Microscopy
International neuroblastoma classification:
4 specific categories:

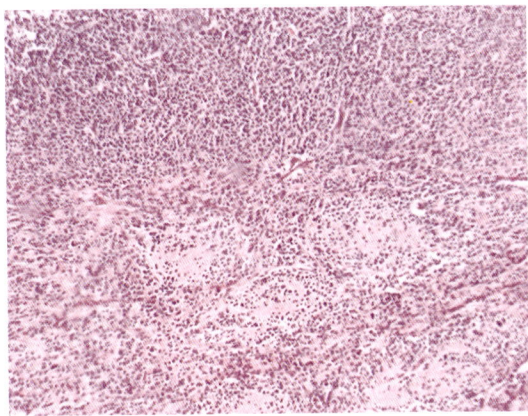

Fig. 12.2a

1. *Neuroblastoma (schwannian stroma-poor):* Groups/nests of neuroblastic cells separated by delicate, often incomplete stromal septa without or with limited schwannian proliferation (comprising <50% of the tumor).

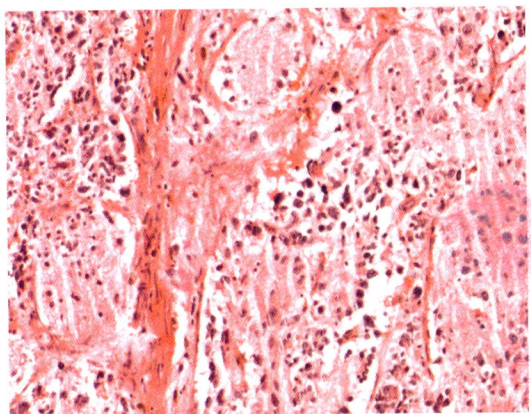

Fig. 12.2b

2. *Ganglioneuroblastoma, nodular:* Maturing or mature ganglion cells with at least one well-circumscribed nodule of neuroblasts.
3. *Ganglioneuroblastoma, intermixed* (schwannian stroma-rich) at least >1 foci neuroblasts intermixed with ganglion cells, intermixed or randomly distributed pattern of microscopic neuroblastic nests. Both have component >50% schwannian stroma.

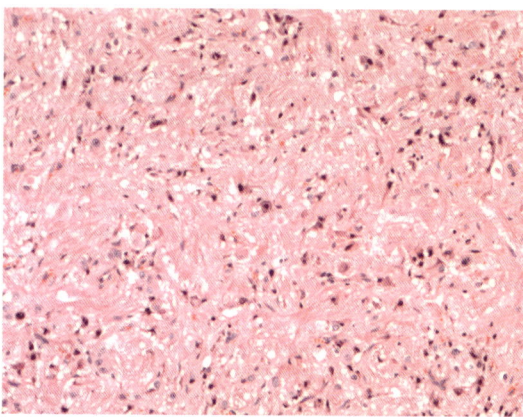

Fig. 12.2c

4. *Ganglioneuroma (schwannian stroma-dominant):* Individually a few scattered neuroblastic cells in schwannian stroma with ganglion cells (maturing and mature subtype).

Degree of Differentiation

Neuroblastoma and neuroblastic component of nodular-type ganglioneuroblastomas are classified into 3 subtypes:
1. **Undifferentiated:** Neuropil absent; no tumor cell differentiation; diagnosis relies on ancillary techniques.
2. **Poorly differentiated:** Neuropil evident in the background; <5% of tumor cells show features of differentiating neuroblasts with synchronous differentiation of nucleus and cytoplasm.
3. **Differentiating:** >5% tumor cells show evidence of the differentiation and neuropil is usually abundant.

Ancillary Studies

- Presence of membrane bound granules in the cytoplasm and neuritic processes with microtubules.
- IHC positive for NSE, synaptophysin, chromogranin, CD57 and other neural antigens.

Molecular Genetics

Gain 17q, amplification of MYC gene, deletion of 1p poor, TRK gene exp—good.

Staging

International neuroblastoma staging system.

Prognosis

- Favorable and unfavorable histology and age
- Mitoses and karyorrhexis index
- Low/intermediate/high risk based on biologic and clinical risk factors.

Differential Diagnosis

For neuroblastoma:
- Ganglioneuroblastoma
- Blastemal predominant Wilms'—epithelial elements (tubule) formation.
- EWS/PNET—perivascular pseudorosettes. CD99
- Rhabdomyosarcoma—strap cells, muscle markers
- Malignant lymphomas
- Desmoplastic small round cell tumor.

Case History: A 70-year-old male with mass lumbar region painless hematuria.

Diagnosis: Papillary renal cell carcinoma

Gross

Cystic, hemorrhagic, with a thick pseudocapsule may be multifocal and bilateral well circumscribed, having a variegated appearance.

Microscopy

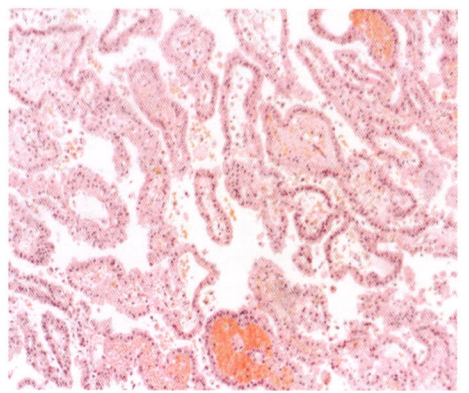

Fig. 12.3

- Circumscribed with pseudocapsule
- Composed of papillae with delicate fibrovascular core neutrophils/foamy macrophages and cholesterol crystals.
- **2 types**
  Type 1: Papillae lined by a single layer of cuboidal cells with scant pale cytoplasm.
  Type 2: Taller, nuclear pseudostratification, high nuclear grade with cells having abundant eosinophilic cytoplasm.

Immunohistochemistry
CK7 and AMACR, CK8/18, CK19, c-kit.

Genetics
- Trisomy and tetrasomy of Ch 7, trisomy of Ch 17, loss of Y Ch.
- No loss of 3p or p53 mutation (in contrast to classical RCC).
- Overexpression of MET mutations.

Differential Diagnosis
- **Clear cell RCC with papillary features:** CK7 negative, CA IX positive
- **Collecting duct carcinoma:** Medullary location, high grade with desmoplasia.
- **MiTF translocation carcinoma:** TFE3 positive.
- **Metanephric adenoma:** CD57 positive.
- **Clear cell papillary RCC:** CK7 and CA IX positive
- **Papillary adenoma** size <15 mm by WHO criteria.

Case History: A 70-year-old male with history of polycythemia vera and mass in lumbar region.

Diagnosis: Chromophobe variant of renal cell carcinoma

Gross
- Large, often 7 cm in diameter, geographic necrosis
- Well-circumscribed, unencapsulated, rarely central scar present.
- Light tan to brown with calcification.

Microscopy

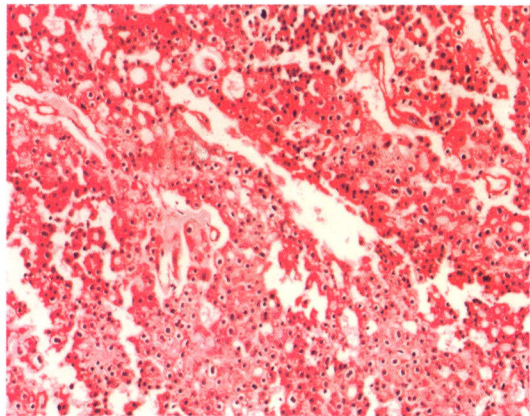

Fig. 12.4

- Tumor cells in solid sheet-like pattern, separated by incomplete hyalinized vascular septa.
- Cells are polygonal with prominent cell border, wrinkled nuclear membrane and perinuclear halo and voluminous cytoplasm.
- *Type 1 cells:* Small cells with solid, slightly granular eosinophilic cytoplasm.
- *Type 2 cells:* Perinuclear halo or translucent zone.
- *Type 3 cells:* Large, polygonal cells with hard cell border, abundant cytoplasm with reticular pattern.

Ancillary Studies
- Hale's colloidal iron (stains acid mucopolysaccharides in micro-vesicles, diffuse, strong and reticular).

- CK7 diffuse and strong and c-kit focal and membranous, others include: Parvalbumin, kidney-specific cadherin, negative for vimentin.

Differential Diagnosis
- **Oncocytoma:** No mitotic figures, no loss of chromosomes 2, 6, 10 or 17.
- **Eosinophilic papillary or clear cell carcinomas:** Hale's colloidal iron negative.

Case History: A 61-year-old male with mass in the kidney.

Diagnosis: (a) Clear cell renal cell carcinoma (b) Clear cell renal cell carcinoma sarcomatoid change (c) Clear cell renal cell carcinoma-rhabdoid change (d) Clear cell renal cell carcinoma with cystic change

Clinical Features
- Pain, hematuria.
- Regional lymph node metastases.
- Some have distant metastasis at presentation.

Gross
- Tumor size: 3 to 25 cm.
- Gray-white areas with an invasive margin.
- Cut surface: Fleshy-to-fibrous with areas of hemorrhage and necrosis.

Microscopy

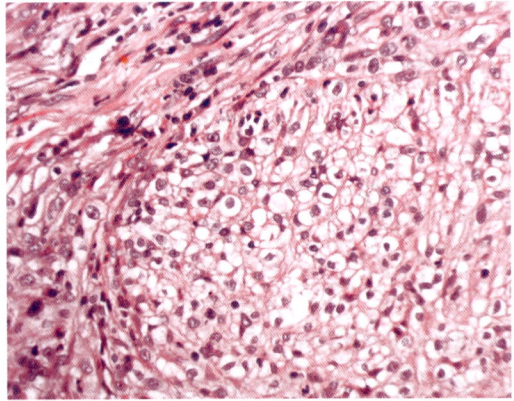

Fig. 12.5a

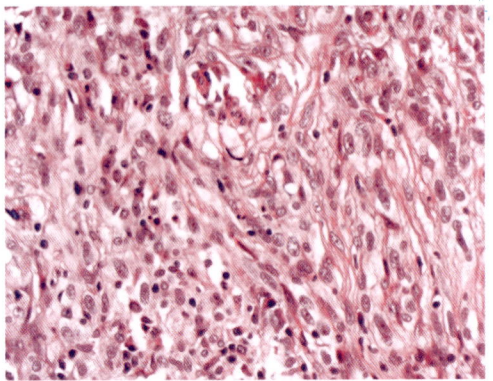

Fig. 12.5b

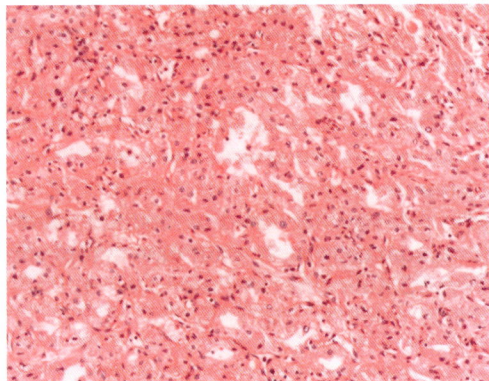

Fig. 12.5c

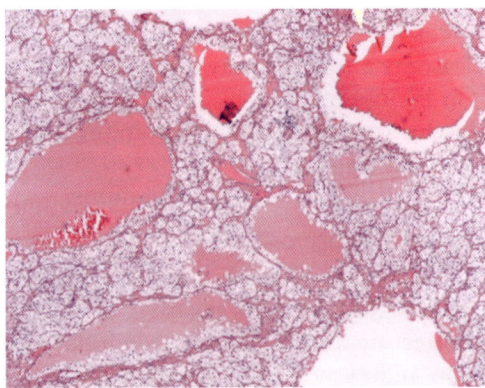

Fig. 12.5d

- Spindle/pleomorphic tumor giant cells.
- Simulate undifferentiated pleomorphic sarcoma, fibrosarcoma, rhabdomyosarcoma or angiosarcoma.
- Can have cartilage and bone differentiation.

Immunohistochemistry

Ki-67 is high in sarcomatoid areas.

Differential Diagnosis

- Retroperitoneal soft tissue sarcoma
- Sarcomatoid urothelial carcinoma
- Rhabdoid transitional cell carcinoma
- Smooth muscle—predominant angiomyolipoma
- Solitary fibrous tumor
- Synovial sarcoma

Case History: A 1-year-old girl baby Nephrectomy specimen.

Diagnosis: Multicystic renal dysplasia

Clinical Features

- Renal failure at birth.
- Abdominal mass mimicking neoplasia in children <1 year of age.
- Associated with congenital urinary tract obstruction in about 50% of cases.

Gross

- Large reniform mass of cysts of various sizes obscuring renal parenchyma.
- In focal and segmental dysplasia, only part of the kidney is involved by the dysplasia and cyst formation.

Microscopy

- Cysts of varying sizes lined by cuboidal epithelial cells surrounded by immature tubules or ducts, islands of immature-appearing cartilage.
- Islands of normal glomeruli and renal tubules between the dysplastic areas.
- Rare cases of Wilms' tumor and renal cell carcinoma (RCC) have been reported in multicystic dysplastic kidneys.

Differential Diagnosis

- Polycystic kidney disease adult and childhood.
- Cystic nephroma.
- Cystic partially differentiated by Wilms.

Case History: A 40-year-old female with tuberous sclerosis. Renal mass removed at laparotomy.

Diagnosis: Angiomyolipoma

Clinical Features

- Usually asymptomatic. Discovered on radiology
- Flank pain, hematuria, palpable mass, retroperitoneal haemorrhage.
- May co-exist with RCC, particularly clear cell carcinoma. Usually benign but may be complicated by hemorrhage, invasion of contiguous organs or non-contiguous involvement of other organs.

Gross

- Usually unilateral and unifocal
- Multiple (1/3) or bilateral (15%) tumors suggest underlying tuberous sclerosis
- Well demarcated, non-encapsulated
- Red (vascular component), gray-white (smooth muscle component) and yellow (adipose component)
- May invade local lymph nodes and renal vein even though benign capsular invasion in 25%.

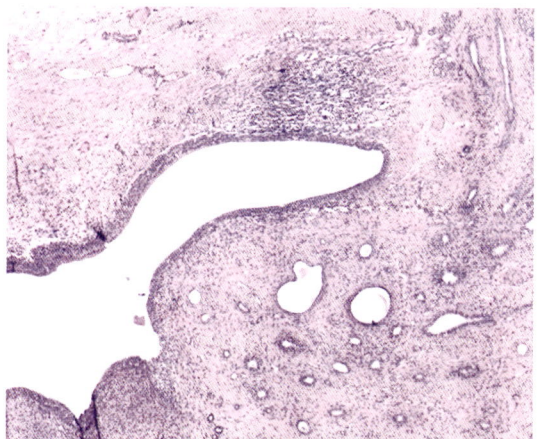

Fig. 12.6

Microscopy

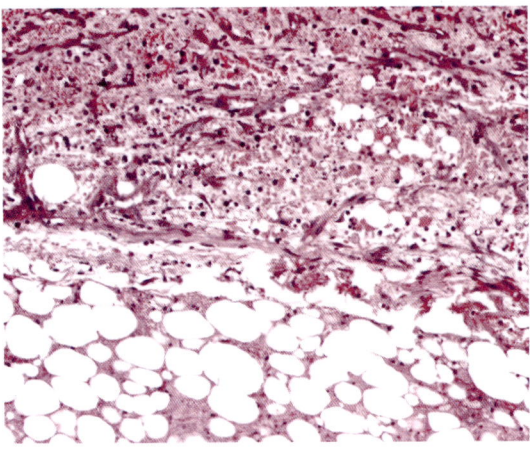

Fig. 12.7

- Triphasic with myoid spindle cells, islands of mature adipose tissue and dysmorphic thick-walled blood vessels without elastic lamina.
- Smooth muscle component appears to originate from vessel walls and may be hypercellular, atypical, pleomorphic or epithelioid.
- May resemble a high-grade sarcoma, if it metastasizes.

Ancillary Studies

- In adipose, myoid and epithelioid cells: HMB45 (100%), MART1/melan-A, muscle specific actin (HHF35, 100%), calponin (100%).
- Belongs to PECOMA family of tumors.

Differential Diagnosis

- **Leiomyoma:** Usually no prominent vascular or adipose component, negative for melanocytic markers
- **Leiomyosarcoma:** Prominent atypia, infiltrative, usually no prominent vascular or adipose component, negative for melanocytic markers
- **Melanoma:** Prominent atypia, infiltrative, usually no prominent vascular or adipose component, negative for melanocytic markers
- **Oncocytoma:** Oncocytes are prominent; no prominent adipose or vascular component, negative for melanocytic markers.
- **Pleomorphic rhabdomyosarcoma:** Smooth muscle component is markedly atypical, tumor is infiltrative, no prominent adipose or vascular component, negative for melanocytic markers.
- **Renal cell carcinoma:** Usually marked atypia and infiltrative margins, not triphasic, negative for melanocytic markers.

Case History: A 1-year-old male with mass abdomen.

Diagnosis: Clear cell sarcoma kidney

Clinical Features

- Mean age of diagnosis: 36 months
- Frequent recurrence/relapse with metastases to bone. Other sites of metastases—lymph nodes, CNS, lung, liver and muscle.

Gross

- Unifocal with irregular but sharp tumor-kidney interface.
- Large (mean: 11 cm); centered in renal medulla
- Cut surface: Homogenous tan/gray or gelatinous and firm with occasional cysts.

Microscopy

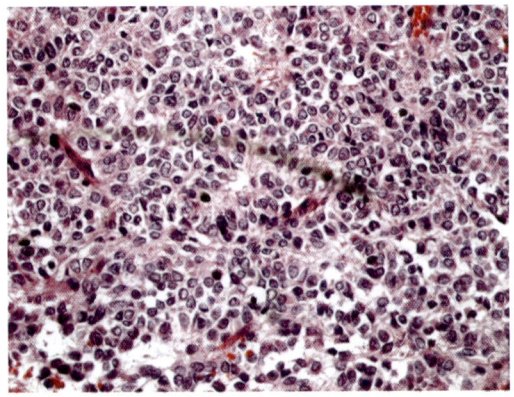

Fig. 12.8

Classic pattern
- Nests or cords of small, polygonal cells with indistinct cell margins, light staining cytoplasm and round nuclei with fine chromatin and grooves.
- No nucleoli, rare mitoses; 20% have clear cells (due to vacuoles); cords are created by an arborizing network of vascular septae high power reveals infiltration of the cells around the normal tubules/glomeruli at the periphery. Vascular invasion common.
- Other patterns (PASS, MSCE)
  - Palisading
  - Anaplastic
  - Spindle/storiform
  - Myxoid
  - Sclerosing
  - Cellular
  - Epithelioid

Ancillary Tests
CD10, BCL-2 Positive and WT1 Negative.

Differential Diagnosis
Wilms' tumor: Pushing border, more aggressively invasive, cells are less uniform and more hyperchromatic and epithelioid areas are keratin positive.

Case History: A 34-year-old male with fever and pus cells in urine.

Diagnosis: Xanthogranulomatous pyelonephritis

Gross
Unilateral with yellow irregular masses diffusely replacing the renal architecture.

Microscopy

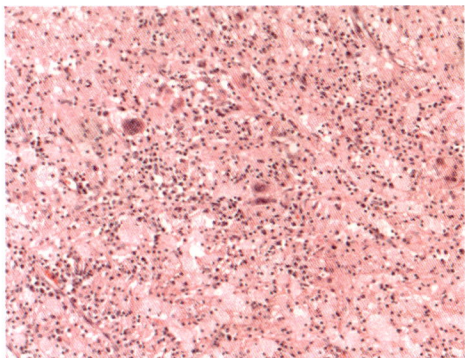

Fig. 12.9

Diffuse granulomatous inflammatory infiltrate—foamy histiocytes, multinucleated giant cells, inflammatory cells. Mimics RCC both gross and microscopy.

Immunohistochemistry
CD68—histiocytes.

Differential Diagnosis
- **Malakoplakia:** Michaelis-Gutmann bodies.
- **Renal clear cell carcinoma:** Cells with clear cytoplasm may resemble histiocytes, but are keratin+, CD68 negative, arranged in compact, tubulocystic, alveolar or rarely papillary patterns; often glassy hyaline globules; usually nuclear grade 2 or higher; chicken wire/delicate vasculature is common (sinusoids near each packet of cells)
- **Renal replacement lipomatosis:** Atrophic renal parenchyma is replaced by fatty tissue, not xanthoma cells.

Case History: A 60-year-old male with history of hematuria.

Diagnosis: Low grade noninvasive papillary urothelial carcinoma

Clinical Features
Painless intermittent hematuria.

Gross

Exophytic, single or multiple, vary greatly in size.

Microscopy

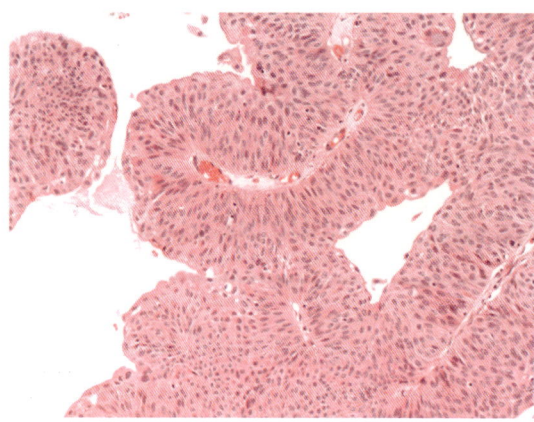

Fig. 12.10

- Delicate papillae with extensive branching.
- Low power: Ordered arrangement of cells.
- Medium power: Some loss of polarity with mild nuclear irregularity and nuclear pleomorphism.
- Mitosis may or may not be found but are usually away from the basement membrane.

Immunohistochemistry

CK20, GATA3, p63, CK5/6.

Differential Diagnosis

- Papillary-polypoid cystitis.
- Papillary urothelial neoplasm of low malignant potential
- High grade papillary urothelial carcinoma
- Papillary nephrogenic adenoma.

Case History: A 52-year-old male with pain lower abdomen and hematuria.

Diagnosis: High grade papillary urothelial carcinoma

Clinical Features

- Painless gross or microscopic hematuria is common
- Urgency, nocturia and dysuria.

Gross

Sessile or cauliflower-like with necrosis and ulceration. Exophytic papillary growth.

Microscopy

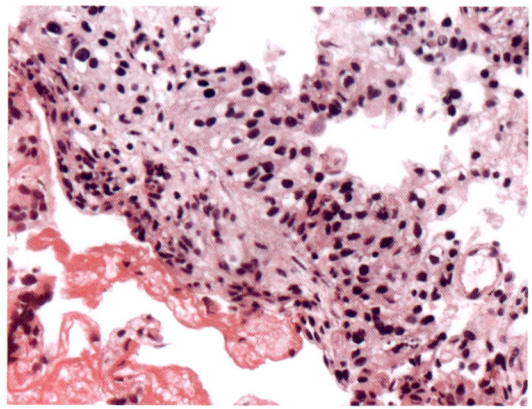

Fig. 12.11

- Irregular fused papillae with cellular disorder, nuclear size variation, pleomorphic nuclei appreciated at low to moderate magnification. Irregular prominent nucleoli can be seen.
- Atypical mitotic figures at all levels.
- Associated with carcinoma *in situ* or dysplasia in adjacent nonpapillary urothelium.
- Invasion must be ruled out.

Differential Diagnosis

- Inverted urothelial papilloma—cytology bland
- Low grade papillary urothelial carcinoma
- Papillary nephrogenic adenoma/metaplasia
- Infiltrating prostatic adenocarcinoma
- Villoglandular differentiation in elderly.

Case History: A 46-year-old male with urine cytology positive for malignant cells.

Diagnosis: Urothelial carcinoma

Clinical Features

- Higher likelihood of locally advanced disease with a few reports showing reduced responsiveness to chemotherapy and radiotherapy.

Microscopy

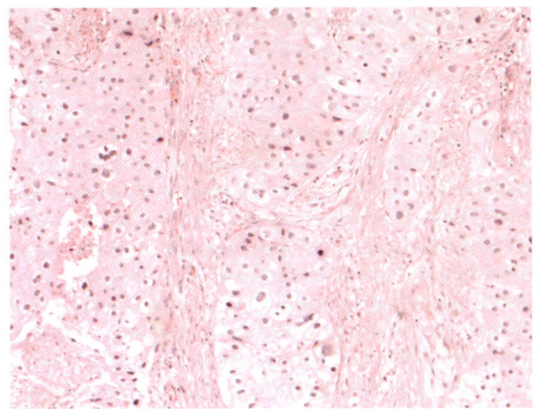

Fig. 12.12a: Infiltrating urothelial carcinoma

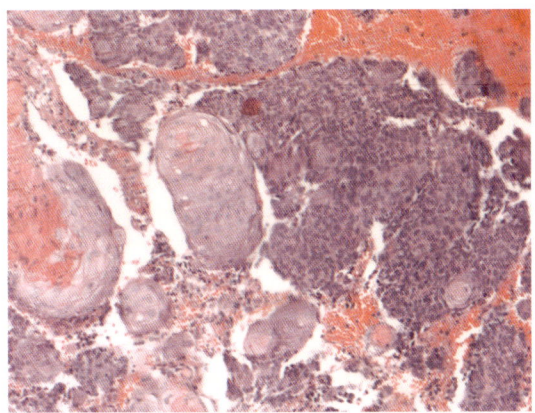

Fig. 12.12b: With squamous differentiation

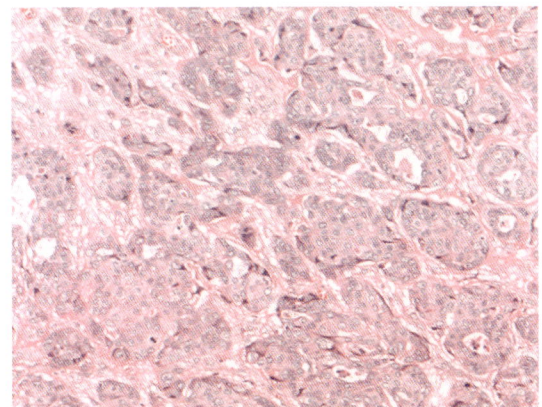

Fig. 12.12c: With glandular differentiation

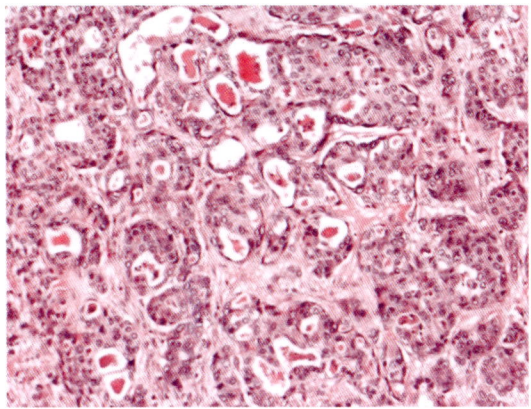

Fig. 12.12d: Microcystic variant

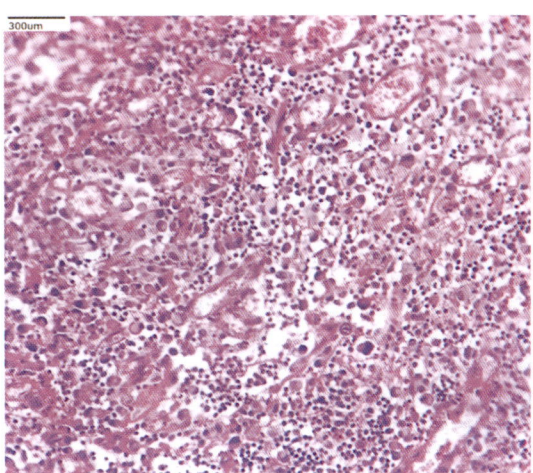

Fig. 12.12e: Lymphoepithelial variant

- Associated with high grade urothelial carcinoma.
- Squamous component has nests of malignant squamous epithelium, characterized by polygonal cells with evidence of keratinization and intercellular bridges.

Note: Recommended to report percentage of squamous component.

Immunohistochemistry

- Positive stains—squamous component: CK14, Mac387. Also CK5/6, CK5/14
- CK20 negative

Divergent differentiation in infiltrating urothelial carcinoma

- Squamous
- Trophoblastic
- Microcystic
- Lymphoepithelioma like
- Clear cell
- Poorly differentiated
- Glandular
- Nested
- Micropapillary
- Plasmacytoid
- Giant cell
- Sarcomatoid

Case History: A 52-year-old male with single lesion in bladder by cystoscopy.

Diagnosis: B cell lymphoma bladder

Gross

Discrete tumors, usually large and centered in dome or lateral walls with overlying epithelium intact and unremarkable.

Microscopy

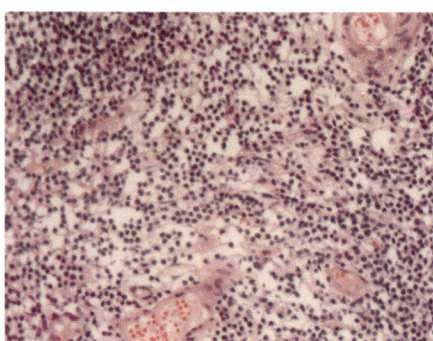

Fig. 12.13a

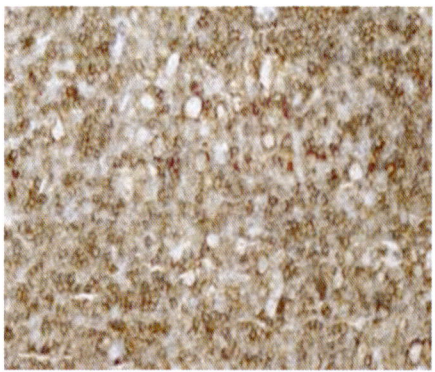

Fig. 12.13b: Immunohistochemistry CD20(positive)

Sheets of low grade, uniform cells that surround and separate, but never destroys muscle fascicles.

Immunohistochemistry

- B cell lymphomas are CD20+
- MALT lymphoma: CD20+, CD19+, CD5–, CD23–, CD10–, CD11c–
- Pan-keratin, vimentin, CK20, CK7 are negative.

Differential Diagnosis

- Urothelial carcinoma with prominent lymphoid infiltrate.
- Undifferentiated carcinoma.

Case History: A 63-year-old female with a single lesion in right kidney.

Diagnosis: Collecting duct carcinoma

Clinical Features

- Back or loin pain, hematuria, weight loss, lymph node involvement.
- Metastasis to lung, liver, bone, adrenal and brain common.

Diagnostic Criteria

- Medullary involvement.
- Predominant tubular morphology.
- Desmoplastic stromal reaction.
- Cytologically high grade.
- Infiltrative growth pattern.
- Absence of other renal cell carcinoma subtypes or urothelial carcinoma.

Gross

- Large tumors located in deep medulla.
- White and firm, hemorrhage and necrosis with an irregular poorly defined tumor margin extending into the cortex and beyond the kidney.

Microscopy

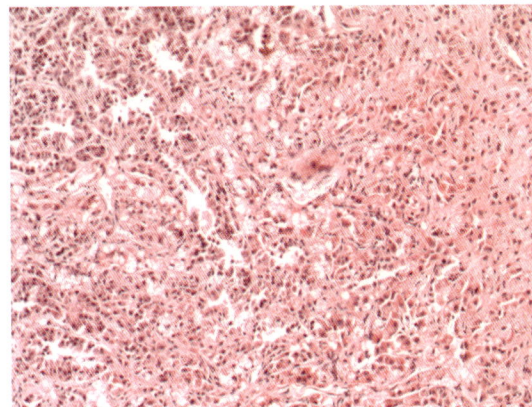

Fig. 12.14

- Tubular, tubulopapillary or tubule cystic tumor with invasive ductal pattern in a desmoplastic stroma.
- Tubules and papillae lined by tumor cells which are cuboidal/columnar/hobnail with eosinophilic or clear cytoplasm with distinct cell membranes having a high-grade nuclei and prominent nucleoli.

Immunohistochemistry

PAX2, PAX8, OCT3/4, SMARCB1, p63, high molecular weight keratin, CK7, Ulex-europaeus, lectins/peanut agglutinin, mucin positive

Differential Diagnosis

- **Papillary RCC:** Not necessarily central, more circumscribed, often psammoma bodies and foamy macrophages within papillae, usually no angiolymphatic invasion, no desmoplasia or inflammation, no dysplasia of collecting duct epithelium, LeuM1+, mucin-, Ulex europaeus-, E-cadherin-, CD117-, trisomy 7 or 17.
- **Renal medullary carcinoma:** Sickled blood cells. Loss of nuclear expression of INI1/SMARCB
- **Urothelial carcinoma:** PAX 8 –/p63 +
- **Adenocarcinoma from urothelium of renal pelvis:** Usually mucinous, resembles colon, vimentin negative
- **Metastatic carcinoma from GI or lung:** Usually well defined borders, multiple. Collecting duct carcinoma is a diagnosis of exclusion.

Case History: A 70-year-old male with abdominal mass.

Diagnosis: Renal oncocytoma

Clinical Features

- 5–9% of renal cell neoplasms with peak in 5th decade.
- Asymptomatic detected on radiological investigations for unrelated symptoms.

Gross

- Cut surface: Mahogany brown to tan or yellow
- Central stellate scar located eccentrically or periphery
- Haemorrhage present, but no necrosis

Microscopy

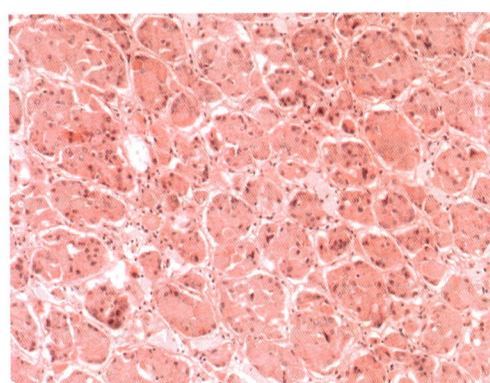

Fig. 12.15

- Solid nests of oncocytic cells
- Large, round eosinophilic cells with densely granular cytoplasm, round regular nuclei, small but visible nucleoli
- Small population of cells with scanty cytoplasm (oncoblasts) present around the scar or at the edge of epithelial islands.

Immunohistochemistry

Diffuse positive for KIT, E-cadherin, S-100A, pancytokeratin, LMWK. Negative for CK7.

Case History: A 60-year-old female with polypoidal lesion urethra.

Diagnosis: Urethral caruncle

Clinical Features

- Only in female urethra. Resembles small raspberry protruding from external urethral meatus.
- Dysuria, increase in urinary frequency and obstructive symptoms.
- Bleeds easily, may become infected.
- Often recurs, perhaps due to persistence of inciting factors.

Gross

Highly vascular, polypoidal lesions having a small raspberry appearance.

Microscopy

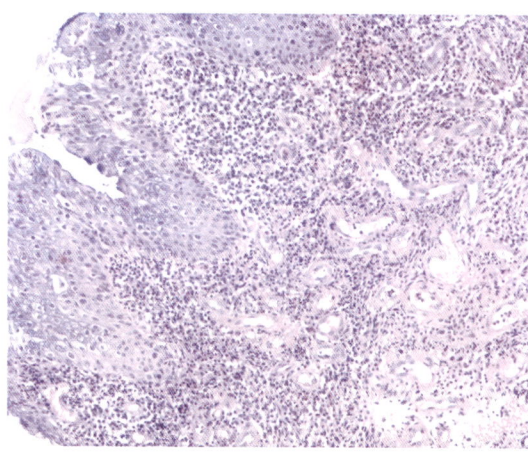

Fig. 12.16

- Acute and chronic inflammatory cellular infiltrate.
- Overlying urothelium may be hyperplastic, ulcerated or exhibit squamous or glandular metaplasia.
- Papillomatous, angiomatous and granulomatous.

Case History: A 3-year-old boy baby with abdominal mass.

Diagnosis: Multicystic nephroma (paediatric cystic nephroma)

Gross

- Lesion can be focal or can replace the entire renal parenchyma.
- Large (5–10 cm), unilateral and solitary multiloculated tumor composed of multiple non-communicating thin-walled cysts of varying size that are filled with clear fluid.
- Sharply demarcated from adjacent kidney by thick fibrous capsule.
- Surface is nodular.
- No solid areas or necrosis is seen.

Microscopy

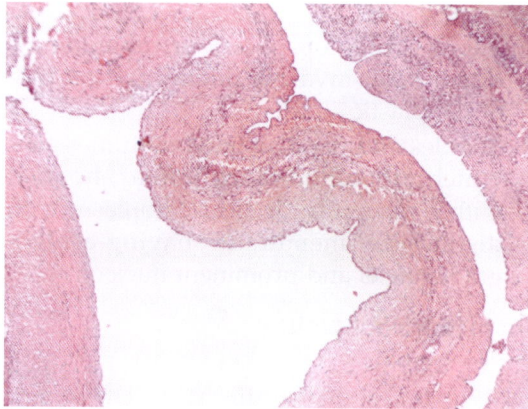

Fig. 12.17

- Unilateral, solitary and multiloculated benign tumor with small non-communicating cysts containing clear colorless fluid
- Cysts lined by flat to hobnail epithelium
- Ovarian stroma-like appearance, no renal tissue
- Fall under the mixed epithelial and stromal tumor.
- Stroma may contain smooth muscle, skeletal muscle, cartilage or microscopic cysts lined by bland cuboidal cells that appear to be abortive tubules.

Molecular Genetics

A sizable portion of PCN carry a DICER1 mutation, either loss of function or missense mutations.

Differential Diagnosis
- Polycystic disease
- **Cystic partially differentiated nephroblastomas (CPDN) and cystic Wilms' tumour (CWT):** CWT has immature nephrogenic elements plus solid nodules distorting the septal; CPDN and CWT lack DICER1 mutations.

Case History: A 70-year-old female with dysuria, a yellow nodule fond on cystoscopy

Diagnosis: Malakoplakia

Clinical Features
- More common in immunocompromised (HIV, renal transplant recipients) and women
- Mean age at diagnosis is fifth decade
- Rare in children
- Patients usually present with urinary symptoms and urinary tract infection

Microscopy

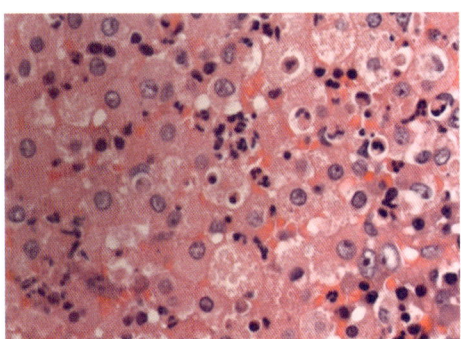

Fig. 12.18a

- Initial inflammatory stage followed by classic stage with numerous Michaelis-Gutmann bodies and later progresses to fibrosis and scarring.
- Foamy epithelioid histiocytes with PAS+ granular eosinophilic cytoplasm in lamina propria, some lymphocytes and occasional giant cells
- Histiocytes have increased number of phagosomes containing non-digested bacteria (usually *E. coli* or proteus), contain Michaelis-Gutmann bodies (iron containing, cytoplasmic laminated mineralized concretions)

Case History: A 40-year-old male with recurrent UTI

Diagnosis: (a) Cystitis cystica (b) Cystitis cystica intestinalis

Clinical Features
- Usually asymptomatic, may cause recurrent urinary tract infections; often benign incidental findings in biopsies done for other reasons
- May occasionally appear as nodular, irregular mass on cystoscopic examination

Microscopy

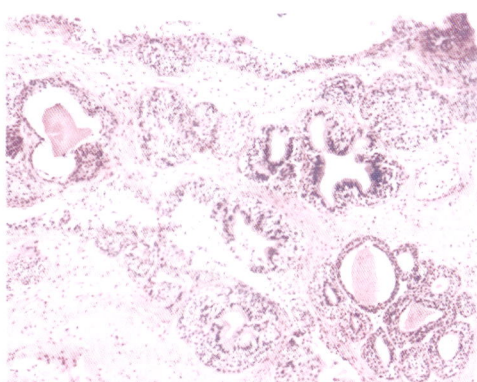

Fig. 12.18b

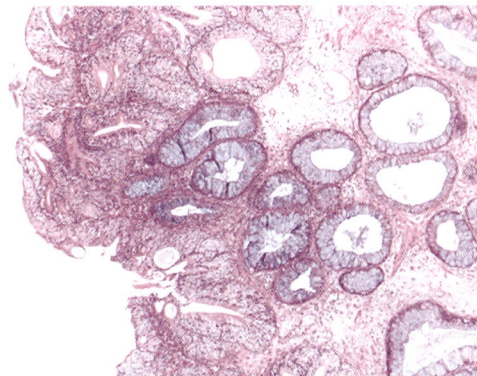

Fig. 12.18c

- **Cystitis cystica:** Brunn nests that grow into lamina propria and are transformed into urothelium lining slit-like or cystic spaces with pink fluid; present in up to 60% of bladders.

- **Cystitis glandularis of intestinal type:** Cystitis glandularis of intestinal type is usually confined to lamina propria, may have mucin extravasation with dissecting mucin pools.

Differential Diagnosis
- **Bladder adenocarcinoma:** Misdiagnosed as adenocarcinoma but no significant atypia, no glandular disarray, no desmoplasia, no muscular invasion, no signet ring cells, no necrosis, no/minimal mitotic activity, no carcinoma *in situ*, no single cells floating in mucin.
- **Endocervicosis**

Case History: A 50-year-old male with painless visible haematuria and debris in urine.

Diagnosis: (a) Urachal villous adenoma with adjacent mucinous adenocarcinoma (b) Tubulovillous adenoma with high grade dysplasia and focal signet ring cells

Clinical Features
- Hematuria and irritative symptoms
- May be associated with *in situ* or invasive adenocarcinoma at diagnosis, less often with *in situ* or invasive urothelial carcinoma.

Gross
Papillary neoplasm.

Microscopy

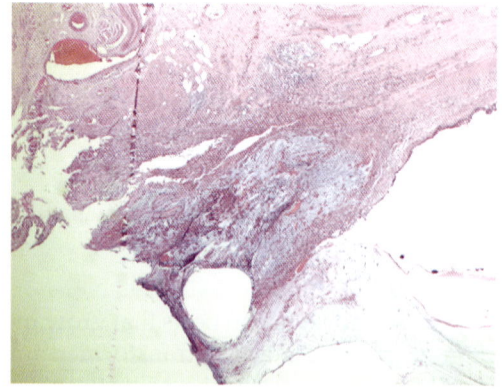

Fig. 12.19a

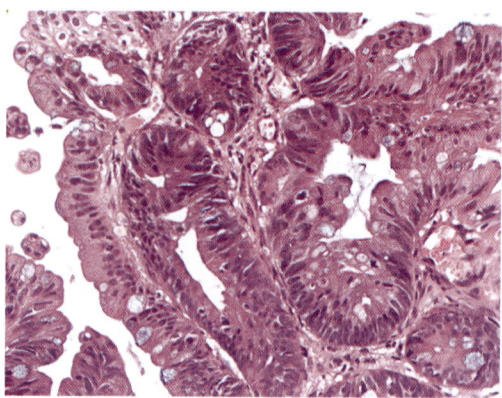

Fig. 12.19b

- It may resemble colonic villous adenoma with pseudostratified columnar epithelium showing nuclear stratification, nuclear crowding, nuclear hyperchromasia, occasional prominent nucleoli and occasional mitoses.
- Associated with cystitis glandularis and cystitis cystica
- MUST sample entire lesion to rule out adenocarcinoma (*in situ* or invasive)

Immunohistochemistry
Positive for CK20 and CEA

Differential Diagnosis
- **Well-differentiated colonic adenocarcinoma extending into bladder:** Clinical history, definite invasion
- **Florid cystitis glandularis:** Lacks well-formed villous structure.

Case History: A 68-year-old female with renal sinus mass by imaging

Diagnosis: Chronic pyelonephritis with actinomycosis

Clinical Features
- Causes 10–20% of end stage renal disease in transplant or dialysis units
- Associated with pyelitis and ureteritis cystica
- Some patients with pyelonephritic scars develop focal and segmental glomerulo-

sclerosis with proteinuria in nephrotic range, perhaps due to renal ablation nephropathy
- Types: Reflux (chronic reflux-associated pyelonephritis) and obstruction (chronic obstructive pyelonephritis)

Gross
- Irregular scarred cortical surface usually at poles, dilated and blunted calyces
- Dilated ureter; retraction and destruction of papillae with "U"-shaped scars.

Microscopy

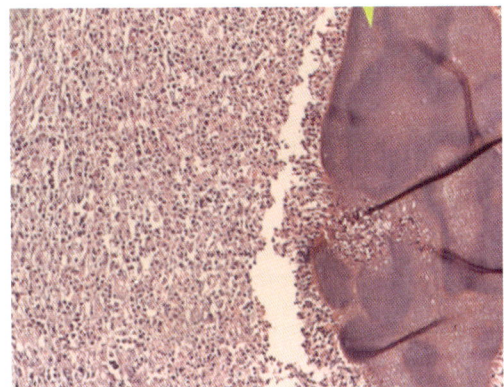

Fig. 12.20

- Tubular thyroidization (filled with colloid casts), tubular atrophy
- Interstitial fibrosis and inflammation (intense diffuse lymphoplasmacytic inflammatory infiltrate with germinal centers)
- Obliterative endarteritis of vessels, interstitial Tamm-Horsfall protein (amorphous, fibrillary, PAS+ material surrounded by inflammatory cells)
- Normal glomeruli early in disease course.

Differential Diagnosis
- **Chronic glomerulonephritis:** Diffusely scarred cortex
- **Vascular disease:** Can cause wedge-shaped cortical scars, but underlying medullary and calyceal areas are normal

Case History: A 70-year-old male with gross hematuria. Ultrasound shows plaque like soft tissue mass at bladder base and cystoscopy revealed sessile indurated tumor on posterior wall bladder.

Diagnosis: Micropapillary carcinoma of bladder

Clinical Features
- Adults, 80% men
- Usually high grade and high stage at presentation with marked nodal metastases with extensive lymphovascular invasion.

Microscopy

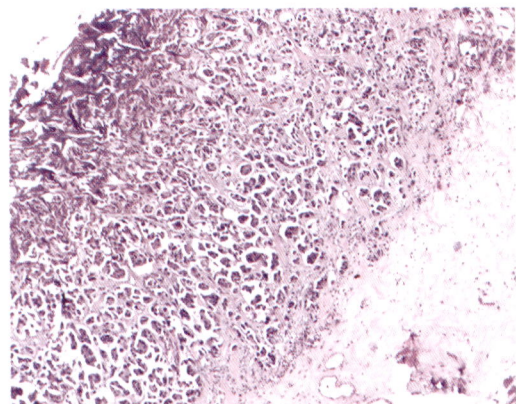

Fig. 12.21

- Small nests and papillae with surrounding retraction spaces, resembling ovarian serous borderline tumors, but without psammoma bodies
- Delicate papillae 1–4 cell layers thick with thin stromal cores and numerous secondary micropapillae
- Micropapillae may lack fibrovascular cores and show hierarchical branching
- Confluent retraction spaces are characteristic.
- Nuclear grade is typically high in deeper portions; may have lower grade appearance at surface
- Most tumors are muscle invasive. Numerous mitoses and frequent true lymphovascular invasion

- Often mixed with urothelial carcinoma in primary, but metastases usually have only micropapillary pattern.

Immunohistochemistry
Positive stain: MUC 1

Differential Diagnosis
- Ovarian borderline tumors: clinical history; no urothelial component; psammoma bodies are common
- Invasive urothelial carcinoma with stromal retraction: No micropapillae; stromal retraction is negative for CD31, CD34, D2-40
- Papillary nephrogenic adenoma

Case History: A 70-year-old female with painless hematuria for past 6 months. Ultrasound showed an hypoechoic lesion in right renal pelvis and the intravenous pyelogram revealed poor functioning of right kidney.

Diagnosis: Urothelial carcinoma of renal pelvis

Clinical Features
- Risk factors: Tobacco use, phenacetin use, industrial carcinogen exposure (coal, asphalt, petrochemicals, tar), thorium containing radiologic contrast material, Balkan endemic nephropathy
- Present with hematuria, flank pain.

Microscopy

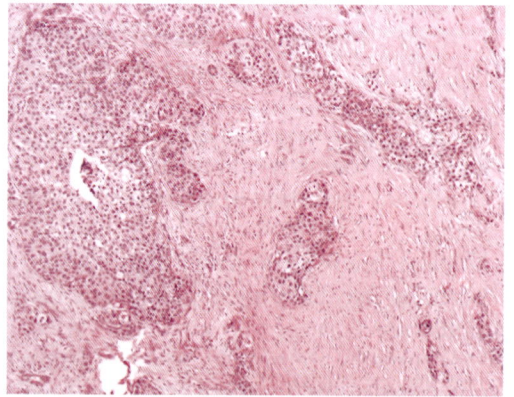

Fig. 12.22

- Similar to urothelial neoplasia in bladder: Nests, clusters or single neoplastic cells
- Grading for papillary neoplasms same as in bladder.

Immunohistochemistry
Positive stains: p63, GATA3, thrombomodulin, 34βE12, CK7, CK20 and may express uroplakin II/III, CK5/6, CAIX and PAX8

Molecular Genetics
- Aberrations of p53, chromosome 9
- Microsatellite instability in 20–30%, associated with inverted growth patterns and hereditary nonpolyposis colorectal cancer syndrome.

Differential Diagnosis
- **Any high grade neoplasm in renal pelvis with unusual morphologic features**
- **Clear cell renal cell carcinoma:** p63 negative, CK7 negative and GATA3 negative
- **Collecting duct carcinoma (CDC):** Both may have desmoplastic stroma, glandular differentiation. Immunohistochemistry may be useful, but has overlap: PAX8 is expressed in almost all CDCs, and 17–20% of upper tract urothelial CAs. Conversely, p63 is expressed in nearly all urothelial CAs, and 14% of CDCs.
- **Renal medullary carcinoma:** It is associated with sickle cell trait, has loss of INI-1

Case History: A 67-year-old female with ultrasound detected mass in the kidney

Diagnosis: Renal lymphoma

Clinical Features
- Less than 1% of renal tumors
- More often secondary involvement than primary; usually bilateral, usually B cell
- Diffuse large cell lymphoma is most common subtype
- High rate of CNS relapse in patients with kidney involvement by diffuse large B cell lymphoma
- May occur in transplanted kidney

Microscopy

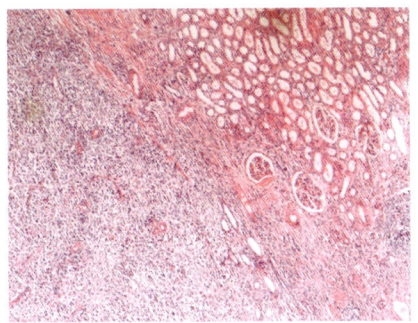

Fig. 12.23

Glomeruli and other structures are usually intact.

References

1. WHO classification of tumors of the urinary system and male genital organs, 4th edition.
2. Sternberg's diagnostic surgical pathology, 6th edition.
3. Rosai and Ackerman's surgical pathology, 11th edition.

APPROACH TO KIDNEY LESIONS

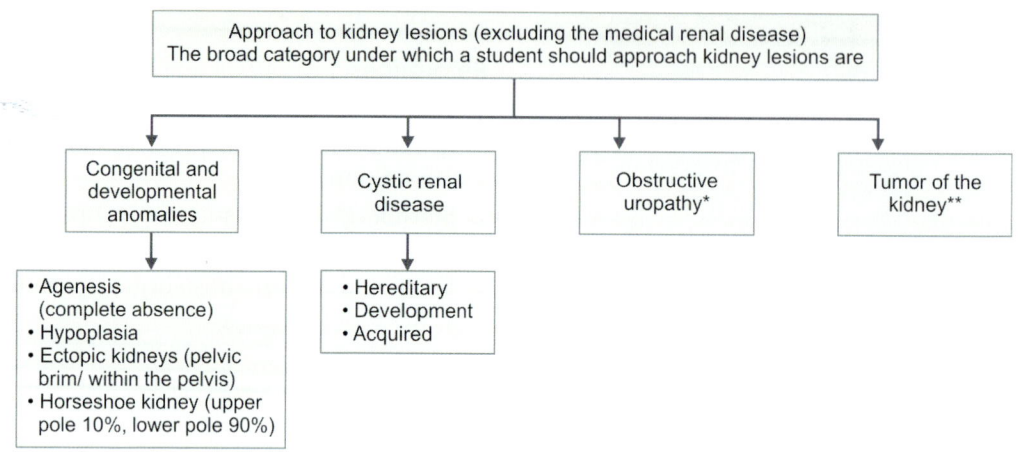

***Obstructive uropathy**
- Congenital anomalies
- Urinary calculi
- Benign prostatic hypertrophy
- *Tumors:* Carcinoma of the prostate, bladder tumors, contiguous malignant disease (retroperitoneal lymphoma), carcinoma of the cervix or uterus
- *Inflammation*: Prostatitis, ureteritis, urethritis, retroperitoneal fibrosis
- Functional disorders: Neurogenic (spinal cord damage or diabetic nephropathy) and other functional abnormalities of the ureter or bladder (often termed dysfunctional obstruction)

** **Renal tumors**
- Clear cell renal cell carcinoma
- **Multilocular cystic renal neoplasm of low malignant potential**
- Papillary renal cell carcinoma
- **Hereditary leiomyomatosis renal cell carcinoma syndrome**
- Chromophobe renal cell carcinoma

Hybrid Oncocytic Chomophobe RCC
- Collecting duct carcinoma
- Renal medullary carcinoma
- **MITF family associated carcinoma (Xp11 translocation carcinomas)**
- **SDH deficiency associated renal cell carcinoma**

- Mucinous tubular and spindle cell carcinoma
- **Tubulocystic carcinoma**
- **Acquired cystic disease associated carcinoma**
- **Clear cell papillary RCC**
- Renal cell carcinoma, unclassified...
- **Papillary adenoma (<15 mm)** and **oncocytoma**

NONEPITHELIAL TUMORS
- Metanephric tumors
- Nephroblastic and other cystic tumors occurring mainly in children
- Mesenchymal tumors
  - Mesenchymal tumors occurring in children
  - Mesenchymal tumors occurring in adults
- Mixed epithelial and stromal tumor family
- **Neuroendocrine tumors** (carcinoid not used)
- Renal hematopoietic tumors
- Germ cell tumors
- Metastatic tumors

Provisional entities
- Oncocytic RCC occurring after neuroblastoma
- Thyroid like follicular RCC
- ALK rearrangement associated RCC
- RCC with angioleiomyomatous stoma

NOT yet included in routine WHO 2016

Contributed by Sandhya Sundaram

CHAPTER 13
Male Genital Tract Lesions Including Prostate

CN Sai Shalini

Case History: A 40-year-old male with complaints of right testicular swelling.

Diagnosis: Seminoma

Clinical Features
- Age: 35–45 years.
- Rare in children and uncommon >50.
- Testicular enlargement with or without pain.

Laboratory Investigations
Increased serum PLAP and hCG.

Gross
- Well demarcated, homogeneous, firm mass, gray white, lobulated and bulging appearance.
- Hemorrhage and necrosis uncommon.

Microscopy

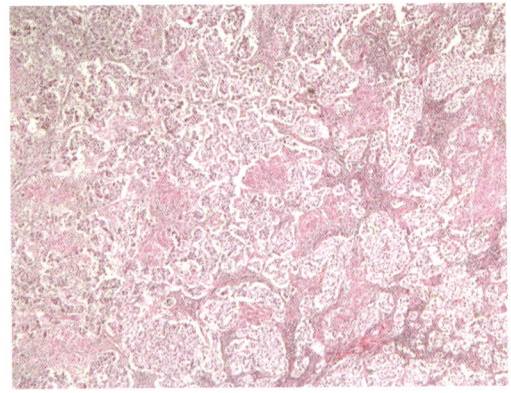

Fig. 13.1

- Diffuse proliferation of large cells arranged in sheets, nests or cords.
- *Patterns:* Tubular, reticular, cystic, microcystic and cribriform.
- Tumor cells are evenly spaced with uniform cells, distinct cell membrane, fine chromatin and prominent nucleoli.
- Cytoplasm is abundant eosinophilic or clear.
- Mitotic figures can also be seen.
- Tumor cells are separated by stroma into lobules and the stroma is infiltrated by lymphocytes.
- Burnt out seminoma: Tumor cells are replaced by hyalinised fibrotic tissue.

Ancillary Tests
- **Special stains:** PAS and PAS-D.
- **Immunohistochemistry:** PLAP, NSE, Oct-4, vimentin, c-kit and angiotensin I-converting enzyme hCG positive in syncytiotrophoblast giant cells.
- **Molecular genetics:** Common—isochromosome 12p mapped by hiwi gene. MAGE-1 Ag VASA mRNA.

Differential Diagnosis
- Malignant melanoma
- Embryonal carcinoma
- Endodermal sinus tumor
- Spermatocytic seminoma

- Choriocarcinoma
- Granulomatous orchitis
- Sertoli cell tumor

Case History: A 19-year-old male with complaints of left loin pain came for renal stone evaluation.

Diagnosis: Mixed germ cell tumor (EC+YST+ teratomatous component)

Clinical Features
- 3rd to 4th decades.
- Present with testicular enlargement.

Gross
- Variegated appearance with solid and cystic areas.
- If lobulated, gray yellow/gray white with mucinous texture—YST. If hemorrhage + necrosis and invade adjacent epididymis and tunica—embryonal carcinoma/choriocarcinoma.
- Cystic and cartilaginous or bony areas: Teratomatous component.

Microscopy

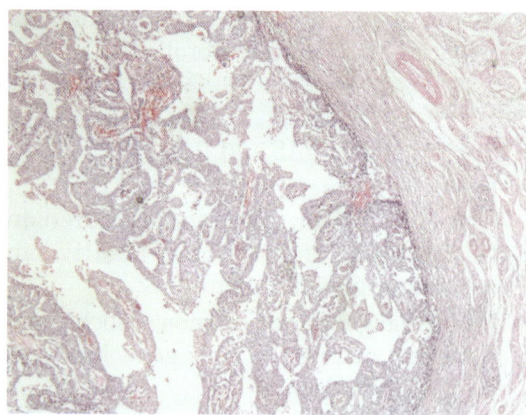

Fig. 13.2

- All components are appreciated by their architectural patterns.
- *Non-seminomatous germ cell tumor (NSGCT)*

Embryonal Carcinoma
Microscopy
- *Patterns:* Acinar, tubular, papillary, solid/syncytial.
- Cellular pleomorphism, with overlapping of cells.
- Large prominent irregular vesicular nuclei, coarse chromatin, and prominent nucleoli.
- Abundant granular eosinophilic to amphophilic cytoplasm with indistinct cell membrane.
- Mitotic activity is increased. Infrequent lymphocytic infiltrate.
- Peritumoral vascular/lymphatic invasion.

Ancillary Tests
- **Immunohistochemistry:** CK cocktail, PLAP, OCT-4, CD30, AFP positive, hCG positive in syncytiotrophoblast cells.
- **Electron microscopy:** Glandular differentiation noted.
- **Molecular genetics:** Isochromosome 12p.

Differential Diagnosis
- Seminoma
- Malignant lymphoma
- Endodermal sinus tumor
- Metastatic carcinoma
- Malignant Sertoli cell tumor
- Choriocarcinoma.

Yolk Sac Tumor
Endodermal sinus tumor.

Clinical Features
- Pure form—commonly in infants and young children.
- Mixed form—common in adults, rare in childhood. Presents with rapid testicular enlargement.

Imaging
Solid intratesticular lesion.

Laboratory Investigations
- Raised serum AFP level.

Microscopy

- Patterns: Reticular—microcystic, macrocystic, polyvesicular vitelline, solid, papillary, spindle cell, enteric, hepatoid, myxomatous.
- Schiller-Duval bodies.
- Extracellular hyaline material.
- YST associated with intratubular germ cell neoplasia.

Ancillary Tests

- **Special stains:** Hyaline globules—PAS+, PAS–, D resistant.
- **Immunohistochemistry:** AFP, CK, PLAP positive
- **CD30, hCG negative.**
- **Molecular genetics:** Loss of chromosome 1, chromosome 6. Gain of chromosome 1, chromosome 20 and chromosome 22.

Polyembryoma: Rare

Microscopy

Numerous embryoid bodies (EC+, YST+, teratoma arranged in a pattern resembling embryo).

Teratoma

Clinical Features

- 1st and 2nd decades.
- 2nd most common tumor of infancy and childhood.
- Gradual testicular swelling with or without pain.

Imaging

Well-circumscribed mass, variable degree of shadowing, cyst formation.

Gross

- Well demarcated, solid or multicystic.
- Cysts filled with gelatinous material.
- Cartilage, bony spicules noted.

Microscopy

- Tumor composed of tissue from different layers—ectoderm, mesoderm, endoderm.
- Immature elements—spindle mesenchymal component, neural, epithelial, embryonic kidney/lung, embryonic rhabdomyoblastic tissue, PNET areas.
- Granulomas—8% of teratomas.
- Monodermal teratomas—struma testis.

Ancillary Tests

- **Immunohistochemistry:** AFP—19–36% +, α_1-antitrypsin +, CEA, ferritin +, PLAP +, hCG +
- **Molecular genetics:** Infantile teratoma—diploid. Adult—hypotriploid.

Differential Diagnosis

- Dermoid cyst of testis
- Epidermoid cyst
- Carcinoma/sarcoma in other organs
- PNET

Choriocarcinoma

Clinical Features

- Due to hematogenous spread presents with hemoptysis, dyspnea, hematemesis, malena, anemia.
- Gynecomastia

Imaging

Hypoechoic to hyperechoic.

Gross

- Testis small/normal in size.
- Present as a hemorrhagic nodule surrounded by grey tan tumor.

Microscopy

- Sheets of syncytiotrophoblast, cytotrophoblast.
- Hemorrhage: Hallmark of choriocarcinoma.

Ancillary Tests

- **Immunohistochemistry:** hCG, HPL, CK, inhibin: Positive in syncytiotrophoblast.

Case History: A 55-year-old male with complaints of painless testicular enlargement.

Diagnosis: Diffuse large B cell lymphoma

Clinical Features
- Primary lymphoma—rare.
- Painless testicular enlargement associated with skin, CNS and Waldeyer's ring involvement.

Gross
- Multiple confluent nodules. Firm, fleshy, homogeneous resembling seminoma.
- No necrosis.

Microscopy

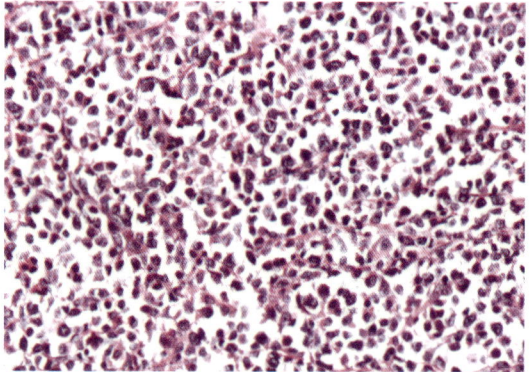

Fig. 13.3

- Tumor cells are infiltrating the interstitium. Seminiferous tubules are spared or involved.
- Vascular invasion—present.

Immunohistochemistry
- LCA, CD3, Tdt positive in T cell lymphoma
- LCA, CD20 positive in B cell lymphoma
- LCA, CD56 positive in NK-cell lymphoma.

Case History: A 22-year-old male with complaints of right testicular swelling and gynecomastia.

Diagnosis: Leydig cell tumor

Clinical Features
- Occurs in 2nd and 6th decades.
- Mostly unilateral, 3% bilateral.
- Testicular swelling, gynecomastia.
- 10% turn malignant.

Gross
Circumscribed, solid mass, yellow-mahogany brown to grey-white with focal hemorrhage/necrosis.

Microscopy

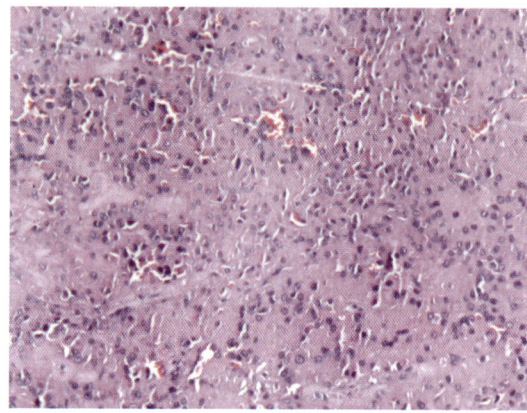

Fig. 13.4

- *Patterns:* Diffuse, nodular, trabecular, tubular, pseudofollicular and rare microcystic.
- Tumor cells are separated by hyalinized, myxoid stroma and numerous thin-walled vessel.
- They are large have round nuclei with abundant eosinophilic cytoplasm or vacuolated cytoplasm and prominent nucleoli.
- Reinke crystalloids, lipofuscin pigments are seen with rare psammoma bodies.

Malignant Features
- Large size
- Infiltrative margin
- Vascular invasion
- Atypia, necrosis
- Lack of pigment

Immunohistochemistry
Inhibin, calretinin, vimentin positive.

Differential Diagnosis
- Leydig cell hyperplasia
- Large cell calcifying Sertoli cell tumor

- Extratesticular growth
- Sarcoma
- Tumor of adrenogenital syndrome
- Malignant melanoma
- Lymphoma
- Metastatic carcinoma
- Hepatoid YST
- Malakoplakia

Case History: A 30-year-old male with history of infertility.

Diagnosis: Sertoli cell-only syndrome (Syn: Germ cell aplasia)

Microscopy

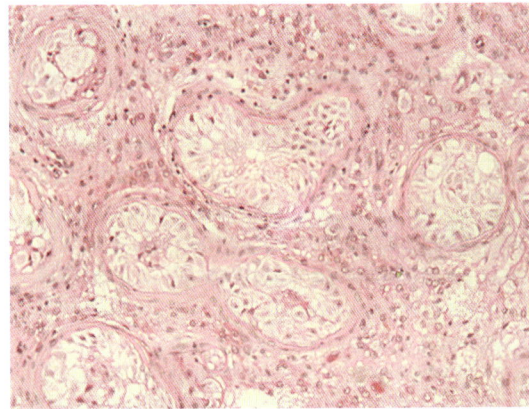

Fig. 13.5

- Tubules are normal or minimally decreased in diameter.
- Tunica and tubular basement membranes do not show hyalinization.
- Germ cells are totally absent. Tubules contain only Sertoli cells.

Ancillary Tests

- **Special stains:** PAS—cytoplasmic glycogen. Masson trichrome—collagen (blue), Reinke crystals (red).
  Elastic stain: Post-pubertal tubules.
- **Immunohistochemistry**
  Sertoli cells: Vimentin, keratin
  Desmin: Positive.
  Leydig cells: Inhibin, melan-A positive.

Differential Diagnosis
- Seminiferous tubule hyalinization.
- Maturation arrest
- Hypospermatogenesis

Case History: A 31-year-old male with complaints of right testicular swelling.

Diagnosis: TB epididymo-orchitis

Gross
Solid nodular enlargement of the testis.

Microscopy

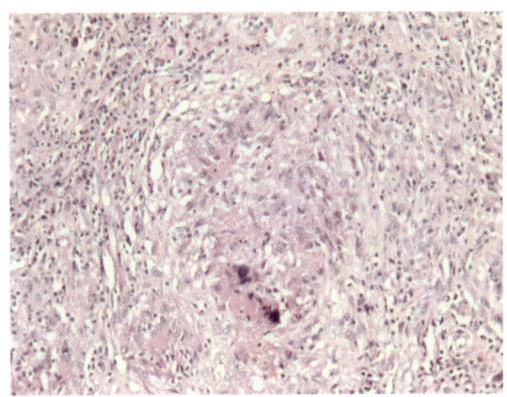

Fig. 13.6

Granulomatous lesion composed of epithelioid cells, multinucleated giant cells, lymphocytes and plasma cells.

Case History: A 75-year-old male with complaints of difficulty in voiding urine. PR-enlarged prostate.

Diagnosis: Prostatic adenocarcinoma, Gleason score 7(4 + 3)

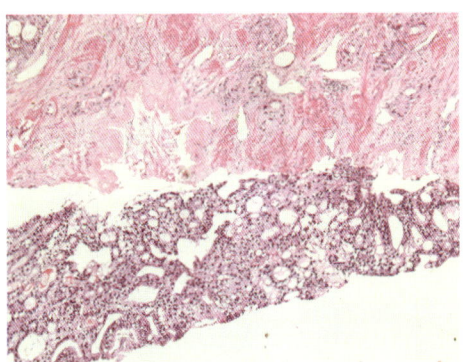

Fig. 13.7

Table 13.1

Pattern	Tumor shape and borders	Stromal invasion	Tumor cell arrangements	Gland size
1	Nodular, well defined and smooth edges	Pushing	Single, round to oval, closely packed, but separate glands	Medium
2	Masses less well defined and less well circumscribed	Some gland separation at tumor edge	Single, separate, round to oval glands, with more variation in gland size and shape, and loosely packed with stromal separation (up to one gland diameter, on average)	Medium
3A	Ill-defined infiltrating edges	Irregular extension	Single separate glands of variable shape and size, with elongated, angular and twisted forms, usually with wide stromal separation	Medium
3B	Ill-defined infiltrating edges	Irregular extension	Same as 3A but glands are smaller	Small to very small
3C	Masses and cylinders with smooth rounded edges	Expansile	Papillary and cribriform epithelium, without necrosis	Medium to large
4A	Raggedly infiltrative	Diffusely permeative	Fused glands, creating masses, cords, or chains	Small, medium, or large
4B	Raggedly infiltrative	Diffusely permeative	Similar to 4A, but cells have cleared cytoplasm: Hypernephromatoid variant	Small, medium, or large
5A	Smooth, rounded cylinders	Expansile	Papillary, cribriform or solid masses with central necrosis: Comedocarcinoma	Variable
5B	Raggedly infiltrative	Diffusely permeative	Masses and sheets of anaplastic carcinoma, with a few tiny glands or signet ring cells	Small

Case History: A 20-year-old male with enlarged prostate. Case of dysuria.

Diagnosis: Embryonal rhabdomyosarcoma of prostate

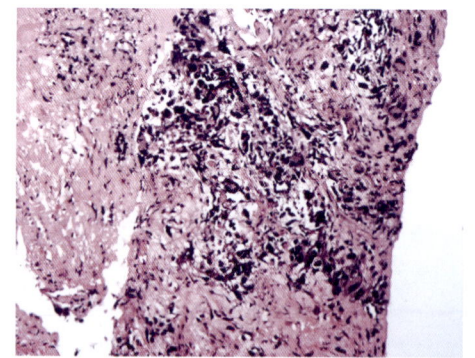

Fig. 13.8

Clinical Features
- Present early when compared to extra-prostatic.
- When growing beneath a mucosal membrane, it forms a polypoid mass resembling bunch of grapes.

Gross
Tumor is poorly circumscribed, white and soft.

Microscopy
- Tumor cells are small and spindle-shaped with acidophilic cytoplasm.
- Highly cellular areas surrounding blood vessels, alternating with paucicellular region with abundant mucoid material.

- Beneath the epithelium, dense zone of undifferentiated tumor cells (Nicholson's cambium layer).
- Cross striations may or may not be present.

Ancillary Tests
- **Immunohistochemistry** Myo-D1, myogenin, desmin, SMA positive.
- **Molecular genetics:** Embryonal—gain of chromosome 2, 8, 13. Alveolar—t(2;13), t(1;13).

Differential Diagnosis
- Pseudosarcomatous fibromyxoid tumor
- Small cell carcinoma
- Lymphoma

Case History: A 50-year-old male with complaints of dysuria.

Diagnosis: Urothelial carcinoma prostate

Clinical Features
- Primary in proximal prostatic duct.
- CIS in urethra and serum PSA increased in some.

Microscopy

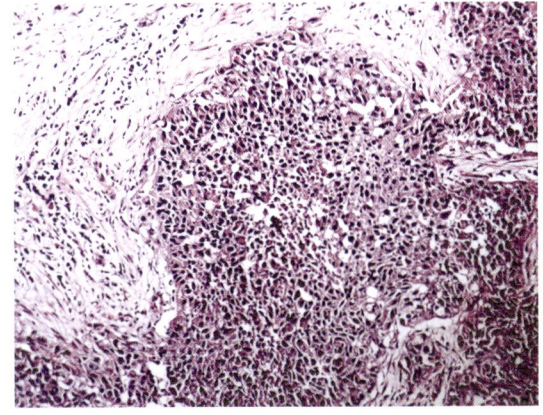

Fig. 13.9

- Carcinoma *in situ* marked nuclear pleomorphism, frequent mitosis, apoptotic bodies.
- Pagetoid spread between basal cells and secretory.

Immunohistochemistry
- Poorly differentiated adenocarcinoma prostate:
  - *Positive stain:* PSA and PRAP
  - *Negative stain:* HMWCK (34βE12 clone), p63, CK7, CK20
- Urothelial carcinoma:
  - *Positive stain:* CK7, CK20, HMWCK, p63
  - *Negative stain:* PSA and PRAP.

Differential Diagnosis
- Poorly differentiated adenocarcinoma prostate arising from bladder neck.
- Poorly differentiated urothelial carcinoma bladder with prostatic extension.

Case History: A 57-year-old male with complaints of difficulty in voiding urine and penile pain.

Diagnosis: Squamous cell carcinoma penis

Clinical Features
- 20–90 years.
- Present with exophytic/ulcerated mass.
- Penile pain, difficulty in voiding.

Gross
Exophytic/ulcerated mass.

Microscopy

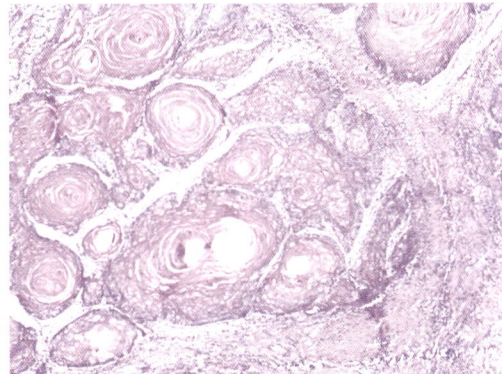

Fig. 13.10

- Well moderately to poorly differentiated carcinoma.
- Superficially invasive tumor—well differentiated.

- Deeply invasive tumor—poorly differentiated.
- Tumor can show spindle, pleomorphic, acantholytic, giant, basaloid or clear cells.

Variants
- Verrucous carcinoma
- Warty carcinoma
- Papillary carcinoma NOS
- Basaloid carcinoma
- Pseudohyperplastic non-verruciform
- SCC
- Sarcomatoid carcinoma
- Adenosquamous carcinoma
- Mixed carcinoma

Differential Diagnosis
Pseudoepitheliomatous hyperplasia.

Case History: A 54-year-old male with complaints of difficulty in voiding urine.

Diagnosis: Verrucous carcinoma

Clinical Features
- Middle aged
- Site: Foreskin, glans

Gross
Large, fungating, ulcerated warty lesion starts at coronal sulcus and spread to glans and preputial skin.

Microscopy

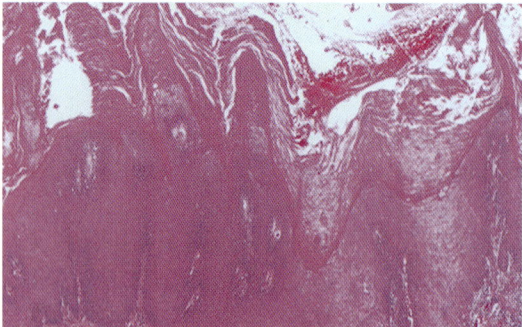

Fig. 13.11

- Exophytic/endophytic papillary growth.
- Well-differentiated papillary neoplasm with acanthosis and hyperkeratosis.
- Broad-based bulbous lesion. No fibrovascular core.
- Bland vesicular nuclei.
- Mitosis confined to the base.

Differential Diagnosis
- Condyloma acuminatum
- Warty carcinoma
- Keratinizing SCC.

Case History: A 50-year-old male with complaints of difficulty in voiding urine.

Diagnosis: High grade dysplasia and carcinoma *in situ* penis

Erythroplasia of Queyrat
Site
- Occurs in glans/prepuce
- Rare in urethral meatus.

Gross
Shiny, elevated, reddish, velvety, erythematous plaque. Can be solitary or multiple.

Microscopy

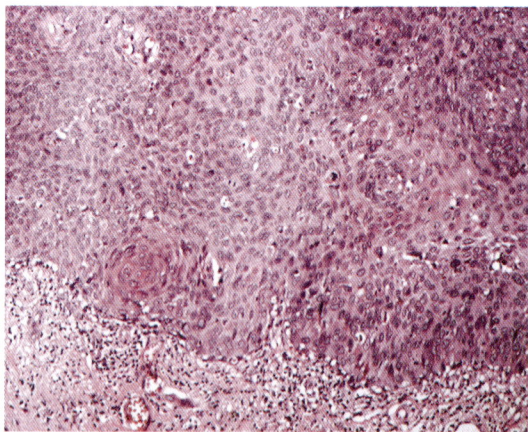

Fig. 13.12

Loss of polarity. Proliferation of large hyperchromatic cells, dyskeratosis and numerous mitosis.

Bowen's Disease
Site
Shaft of penis.

Gross

Demarcated scaly plaques.

Microscopy

- Hyperkeratosis
- Involves pilosebaceous unit.

Bowenoid Papulosis

Site

Penile shaft, perineum.

Gross

Multicentric, involves sweat gland.

Microscopy

Hyperkeratosis, parakeratosis, papillomatosis. Surface maturation more than Bowen's disease and EQ.

Case History: A 31-year-old male with complaints of difficulty in voiding urine with high PSA.

Diagnosis: Granulomatous prostatitis

Definition

Granulomas involving the prostate can be due to:
- Tuberculosis
- Non-specific due to foreign body reaction to ruptured prostatic secretions.
- Post-biopsy granulomas
- Allergic causes
- Post-BCG (immunotherapy) for bladder carcinoma.

Microscopy

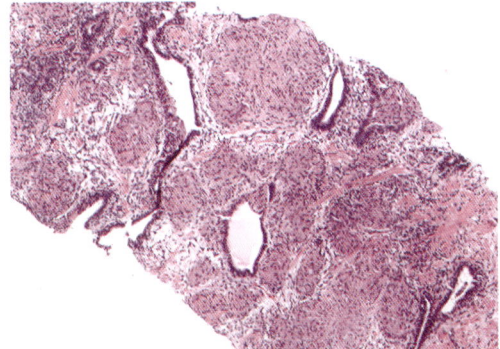

Fig. 13.13

- Lobular, dense infiltrate of lymphocytes, plasma cells, histiocytes and multinucleated giant cells mixed with neutrophils and eosinophils.
- Caseating or non-caseating granulomas.
- Post-biopsy and allergic granulomas can have necrobiotic granulomas.

Case History: A 38-year-old male with complaints of scrotal swelling.

Diagnosis: Adenomatoid tumor

Clinical Features

- 30% of testicular adnexal tumors.
- Usually 3rd to 5th decades.
- Most commonly lower pole of epididymis; also tunica vaginalis, spermatic cord.
- Presents as solid, well-circumscribed mass in scrotum, often associated with pain.
- Usually 1–5 cm, rarely larger benign, even if it extends into testis.

Gross

- 1–5 cm, well-circumscribed solid tumor, adherent to testis/testicular adnexa.
- Cut surface may have small cystic spaces.

Microscopy

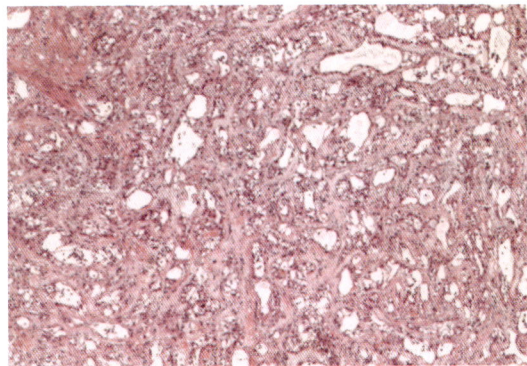

Fig. 13.14

- No distinct growth pattern.
- Unencapsulated, cuboidal to flat cells forming cords that are either epithelial-like or form channels with dilated lumina simulating vessels.

- Cells have acidophilic cytoplasm with cytoplasmic vacuoles.
- Nuclei lack nucleoli. Mitoses and necrosis are usually absent.
- Intervening stroma may have smooth muscle and elastic fibers, desmoplastic quality and inflammatory cells.
- Rarely, tumor may extend into testicular parenchyma or even rarer, be totally inside the testis.
- *Most tumors show a mixture of* adenomatoid (tubular), angiomatoid (canalicular), solid (plexiform) and cystic (mixed).

Immunohistochemistry
- **Positive stains:** Calretinin, pan cytokeratins (EMA, AE1/AE3, CAM 5.2)
- **Variable, focal to diffuse:** CK5/6, CK7.

Differential Diagnosis
- **Malignant mesothelioma:** HBME1+, mitoses and necrosis.
- **Metastatic adenocarcinoma:** Positive for one or more of CEA, PSA, MOC31/BerEP4 and CD15 are useful.
- **Papillary cystadenoma of epididymis.**

CHAPTER 14

Diseases of the Female Genital Tract

MP Kanchana, Divya D

Case History: A 14-year-old female with left ovary.

Diagnosis: Gonadal dysgenesis

Terminology
- *Streak testis:* Streak tissue identified at periphery of differentiated testis.
- *Streak gonad:* Ovarian-type stroma without differentiated gonadal structures.

Microscopy

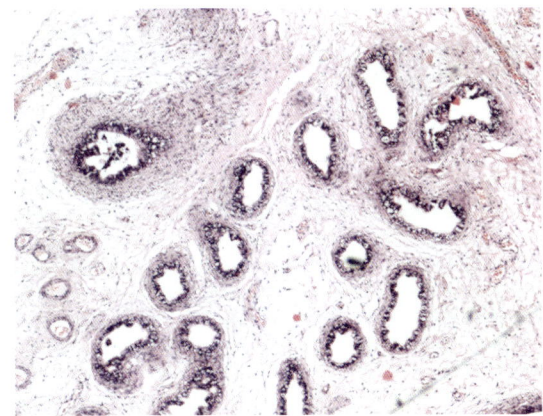

Fig. 14.1

- Prepubertal patients show normal immature testis.
- At/after puberty, tubules exhibit mild hypospermatogenesis to total sclerosis.
- Streak gonad has ovarian stroma without primordial ovarian follicles.
- Streak ovary is streak gonad with primordial follicles and primitive sex cord-like structures with or without germ cell components within the ovarian-type stroma, mimicking gonadoblastoma, granulosa cell tumor or Sertoli cell tumors.

Differential Diagnosis
True hermaphroditism.

Case History: A 65-year-old female with abdominal pain since one year. CECT—solid cystic mass (M) 4 × 4 cm in left ovary. CA 125–85.9 U/ml. Clinical diagnosis—Ca ovary. TAH with BSO: Left ovarian mass.

Diagnosis: Borderline papillary serous cystadenofibroma—ovary

Gross
- Partially cystic with watery or mucinous cyst fluid with intracystic or surface soft white to tan cauliflower-like papillary projections.
- Gross examination is not reliable to distinguish benign, borderline and malignant.

Microscopy

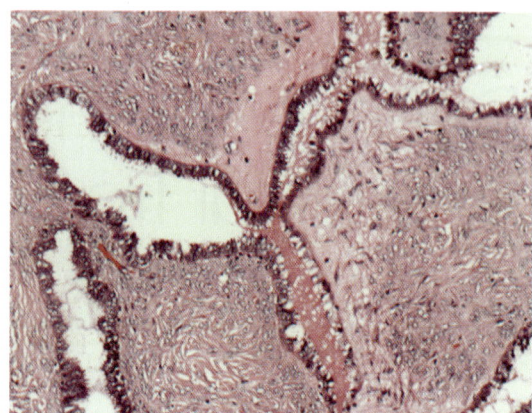

Fig. 14.2

- Broad, branching papillae (hierarchical branching) focally covered by stratified epithelium with mild to moderate atypia with a few mitoses.
- Some cells appear free floating as an artifact of sectioning.
- Epithelial cells may be columnar, polygonal or round with moderate to abundant eosinophilic cytoplasm.
- Cilia or surface snouts may be present.
- Intracystic spaces may be clear or contain mucin.
- Stroma is fibrous and edematous with variable psammoma bodies.
- Various patterns: Cribriform, individual eosinophilic cells and cell clusters, simple and non-complex branching papillae, inverted macropapillae and micropapillae.
- No stromal invasion; but may be associated with low-grade serous carcinoma, which does have destructive stromal invasion with an associated stromal reaction.
- Be careful not to confuse tangential sectioning with invasion.
- Pathology reports should describe surface involvement, microinvasion, micropapillary or cribriform growth, nodal metastases, invasive implants.

Differential Diagnosis

- Benign serous papillary cystadenoma
- Serous carcinoma
- Mucinous borderline tumors
- Ovarian clear cell carcinoma.

Case History: A 60-year-old female with left ovarian mass (M) 20 × 15 cm with ascites. TAH with BSO. Left ovarian mass.

Diagnosis: Borderline mucinous neoplasm with Brenner's component

Clinical Features

- Pure borderline tumors and borderline tumors with intraepithelial carcinoma or microinvasion are almost always stage I and clinically benign, but must sample tumor extensively to rule out more extensive invasion.
- High stage borderline tumors with abdominal cavity mucin may represent ovarian metastases rather than primary borderline tumors—must examine appendix to correctly interpret.

Microscopy

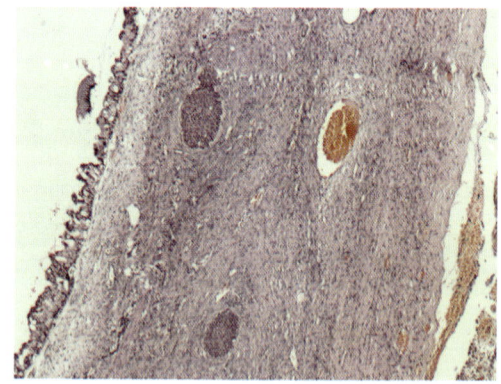

Fig. 14.3

Intestinal Type

- Resemble dysplastic intestinal epithelium with goblet cells, neuroendocrine cells and occasional Paneth cells.
- Neoplastic cells have hyperchromasia, crowding, increased mitosis, stratification forming papillae with thin fibrous cores.

- Lumens contain mucin.
- Stroma may have a brisk inflammatory reaction with histiocytes and large areas of necrosis.

Endocervical Type
- Contain broad papillae lined by benign appearing stratified mucinous and eosinophilic endocervical-like cells.
- Brisk neutrophilic response.
- Intraepithelial carcinoma and microinvasion are rare.

Case History: A 45-year-old female with ovarian mass.

Diagnosis: Clear cell carcinoma

Clinical Features
- Clear cell carcinoma most commonly associated with vascular thrombotic events and paraneoplastic hypercalcemia.
- Fifth to seventh decades.

Gross
- Thick-walled unilocular cyst with multiple yellow beigè fleshy nodules.
- May present as single fleshy nodule in an endometriotic cyst (25%) with chocolate brown fluid.

Microscopy

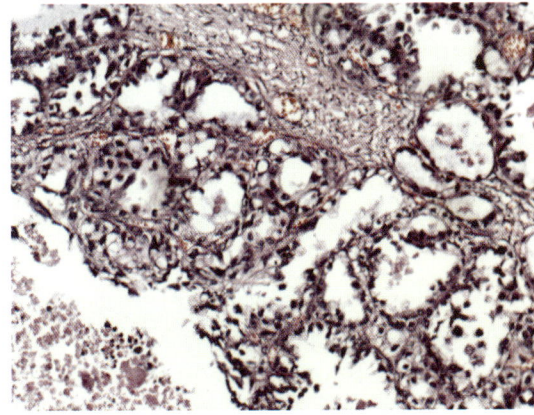

Fig. 14.4

Architecture
- Tubulocystic
- Papillary
- Solid
- CCC may arise from cyst in the background.
- Papillary pattern is more associated with endometriosis.
- Adenofibroma background is seen in tubulocystic pattern.
- Solid pattern shows polyhedral or hobnail cells with abundant clear and/or eosinophilic granular cytoplasm.

Ancillary Tests
- **Special stain:** PAS positive in hyaline globules.
- **Immunohistochemistry:** CK7, CK20, EMA and CD15 positive.
- Clear cell carcinoma may express AFP.
- **Electron microscopy:** Epithelial cells with abundant glycogen granules and ER. Stubby microvilli on apical surface.

Differential Diagnosis
- Dysgerminoma.
- Rarely struma ovarii.

Case History: A 75-year-old female with abdominal pain and lump since 6 months. MRI suggestive of malignant ovarian mass. CA 125–190 U/ml. Ovarian mass for HPE.

Diagnosis: Fibrothecoma

Clinical Features
- Common; benign; arise after puberty.
- 40% of tumors >6 cm are associated with ascites.
- Also associated with right-sided hydrothorax, Meigs syndrome and basal cell nevus syndrome.

Gross
Mean 6 cm, usually unilateral, solid, lobulated, firm, white and may have myxoid change.

Microscopy

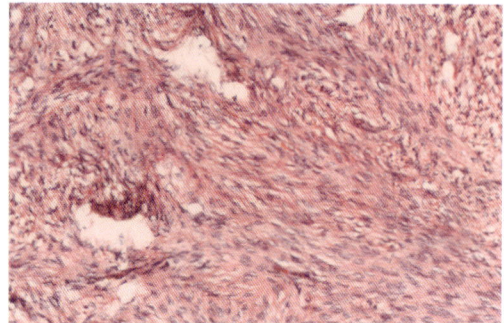

Fig. 14.5

- Closely packed spindle cells in "feather-stitched" or storiform pattern.
- May have hyaline bands and edema; no atypia.
- Spindle cells with moderate pale cytoplasm containing lipid droplets and central nuclei.
- Intervening stroma has collagen deposition and focal hyaline plaque formation.

Positive Stains

- WT1, ER, PR, SMA, occasional S-100 and CD34.
- Oil red O or Sudan black (fat stains) on fresh/frozen tissue.

Differential Diagnosis

- Brenner tumor
- Cellular fibroma
- Fibromatosis
- Fibrosarcoma
- Krukenberg tumor
- Massive edema

Case History: A 48-year-old female with ovarian mass (M) 12 × 10 cm with ascites. CA125–4.08 U/ml.

Diagnosis: Granulosa cell tumor with Sertoli cell component

Gross

- Size: 1 to 30 (average 12) cm.
- Predominantly solid or solid and cystic.
- Rarely uni- or multilocular cyst. Yellow-white cut surface.
- Frequent areas of hemorrhage.

Microscopy

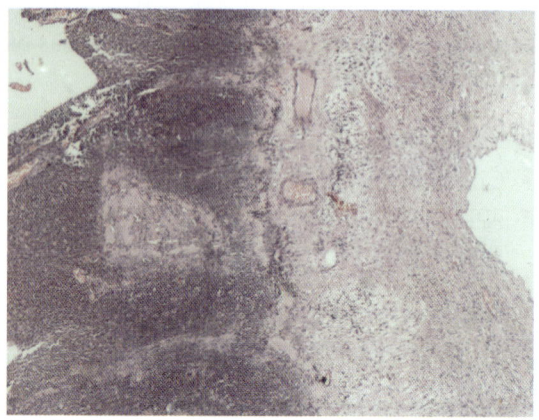

Fig. 14.6

- *Patterns:* Diffuse, trabecular, microfollicular (Call-Exner bodies), macrofollicular, insular, gyriform, and watered-silk growth patterns.
- Proliferation of granulosa cells in a fibro-thecomatous background. Cells with scant cytoplasm and round to oval nuclei with a longitudinal groove.
- Minimal cytologic atypia and low mitotic rate (typically 5/10 HPFs).
- *Sertoli cell component:* Closely packed solid or hollow tubules lined by well-differentiated cuboidal to columnar epithelial cells. Other patterns include cord-like and diffuse; variable stroma. Occasional cells with bizarre nuclei; minimal mitoses, minimal atypia.

Ancillary Tests

- **Histochemistry:** Reticulin surrounds groups of cells.
- **Immunohistochemistry:** Inhibin, calretinin, CD99, CD56, and vimentin positive. Keratin, CD10, S-100, WT-1, smooth-muscle actin, and desmin can be positive EMA and CK7 negative.

Case History: A 68-year-old female with ovarian mass, CA ovary.

Diagnosis: Dysgerminoma

Laboratory Investigations

Elevation of serum hCG levels.

Gross
- Well-encapsulated tumor.
- Unilateral in 90% cases.
- Tumors average 15 cm in maximal dimension.
- *Cut surface:* Solid, uniform or lobular and creamy white or light tan. Irregular areas of coagulative necrosis may be present.
- May be associated with cystic change or macroscopic calcification.

Microscopy

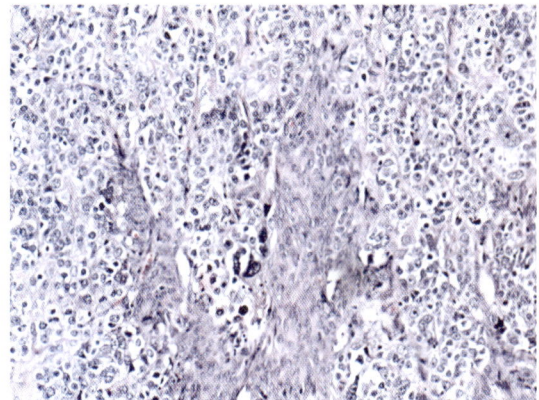

Fig. 14.7

- Proliferating germ cells have a monotonous appearance with polygonal shape, abundant pale cytoplasm and fairly uniform nuclei.
- They aggregate in cords and clumps, although sometimes the lack of cohesion between cells may lead to the formation of pseudoglandular spaces.
- Stroma is usually reduced to thin perivascular sheaths, occasionally it can be abundant.
- It always contains variable amounts of chronic inflammatory infiltrate, mainly T lymphocytes and macrophages.
- Epithelioid granulomas are a prominent feature in a quarter of cases.

Immuohistochemistry
Vimentin, PLAP, CD117.

Case History: A 20-year-old female with abdominal pain and distension—20 days, abdominal mass occupying M/S 19 × 15 × 7 cm. CA 125–57 U/ml. AFP and β-hCG are WNL. Clinical diagnosis—dermoid ovary. Right oophorectomy done.

Diagnosis: Mature cystic teratoma with gliomatosis peritonei

Gross
- Usually 10 cm.
- Cystic cut section with abundant hair and sebaceous material.
- Solid mural nodule (Rokitansky protuberance) associated with teeth and bone. 10% bilateral.

Microscopy

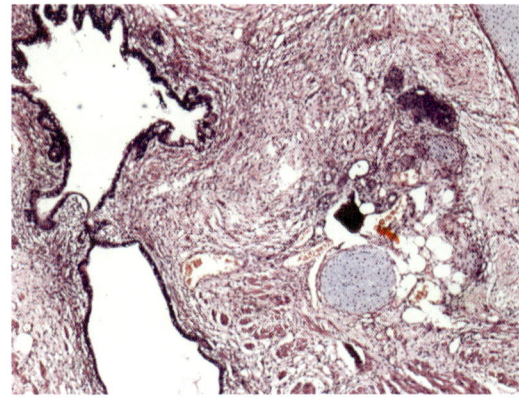

Fig. 14.8

- Mature tissue from all germ layers recapitulating normal composition of different organs—sieve-like pattern resulting from lipogranulomatous reaction.

Unusual Findings
These include:
- Prominent vascular proliferation.
- Microscopic foci of immature neural tissue.
- Granulomatous peritonitis.
- Melanosis peritonei.
- Benign tumors and secondary malignancies.
- Gliomatosis peritonei.

Differential Diagnosis
Immature teratoma.

Case History: A 16-year-old female with lower abdominal pain since last 2 months. CECT: Right adnexal mass. AFP levels. β-hCG and LDH were WNL.

Diagnosis: Yolk sac tumor

Lab Investigations
Elevated serum levels of AFP and CA 125.

Gross
- Unilateral, large, solid gray to tan.
- Honeycomb (microcystic) appearance in polyvesicular vitelline variant. Associated with mature cystic teratoma often identified by calcifications (15%).
- Unilateral, large, solid gray to tan.

Microscopy

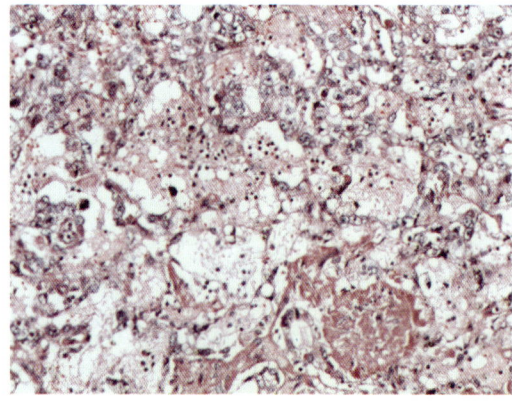

Fig. 14.9

- *Patterns:* Reticular or microcystic patterns formed by a loose network of flat/cuboidal cells.
- *Polyvesicular vitelline pattern* in 25%; vesicular structures with eccentric constrictions surrounded by a dense spindle cell stroma; may have better prognosis in pure form.
- *Other patterns:* Endometrioid (rare), hepatoid, glandular, intestinal differentiation, parietal, solid, undifferentiated.
- *Schiller:* Duval body is pathognomonic—central blood vessel enveloped by germ cells within a space similarly lined by germ cells, resembles glomerulus. Hyaline droplets present in all tumors.

Ancillary Studies
- PAS positive
- AFP and 1-antitrypsin positive, typically only focal
- Cytokeratin and CD34 positive
- CEA positive in glandular and hepatoid variant
- Hyaline globules PAS-diastase positive, AFP and 1-antitrypsin negative.

Differential Diagnosis
- Clear cell carcinoma
- Endometrioid carcinoma, secretory variant
- Dysgerminoma
- Hepatoid carcinoma and hepatocellular carcinoma
- Sertoli-Leydig cell tumor, retiform variant.

Case History: A 21-year-old female with abdominal pain since 1 year. Serum AFP levels TAH with BSO; ovarian mass.

Diagnosis: Immature teratoma

Clinical Features
- Usually prepubertal or young women (mean 18 years).
- Most recurrences within 2 years.

Gross
Bulky, solid or cystic with necrosis, hemorrhage.

Microscopy

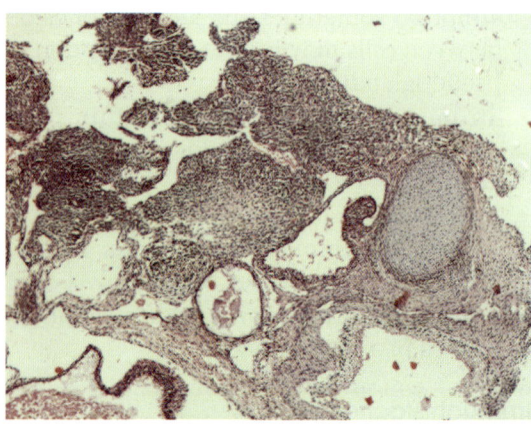

Fig. 14.10

- Usually neurogenic elements (GFAP+); mesodermal elements common; some tumors derived primarily of esophageal, liver and intestinal structures (endodermal).
- *Grading:* Norris grading system (correlates best with extraovarian spread, survival)
  1. Abundant mature tissue, loose mesenchymal tissue with occasional mitoses, immature cartilage and tooth anlage.
  2. Less mature tissue than grade 1, rare foci of neuroepithelium with mitoses, <4 low power fields in any one slide.
  3. A little/no mature tissue; numerous neuroepithelial elements merging with cellular stroma occupying 4+ low power fields.

Case History: A 36-year-old female with abdominal pain since last 1 month. CECT: Ovarian mass with calcification. CA125–62 U/ml staging laparotomy done.

Diagnosis: Struma ovarii

Clinical Features
- May show pathologic changes of thyroid gland including hyperfunctioning.
- Malignancies are usually papillary thyroid carcinoma.
- Associated with mucinous cystadenoma, Brenner tumor, carcinoid tumor and dermoid cyst.

Gross
Resembles red-brown thyroid tissue but usually multilocular cystic; usually unilateral.

Microscopy

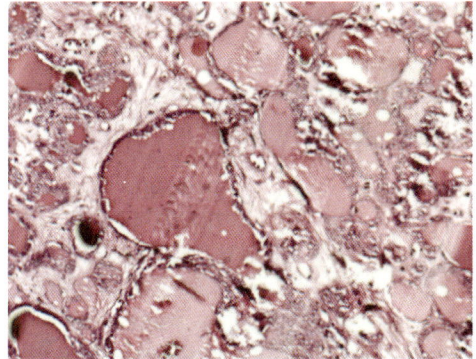

Fig. 14.11

- Thyroid follicles with colloid; other teratomatous elements may be present.
- Rarely has solid or pseudotubular patterns, microfollicles, abundant eosinophilic cytoplasm, abundant clear cytoplasm or minimal thyroid follicles.

Positive Stains
Thyroglobulin.

Differential Diagnosis
Metastatic thyroid carcinoma to ovary.

Case History: A 53-year-old female, known case of carcinoma stomach post-surgery and chemotherapy in 2012 with case of bleeding per vagina and right adnexal mass.

Diagnosis: Signet ring cell carcinoma

Clinical Features
- The term Krukenberg tumor refers to a metastatic mucinous/signet ring cell adenocarcinoma of the ovaries which typically originates from primary tumors of the GI tract, most often colon and stomach.

Tumors can spread to the ovary by several pathways:
- Direct spread
- Transcoelomic dissemination
- Hematogenous spread
- Lymphatic spread.

Gross
- *Laterality:* Mostly bilateral.
- *Size:* Mostly <10 cm.
- *Surface involvement:* Mostly multiple small nodules on surface.
- *Extensive intra-abdominal spread:* Mostly true for metastatic mucinous tumor.
- Hilar involvement common in hematogenous spread.

Microscopy

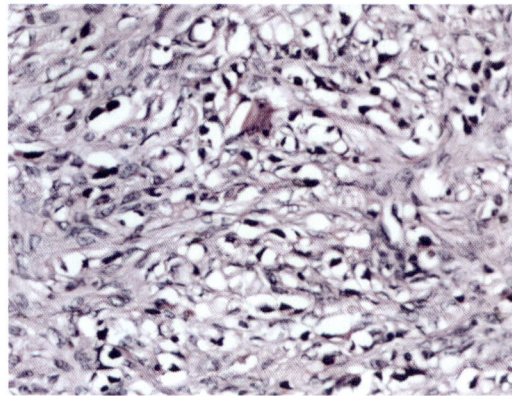

Fig. 14.12

- Multinodular growth pattern with intervening normal ovarian parenchyma.
- Sheets of signet ring cells. Multiple vascular emboli.

Differential Diagnosis

Primary endometrioid or mucinous carcinoma.

Case History: A 57-year-old female with fever and watery discharge per vagina. Section from fallopian tube and ovary.

Diagnosis: Granulomatous inflammation

Clinical Features

- Usually involves both fallopian tubes.
- Hematogenous spread occurs.

Microscopy

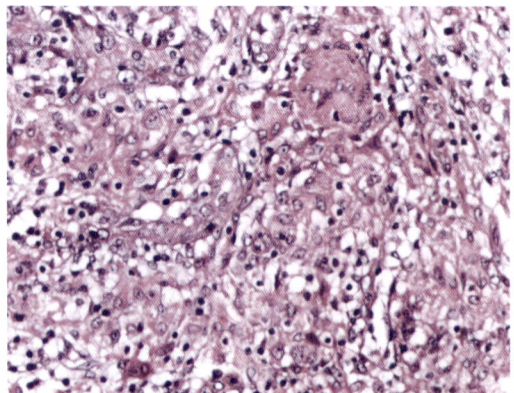

Fig. 14.13

- Caseating granulomas within mucosa.
- Extreme adenomatous proliferation may resemble carcinoma.
- Chronic inflammation and fibrosis in the muscle layer.

Case History: A 23-year-old female with abdominal pain and hemoperitoneum. Left salpingectomy specimen.

Diagnosis: Ectopic pregnancy

Sites

Ampulla (~80%), isthmus (12%), fimbriae (5%), cornu (2%).

Gross

Distension of tube with thin or ruptured wall, dusky red serosa and hematosalpinx, possibly with fetal parts identified.

Microscopy

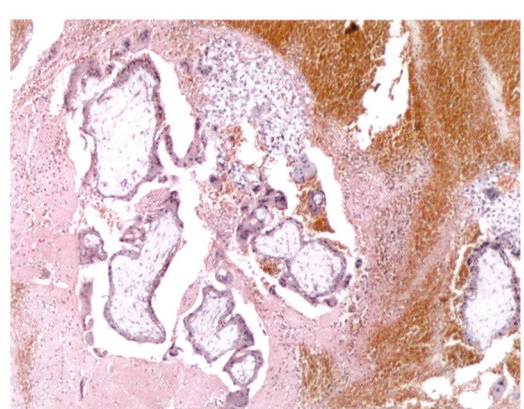

Fig. 14.14

- Intraluminal chorionic villi and extravillous trophoblast (may be degenerated); variable fetal parts.
- Decidual change in lamina propria in 1/3rd; mesothelial reactive proliferation with papillary formation and psammoma bodies.
- *Uterus:* Gestational hyperplasia with Arias-Stella reaction, no enlarged, hyalinized spiral arteries, no fibrinoid matrix.

Differential Diagnosis

- Missed abortion
- Incomplete abortion.

Case History: A 29-year-old female, products of conception for histopathological examination.

Diagnosis: Partial mole

Clinical Features
- Vaginal bleeding is the presenting symptom.
- β-hCG is usually increased but some patients have normal or decreased levels.

Gross
- Volume of tissue is small.
- Villi are smaller than complete mole.
- Fetal parts or fetal membranes may be present.

Microscopy

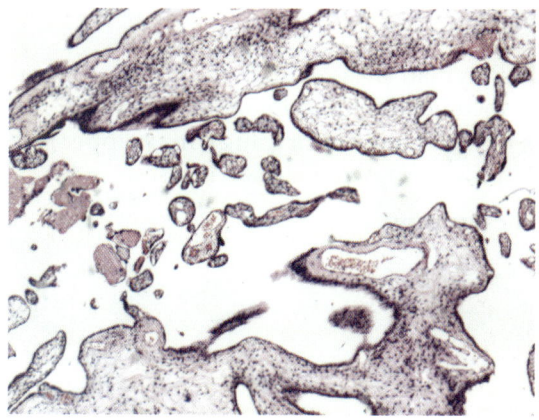

Fig. 14.15

- Molar changes are focal.
- Mixture of edematous and normal shaped villi.
- Trophoblastic hyperplasia is less marked, scalloped pattern of the enlarged villi yielding a pattern of trophoblastic invagination into villous stroma.
- Presence of fetal structures.

Differential Diagnosis
- Complete mole
- Nonmolar hydropic abortion
- Hydropic abortus
- Choriocarcinoma
- Placental site trophoblastic tumor.

Case History: A 55-year-old female, uterine mass M/S 20 × 15 cm. Hysterectomy done.

Diagnosis: Symplastic leiomyoma

Clinical Features
- Also called bizarre or atypical leiomyoma.
- Associated with progestin use.
- Benign behavior, but rarely leiomyosarcomas may arise from them.

Microscopy

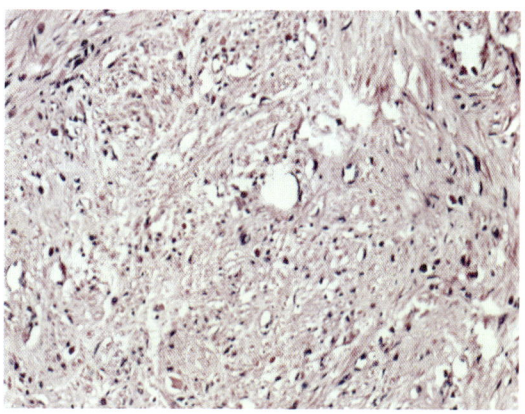

Fig. 14.16

- Large, bizarre multinucleated tumor cells, atypical nuclei in otherwise normal appearing leiomyoma.
- No/rare mitotic figures.
- Moderate/severe atypia, less than 10 mitotic figures/10 HPF and NO tumor cell necrosis.

Immunohistochemistry
Vimentin, desmin and SMA.

Case History: A 51-year-old female with friable mass in the endometrial cavity M/S 4.5 × 3.2 × 2.8 cm. Radical hysterectomy done.

Diagnosis: Endometrioid adenocarcinoma

Clinical Features
- Most women are postmenopausal as the disease is relatively uncommon in young women.
- The initial manifestation of endometrial carcinoma usually is abnormal vaginal bleeding.

Gross

- The endometrial surface is shaggy, glistening and tan and may be focally hemorrhagic.
- It is almost uniformly exophytic even when deeply invasive.
- The neoplasm may be focal or diffuse.
- Sometimes, it can present as polypoidal masses.
- Myometrial invasion by carcinoma results in enlargement of uterus.
- Myometrial invasions appear as well demarcated, firm, grey white tissue with linear extensions beneath an exophytic mass or as multiple white nodules with yellow areas of necrosis.

Microscopy

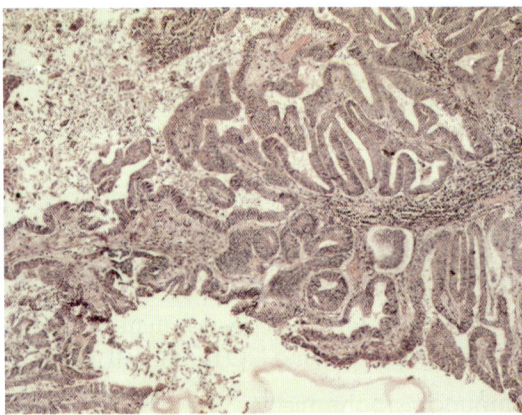

Fig. 14.17

- Crowded, complex branching glands with cribriform architecture and back-to-back glands without intervening stroma.
- Loss of polarity and cytologic atypia: Large, round nuclei with prominent nucleoli, nuclear membrane condensation.
- Glands may infiltrate into the myometrium, inducing a desmoplastic response.
- The microscopic appearances of endometrioid carcinoma are determined by the grade of the tumor.
- Grade of tumor is based on architectural pattern, nuclear features.
  Grade 1: No more than 5% of the tumor is composed of solid masses.
  Grade 2: 6 to 50% of the tumor is composed of solid masses.
  Grade 3: More than 50% of the tumor is composed of solid masses.

Differential Diagnosis

- Endometrial hyperplasia
- Metastatic adenocarcinoma
- Atypical polypoid adenomyoma

Case History: A 42-year-old female with case of dysmenorrhea. USG suggestive of fibroid uterus.

Diagnosis: Endometrial stromal sarcoma

Gross

- Polypoid mass extending into broad ligament, ovaries and fallopian tubes.
- Lymphatic tumor plugs may appear as yellow, ropy or ball-like masses.

Microscopy

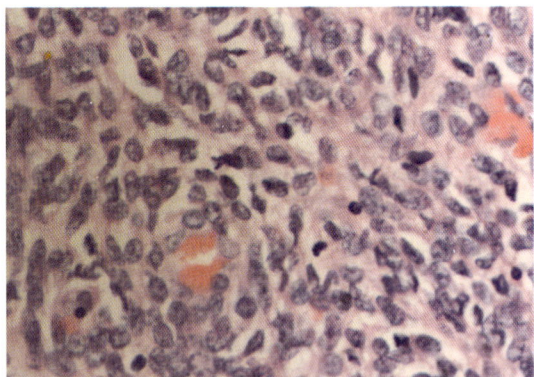

Fig. 14.18

- Monotonous ovoid to spindly cells with minimal cytoplasm intimately associated with prominent arterioles, closely resembles proliferative endometrial stroma.
- Up to 10–15 mitotic figures per 10 HPF in most active areas. Tongue-like infiltration between muscle bundles of myometrium.
- Angiolymphatic invasion common.

Immunohistochemistry

- *Positive stains:* CD10 and vimentin positive. Cytokeratin shows focal positivity.
- EMA, SMA and desmin are negative.

Differential Diagnosis

- Stromal nodule
- Adenomyosis with sparse glands
- Cellular leiomyoma
- Metastatic lobular carcinoma
- Pseudosarcomatous changes in the stroma.
- Fragmented lymphoid follicles in biopsies or curettings.
- Intravascular leiomyomatosis.

Case History: A 46-year-old female with case of pain abdomen and menorrhagia. CECT: Suggestive of fibroid uterus.

Diagnosis: Leiomyosarcoma

Clinical Features

Peaks at ages 40–69 years; mean is 54 years.

Gross

- Bulky fleshy tumor invading into myometrial wall or polypoid tumor projecting into lumen.
- Often hemorrhagic or necrotic.
- Grossly appears invasive/infiltrative. Usually 5 cm or more, but not multiple.

Microscopy

- Hypercellular with spindle cells resembling smooth muscle with moderate to severe pleomorphism. Infiltrative border is most helpful feature for diagnosis.
- 10+ mitotic figures per 10 high power fields (HPF) in most mitotically active area with abundant abnormal mitotic figures.
- Coagulative tumor cell necrosis is common.
- Rarely contains osteoclast-like giant cells.
- Epithelioid and myxoid leiomyosarcomas are rare variants with mild nuclear atypia and often <3 mitotic figures/10 HPF.
- Smooth muscle tumors of uncertain malignant potential (STUMP): Tumor cell necrosis in a typical leiomyoma; necrosis of uncertain type with ≤10 MF/10 HPFs or marked diffuse atypia; marked diffuse or focal atypia with borderline mitotic counts and necrosis difficult to classify.

Immunohistochemistry

Positive stains: Smooth muscle actin, myosin, desmin, Ki-67, ER, PR, EMA, h-caldesmon, keratin, p53, focal CD10, histone deacetylase 8, androgen receptor (variable), and c-kit (variable).

Differential Diagnosis

- Endometrial stromal sarcoma with smooth muscle metaplasia.
- Mitotically active leiomyoma
- Cellular leiomyoma
- Hemorrhagic leiomyoma and hormone-induced changes
- Leiomyoma with bizarre nuclei (atypical leiomyoma)
- Myxoid leiomyoma
- Epithelioid leiomyoma
- Leiomyoma with massive lymphoid infiltration

Case History: A 59-year-old female with pain abdomen and vomiting since last 3 days. CECT: Ovarian mass with ascites and omental thickening. CA125–600 U/ml.

Diagnosis: MMMT predominantly epithelial with heterologous component

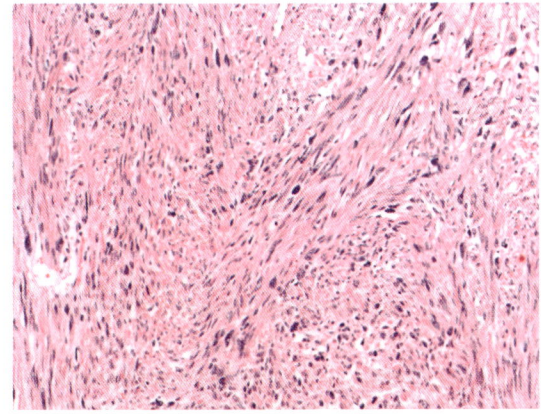

Fig. 14.19

Clinical Features

- Rare, almost always in postmenopausal women (median age 65 years).
- Associated with chronic estrogen stimulation and radiation therapy.
- Other predisposing factors include nulliparity, diabetes, obesity.

Gross

- MMMTs are frequently polypoidal and usually fills the entire endometrial cavity.
- Many invade the myometrium and some are confined to polyps.
- The protruding tip of the tumor is necrotic.
- The tumors are soft to firm with necrosis and hemorrhage.

Microscopy

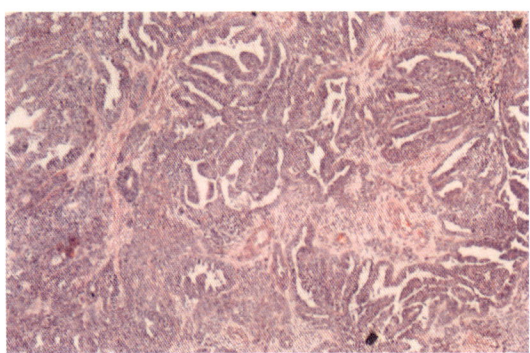

Fig. 14.20

- MMMTs are composed of intimate admixtures of histological malignant epithelial and mesenchymal components.
- The most common type of epithelial component is endometrioid carcinomas which is often accompanied by squamous differentiation.
- Half the cases demonstrate the homologous type of stromal component, which is high grade endometrial stromal sarcoma or fibrosarcoma in most and occasionally leiomyosarcoma.
- When heterologous elements present rhabdomyosarcoma and chondrosarcoma are the most common types encountered.

Ancillary Tests

- **Immunohistochemistry:** Positive for cytokeratin and epithelial membrane antigen.
- **Molecular genetics:** p53 alteration occurs early before clonal expansion. Loss of heterozygosity involving 17p, 17q, 11q, 15q and 21q. Overexpression of c-myc. Altered methylation of H19 gene. Mutations (loss of immunostaining): PTEN (39%), MLH1 (33%), MSH2 (22%), MSH6 (21%); p53 overexpression.

Differential Diagnosis

Squamous cell carcinoma with sarcoma like stroma.

Case History: A 57-year-old female with case of white discharge per vagina since 1 week and post-menopausal bleeding. Cervical biopsy for interpretation.

Diagnosis: Amoebic cervicitis

Clinical Features

Most patients present with foul-smelling, bloody, purulent, or serosanguineous vaginal discharge.

Microscopy

- The diagnosis can be made by cervical smear, wet preparation, culture, or biopsy.
- Cervical cytology and wet preparation are convenient and reliable for screening purposes especially in endemic zones.
- The characteristic morphology of amoebic trophozoite is spherical to oval (15–20 m diameter), with a thin cell membrane and single nucleus having a prominent nuclear border and karyosome.
- The cytoplasm is vacuolated, which leads to confusion with macrophages. The presence of trophozoites containing red blood cells is indicative of tissue invasion.
- Cytochemistry with periodic acid–Schiff stains the cytoplasm of the trophozoites magenta red in tissue sections.

- Heidenhain's iron hematoxylin can also be done, a process that stains the trophozoites black.
- Immunoperoxidase staining is also helpful in making a diagnosis.
- Sensitive serological tests and nucleic acid amplification tests are now available to diagnose amoebiasis.

Case History: A 35-year-old female with cervical growth. Epithelioid trophoblastic tumor. Biopsy from the mass.

Diagnosis: Decidual reaction

Clinical Features
- Also called cervicitis decidualis, deciduosis.
- Multiple small, yellow/red elevations of cervical mucosa.
- Soft, friable, bleed easily; rarely are fungating and resemble carcinoma.

Microscopy

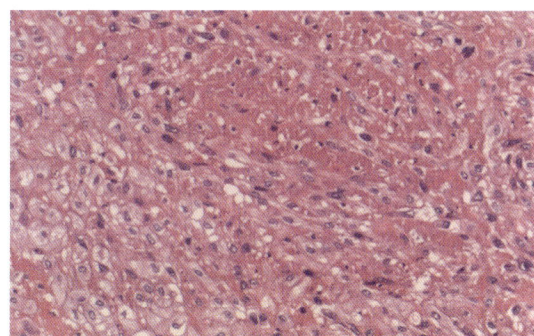

Fig. 14.21

Decidual cells with abundant pale granular cytoplasm, bland nuclei.

Immunohistochemistry
- *Positive stains:* Vimentin, desmin, α_1-antitrypsin. Variable PLAP, β-hCG.
- *Negative stains:* Keratin.

Case History: A 42-year-old female with endocervical polyp. Polypectomy done.

Diagnosis: Microglandular adenosis

Clinical Features
- Common cervical lesion associated with birth control pills or pregnancy in young women, although also in postmenopausal women.
- Usually incidental, may grow as a polypoid mass.

Gross
Polypoid, single or multiple. Early lesions are sessile.

Microscopy
- Complex proliferation of small back-to-back glands lined by cuboidal, columnar or flattened cells with prominent vacuoles above/below vesicular nuclei.
- Indistinct nucleoli, usually no atypia.
- May be associated with immature or mature squamous metaplasia.
- May have areas of solid growth, mucin pools, pseudoinfiltrative pattern, signet ring cells, focal atypia, occasional mitotic figures, acute and chronic inflammation, hobnail cells.

Ancillary Tests
- *Positive stains:* Mucin (vacuoles and lumina).
- *Negative stains:* CEA (usually), CD10, vimentin.

Differential Diagnosis
- Microglandular adenocarcinoma
- Clear cell carcinoma.

Case History: A 46-year-old female with case of bleeding per vagina. O/E ulceroproliferative friable growth cervix M/S 2.5 × 2.5 × 2 cm.

Diagnosis: Adenosquamous carcinoma.

Clinical Features
More common during pregnancy.

Microscopy
- Usually defined as biphasic pattern of well-defined malignant glandular and squamous components clearly identifiable without special stains.

- Glandular component is usually endocervical and poorly differentiated with cytoplasmic vacuoles or luminal mucin; squamous component also is poorly differentiated; if endometrioid it is named as endometrioid carcinoma with squamous differentiation.

Immunohistochemistry

p63 (squamous component), CK7.

Differential Diagnosis

- Squamous cell carcinoma with focal mucin droplets.
- Adenoid basal carcinoma.
- Extension of endometrial adenocarcinoma.
- Adenocarcinoma with coexisting SIL.

Case History: A 38-year-old female with abdominal pain since 6 months. P/S polyp (m) 0.5 × 0.5 cm extending through the OS. Do not bleed on touch. Polypectomy done.

Diagnosis: Glassy cell carcinoma

Clinical Features

- Younger age group (mean 41 years), associated with pregnancy, HPV 18 and 16.
- Historically considered more aggressive with poorer prognosis.
- May have peripheral blood eosinophilia.

Gross

Exophytic mass or barrel-shaped cervix.

Microscopy

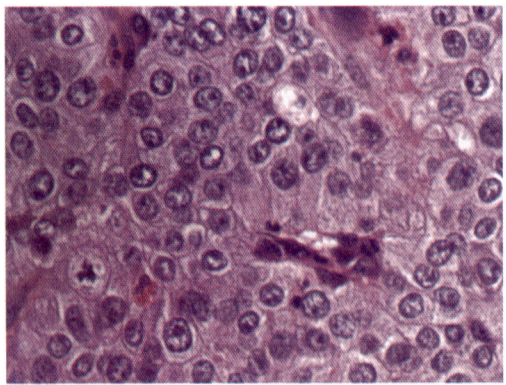

Fig. 14.22

- Solid nests of markedly pleomorphic, polygonal tumor cells with prominent cell membrane, glassy and eosinophilic cytoplasm, large eosinophilic nuclei, prominent nucleoli, surrounded by heavy inflammatory infiltrate containing eosinophils.
- Frequent mitotic figures.
- Pure cases have no histologic evidence of glandular or squamous differentiation (i.e. no intracellular bridges, no dyskeratosis, no intracellular glycogen), which is detectable only by EM.
- Often less invasion that is suspected.

Ancillary Tests

Immunohistochemistry

- *Positive stains:* PAS+ cell wall, vimentin, focal mucin, focal CEA.
- *Negative stains:* p63, HMB45, ER and PR.

Differential Diagnosis

Non-keratinizing squamous cell carcinoma.

Case History: A 40-year-old female with bulky cervix, bleeds on touch. Biopsy taken from the cervical growth.

Diagnosis: Neuroendocrine carcinoma small cell type.

Clinical Features

- Clinically aggressive with rapid metastases; frequently presents with parametrial invasion and pelvic lymph node metastases.
- Mean age 43 years, range 23 to 63 years.
- Associated with HPV 18 occasionally associated with Cushing syndrome or symptoms of other peptide hormones.

Gross

- May be ulcerative and infiltrative.
- Often barrel-shaped cervix.

Microscopy

- Loose aggregates of uniform small cells with indistinct cell borders, scant cytoplasm, hyperchromatic nuclei with fine granular chromatin, nuclear molding,

indistinct nucleoli, extensive mitotic activity, single cell necrosis.
- May form sheets with small acini resembling rosettes.
- Necrosis common
- Vascular invasion in 9%

Ancillary Tests
Immunohistochemistry
Positive stains: NSE (80%), chromogranin (60%), synaptophysin (70%), serotonin, CEA, p16, S-100, keratin (variable). CD56 is sensitive but not specific.
Negative stains: CK20, Rb, p53, p63, CD117/c-kit.

Differential Diagnosis
- Carcinoid tumor.
- Metastatic carcinoma
- Small cell, squamous cell carcinoma.

Case History: A 50-year-old female with bleeding per vagina—1 month. On examination, ulceroproliferative friable growth in the anterior lip of cervix involving the upper 2/3rds of anterior vaginal wall.

Diagnosis: Malignant melanoma

Clinical Features
- Usually presents with vaginal bleeding
- Poor prognosis with historical 5-year survival of 40% with stage I disease.

Gross
Gray-blue-black nodule.

Microscopy
- Often small cell and spindle cell variants.
- Junctional activity present in <50%, variable melanin pigment.
- Stromal infiltration by malignant cells.

Immunohistochemistry
- *Positive stains:* S-100, HMB45, vimentin, Ki-67 (high percentage).
- *Negative stains:* Keratin, CD45, ER, PR.

Differential Diagnosis
Metastatic melanoma.

Case History: A 29-year-old female with G3P2L2, gestational age 36 weeks. Placenta specimen.

Diagnosis: Chorangioma

Gross
- Well circumscribed, purple-red, homogenous mass lesion usually <0.5 cm.
- Often located under chorionic plate and at placental margin.

Microscopy

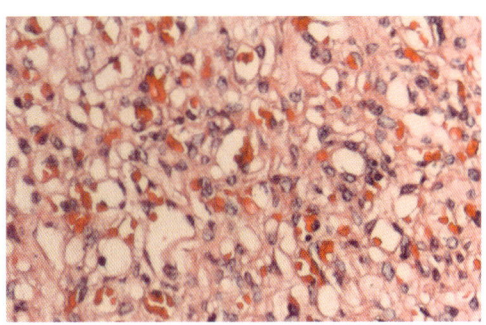

Fig. 14.23

- Well-circumscribed mass of small capillaries lined by benign endothelium, may demonstrate mitoses or degenerative changes.
- May be associated with non-specific trophoblast hyperplasia similar to partial moles, but lesions are not composed of trophoblastic tissue.
- May be capillary, cavernous, cellular, angiomatous, degenerative or atypical.
- Atypical chorangioma: Rare; characterized by increased cellularity and mitotic activity; variable nuclear atypia, necrosis and solid areas; may resemble sarcoma, but benign behavior.
- Positive stains—CK18 (indicates origin from chorionic plate and anchoring villi), CD31, CD34, factor VIII, GLUT1.

Case History: A 25-year-old female premature rupture of membranes.

Diagnosis: Chorioamnionitis

Clinical Features
- Maternal inflammatory response usually due to ascending bacterial infection by

group B streptococci, *Listeria monocytogenes* and fusobacterium.
- Two or more microbes are common.
- May cause premature rupture of membranes.
- Major cause of fetal/neonatal infection, stillbirth, prematurity and perinatal morbidity and mortality.

Gross

- Dull, opaque membranes with yellow-green discoloration and cloudy amniotic fluid, possibly with purulent exudates.
- May be grossly normal.

Microscopy

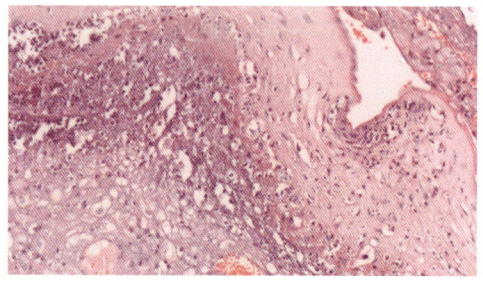

Fig. 14.24

- Neutrophilic infiltrate of free membranes and those overlying the chorionic plate.
- Variable fetal response including funisitis and chorionic plate vasculitis.
- May have acute intervillositis (often due to *Listeria monocytogenes*) or peripheral funisitis (often due to Candida).

Grading

Stage 1 (mild): Acute subchorionitis/acute chorionitis:
- Neutrophils in subchorionic fibrin or interface between decidua and chorion.

Stage 2 (moderate): Acute chorioamnionitis:
- Neutrophils in connective tissue plane between chorion and amnion.

Stage 3 (severe): Necrotizing chorioamnionitis:
- Necrosis, amnion sloughing, thickening of amnion basement membrane and neutrophilic karyorrhexis. Multifocal abscesses may be present.

CHAPTER 15

Soft Tissue Tumors and Tumor-like Lesions

Shalinee Rao, M Susruthan

Soft tissue lesions are better approached by the predominant cell as follows:
- Spindle cell
- Epithelioid
- Pleomorphic
- Round cell
- Biphasic/mixed
- Myxoid

Spindle Cell Nuclear Pattern

Cigar-shaped nuclei—smooth muscle
Pointed ends—fibroblast
Wavy nuclei—nerve

Epithelioid

Granular cell tumor, ASPS, clear cell sarcoma, epithelioid sarcoma, malignant rhabdoid tumor, glomus tumor, GIST.

Pleomorphic

Pleomorphic LMS, RMS, LPS, MFH (NOS), myxofibrosarcoma.

Round cell

Ewing's sarcoma, RMS, round cell LPS, DSCRT, mesenchymal chondrosarcoma.

Biphasic

Synovial sarcoma, myoepithelial carcinoma, GIST, glandular MPNST, dedifferentiated LPS.

The architectural patterns best characterised are:
- Fascicular
- Storiform
- Lobulated
- Plexiform
- Nuclear palisading
- Hemangiopericytoma

Additional Characters

Collagenous stroma, collagen bundles, prominent inflammation, distinctive giant cells, calcification/osteoid, distinct blood vessels.

Immunohistochemistry

General Markers

Vimentin: Antigen integrity

Cytokeratin: Epithelioid sarcoma, synovial sarcoma, DSCRT

Desmin: RMS, LMS, DSCRT

CD99: Ewing's sarcoma, synovial sarcoma, mesenchymal chondrosarcoma, SFT

CD34: SFT, DFSP, spindle cell lipoma

Specific Protein Correlates

Beta catenin: Desmoid type fibromatosis
MDM2: LPS
INI1 loss: Malignant rhabdoid tumor, epithelioid sarcoma.

Translocon Associated Tumors

TFE 3: Alveolar soft part sarcoma
FLI 1: Ewing's sarcoma
ERG: Ewing's sarcoma (small subset)
ALK: Inflammatory myofibroblastic tumor.

Novel Markers

DOG1: GIST
TLE 1: Synovial sarcoma
MUC 4: Low grade fibrosarcoma, sclerosing epithelioid sarcoma.

Case History: A 39-year-old male with painless mass in the lower thigh region.

Diagnosis: Synovial sarcoma

Clinical Features

- Affects young adults.
- 60% are males.
- Long-standing pain and palpable mass.

Imaging

X-ray shows lesional focal calcifications.

Gross

- Well circumscribed, firm and gray pink.
- Bulging and fish flesh appearance.

Microscopy

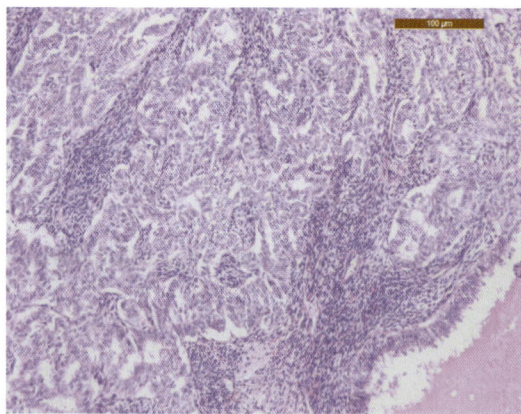

Fig. 15.1

- Biphasic, monophasic and poorly differentiated form.
- *Biphasic form:* Classic type. Distinct 2 components with sarcomatous spindle cells with fibroblasts like appearance and epithelial component made up of plump epithelial-like cells forming glands/nests/cords.
- *Monophasic form:* Lack the epithelial cells. Spindle cells are arranged in plump fascicles with hyalinization and distinct lobulation accompanied by mast cells, occasional osseous or cartilaginous metaplasia, focal whorling.
- *Poorly differentiated form:* Common in elderly. More cellular atypia and mitotic activity. Tumor cells are spindle, small, large or clear. May resemble round cell tumor-like Ewing's sarcoma.

Ancillary Tests

- **Immunohistochemistry**
  Positivity: Vimentin, cytokeratin 7 and 19, EMA, S-100, CD99, BCL-2, TLE-1.
- **Electron microscopy:** Epithelial areas have true glandular epithelium intercellular spaces within processes and specialized cell junctions.
- **Molecular genetics:** All histologic types demonstrate tumor-specific chromosomal translocation t(X; 18) (p11.2; q11) produces fusion genes SYT-SSX1 and SYT-SSX2.
- SYT-SSX1 is biphasic while SYT-SSX2 is monophasic.

Differential Diagnosis

- **Spindle variant resembles other sarcomas.**
- **Metastatic adenocarcinoma:** If primarily epithelial component.
- **MPNST:** Usually negative for CK7 and CK19; negative for SYT-SSX fusion products.

Case History: A 31-year-old female with painful tiny nodule of nailbed of left ring finger.

Diagnosis: Glomus tumor

Epidemiology

Seen in young adults. No sex predilection. Digital and subungual lesions predominant in women. Present in skin in dermis; or subcutis of the upper and lower extremities especially hands and GIT. Rarely occurs in head and neck.

Origin
Arises from modified smooth muscle cell located in the walls of specialized arteriovenous anastamosis (the Sucquet-Hoyer canal) involved temperature regulation.

Clinical Features
Painful red-blue nodules. Can also present clinically as varicosities of the lower extremities. Cutaneous lesions are associated with paroxysmal pain in relation to tactile stimulation. Subungual tumors are exquisitely painful due to abundant nerve fibers. In children, it can be multiple and of infiltrative nature. Solitary and multiple glomus tumor involving digits are associated with von Recklinghausen disease (NF type I).

Gross
Well circumscribed usually <1 cm in diameter.

Microscopy

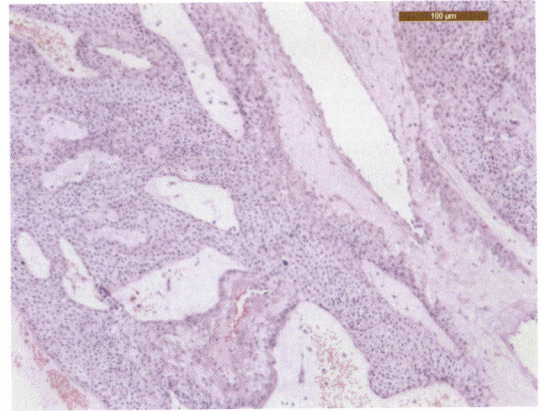

Fig. 15.2

Usually benign in nature and composed of glomus cells, blood vessels and smooth muscles. Glomangiomas are most common accounting for 60% of glomus tumors followed by solid glomus tumors and glomangiomyomas. Glomus cells are round with pale eosinophilic cytoplasm and a large central round or oval punched out uniform nucleus. Cell borders are sharply defined and PAS positive. Surrounding stroma appears edematous can show myxoid degeneration. Small blood vessels are scattered between tumor cells.

Glomangioma: Glomus tumors that resemble cavernous hemangiomas.

Glomangiomyoma: Combines features of glomus tumor and angioleiomyoma.

Glomangiomatosis: Diffuse angiomatosis resembling angiomatosis with excess glomus cells. Often associated with considerable fat and pain. Probably represents vascular malformations.

Infiltrating glomus tumor: It is a rare variant, deep seated with diffuse infiltration of surrounding soft tissue and has a high recurrence rate.

Symplastic: Lesion with marked nuclear atypia with no other malignant features.

Glomus tumor of uncertain malignant potential: High mitotic activity (5+/50 HPF) and superficial or 2 cm + only or deep only.

Criteria for malignant lesions: Deep location; size >2 cm; atypical mitotic figures; moderate to high nuclear grade; mitosis 5+/50 HPF.

Ancillary Tests

Immunohistochemistry
Positivity: SMA; muscle-specific actin; focal positive for desmin; CD34.

Molecular genetics: Genetic aberration associated with multiple inherited glomangiomas has been linked to 1p21–22. Gene is named glomulin. BRAF mutations have been identified in some glomus tumors.

Differential Diagnosis
- **Cutaneous adnexal neoplasm especially eccrine spiradenoma:** Focal ductal differentiation, two population of cells and positivity for epithelial markers are present in eccrine spiradenoma.
- **Intradermal nevus:** With pseudovascular spaces, show focal nesting, evidence of maturation and positivity for S100.

Case History: A 29-year-old lady with a 2 cm nodule on abdominal wall near suprapubic region.

Diagnosis: Scar endometriosis

Clinical Features

- Mass near the previous surgical scars, accompanied by increasing colicky-like pain during the menstruation.
- Can easily be mistaken clinically for hematoma, neuroma, hernia, granuloma, abscess, scar tissue, neoplastic tissue, or even metastatic carcinoma.

Gross

Bluish cystic nodule surrounded by fibrosis.

Microscopy

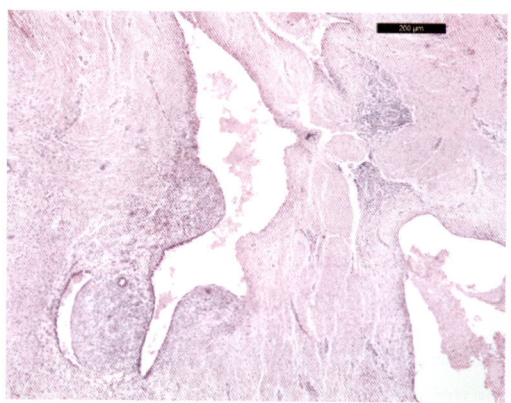

Fig. 15.3

- Endometrial glands and stroma are seen embedded in dense fibrous mass exhibiting signs of fresh and old hemorrhage.
- Stromal component can undergo smooth muscle metaplasia.

Case History: A 45-year-old lady with swelling forehead right side for 2 months.

Diagnosis: Dermatofibrosarcoma protuberance (DFSP)

Clinical Features

- Slow growing lesion involving skin and subcutaneous tissue.
- Sarcomatous change in lesion is associated with clinically aggressive course.

Gross

- Plaques, exophytic solitary lesions to nodular clusters.
- Measures a few cm to massive pedunculated tumors >20 cm in size.
- Hypopigmented/hyperpigmented lesion with or without skin ulceration can be seen.

Microscopy

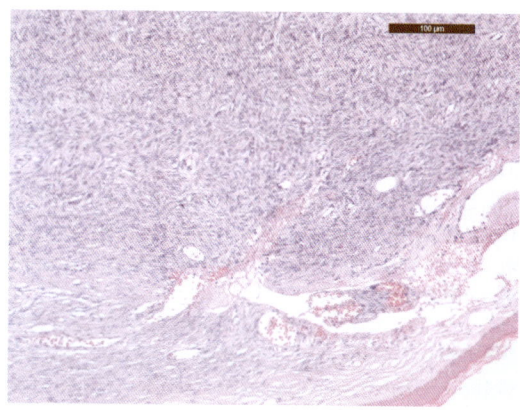

Fig. 15.4

- Usually located in dermis, with prominent storiform pattern having monomorphic fibroblast-like cells that can invade into subcutis.
- Tumor cells are fusiform with amphophilic to eosinophilic cytoplasm and elongated nuclei.
- Minimal nuclear hyperchromasia seen.
- Rarely foam cells and Touton cells and granular cells can feature.
- Mitotic index is low <5 mitosis/HPF.
- Bednar tumor is pigmented variant due to dendritic cells with melanin, S-100 + only in pigmented cells, HMB45 negative. Common in blacks.

Ancillary Tests

- **Immunohistochemistry:** Positivity for CD34 and vimentin.
- **Molecular genetics:** t(17;22) and COL1A1-PDGFB gene fusion.

Differential Diagnosis
- Cellular dermatofibroma
- Atypical fibroxanthoma
- Histoid Hansen.

Case History: A 29-year-old male with large mass in right thigh.

Diagnosis: Myxoid liposarcoma

Clinical Features
Presents as large painless mass in limb or thigh in muscle or deep tissue.

Gross
Well-circumscribed multinodular usually intramuscular tumors with gelatinous and fleshy cut surface.

Microscopy

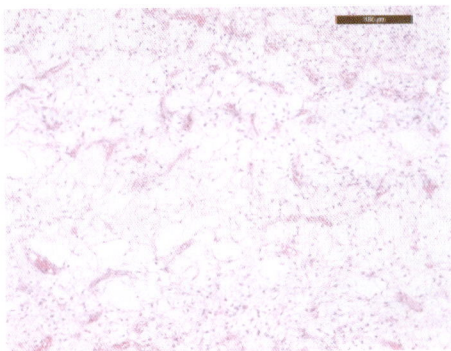

Fig. 15.5

- Tumor is paucicellular and composed of stellate or fusiform cells without atypia.
- There is prominent chicken-wire type of vasculature within tumor tissue.
- Many signet ring lipoblasts are seen particularly at periphery of lobules.
- Tumor characteristically shows mucoid matrix-rich in hyaluronidase sensitive acid mucopolysaccharides and may have large mucoid pools.
- Lymphangioma-like cystic degeneration is relatively specific.

Ancillary Tests
- **Molecular genetics:** t(12;16) (q13;p11) seen in more than 90% of cases
- **Immunohistochemistry:** Positive for vimentin, S-100, CD36.

Differential Diagnosis
- **Extraskeletal myxoid chondrosarcoma:** Malignant chondrocytes, no cytoplasmic fat vacuoles, no prominent vasculature
- **Lipoblastoma:** Similar histology but age 5 years or less
- **Myxofibrosarcoma:** Older adults, often superficial, infiltrative, no cytoplasmic fat vacuoles, more nuclear atypia, thicker curvilinear vessels, frequent mitotic figures
- **Myxoma:** Extremely paucicellular, lacks a prominent vascular component.

Case History: A 32-year-old male with epigastric pain and retroperitoneal mass.

Diagnosis: Malignant triton tumor

Criteria
There are three diagnostic criteria proposed:
- Tumor arises along a peripheral nerve, or in a ganglioneuroma or in a patient with neurofibromatosis type 1 (NF1) or has a metastatic character.
- Growth characteristics of the tumor is typical for a Schwann cell tumor.
- Rhabdomyoblasts arise within tumor tissue.

Gross
Large mass producing fusiform enlargement of major nerve.

Microscopy

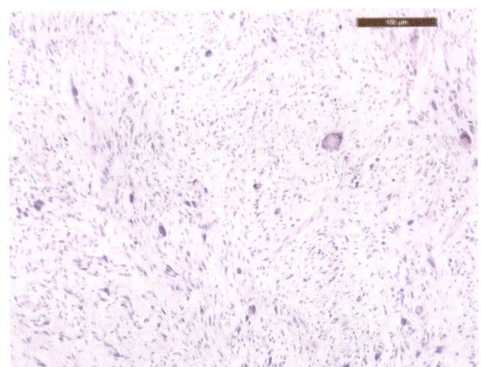

Fig. 15.6

- Monomorphic serpentine cells, palisading, large gaping vascular spaces, perivascular plump tumor cells, geographic necrosis

with tumor palisading at edges, resembling glioblastoma multiforme.
- Frequent mitotic figures. May have bizarre cells and cells resembling rhabdomyoblasts.

Ancillary Tests

Immunohistochemistry: S-100 protein or Leu-7 positivity in nerve sheath differentiation. Desmin, muscle-specific actin, myosin, vimentin, and myoglobulin: Rhabdomyoblastic cells.

Differential Diagnosis

Malignant spindle cell tumors.

Case History: A 6-year-old girl with nasal congestion, tenderness right maxillary and frontal paranasal sinuses and right eye prominence with diplopia.

Diagnosis: Rhabdomyosarcoma—embryonal

Clinical Features

- Generally related to mass effects and obstruction.
- Head and neck lesions can cause proptosis, diplopia, sinusitis, or unilateral deafness, depending on their location.

Gross

- Poorly circumscribed mass, white, soft or firm, infiltrative.
- Characteristic polypoid appearance in botryoid sarcoma with clusters of small, sessile or pedunculated nodules that abut an epithelial surface.

Microscopy

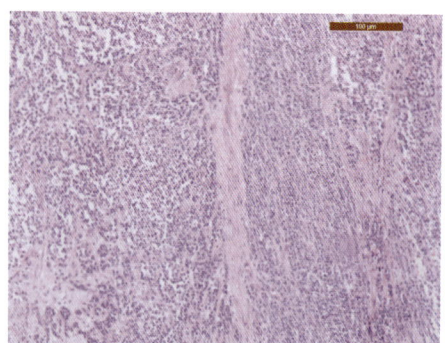

Fig. 15.7

- Varying degree of cellularity with alternating hypercellular areas and stromal areas with myxoid appearance.
- Composed of primitive mesenchymal cells in various stages of myogenesis.
- Sheets of small, spindled or moderate to poorly differentiated round cells with scant or deeply eosinophilic cytoplasm and eccentric, small oval darkly stained nuclei.
- Highly cellular areas around blood vessels alternate with paucicellular regions.

Ancillary Tests

- **Special stain:** PAS stain highlights glycogen in tumor cells.
- **Immunohistochemistry:** Positivity for vimentin in all cells. Some cells should stain for desmin, Myo-D1 or myogenin.
- **Molecular genetics:** Loss of heterozygosity at chromosome 11p15.5 and trisomy 8.

Differential Diagnosis

- Desmoplastic round cell tumor
- Ewing/PNET
- Non-Hodgkin lymphoma
- Neuroblastoma

Case History: A 49-year-old lady with epigastric discomfort and regurgitation underwent endoscopy and esophageal biopsy.

Diagnosis: Granular cell tumor

Clinical Features

Slow growing tumor, rarely tender.

Location

Commonly arise in skin or subcutaneous tissue preferably in trunk and tongue.

Gross

- Usually measure 3–5 cm in size.
- Hard consistency and ill-defined margins.

Microscopy

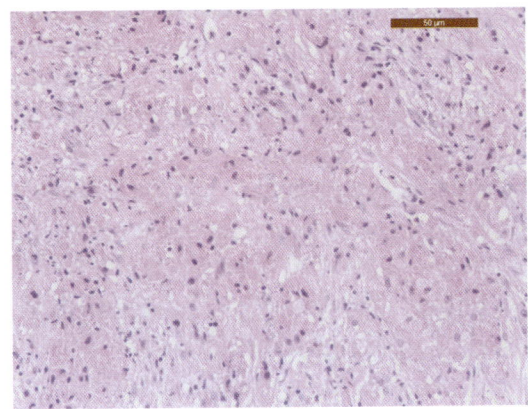

Fig. 15.8

- Uniform appearance with poorly defined margins in 50% of cases.
- Tumor cells are arranged in nests and trabeculae. These cells are rounded to polygonal with abundant granular eosinophilic cytoplasm and centrally placed pyknotic nulcei.
- Large droplets or granules can also feature.

Variants of Granular Cell Tumor

- Gingival granular cell tumor of newborn infants.
- Malignant granular cell tumor.

Ancillary Tests

- **Special stain:** Diastase resistant PAS positivity.
- **Immunohistochemistry:** S-100, CD68, NSE.
- **Electron microscopy:** Numerous secondary lysosomes containing prominent myelin figures.
- **Molecular genetics:** Expression of HLA-DR.

Differential Diagnosis

- Hibernoma
- Fibroxanthoma

Case History: A 40-year-old female with pelvic mass presented with recurrent suprapubic and right flank pain and dysuria.

Diagnosis: Hemangiopericytoma (HP)

Clinical Features

- Occurs in soft tissues of the extremities especially distal lower limb, retroperitoneum, pelvic fossa and thigh.
- Deep seated lesions.
- Slowly enlarging painless mass but can be painful.

Gross

- Can be solitary or multiple lesions and are fairly circumscribed masses covered with thin vascular pseudocapsule.
- Tumor is gray/white to red/brown on cut surface, fleshy or spongy with hemorrhage, cystic degeneration, variable necrosis.
- Averages 4–8 cm in size.

Microscopy

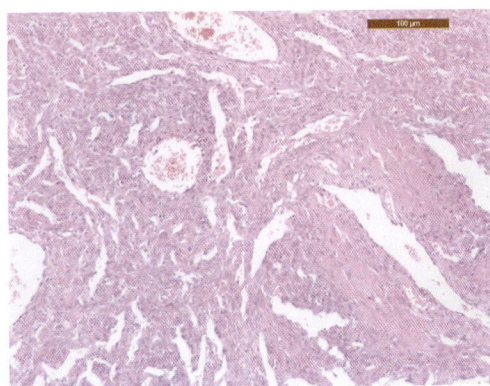

Fig. 15.9

- Tumor cells area arranged in lobules and patternless pattern with thin-walled ramifying blood vessels in a staghorn pattern.
- Tumor cells are uniform small bland oval to spindle with oval nucleus and ill-defined minimal cytoplasm.
- Focal and diffuse myxoid change and stromal fibrosis can also be seen.

Ancillary Tests

- **Special stain:** Silver stain highlights tumor cells that are located outside vascular spaces and each is surrounded by reticulin fibers.
- **Immunohistochemistry:** Positivity for vimentin, CD34, factor VIII.

Differential Diagnosis
- Synovial sarcoma
- Mesenchymal chondrosarcoma
- Juxtaglomerular tumor
- Phosphaturic mesenchymal tumor.

Case History: A 55-year-old male with swelling left calf region with prominent vascularity.

Diagnosis: Malignant fibrous histiocytoma-storiform pleomorphic

Clinical Features
- Progressive painless mass lesion.
- Fever, leukocytosis with neutrophilia or eosinophilia may also feature.

Gross
Solitary, large multilobulated, fleshy firm tumor with areas of cystic change, hemorrhage and necrosis.

Microscopy

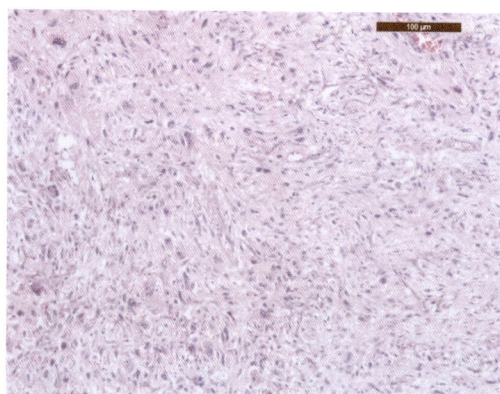

Fig. 15.10

- Tumor cells are characteristically arranged in fascicles and storiform pattern around slit-like vessels.
- Cells are spindle to highly pleomorphic.
- Histiocytic cells, xanthoma cells and chronic inflammatory cells are also present.
- Hyaline globules can be seen in cytoplasm of tumor giant cells; related apoptosis and are known as thanatosomes.

Ancillary Tests
- **Immunohistochemistry:** Vimentin, α_1-antrypsin, α_1-chymo-trypsin, CD68.
- **Electron microscopy:** Fibroblasts, myofibroblasts, histiocytes and primitive mesenchymal cells.

Differential Diagnosis
- Pleomorphic liposarcoma
- Fibrosarcoma
- Synovial sarcoma
- MPNST
- Leiomyosarcoma
- Pleomorphic rhabdomyosarcoma.

Case History: A 22-year-old male with chest pain underwent chest X-ray which showed anterior mediastinal mass.

Diagnosis: Alveolar soft part sarcoma

Clinical Features
- Presents typically in adolescents and young adults.
- In children more common in head and neck region.
- Often long history of slow growth can be seen.

Gross
- Well circumscribed, large firm grey or yellowish.
- Areas of necrosis and hemorrhage can also be seen.

Microscopy

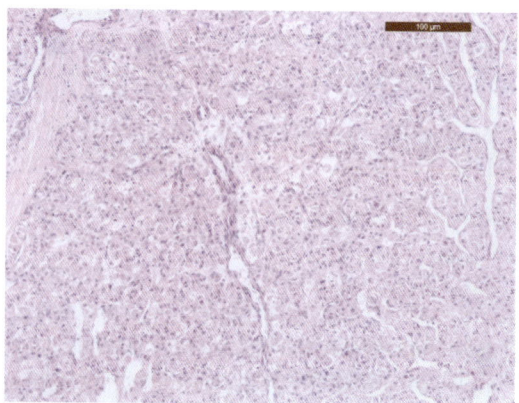

Fig. 15.11

- Tumor cells are separated into nests by fibrous bands.
- Detachment of cells in central area reflects a typical alveolar pattern.
- Individual cells are large round to oval have abundant granular eosinophilic cytoplasm with eccentric rounded nuclei and prominent nucleoli.

Ancillary Tests
- **Special stain:** In about 50% cases PAS diastase stain reveals intracytoplasmic granules and crystalline rods.
- **Immunohistochemistry:** Positivity for NSE, S-100, MyoD1, CD147, desmin and TFE-3.
- **Electron microscopy:** Membrane bound crystalline/filamentous material originates close to Golgi apparatus and takes geometric shapes.
- **Molecular genetics:** Re-arrangement of 17q25, unbalanced translocation t(x;17), TFE-3-ASPL fusion gene.

Differential Diagnosis
- Metastatic renal cell carcinoma
- Metastatic amelanotic melanoma.

Case History: A 21-year-old male presented with right iliac fossa pain and intra-abdominal mass.

Diagnosis: Desmoplastic round cell tumor

Clinical Features
- Presentation depends on site of involvement.
- Peritoneum involvement can present as abdominopelvic mass and ascites.
- Pressure effects on neighboring structures (intestines, ureters) have been described.

Location
- Peritoneum, pleura and tunica vaginalis
- Solid organs such as liver ovary, bone, pancreas, kidney
- Non-abdominal locations like the nasal sinus and posterior cranial fossa.

Imaging
Show large confluent masses over the parietal peritoneum, nodules over the mesentery, and ascites, usually with no organ involvement.

Gross
- Multiple nodules at the affected site, with sometimes a larger dominant nodule.
- Cut surface of the tumor is firm, grey-white showing areas of necrosis and hemorrhage.

Microscopy

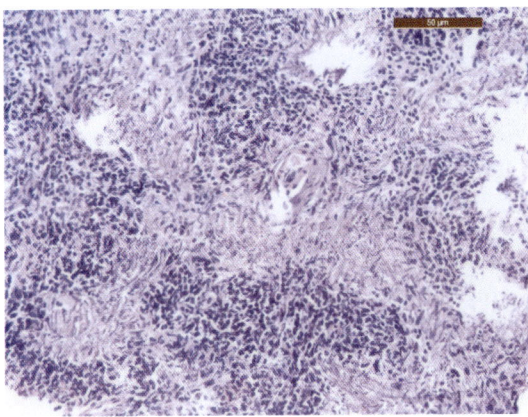

Fig. 15.12

- Characteristic patterns noted on histology include islands of neoplastic cells arranged in diffuse sheets surrounded by a dominant desmoplastic stroma.
- Other patterns include infiltrative (Indian—file appearance), rosetting, and gland formation.
- Tumor cells appear uniformly small, round to elongated, with scanty cytoplasm.
- Nuclei typically are round hyperchromatic with inconspicuous nucleoli.
- The desmoplastic stroma is composed of fibroblasts and myofibroblasts embedded in loose collagenous tissue.

Ancillary Tests
- **Immunohistochemistry:** Immunopositivity for cytokeratin (CK), epithelial membrane antigen, vimentin, and neuron-specific enolase. Immunoexpression of WT1 antigen

by tumor cells serves as a sensitive and specific marker for DSRCT.
- **Molecular genetics:** A recurrent specific chromosomal abnormality that has been reported in DSRCT is t(11;22) (p13:q12: EWS-WT1) chimeric transcripts.

Differential Diagnosis
- Non-Hodgkin's lymphoma (NHL)
- Ewing's sarcoma/primitive neuroectodermal tumor (PNET)
- Wilms' tumor
- Embryonal rhabdomyosarcoma.

Case History: A 40-year-old lady with rapidly growing right forearm swelling.

Diagnosis: Nodular fasciitis

Clinical Features
- Common lesion that typically presents as a rapidly growing mass on the flexor forearm, chest, back or elsewhere.
- Arises from superficial fascia, occasionally intramuscular or intravascular.

Gross
- Tan-white-gray, myxoid appearance, usually 3 cm or less.
- Relatively well circumscribed, no definite capsule.
- May be centered in subcutis and may grow into skeletal muscle.

Microscopy

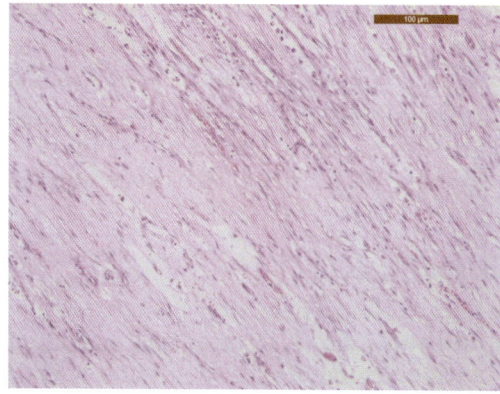

Fig. 15.13

- Zonation effect with hypocellular central region and hypercellular periphery.
- Composed of uniform, plump, immature, spindled to stellate fibroblasts or myofibroblasts without atypia, with a feathery, "tissue culture" like growth pattern due to abundant ground substance.
- Uniform elongated nuclei with punctate nucleoli and without significant nuclear atypia.
- Cellular areas may have storiform or fascicular patterns.
- Vasculature is usually prominent.

Ancillary Tests
- **Immunohistochemistry:** SMA vimentin and calponin.
- **Electron microscopy:** Cells resemble myofibroblasts, are elongated with abundant, often dilated rough endoplasmic reticulum.
- **Molecular genetics:** Balanced translocation t(17;22) (p13; q13) resulting in MYH9-USP6 gene fusion.

Differential Diagnosis
- Benign fibrous histiocytoma
- Fibromatosis
- Inflammatory myofibroblastic tumor
- Myositis ossificans
- Myxofibrosarcoma

Case History: A 20-year-old male presented with headache and rapidly progressive painless proptosis.

Diagnosis: Inflammatory myofibroblastic tumor

Clinical Features
- Fever, growth failure, malaise, weight loss, anemia, thrombocytosis, polyclonal hyperglobulinemia and elevated sedimentation rate.
- Symptoms disappear after excision of mass.
- In children and young adults (mean age 10 years)

Location
- Head and neck, lung, salivary glands, CNS, mediastinum, orbit, bladder and bone.
- Found in retroperitoneum (omentum) and mesentery.

Gross
- Circumscribed, not encapsulated, white tan mass with whorled fleshy or myxoid cut surface.
- May have focal hemorrhage, necrosis or calcification, mean size 6 cm.

Microscopy

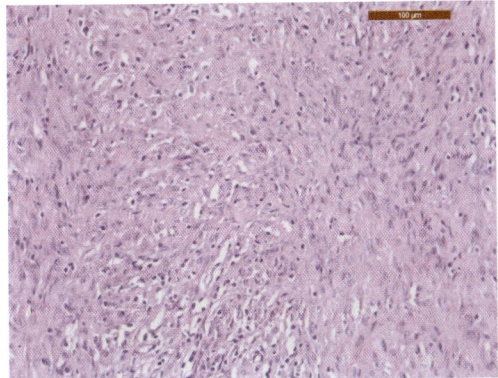

Fig. 15.14

- Myofibroblastic and fibroblastic spindle cells with inflammatory infiltrate of lymphocytes, plasma cells, eosinophils, histiocytes in a background of abundant blood vessels.
- May have ganglion cell-like myofibroblasts.

Mixture of Three Patterns
- Resembling nodular fasciitis with elongated myofibroblasts
- Cellular with spindled myofibroblasts and fibroblasts
- Densely hyalinized stroma
- All 3 patterns have no nuclear pleomorphism, no atypical mitotic figures.

Malignant Behavior
Associated with highly atypical polygonal cells with oval nuclei, prominent nucleoli, Reed-Sternberg-like cells, atypical mitotic figures.

Ancillary Tests
- **Immunohistochemistry:** Vimentin, α-SMA, MSA and calponin. ALK 1/p80 in 40% cases.
- **Electron microscopy:** Myofibroblastic cells and activated fibroblasts.
- **Molecular genetics:** Clonal abnormalities of 2 p23 including t(2;5) (p23; q35). Associated with ALK deregulation and younger patients.

Differential Diagnosis
- Low grade myofibroblastic sarcoma
- Nodular fasciitis

Case History: A 70-year-old lady with bleeding ulcerated nodule over the occipital region of scalp.

Diagnosis: Angiosarcoma

Clinical Features
Presentation and behavior depends on location of tumor.

Location
Older adults in skin (scalp, face) and soft tissue of extremities; also bone, breast, heart, lung, liver, spleen, and thyroid.

Gross
- **Early:** Small, sharply demarcated, asymptomatic, multiple red nodules.
- **Late:** Fleshy, gray-white with hemorrhage, necrosis, deeply invasive.

Microscopy

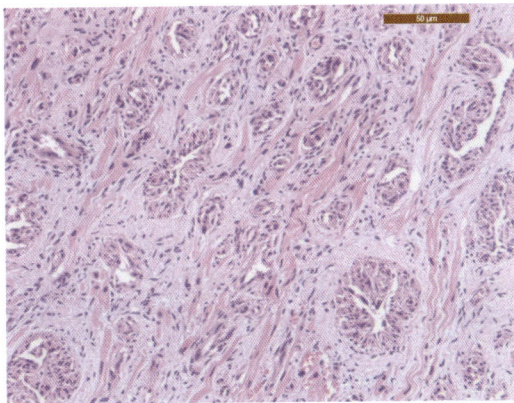

Fig. 15.15

- Atypical vascular spaces lined by endothelial cells with cytologic atypia, multilayering.
- In more solid areas are intracytoplasmic lumina containing red blood cells.
- Multinucleated cells may have prominent hyaline globules containing α_1-antitrypsin and α_1-antichymotrypsin.
- Brisk mitotic activity and necrosis are common.
- Post-radiation lesions usually high grade.

Ancillary Tests
- **Immunohistochemistry:** Positivity for factor 8 related protein, CD31, thrombomodulin, CD34, c-kit (50%). Variable positivity for VEGFR-3.
- **Molecular genetics:** Amplifications of MYC.

Case History: A 40-year-old lady with 3 months of epigastric pain and ultrasound abdomen showed retroduodenal mass in close proximity with aorta and left kidney.

Diagnosis: Paraganglioma

Gross
- Rubbery, firm, may have pseudocapsule.
- Brown cut surface; variable central scar.

Microscopy

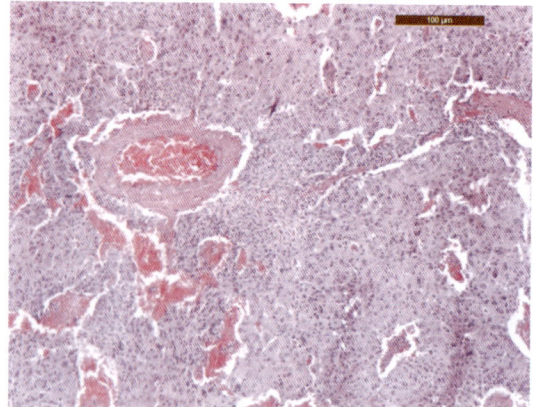

Fig. 15.16

- Nesting (Zellballen) or trabecular pattern of cells within a prominent vascular network.
- Nests composed of round/oval cells and giant multinucleated cells with abundant granular eosinophilic or basophilic cytoplasm, may have nuclear atypia and vascular invasion (do not indicate malignancy).
- May have dysmorphic vessels, melanin-like pigment, abundant stroma and osseous metaplasia. Intracytoplasmic hyaline globules are present in sympathoadrenal paragangliomas.
- No mitotic figures except in obviously malignant tumors.

Specific Types
- Aorticopulmonary paraganglioma
- Carotid body paraganglioma
- Cauda equina paraganglioma.

Jugulotympanic Paraganglioma
- Laryngeal paraganglioma
- Mediastinal paraganglioma
- Organ of Zuckerkandl paraganglioma
- Pigmented paraganglioma
- Vagal paraganglioma.

Ancillary Tests
- **Immunohistochemistry:** Positivity for synaptophysin and chromogranin; sustentacular cells S-100 positivity.
- **Molecular genetics**

  Familial cases: Autosomal dominant with paternal imprinting, linkage to 11q23 and 11q13 and usually carotid body paragangliomas. Sympathoadrenal—associated with MEN 2a and 2b.

Differential Diagnosis
- Alveolar rhabdomyosarcoma
- Alveolar soft part sarcoma
- Carcinoid tumor
- Liposarcoma
- Melanoma
- Metastatic carcinoma of kidney.

Case History: A 12-year-old girl with slightly painful large irregular, pendulous swelling present in the right leg extending from knee joint to ankle joint for 1 year duration.

Diagnosis: Plexiform neurofibroma

Clinical Features

- Most common site is head and neck region.
- Superficial soft tissue involvement is more frequent than deep tissue.
- Involvement of entire extremity gives appearance termed elephantiasis neuromatosa.

Gross

Large lesions involving large segment of nerve, distorting and contorting into bag of worms.

Microscopy

Fig. 15.17

- Tumor tissue has nodular or diffuse arrangement.
- Consists of tortuous mass of expanded nerve branches which are seen cut in various planes of section with increased endoneural matrix.
- Tumor is hypocellular with myxoid background and consists of Schwann cells, fibroblasts and mast cells.
- Presence of increased cellularity, mitotic activity and nuclear atypia indicates malignant change.

Immunohistochemistry

- S-100 in scattered cells.
- Perineurial cells are EMA + in plexiform but not in ordinary neurofibromas.

Differential Diagnosis

Plexiform schwannoma.

Case History: A 25-year-old female with polypoidal mass arising from the right anterior labia minora of 6 months duration.

Diagnosis: Aggressive angiomyxoma

Clinical Features

- Reproductive age females with peak in the 3rd decade.
- In women, vulvar region most common site.
- In men, it arises from inguinal region, along the spermatic cord, or in scrotum.

Gross

- Soft, partially circumscribed or polypoid.
- *Cut surface:* Glistening, homogenous, gelatinous appearance ranging in size from a few centimetres to 20 cm or more.

Microscopy

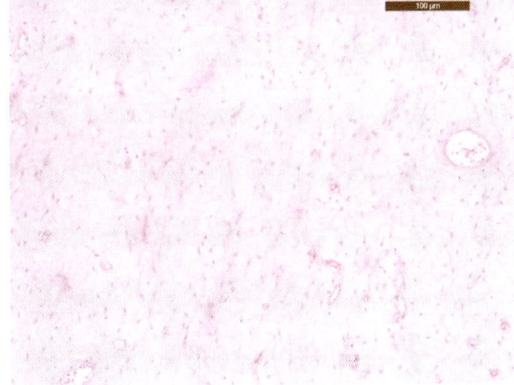

Fig. 15.18

- Widely scattered spindled to stellate-shaped cells with ill-defined cytoplasm with centrally located nuclei.
- Characteristic feature is the presence of variable sized vessels that range from small thin-walled capillaries to large vessels with

secondary changes including perivascular hyalinization and medial hypertrophy.
- Mitosis is rare or absent and is not atypical.

Immunohistochemistry
Vimentin, SMA, muscle specific actin, ER, PR positive.

Differential Diagnosis
- **Angiomyofibroblastoma:** Plump epithelioid cells in perivascular pattern. Bi and multinucleated cells present. Rarely myxoid
- **Intramuscular myxoma and juxta-articular myxoma:** Less cellular, less vascular
- **Cutaneous myxoma:** Lobular or multinodular and is sparsely cellular proliferation of stellate and spindle shaped
- **Myxoid neurofibroma:** Composed of cells with wavy or buckled nuclei
- **Myxoid leiomyoma**
- **Fibroepithelial stromal polyps.**

Case History: A 10-year-old girl with painless fluctuant labial swelling involving the lower lip for 2 months.

Diagnosis: Cysticercosis

Clinical Features
Presents as a palpable, subcutaneous nodule.

Gross
- Circumscribed, white to tan, cystic nodules of size 1 to 2 cm containing a clear fluid.
- Larval forms identified within the cystic cavity.

Microscopy

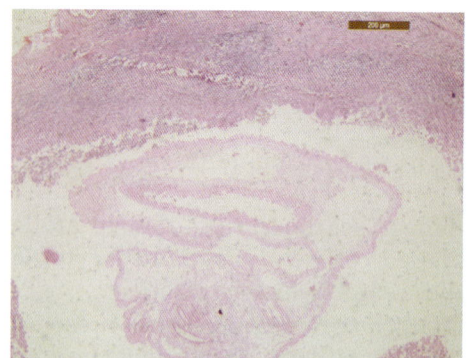

Fig. 15.19

- Cystic cavity contains the larval form.
- Scolex with hooklets and two pairs of suckers.
- Larval form has duct-like invaginations lined by double-layered, eosinophilic membrane.
- Body wall exhibits a myxoid matrix and calcareous bodies (called concretions). Birefringent hooklets may be identified.
- Granulomatous reaction, inflammatory infiltrate with lymphocytes and eosinophils, fibrosis and calcification.

Case History: 39/M, Painless swelling in right thigh

Diagnosis: Angiomatoid fibrous histiocytoma

Introduction
It is a rare subcutaneous tumor more commonly affecting the limbs with equal sex distribution and peak incidence in first two decades.

Gross
- Median size –2 cm (ranging from 0.7 to 12 cm), well-circumscribed lesion, firm in consistency.
- Cut surface may have multilocular hemorrhagic appearance.

Microscopy

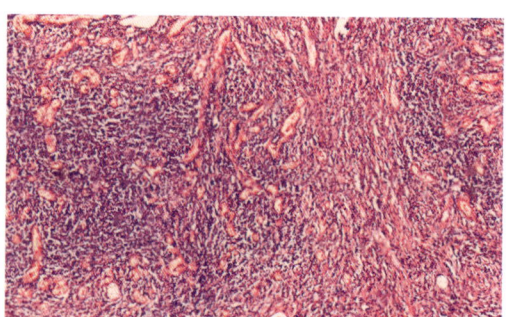

Fig. 15.20

4 key features:
i. Thick Fibrous pseudocapsule containing hemosiderin laden macrophages.

ii. Peri capsular cuffing of lympho-plasmacytic cells with or without germinal center formation.
iii. Nodules composed of spindle or histiocytoid cells with distinctive syncytial growth pattern.
iv. Pseudo-angiomatoid spaces filled with blood and surrounded by tumor cells.

Immunohistochemistry
- Positive for EMA, CD68, CD99.
- Negative for S100, CD34

Differential Diagnosis
- Angiosarcoma
- Aneurysmal variant of benign fibrous histiocytoma

Case History: A 39-year-old female with history of chronic rhino-sinusitis

Diagnosis: Perineuriomas

Introduction
Benign peripheral nerve sheath tumors composed entirely of perineural cells and are of two types: Sclerosing and reticular perineuriomas. Females are commonly affected than males. Site : Lower limb > upper limb > trunk.

Gross
- Unencapsulated but well-circumscribed lesion. Size ranging from <1 cm to 20 cm.
- Cut surface: Yellow/tan/white, firm or rubbery in consistency.

Microscopy

Spindles cells arranged in storiform pattern and having wavy or tapering nuclei, indistinct nucleoli and delicate bipolar cytoplasmic processes.

Immunohistochemistry
- Positive for EMA, focal staining for SMA may be seen.
- Negative for S100 and GFAP.

Differential Diagnosis
- Benign fibrous histiocytoma (because of storiform pattern).
- For sclerosing perineurioma—epithelioid hemangioendothelioma, fibroma of the tendon sheath, calcifying fibrous pseudotumor, fibrosing tenosynovial giant cell tumor.

Case History: A 71-year-old female has retro-peritoneal mass

Diagnosis: Fibrosarcomas

Introduction
Malignant neoplasms composed of fibroblasts with variable collagen production. Affects middle to old age people with no sex predilection. Most common site - deep soft tissues of extremities, trunk, head and neck.

Gross
- Circumscribed, firm, white/tan mass.
- High grade tumors show areas of hemorrhage and necrosis.

Microscopy

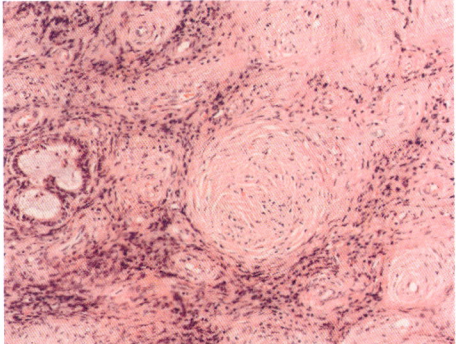

Fig. 15.21

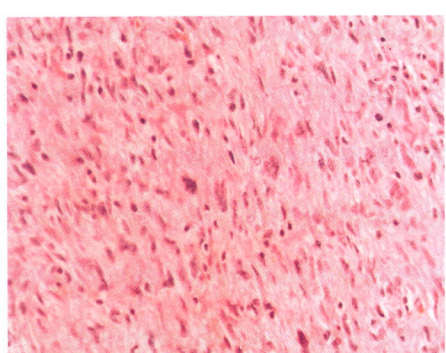

Fig. 15.22

- Lesion composed of monomorphic spindle cells arranged in Herringbone pattern with scant cytoplasm, tapered and darkly staining nuclei and variably pleomorphic nucleoli.
- Stroma has variable collagen.

Immunohistochemistry

Focal positivity for SMA indicating myofibroblastic differentiation.

Differential Diagnosis

- Monophasic fibrous synovial sarcoma
- MPNST

Case History: A 78-year-old male has swelling in right trapezius muscle

Diagnosis: Desmoid type fibromatosis

Introduction

- Locally aggressive neoplasm having infiltrative growth but do not metastasize.
- *Site:* Abdominal and extra-abdominal. Usually deep seated, firm.

Gross

- Poorly circumscribed lesion with size ranging from 5 to 10 cm.
- Cut surface—firm, gritty, glistening white, coarsely trabeculated surface resembling scar tissue.

Microscopy

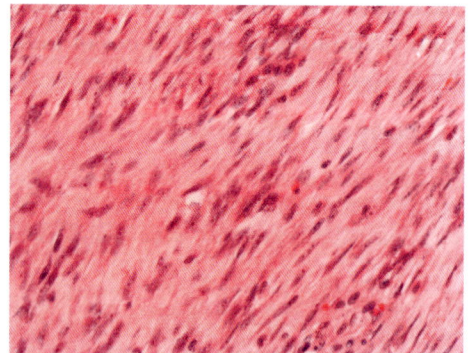

Fig. 15.23

- Poorly circumscribed lesion composed of elongated slender spindle shaped cells of uniform appearance in a collagenous stroma with variably prominent blood vessels.

Immunohistochemistry

- Positive for beta-catenin (nuclear positivity), variably positive for SMA.
- Negative for desmin and S100.

Case History: A 38-year-old male with gluteal swelling.

Diagnosis: Epithelioid sarcoma

Introduction

- Epithelioid cytomorphology and is more common in young adults with a slight male preponderance.
- Two forms are seen:
  1. Conventional/classic (distal) form
  2. Large cell (proximal) variant

Gross

- Classic form—indurated, ill defined subcutaneous or dermal nodules.
- Deep seated tumors—large, multinodular masses involving tendon/fascia.
- C/S—grey-white or grey tan with areas of necrosis and hemorrhage.

Microscopy

- **Classic type:** Cellular nodules of spindle or epithelioid cells with central necrosis/degeneration.
- **Proximal type:** Multinodular growth pattern composed of large epithelioid cells with marked cytologic atypia, large vesicular nuclei, and prominent nucleoli. Paranuclear hyaline inclusions imparting a rhabdoid appearance.

Immunohistochemistry

- Loss of nuclear expression of SMARCB1.
- Positive for HMW-CK, EMA.

Differential Diagnosis

- **Inflammatory lesions:** Necrotizing infectious granuloma, necrobiosis lipoidica, granuloma annulare, or rheumatoid nodule.
- **Malignant lesions:** Malignant epithelioid hemangioma-endothelioma, epithelioid MPNST, epithelioid angiosarcoma.

CHAPTER 16

Lesions of the Bone and Joints

D Prathiba

Case History: A 55-year-old female with increased serum calcium.

Diagnosis: Tumoral calcinosis

Clinical Features
Associated with trauma, hyperparathyroidism, renal failure, metastatic carcinoma, myeloma, scleroderma, sarcoidosis and hypermetabolic state.

Laboratory Findings
Elevated serum calcium, phosphate and vitamin D.

Imaging
Lobulated calcification, separate from associated bone.

Gross
Large, multinodular chalky masses.

Microscopy

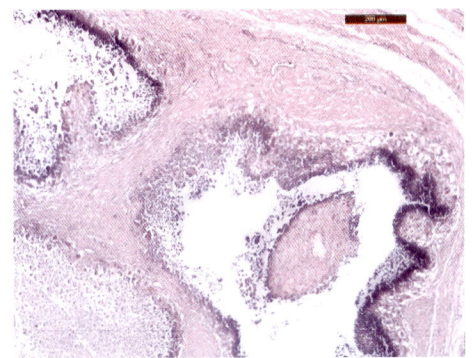

Fig. 16.1

- Lobules of calcified material with histiocytic giant cells.
- Psammomatous calcification may be seen.

Differential Diagnosis
Dystrophic calcification.

Case History: A 15-year-old boy with a history of previous trauma.

Diagnosis: Aneurysmal bone cyst

Clinical Features
- Age: 10–20 years
- Sex: M : F 1 : 1

Site
Vertebrae, flat bones, femur (metaphysis).

Imaging
Eccentric expansion of bone, with erosion and destruction of cortex and a small periosteal new bone formation.

Gross
Spongy hemorrhagic mass covered by thin shell of reactive bone, which may extend to soft tissue.

Microscopy

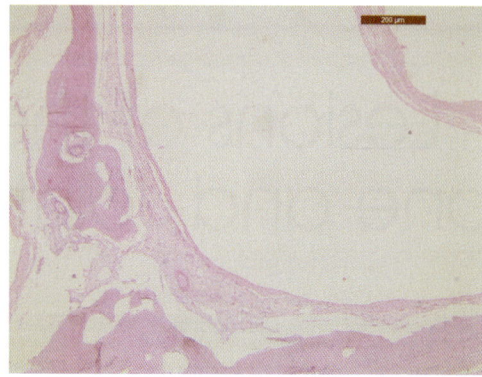

Fig. 16.2

- Large cystic spaces filled with blood and separated by fibrous septa.
- Cysts and septa lined by fibroblasts, myofibroblasts and histiocytes, but not endothelium.
- Degenerated calcifying fibromyxoid tissue present.

Molecular Genetics

Abnormalities of 17p13.2 loci.

Differential Diagnosis

- **Solitary bone cyst:** Vascularised connective tissue, hemosiderin, cholesterol clefts seen. Dense bone with irregular cement lines surrounds the cyst.
- **Giant cell tumor:** Lacks fibroblastic cells.
- **Hemangioma:** Endothelial lining seen lining blood filled spaces.
- **Telangiectatic osteosarcoma:** Pleomorphic malignant cells seen.
- **Giant cell reparative granuloma:** Location in jaw.

Case History: A 17-year-old male with knee pain, with an increased intensity at night.

Diagnosis: Osteoid osteoma

Clinical Features

- Age: 10 to 30 years
- Sex: M : F 2 : 1
- Intense pain which is more intense at night, relieved by NSAIDs.

Site

- Any bone.
- Most commonly femur, tibia, humerus, bones of hands and feet, vertebra.

Imaging

Radiolucent central nidus <1.5 cm, surrounded by a peripheral sclerotic reactive bone.

Gross

Small circumscribed nidus with surrounding sclerosis.

Microscopy

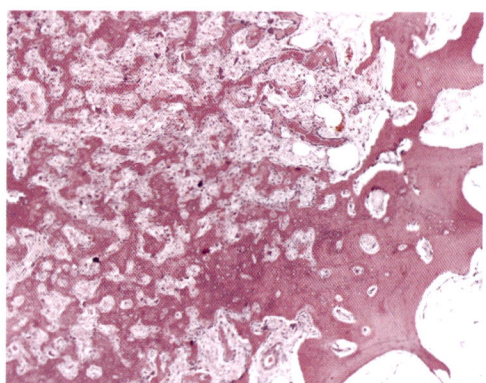

Fig. 16.3

- Sharply delineated central nidus composed of more or less calcified osteoid lined by plump osteoblasts within highly vascular connective tissue.
- Surrounding the nidus, there is a thick layer of dense bone.

Differential Diagnosis

- **Benign osteoblastoma:** Lack of intense pain, absence of surrounding area of dense bone.
- **Reactive bone:** No central nidus
- **Osteosarcoma:** Pleomorphic malignant cells forming osteoid.

Case History: A 20-year-old male with growth in distal femur.

Diagnosis: Osteochondroma

Clinical Features
- Age: 10–30 years
- Sex: M : F 1 : 1
- Usually asymptomatic.

Site
Femur, tibia, humerus, and pelvis.

Location
Cortex of metaphysis.

Imaging
Metaphyseal lesions which grow in a direction opposite to adjacent joint.

Gross
- Cartilage capped bony outgrowth up to 10 cm, attached by a bony stalk to the bone of origin.
- Cartilaginous cap covered by fibrous membrane which is continuous with periosteum of adjacent bone.

Microscopy

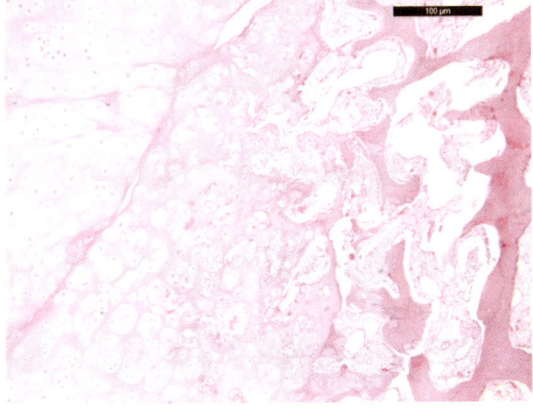

Fig. 16.4

- Lesion made up of mature bony trabeculae located beneath cartilaginous cap.
- Cells resemble those of normal hyaline cartilage.

Molecular Genetics
Mutation in EXT1 or EXT2 gene.

Differential Diagnosis
- **Bizzare parosteal osteochondromatous proliferation:** Enlarged, bizzare, binucleated chondrocytes
- **Periosteal osteosarcoma:** Neoplastic spindle cells seen between bony trabeculae
- **Secondary well-differentiated chondrosarcoma:** Invasion into surrounding tissue seen

Case History: A 15-year-old girl with a well-circumscribed mass in tibia.

Diagnosis: Chondromyxoid fibroma

Clinical Features
- Age: 10–25 years
- Sex: M : F 1 : 1

Site
Tibia, femur, feet, and pelvis.

Imaging
Well circumscribed, purely lytic defect in the metaphysis.

Gross
Solid, yellowish white or tan, replaces bone and thins cortex.

Microscopy

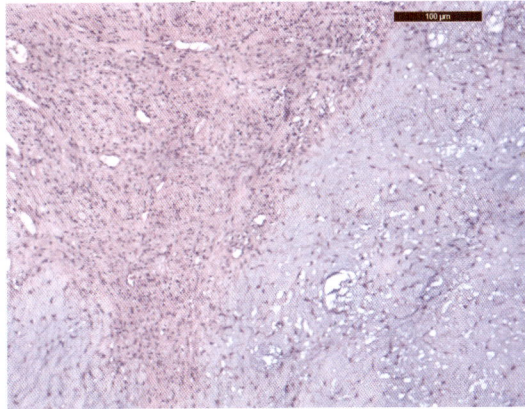

Fig. 16.5

- Hypocellular lobules with a myxochondroid appearance, separated by intersecting

bands of highly cellular tissue composed of fibroblast-like spindle cells and osteoclasts.
- Extensive vascularity is present in peripheral areas.

Ancillary Tests
- **IHC:** S-100 positive.
- **Molecular genetics:** Rearrangement of chromosome 6 at q13 or q25.

Differential Diagnosis
- **Chondroblastoma:** Cells are similar but not lobulated.
- **Chondrosarcoma:** Similar histology but malignant radiologically, no hypocellular center. It infiltrates surrounding tissue.
- **Fibrous dysplasia:** may show myxoid change but not lobulated.
- **Fibromyxoma:** No cartilaginous areas.

Case History: A 35-year-old male with painful swelling in the leg.

Diagnosis: Chondrosarcoma

Clinical Features
- Age: 30–60 years
- Sex: M : F 3 : 1

Site
Pelvis, ribs, femur, humerus, and vertebrae.

Types According to Location
- Central chondrosarcoma
- Peripheral chondrosarcoma
- Juxtacortical chondrosarcoma.

Imaging
- Osteolytic lesion with splotchy calcification.
- Ill-defined margin, fusiform thickening of shaft, perforation of cortex.

Gross
Pearly white or light blue appearance of cartilage.

Microscopy

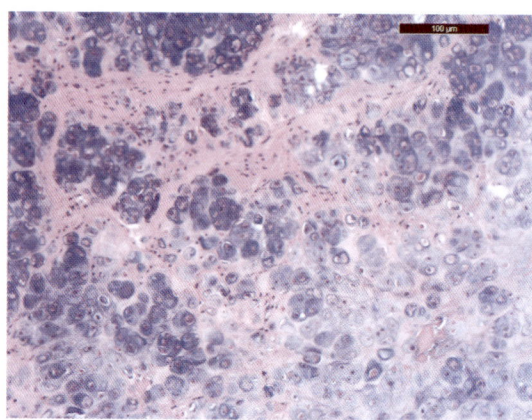

Fig. 16.6

- Not well circumscribed, malignant cartilage, permeates marrow spaces entrapping trabecular bone.
- Myxoid change in matrix noted.
- Crowding of nuclei seen.

Variants
- Clear cell CS
- Myxoid CS
- Dedifferentiated CS
- Mesenchymal CS

Ancillary Tests
- **IHC:** ER, S-100 and SOX 9 are positive.
- **Molecular genetics:** Inactivation of CDKN2A.
- Hemizygous deletion of EXT1 or EXT2.
- Overexpression of p53.

Case History: A 25-year-old female with a mass in the right knee.

Diagnosis: Giant cell tumor/osteoclastoma

Clinical Features
- Age: 20–30 years
- Sex: M : F 4 : 5

Site
Femur, tibia, and radius.

Imaging
Entirely lytic, expansile lesion in epiphysis.

Gross
- Variable size.
- Cut surface—solid, tan or light brown, traversed by fibrous trabeculae and often has hemorrhagic areas. Cortex thinned.

Microscopy

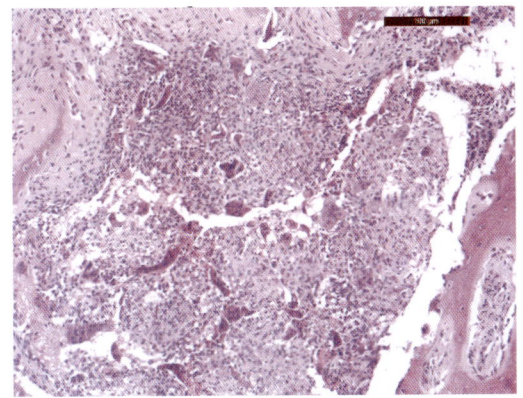

Fig. 16.7

- Two components—stromal cells and giant cells.
- The giant cells have 20 or 30 nuclei resembling osteoclasts, arranged towards the center.
- The stromal cells are mononuclear and they are neoplastic.

Immunohistochemistry
- Giant cells—acid phosphatase, 1-antitrypsin, cyclin D, ER positive
- Stromal cells—Ki-67 is useful in predicting prognosis.

Differential Diagnosis
- **Aneurysmal bone cyst:** They have fibroblastic cells lining the large cysts
- **Chondroblastoma:** Chondroid differentiation, chickenwire matrix surrounds chondroblasts
- **Chondromyxoid fibroma:** Well circumscribed, hypocellular lobules of cartilage.
- **Langerhans cell histiocytosis:** Fewer giant cells and many eosinophils seen.
- **Pigmented villonodular synovitis:** Hemosiderin laden macrophages seen.

Case History: A 20-year-old female with finger nodule.

Diagnosis: Giant cell tumor of tendon sheath

Clinical Features
- Age: <40 years (young and middle aged)
- Sex: Most common in women.
- Monoarticular pain.

Location
- Wrist, fingertips, between ankle and toe tips.
- Flexor surface affected commonly.

Gross
Single mass measuring 1–3 cm with well-defined capsule, lobulated, whitish, gray to yellowish brown in color.

Microscopy

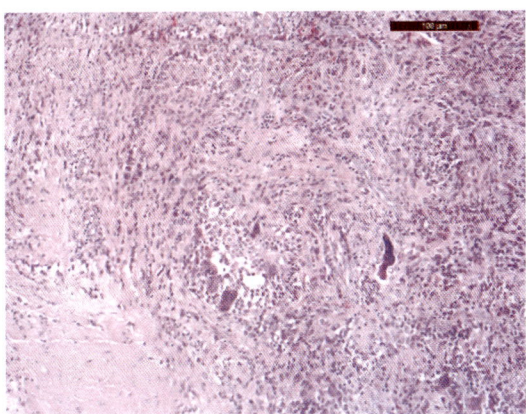

Fig. 16.8

- Closely packed medium-sized polyhedral cells with giant cells containing fat and hemosiderin.
- Mitotic figures may be seen along with focal hyalinised areas.

Differential Diagnosis
Epithelioid sarcoma: Granuloma like formations, necrosis, invasive nature, epithelioid features, keratin+.

Case History: An 11-year-old boy with periostitis in hand, after minor trauma.

Diagnosis: Myositis ossificans

Sites

Flexor muscle of the upper arm, quadriceps femoris, adductor muscles of the thigh, gluteal muscles.

Imaging

Early periosteal reaction with faint soft tissue calcification (3–6 weeks) replaced by mature bone (10–12 weeks).

Gross

Well circumscribed, soft center, gritty periphery.

Microscopy

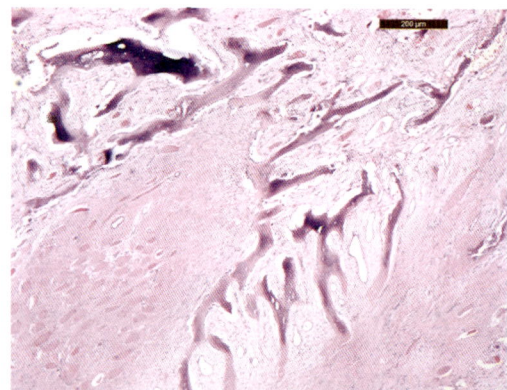

Fig. 16.9

- Highly cellular stroma with new bone or rarely cartilage.
- 'Zonal phenomenon' maturation pattern characterized by central cellular area, followed by an intermediate area of osteoid formation, followed by peripheral shell of highly organized bone.

Differential Diagnosis

- **Extraosseous osteosarcoma:** Elderly patients, malignant cytology, either no zonation or more mature centrally.
- **Juxtacortical osteosarcoma:** Either no zonation or more mature centrally.

Case History: An 8-year-old girl with tumor in the femur.

Diagnosis: Ewing's sarcoma

Clinical Features

- Age: 5 to 20 years
- Sex: M: F 1 : 2
- Pain, fever
- Leukocytosis

Imaging

- Cortical thickening, widening of medullary canal.
- Reactive periosteal bone deposited in layers parallel to cortex (onion skin appearance).
- Widening of medullary canal.

Gross

- White, fleshy, ill-defined with involvement of medulla and cortex with periosteal elevation.
- May be necrotic or resembles pus.

Microscopy

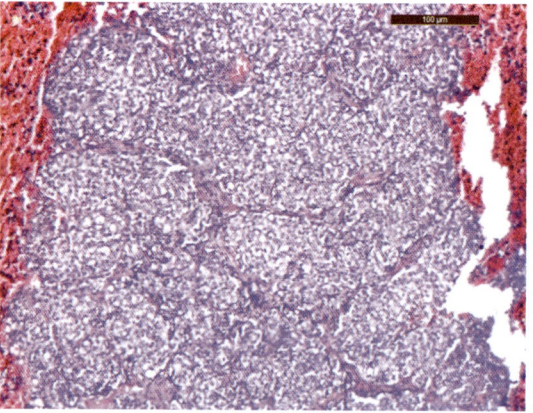

Fig. 16.10

- Sheets of small round uniform cells with scant cytoplasm.
- Round nuclei with indentations, small nucleoli. Pseudorosette (perivascular, Homer Wright) formation.
- Necrosis common.

Ancillary Tests
- **IHC:** CD99, NSE, FLI 1, vimentin.
- **Molecular genetics:** Most commonly t(11;22) (q24;q12) or t(21;22) (q22;q12). Fusion of EWS with FLI gene.

Differential Diagnosis
Small round blue cell tumors
- *Embryonal rhabdomyosarcoma:* Myogenin positive
- *Lymphoma:* CD45 positive
- *Metastatic neuroblastoma:* Patients younger than 5 years, primary should be evident.

Case History: A 36-year-old male with right ankle pain.

Diagnosis: Synovial chondromatosis

Clinical Features
- Always monoarticular.
- Involves large joints (knees and hips).
- Pain, swelling or limited motion.

Imaging
- Non-specific.
- Diffuse swelling in joints or calcific densities within joints.

Gross
Osteocartilaginous bodies confined to synovium or extruded into joint cavity.

Microscopy

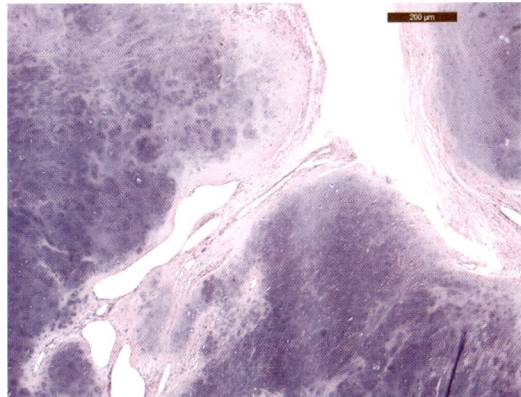

Fig. 16.11

- Nodules of cartilage within the synovium.
- Chondrocytes with moderate atypia.
- Sequence of disease:
  - Active intrasynovial disease with no loose bodies
  - Intrasynovial proliferation and free loose bodies
  - Multiple free osteochondral bodies with no demonstrable intrasynovial disease.

Differential Diagnosis
- **Cartilaginous loose bodies:** Associated with arthritis
- **Chondrosarcoma:** Not within a joint, no characteristic clustering pattern, marked myxoid change, spindling of nuclei
- **Osteochondritis dissecans:** No lobulation, clustering or atypia.

Case History: A 34-year-old male with Ollier disease.

Diagnosis: Enchondroma

Types
- Enchondromas of hands and feet
- Calcifying enchondroma
- Soft tissue enchondroma
- Juxtacortical enchondroma

Clinical Features
- **Ollier disease:** Multiple enchondromas predominantly unilateral, associated with ovarian sex cord stromal tumor.
- **Maffucci syndrome:** Enchondromas with soft tissue hemangiomas.
- **Age:** 10–40 years
- Usually asymptomatic.
- Pain due to pathological fracture.

Site
- Hands and feet, ribs, femur, and humerus.
- Medulla of diaphysis.

Imaging
- Thinning but preservation of cortex.
- Pathologic fractures common.

Gross

Well circumscribed, pale blue, solid, resembles cartilage without myxoid change.

Microscopy

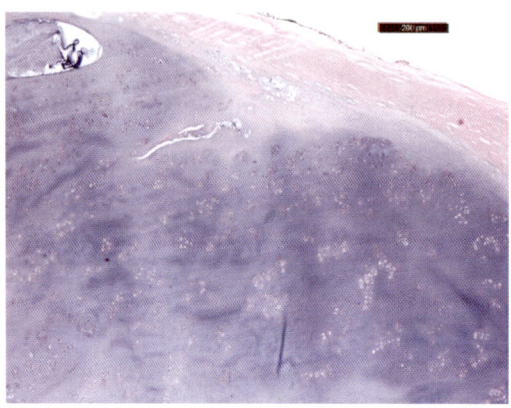

Fig. 16.12

- Mature lobules of hyaline cartilage.
- Foci of myxoid degeneration, calcification and enchondral ossification common.

Differential Diagnosis

- **Epiphyseal dysplasia:** In babies, affects multiple joints.
- **Low grade chondrosarcoma:** Breaks through or erodes cortex, marked myxoid change, large tumors occupy marrow space and entrap bony trabeculae.

Case History: A 14-year-old boy with tender, palpable mass in the right parietal region of skull.

Diagnosis: Langerhans cell histiocytosis

Clinical Features

- Age: 5 to 15 years
- Sex: M : F 3 : 2

Sites

Skull, jaw, humerus, ribs, and femur.

Location

Metaphysis or diaphysis is of 3 types:
- Solitary bone involvement
- Multiple bone involvement
- Multiple organ involvement.

Imaging

Lytic masses that may extend to soft tissues.

Gross

Sharply circumscribed lesion.

Microscopy

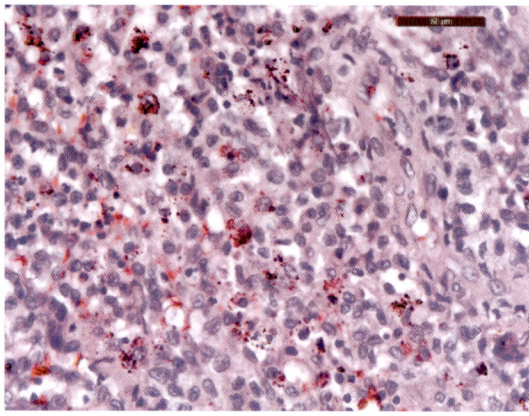

Fig. 16.13

- Infiltration by Langerhans cells which are polygonal cells with eosinophilic cytoplasm, oval nuclei with longitudinal grooves.
- Other features—eosinophils, giant cells, neutrophils, foam cells, lymphocytes, plasma cells, necrosis, mitosis seen.

Ancillary Tests

- **IHC:** CD1a, S-100, vimentin, CD68, Langerin.
- **Electron microscopy:** Intracytoplasmic Birbeck granules with its characteristic tennis racket appearance seen.
- **Molecular genetics:** Loss of DNA sequences involving several chromosomes and 1p.

Differential Diagnosis

- Osteomyelitis
- Rosai-Dorfman disease
- Lymphoma
- Acute myelomonocytic leukemia.

Case History: An 18-year-old boy with a painful mass in the femur.

Diagnosis: Chondroblastoma

Clinical Features
- Age: 10–25 years
- Sex: M : F 2 : 1
- Pain, restricted joint mobility.

Location
Epiphysis of femur, humerus, feet, pelvis, scapula.

Imaging
Well circumscribed with areas of rarefactions.

Gross
Well circumscribed, white-blue-gray with variable necrotic, calcific and cystic areas.

Microscopy

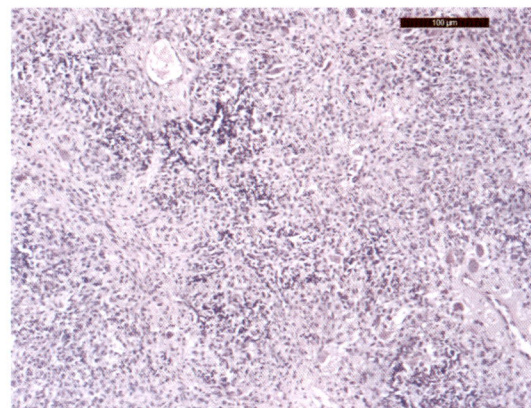

Fig. 16.14

- Pink and blue. Hypercellular areas, fibrous and chondroid areas with occasional spindle cells.
- Compact polyhedral chondroblasts with sharply defined cell membranes. Nuclei are round to indented and lobulated.
- Intracytoplasmic glycogen granules and osteoclast-like giant cells seen.
- Thin lines of calcification (chicken-wire calcification) present.

Ancillary Stains
- PAS-D (glycogen)
- Reticulin (surrounds each cell)
- S-100, vimentin, NSE.

Differential Diagnosis
- **Chondromyxoid fibroma:** Metaphyseal, myxoid with pseudolobular pattern with pleomorphic stellate cells
- **Giant cell tumor:** Numerous clustered giant cells, no chondroid differentiation, no chicken-wire matrix.

Case History: A 45-year-old female with morning stiffness.

Diagnosis: Rheumatoid arthritis

Clinical Features
- Sex: Mostly women
- Age: 10 to 29 years
- Joints of feet and hand
- Malaise, musculoskeletal pain, swollen warm joints, morning stiffness.

Imaging
- Joint effusion, juxta-articular osteopenia, erosions and narrowing of joint space.
- Radial deviation of wrist, ulnar deviation of digits, swan-neck finger abnormalities.

Gross
Joints have edematous, thick, hyperplastic synovium, covered by delicate and bulbous fronds.

Microscopy

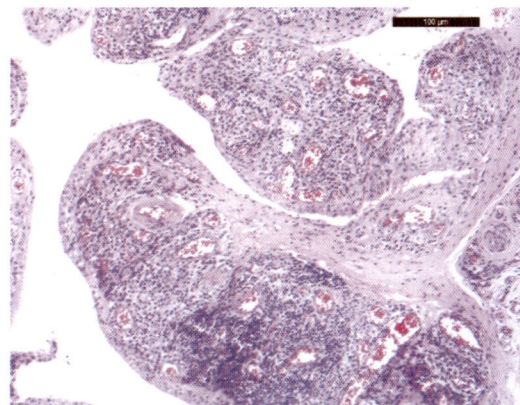

Fig. 16.15

- Hyperemia and proliferation of synovial membrane, infiltration by lymphocytes, plasma cells, macrophages.

- Lymphoid follicles with germinal center formation, pannus formation composed of synovium with inflammatory cells, granulomatous tissue and fibroblasts.
- Rice bodies formation seen.

Molecular Genetics
HLA-DR4, DR1

Case History: A 40-year-old female with a history of thyroidectomy.

Diagnosis: Follicular carcinoma—metastasis to bone

Imaging
Lytic lesions in medulla.

Gross
Usually involves medullary region of bone.

Microscopy

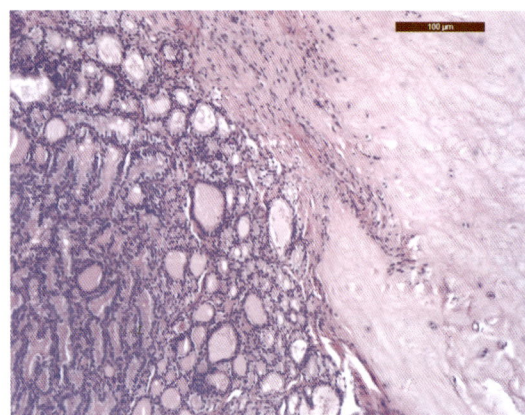

Fig. 16.16

- Thyroid follicular cells with follicle formation within the bone.
- Points for substantiating the diagnosis: History of carcinoma thyroid.

Immunohistochemistry
TTF1 +ve.

Case History: A 63-year-old male with pain in the thigh.

Diagnosis: Neuroendocrine carcinoma metastasis to bone.

Clinical Features
- Pain
- Pathological fractures
- Spinal cord compression (in vertebral metastasis)
- Rarely hypercalcemia.

Imaging
PET and CT, PET is more sensitive.

Gross
Polypoid lesions 2 mm to 4 cm, arising in submucosa.

Microscopy
- Large polyhedral cells with hyperchromatic nuclei.
- Also anaplastic cells, areas of necrosis and mitotic figures.

Differential Diagnosis
- Large cell lymphoma
- Metastatic adenocarcinoma.

Immunohistochemistry
Synaptophysin, chromogranin, TTF-1, PAX8 (duodenal carinoid), CDX2 (ileal carcinoid).

Case History: A 32-year-old male with lesion in the rib and pigmentation of the skin.

Diagnosis: Fibrous dysplasia

Clinical Features
- McCune-Albright syndrome (fibrous dysplasia, precocious puberty and skin hyperpigmentation).
- Mazabraud syndrome (fibrous dysplasia and soft tissue myxomas).
- Age: 10–30 years
- Sex: M : F 3 : 2
- Monostotic and polyostotic
- Ribs, femur, tibia, jaw, skull (monostotic)
- Medulla of diaphysis or metaphysis

Imaging
- Fusiform, expanded mass with thinning of cortex.

- Occasionally lesion protrudes far beyond normal bone contour (fibrous dysplasia protuberans).

Gross
Gritty to cut, grayish color, cortical bone thinned and expanded.

Microscopy

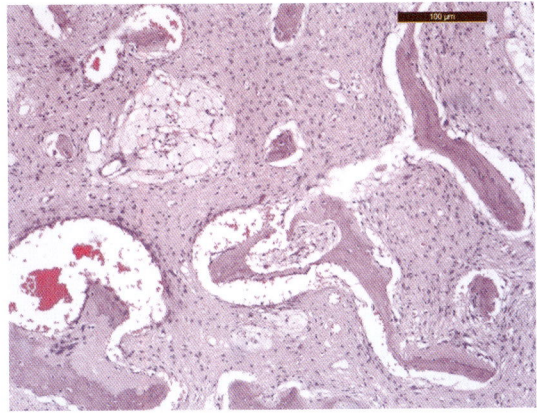

Fig. 16.17

- Curvilinear trabeculae (Chinese letter pattern) of metaplastic woven bone, hypocellular, fibroblastic stroma, no osteoblastic rimming.
- Abrupt transition of normal to abnormal bone.

Stains
Periostin

Differential Diagnosis
Well-differentiated osteosarcoma: Has lacy, malignant bone; intramedullary extension, cortical violation, soft tissue extension.

Case History: A 47-year-old male with severe pain in the left greater toe.

Diagnosis: Gout
- Sex: Males more common
- Metatarsophalangeal joints, often first affected
- Age >30, family history
- Alcohol, obesity and lead

Gross
Chalky white appearance of gouty deposits.

Microscopy

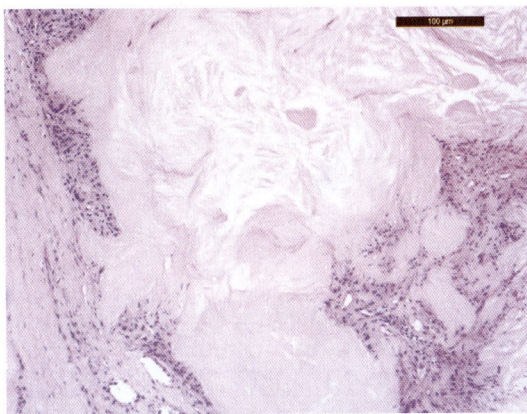

Fig. 16.18

- Fixation in alcohol important for preserving sodium urate monohydrate deposits which appear as needle shaped, doubly refractile crystals.
- Tophi: Urate crystals, granulomatous inflammation and hyperplastic synovium.
- Chronic disease: Deposits in soft tissue, ligament, skin.
- Gouty deposits surrounded by fibrous tissue rimmed by histiocytes and giant cells.

Differential Diagnosis
Crystal deposition Deposition of calcium pyrophosphate (pseudogout), calcium phosphate, talc, methyl methacrylate (prosthetic joints).

Case History: History of radiation therapy.

Diagnosis: Osteosarcoma conventional

Clinical Features
- Age: 10 to 25 years
- Sex: M : F 3 : 2
- Femur, tibia, humerus, pelvis, jaw, fibula
- Medulla of metaphysis
- Paget's disease

- Radiation, chemotherapy
- Pre-existing bone lesions, foreign bodies, trauma and genetic predisposition.

Imaging
- Large destructive lytic or blastic mass.
- May breakthrough cortex and elevate periosteum.
- Sunburst pattern due to new bone formation in soft tissue.

Gross
- Big, bulky, hemorrhagic with cystic degeneration.
- Spreads within medullary cavity, destroys cortex, elevates periosteum, invades soft tissue.
- May form satellite nodules (skip metastasis).

Microscopy

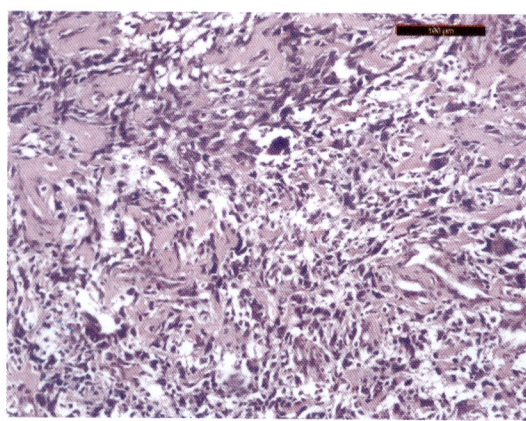

Fig. 16.19

- Tumor destroys pre-existing bony trabeculae.
- Osteoid bone produced by tumor cells without interposition of cartilage.
- Osteoid—eosinophilic, glassy, irregular contour.

Variants
- Osteoblastic
- Fibroblastic
- Chondroblastic

Ancillary Tests
- **IHC:** Alkaline phosphatase, vimentin, S-100, vWF.
- **Molecular genetics:** Aneuploid or hyperploid and p53 mutation.

Differential Diagnosis
- **Exuberant fracture callus:** History of fracture, no atypia
- **Myositis ossificans:** Zonation present, no atypia.

Case History: A 60-year-old male with multiple lesions in the pelvis and skull.

Diagnosis: Paget's disease

Clinical Features
- Age: >55 years
- Sex: 4 : 3 (M : F)
- Lumbosacral, pelvis, skull
- Localised pain.
- Secondary osteoarthritis.
- Leontiasis ossea: Cranium too heavy to lift.
- Platybasia: Invagination of base of skull due to weak bone.

Imaging
- Early—radiolucency
- Late—increased bone density, increased microfracture, sharp demarcation between normal and defective bone, loss of distinction between cortex and medulla.

Microscopy

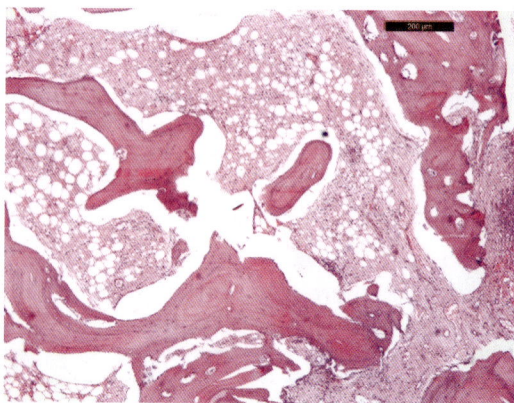

Fig. 16.20

- Increased osteoclastic and osteoblastic activity.
- Acute stage—primary woven bone, focal mosaic pattern of lamellar bone, jigsaw puzzle-like, with prominent irregular cement lines. Osteolytic phase has osteoclasts with up to 100 nuclei.
- Later stage—thick trabeculae, thick bone, marrow fibrosis.

Ancillary Stain
Reticulin highlights disorganization of lamellar bone.

Differential Diagnosis
- **Polyostotic fibrous dysplasia:** Cortical bone has eccentric atrophy
- **Chronic osteomyelitis**
- **Reactive bone adjacent to carcinoma**
- **Radiation effect**

Case History: A 31-year-old female with a painful swelling in the left lower limb.

Diagnosis: Small cell osteosarcoma

Microscopy

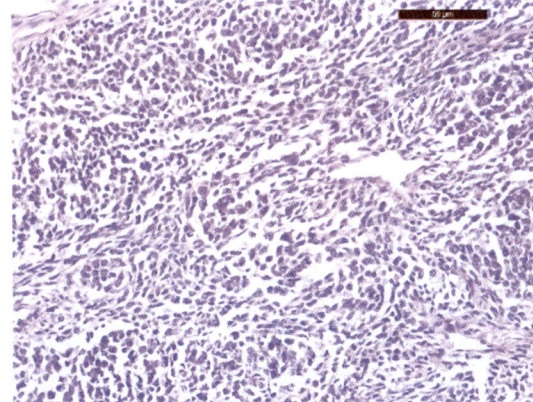

Fig. 16.21

- Diffuse, small, uniform, round, or spindled tumor cells.
- Focally produce osteoid, occasionally with cartilage.

Immunohistochemistry
Vimentin, variable S-100.

Differential Diagnosis
- **Ewing's/PNET:** CD99 positive
- **Lymphoma:** CD45 positive

Case History: A 36-year-old male with slow-growing painless mass in the thigh.

Diagnosis: Parosteal osteosarcoma

Clinical Features
- Age: 30–60 yrs
- Sex: F > M
- Arises from metaphysis of long bones.
- 70% of tumors occur in posterior aspect of distal femur.
- Slow-growing painless mass.

Imaging
X-ray: Prominent extracortical calcified mass that encircles bone. No continuity with bone marrow.

Gross
- Large lobulated mass encircling bone.
- Firm to hard. May contain cartilage.
- Satellite nodules may be present.

Microscopy

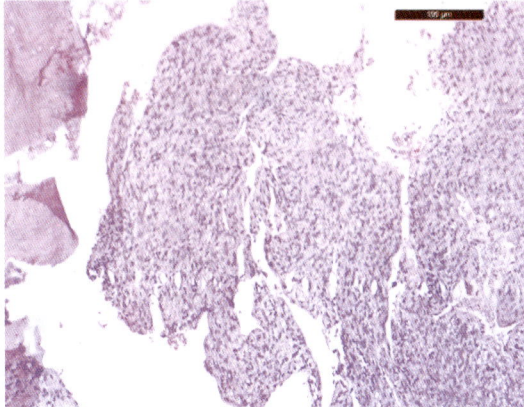

Fig. 16.22

- Low grade neoplasm composed of well-formed bony trabeculae, osteoid, variable cartilage and highly fibrous spindle stroma.

- Stroma is hypocellular but malignant with mild atypia.
- 15% can have coexisting areas of dedifferentiation.
- Rarely osteoclast-like giant cells are seen. No/rare mitotic figures.

Differential Diagnosis

- **Periosteal osteosarcoma** is characterized by lobulated islands of malignant cartilage and areas of moderately high-grade spindle cells located peripherally. Trabeculae of mature osteoid are absent and the lesion shows a little tendency to invade skeletal muscles.
- **High grade surface osteosarcomas:** May be juxtacortical but with cellular pleomorphism and atypia
- **Conventional osteosarcoma with periosteal spread**
- **Myositis ossificans:** Orderly maturation, not attached to underlying bone, more active histologically
- **Osteochondroma:** Tumor continuous with bone, fatty or hematopoietic marrow present.

Case History: A 38-year-old male with pain in the anterior aspect of thigh.

Diagnosis: Extraskeletal mesenchymal chondrosarcoma

Clinical Features

- Can be found in all ages (peak in 2nd and 3rd decades) without a gender predilection.
- Most common in lower extremities.
- Swelling associated with pain.

Imaging

Calcified, eccentric, osteolytic lesion, demonstrating extraosseous extension.

Gross

Pink fleshy mass with calcification.

Microscopy

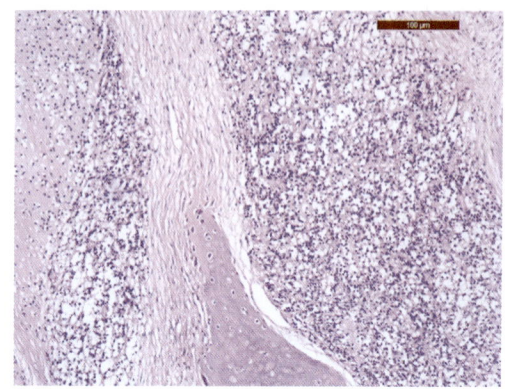

Fig. 16.23

Areas with well-differentiated cartilage mixed with highly cellular areas containing undifferentiated small spindle-shaped or round cells with scant cytoplasm with hemangiopericytoma like vascular pattern.

Molecular Genetics

HEY1-NCOA2 fusion.

Differential Diagnosis

- **Ewing's sarcoma:** No cartilage
- **Small cell osteosarcoma:** Irregular fine trabecular deposition of osteoid
- **Dedifferentiated chondrosarcoma:** Sharp demarcation is present between the cartilage and malignant cellular areas.

Case History: A 6-year-old girl with expansile lytic lesion in the proximal metaphysis of left humerus.

Diagnosis: Telangiectatic osteosarcoma

Clinical Features

Enlarging painful palpable mass. Associated with pathological fracture

Imaging

Lytic lesion with bone destruction

Site

Metaphysis extend into the diaphysis

Gross

Hemorrhagic multicystic lesion with blood clots described as "bag of blood"

Microscopy

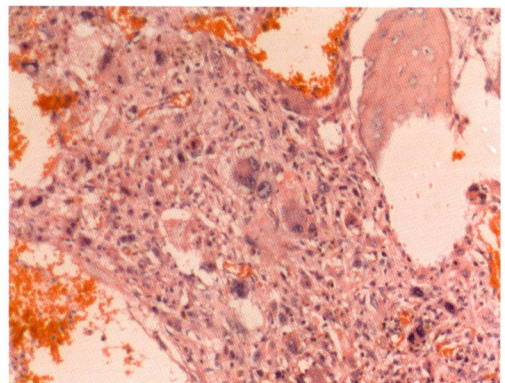

Fig. 16.24

- Blood filled or empty cystic spaces separated by septae
- The septae shows pleomorphic cells with nuclear hyperchromasia, osteoclastic giant cells
- Osteoid formation is focally seen

Differential Diagnosis

- **Aneurysmal bone cyst:** Large cystic spaces filled with blood and separated by fibrous septa.
- **Angiosarcoma:** Atypical vascular spaces lined by endothelial cells with cytological atypia, multilayering.

CHAPTER 17

Skin Lesions

Leena D Joseph

Reaction Patterns in Dermatopathology

Ackerman scheme
1. Superficial perivascular dermatitis
2. Superficial and deep perivascular dermatitis
3. Folliculitis and perifolliculitis
4. Nodular and diffuse dermatitis
5. Fibrosing dermatitis
6. Vasculitis
7. Intraepidermal bullous disease
8. Subepidermal bullous disorders
9. Panniculitis

Immunobullous Disorders

Intraepidermal bullae
1. *Subcorneal:* Subcorneal pustular dermatosis, bullous impetigo, milaria crystallina, staphylococcal scalded skin syndrome, pemphigus foliaceous.
2. *Bullae in stratum malphighi(due to acantholysis):* Pemphigus group, Hailey-Hailey disease.
3. *Bullae in stratum malphighi (due to spongiosis):* Dermatitis, insect bite reaction, incontinentia pigmenti.
4. *Bullae in stratum malphighi (due to cytolysis and ballooning degeneration):* Viral disease such as herpes simplex and zoster.
5. *Bullae in stratum malphighi (due to granular degeneration):* Epidermolytic hyperkeratosis.
6. *Bullae due to basal cell degeneration:* Lichen scleroses et atrophicus, lichen planus, some forms of epidermolysis bullosa.

Subepidermal bullous disease
1. Bullous pemphigoid
2. Herpes gestationis
3. Cicatricial pemphigoid
4. Dermatitis herpetiformis
5. Linear IgA bullous disease of adults and children
6. Epidermolysis bullosa acquisita
7. Porphyria cutanea tarda

Case History: A 28-year-old female with non-palpable purpura over the abdomen for 3 days.

Diagnosis: Leucocytoclastic vasculitis

Clinical Features

Erythematous macules or papules, particularly in lower limb.

Microscopy

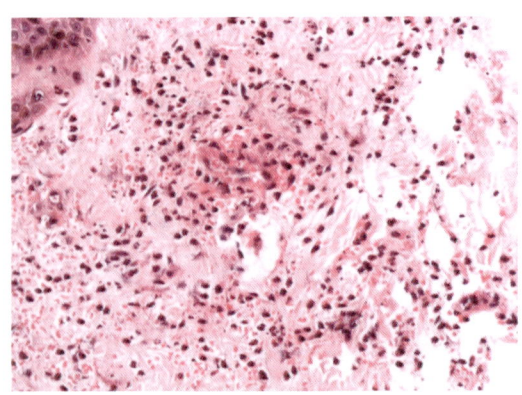

Fig. 17.1

- Reaction pattern of small vessels mainly post-capillary venules with vascular damage and neutrophilic infiltrate.
- Karyorrhexis or leucocytoclasis is seen.
  - Fibrinoid necrosis
  - Extravasated RBC's

Immunofluorescence

Useful to confirm vascular damage as deposition of fibrinogen, C3, IgG and IgM can be seen within vessel walls.

Differential Diagnosis

- **Henoch-Schönlein purpura:** The histology is identical. IgA deposition on immunofluorescence will confirm a clinical diagnosis.
- **Urticarial vasculitis:** While the changes may be very similar in this condition, typically there is more prominent superficial dermal edema, and the density of the inflammatory infiltrate is less. In particular there may be a less neutrophilic component with even a pure lymphocytic vasculitis
- **Septic vasculitis:** Here the clue is vascular occlusion by thrombus. There may be little leukocytoclasis.
- **Sweet syndrome:** The presence of notable papillary dermal edema and a diffuse neutrophilic infiltrate in Sweets should be discriminatory. There should be no significant fibrinoid necrosis.

Case History: A 40-year-old female with single brown sharply demarcated nodule of face.

Diagnosis: Seborrheic keratosis

Clinical Features

- Single or multiple, seen on trunk and face and even extremities excluding palms and soles.
- Sharply demarcated brownish in color, raised with stuck on look.

Microscopy

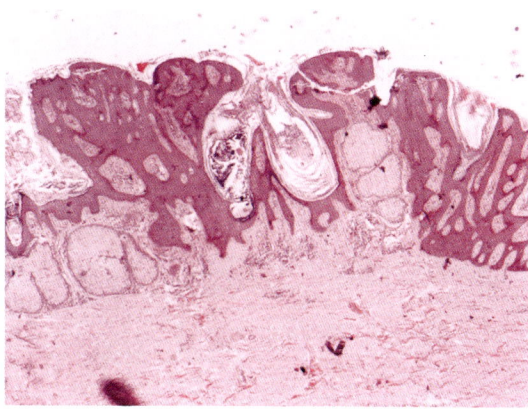

Fig. 17.2

- Hyperkeratosis, acanthosis and papillomatosis.
- Acanthosis is due to upward extension of the tumor.
- Line can be drawn from normal epidermis to the other end.

Two types of cells are seen

Squamous cells and basaloid cells.

Irritated type and inverted follicular keratosis: Squamous cells outnumber the basaloid cells, eddies are present.

Differential Diagnosis

Horn pearls of squamous cell carcinoma.

Case History: A 28-year-old female with warty lesion over the dorsal aspect of the finger.

Diagnosis: Verruca vulgaris

Clinical Features

Located on the dorsal aspect of the fingers and hands as a painless, circumscribed, firm elevated papules with papillomatous, hyperkeratotic surfaces.

Microscopy

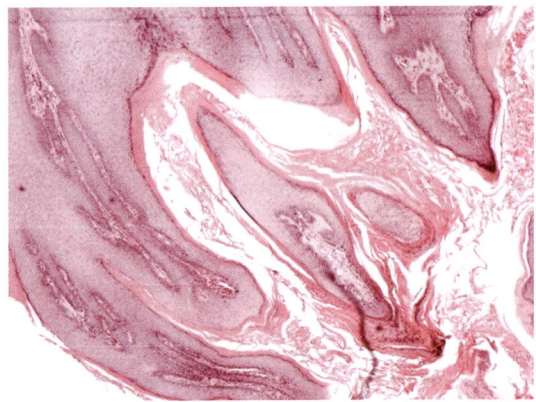

Fig. 17.3

- Acanthosis, papillomatosis and hyperkeratosis.
- Rete ridges are elongated and at the periphery of the verrucae are bent inwards so that they appear to point radially towards the center (arborization).
- Vacuolated cells or koilocytes are present.
- Koilocytes have small round basophilic nuclei surrounded by clear halo and pale staining cytoplasm.

Differential Diagnosis

From other papillomatosis by the presence of koilocytes.

Case History: A 58-year-old male with macule black in color with irregular margin.

Diagnosis: Nodular melanoma, malignant melanoma

Melanoma in situ and nontumorigenic invasive melanomas may be divided into:
- Lentigo maligna
- Superficial spreading
- Acral lentiginous
- Mucosal lentiginous type.

Clinical Features

All melanomas arise from melanocytes at the epidermal dermal junction. Majority of the melanomas are secondary to sun exposure.

Clinical Diagnostic Criteria Include ABCD

- A for lesional asymmetry
- B for border irregularity
- C for color variegation.
- D for diameter greater than 6 mm.

Microscopy

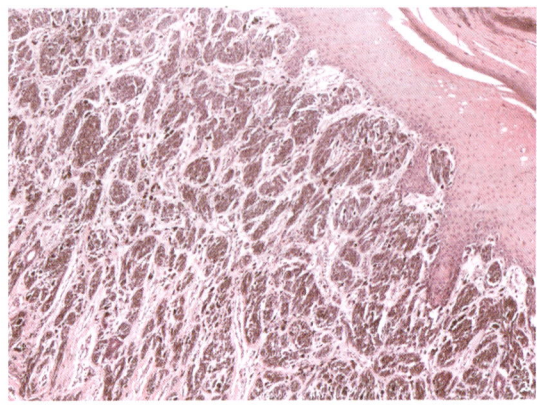

Fig. 17.4

- Most of the lesional cells in nontumorigenic melanomas are located in the epidermis.
- Clinically the tumorigenic vertical growth presents as an expanding papule.
- Proliferation of the melanoma cells in the extracellular matrix of the dermis to form an expansile mass.

Ancillary Tests

- **Special stains:** Fontana Masson, azure blue
- **Immunohistochemistry:** HMB-45, melan A, S-100 positive.

Differential Diagnosis

- Nevus
- Pigmented seborrheic keratosis
- Hemangioma
- Pigmented basal cell carcinoma.

Case History: A 27-year-old female with lesion on the labia majora.

Diagnosis: Hidradenoma papilliferum

Clinical Features

Usually seen in women on labia majora or in the perineal/perianal region.

Microscopy

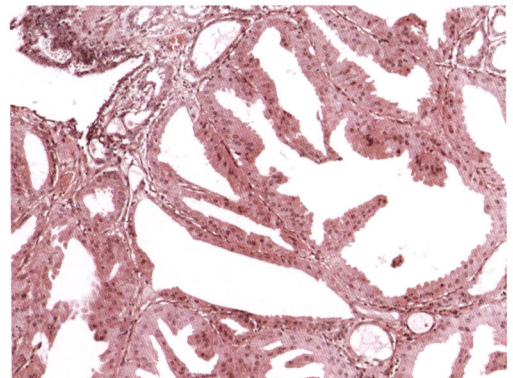

Fig. 17.5

- Adenoma with apocrine differentiation. Located in dermis, well circumscribed, surrounded by a fibrous capsule, no connection with the overlying epidermis.
- Within the tumor, tubular and cystic spaces are seen, with papillary folds projecting into cystic spaces.
- Lumina are lined by only a single row of columnar cells, with oval pale staining nucleus located near the base, eosinophilic cytoplasm and active decapitation secretion.

Differential Diagnosis

- **Syringocystadenoma papilliferum:** Glandular papillary proliferations connected to skin surface with dense plasma cell infiltrate.
- **Tubular apocrine adenoma:** Well- circumscribed dermal neoplasm that may extend into subcutis. Lobular pattern of dermal and subcutaneous tubular apocrine structures often encased by a fibrous, sometimes hyalinized stroma. Lobules have dilated, variably sized tubules lined by two layers of epithelial cells. Pseudopapillae are common. Rare connection with overlying epidermis. Positive for EMA, CEA, Cam 5.2, SMA, GCDFP-15, CK7, S100.

Case History: A 45-year-old female with reddish brown patch on the face.

Diagnosis: Lupus vulgaris

Tuberculosis of Skin

Seen as
- Primary tuberculosis
- Tuberculosis verrucosa cutis
- Lupus vulgaris
- Scrofuloderma
- Tuberculous gumma
- Tuberculosis cutis orificialis.

Clinical Features

- Lesions are seen on the head and neck, mainly around the nose.
- One or a few well-demarcated reddish brown patches containing deep seated nodules, apple jelly nodules are seen.

Microscopy

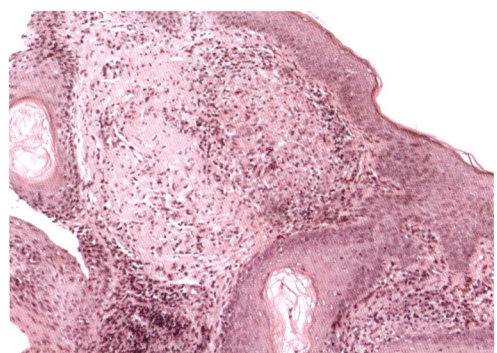

Fig. 17.6

- Tuberculoid granulomas with Langhans giant cells are seen, caseation necrosis is slight or absent.
- Associated infiltrate of lymphocytes

Special Stains

Acid-fast staining.

Differential Diagnosis

- Sarcoidosis
- Mycosis
- Leishmaniasis
- Non-tuberculosis, mycobacteriosis and leprosy
- Syphilis
- Foreign body implantation reaction
- Wegener's granulomatosis
- Rosacea.

Case History: A 23-year-old male with erythematous macule over lower limbs.

Diagnosis: Lepromatous leprosy, Hansen's disease (leprosy)

Clinical Features
- Three clinical types—macular, infiltrative nodular and diffuse.
- Lesion seen as numerous ill-defined confluent, hypopigmented or erythematous macules.
- Infiltrative nodular (leonine facies)—papules, nodules and dull red diffuse infiltrate.

Microscopy

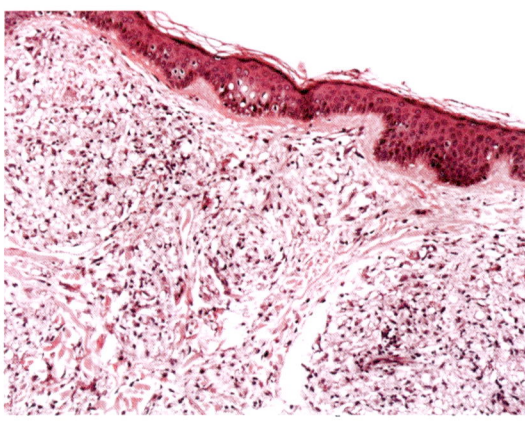

Fig. 17.7

- Extensive cellular infiltrate
- Narrow grenz zone of normal collagen, flattened epidermis
- Destruction of cutaneous appendages; BI—4 or 5
- No granulomas are present, but plasma cells may be seen
- Lepra cells or Virchow cells are present.

Hansen's Histioid
Solid staining bacilli like sheaves of wheat, spindled out macrophages.

Borderline Lepromatous
Lymphocytes are more prominent. Tendency to form poorly to moderately defined granulomas. Perineural fibroblast proliferation (onion skinning).

Borderline Tuberculoid (BT)
Microscopy
- Granulomas with peripheral lymphocytes follow the neurovascular bundles and infiltrate sweat glands and erector pili muscle.
- Langhans giant cells are variable, nerve erosion is present; BI:0–2.

Tuberculoid (TT)
Microscopy
- Compact granulomas along neurovascular bundles and dense peripheral lymphocytes, Langhans giant cells are absent.
- Dermal nerves may be absent or eroded by the dense infiltrate.

Leprosy Reactions
- *Type I reaction:* Upgrading or downgrading reaction (reversal reaction).
- *Type II reaction:* Erythema nodosum leprosum.

Special Stains
- Wade Fites stain (most commonly used).
- Modified Ziehl-Neelsen stain
- Methenamine silver stain (can demonstrate fragmented bacilli).

Differential Diagnosis
- **Tuberculoid leprosy:** To be differentiated from the other granulomatous dermatitides
- **Sarcoidosis:** Naked granulomas are seen
- **Cutaneous syphilis:** In this condition granulomas are seen in dermis and not in the nerves
- **Granuloma annulare:** Intragranuloma necrosis can be confused with granuloma annulare
- **Xanthomas:** These are differential diagnosis for lepromatous leprosy

Case History: A 38-year-old male with ivory colored plaques over the lower limbs.

Diagnosis: Scleroderma

Clinical Features

Two types:
1. Circumscribed scleroderma (morphea)
2. Systemic scleroderma (progressive systemic sclerosis)
3. Hardening of the skin can be seen in genetic, metabolic, neurologic and immunologic disorder.

Morphea is divided into six types based on morphology and distribution of the lesions

1. Guttate
2. Plaque
3. Linear
4. Segmental
5. Subcutaneous
6. Generalised

Microscopy

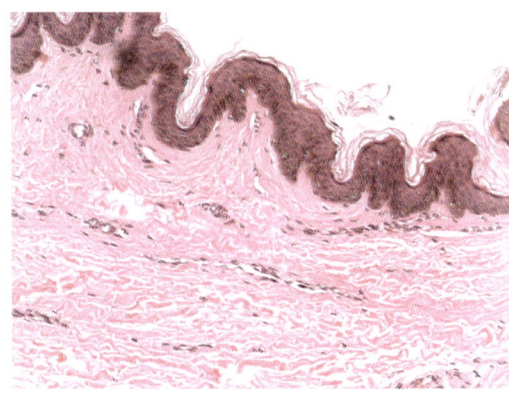

Fig. 17.8

Biopsy should include subcutaneous tissue.
Early inflammatory stage:
- Reticular dermis shows interstitial lymphoplasmacytic infiltrate with slightly thickened collagen bundles.
- Later inflammatory cells surround eccrine coils with more collagen and decreased adipocytes.

Late Sclerotic Stage

- Disappearance of the inflammatory infiltrate except in the subcutis, epidermis is normal.
- Collagen bundles in the reticular dermis appear thickened, closely packed and hypocellular.
- Eccrine glands are atrophied with a few or no adipocytes surrounding them, but only newly formed collagen.

Differential Diagnosis

- **Elastosis:** Due to sunlight and normally seen on thick dermis of fingers and dorsum of hand
- **Eosinophilic fasciitis:** Only deep fascia thickening seen.
- **Lichen sclerosis et atrophicus**

Case History: A 6-year-old girl mole of right eyebrow.

Diagnosis: Intradermal nevus

Clinical Features

Pigmented or non-pigmented lesions usually less than 5 mm in diameter.

Five clinical types are
1. Flat lesions
2. Slightly elevated lesions
3. Papillomatous lesions
4. Dome-shaped lesions
5. Pedunculated lesions

Histopathological types
- Lentigo simplex
- Junctional nevus
- Compound nevus
- Intradermal nevus

Microscopy

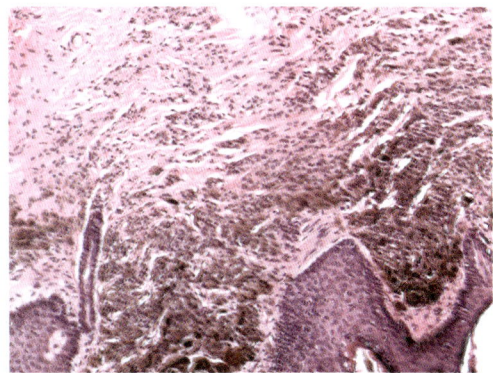

Fig. 17.9

- Intradermal nevus shows no junctional activity.
- The upper dermis contains nests and cords of nevus cells, nevus giant cells may also be seen.
- During tissue processing clefts may form between the tumor nests.

Case History: A 15-year-old boy with skin covered firm papule along the nasolabial fold.

Diagnosis: Trichoepithelioma

Clinical Features

- Solitary or multiple lesions; autosomal dominant inheritance for multiple lesions.
- Numerous rounded skin colored, firm papules and nodules; 2–8 mm size.
- Seen mainly in the nasolabial folds.

Microscopy

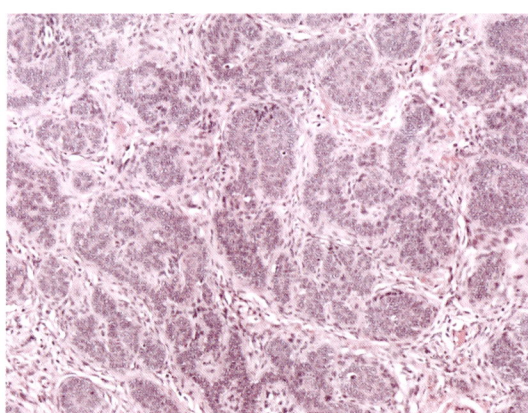

Fig. 17.10

- Superficial dermal lesions, well circumscribed, small and symmetric.
- Horn cysts are most characteristic histologic feature abrupt and complete keratinization.
- Next important feature is tumor islands composed of basophilic cells, with peripheral palisading and surrounded by stroma.
- May show papillary mesenchymal bodies.

Differential Diagnosis

- Syringoma
- Keratotic basal cell carcinoma
- Nevoid BCC.

Case History: A 40-year-old female with nodule on the eyelid.

Diagnosis: Sebaceous gland carcinoma

Introduction

Ocular and extraocular types.
- *Ocular types:* Originate from the meibomian glands in the eyelids.
- *Extraocular types:* Head and neck, vulva, penis.

Microscopy

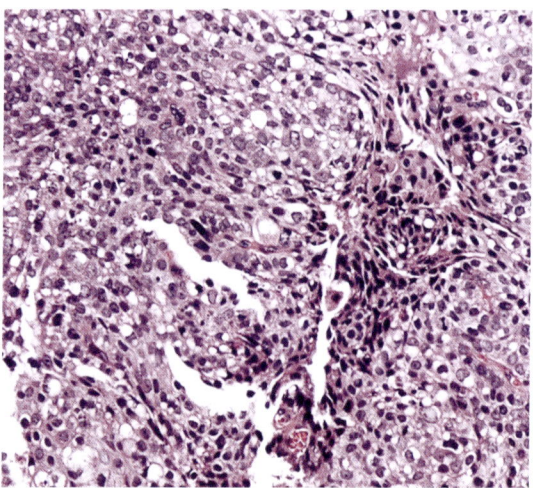

Fig. 17.11

- Irregular lobular formation, great variation in the size of the lobules.
- Undifferentiated cells and sebaceous cell are seen at the center of most lobules.
- Cells with nuclear and nucleolar pleomorphism.
- Cells with fine lipid globules demonstrated by fat stains.
- May have areas of atypical keratinizing cells.

Immunofluorescence

Keratin and EMA positive.

Differential Diagnosis
- Basal cell carcinoma with sebaceous differentiation.
- Squamous cell carcinoma with hydropic changes.
- Malignant neoplasms with clear cells.

Case History: A 40-year-old female with subcutaneous nodule.

Diagnosis: Chondroid syringoma (mixed tumor of the skin)

Clinical Features
- Firm intradermal or subcutaneous nodules.
- Usually on head and neck, 0.5–3 cm.

Microscopy

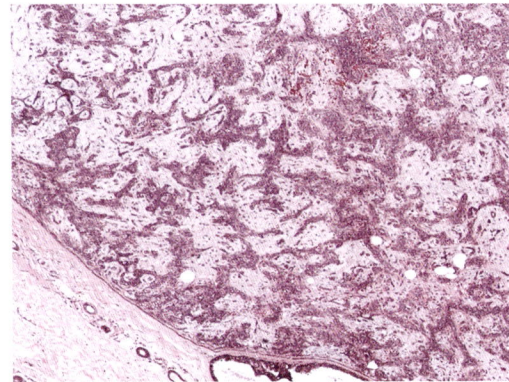

Fig. 17.12

Two types of chondroid syringomas are recognized
- Tubular, cystic partially branching lumina.
- Small tubular lumina.
- Stroma has mucoid, faintly basophilic appearance.
- Malignant chondroid syringoma—anaplastic changes, aggressive behavior.

Special Stain
Tubular lumina contain small amount of amorphous, eosinophilic material that is PAS positive and diastase resistant.

Case History: A 50-year-old female with nodular lesion over the outer canthus of eye.

Diagnosis: Basal cell carcinoma

Clinical Features
Seen exclusively on hair bearing skin mainly face, usually single lesion.

Clinical Types
- Superficial BCC
- Nodular BCC
- Micronodular BCC
- Infiltrating BCC
- Fibroepithelioma

Microscopy

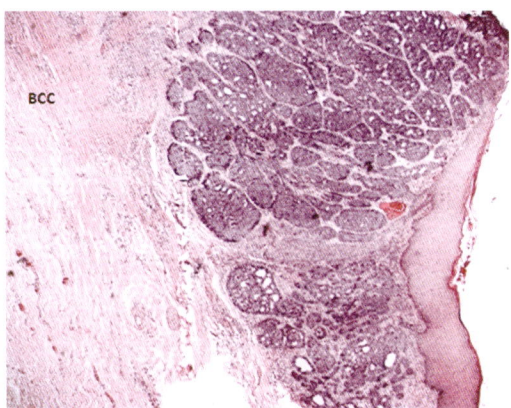

Fig. 17.13

- Predominant basal cell type, peripheral palisading of lesional cell nuclei, a specialised stroma, and clefting artefact between the epithelium and the stroma.
- Variable degree of cytologic atypia and mitotic activity.

Histologic Variants
- Keratotic BCC
- BCC with sebaceous differentiation: Adenoid BCC
- Adamantinoid type
- Granular type
- Clear cell type with matrical differentiation.

Immunohistochemistry
- *Positive stains:* p53, BCL-2, p63, MNF116
- *Negative stains:* EMA, CEA, CK20.

Differential Diagnosis
- Merkel cell carcinoma
- Microcystic adnexal carcinoma
- Squamous cell carcinoma
- Trichoblastoma/trichoepithelioma

Case History: An 8-year-old boy with nodule over the nape of neck.

Diagnosis: Pilomatricoma

Clinical Features
- Solitary lesion, face and upper extremities are most common sites.
- Deep seated nodule covered with skin 0.5 to 3 cm in greatest dimension.
- More in children and adolescents.

Microscopy

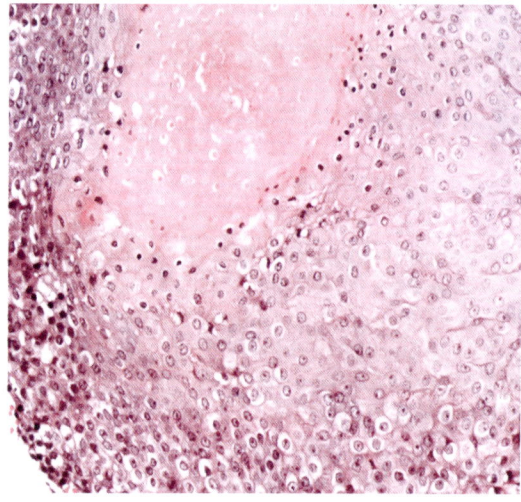

Fig. 17.14

- Tumor is sharply demarcated, surrounded by capsule, located in the lower dermis and extends into subcutaneous fat.
- Islands of epithelial cells are embedded in a cellular stroma.
- Islands are composed of basophilic cells and shadow cells.

Special Stains
Shadow cells may have calcium deposits which can be demonstrated by von Kossa stain.

Differential Diagnosis
- Trichilemmal cysts
- BCC with foci of matrical differentiation.

Case History: A 28-year-old male with pink to red scaly papules and plaques over the entire body.

Diagnosis: Psoriasis

Three Types of Psoriasis
1. Psoriasis vulgaris
2. Generalised pustular psoriasis
3. Localised pustular psoriasis.

Psoriasis Vulgaris
- Common inflammatory skin disorder.
- Pink to red scaly papules and plaques, variable sized, sharply demarcated dry and covered with fine silver scales, Auspitz sign is positive.

Sites of Predilection
Scalp, sacral region, extensor aspects of the extremities.

Microscopy

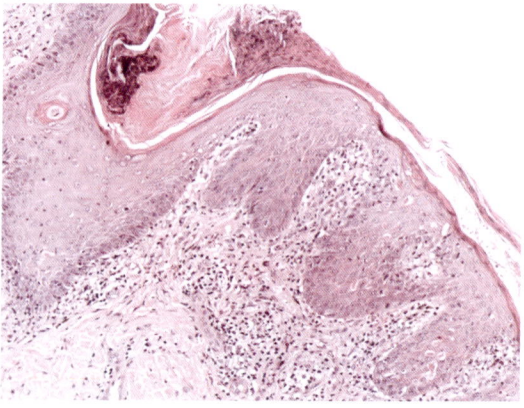

Fig. 17.15

- Diagnostic features vary with the stage of the lesion.
- Earliest change is capillary dilation and edema in the papillary dermis with lymphocytes surrounding the capillaries.
- Fully developed lesion shows acanthosis with regular elongation of the rete ridges with thickening and clubbing in the lower portions (resembling camel feet), increased mitosis in the rete ridges.
- Thinning of the suprapapillary dermis with the occasional presence of spongiform pustules of Kogoj.
- Pallor of the upper layer of the epidermis.
- Diminished to absent granular layer, confluent parakeratosis, presence of Munro microabscesses, elongation and edema of the dermal papillae, dilated and tortuous capillaries.

Differential Diagnosis

- **Chronic eczematous dermatitis:** (Psoriasiform dermatitis) uneven elongation of rete ridges, marked spongiosis, crusting in the cornified layer.
- **Lichen simplex chronicus**
- **Seborrheic dermatitides:** Accentuated spongiosis, mounds of parakeratosis, irregular acanthosis with neutrophil in follicular ostia.
- **Pityriasis rubra pilaris:** Thick suprapapillary plates, broader and shorter rete ridges, preserved granular layer. It lacks Munro micro—abscess.
- **Spongiform pustules**

Case History: A 45-year-old male with violaceous papules over skin.

Diagnosis: Lichen planus

Clinical Features

- Skin lesions are small, flat topped, shiny polygonal violaceous papules that may coalesce to plaques.
- White lines on the plaques are called Wickham's striae. Pronounced pruritis.

Microscopy

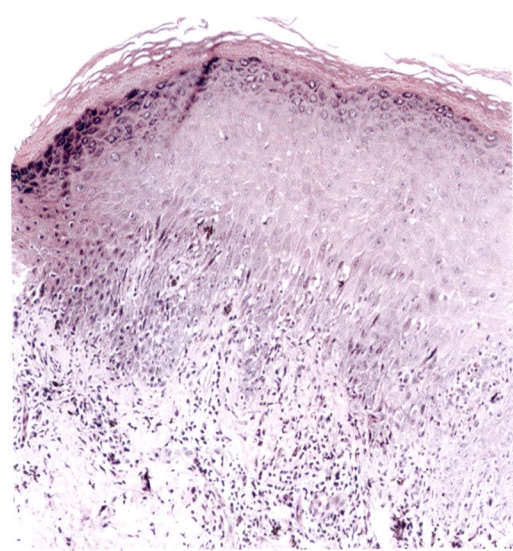

Fig. 17.16

- Compact orthokeratosis. Wedge-shaped hypergranulosis, irregular acanthosis.
- Vacuolar alteration of the basal layer.
- Band-like dermal lymphocytic infiltrate, saw-toothed appearance of the rete ridges.
- Dome-shaped papillae between the rete ridges, pigment incontinence.
- Civatte bodies
- Max Joseph spaces may be present.

Differential Diagnosis

- GVHD
- Lichen nitidus
- Lupus erythematosus
- Drug reactions
- Lichenoid actinic keratosis
- Lichen planus like keratosis.

Case History: A 48-year-old male with solitary nodular lesion over the arm.

Diagnosis: Nodular hidradenoma

Clinical Features

Solitary, intradermal tumor, 0.5 to 2 cm.

Gross

Presence of cysts.

Microscopy

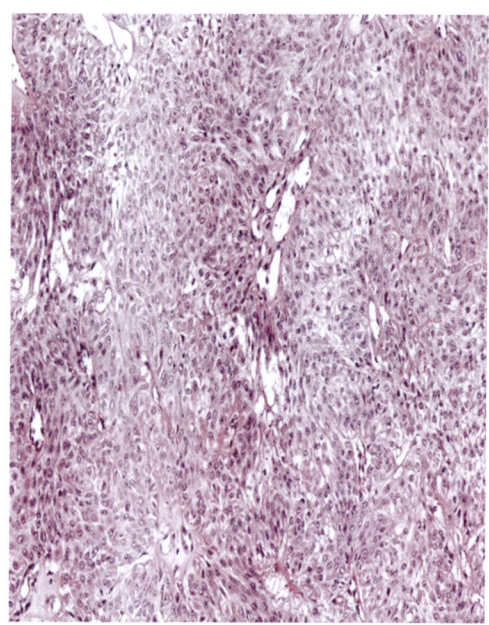

Fig. 17.17

- Well circumscribed, may appear encapsulated.
- Epithelial lobules in the dermis, within the lobules tubular lumina of various types are present.
- If absent step sectioning is needed to identify the lumina.
- Presence of cysts with eosinophilic material.
- Tubular lumina are lined by cuboidal to columnar epithelium.

Two types of cells are seen in the solid portions:
- Polyhedral cells with rounded nucleus and basophilic cytoplasm.
- Round with clear cytoplasm, distinctly visible cell borders.
- Squamous differentiation with horn pearls may be present.

Special Stains

Clear cells contain PAS positive diastase resistant material along the periphery.

Immunohistochemistry

Keratin, EMA, S-100, vimentin.

Differential Diagnosis

- **Trichilemmoma:** Also shows presence of clear cells rich in glycogen and foci of keratinisation (only nodular hidradenoma shows presence of cysts and tubular lumina, whereas trichilemmoma shows peripheral palisading of tumor cells)
- **Malignant nodular hidradenoma:** Larger asymmetric with invasion, atypical mitosis, tumor necrosis, areas of high cellularity, marked cytologic atypia.

Case History: A 42-year-old male with solitary intradermal painful lesion.

Diagnosis: Eccrine spiradenoma

Clinical Features

Seen as a solitary intradermal nodule measuring 1–2 cm in diameter.

Microscopy

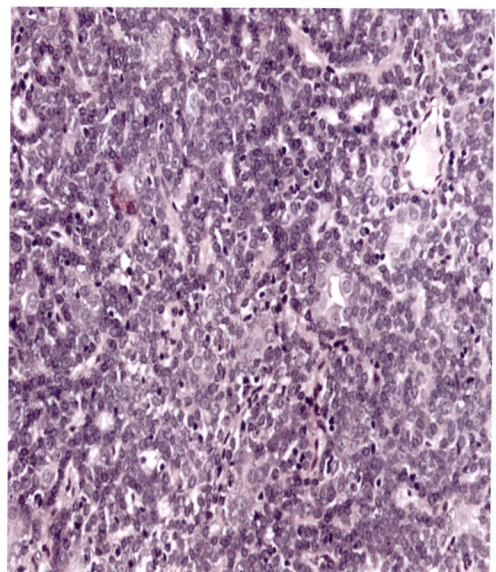

Fig. 17.18

- The tumor consists of one large, sharply demarcated lobule, may display a fibrous capsule.
- Tumor lobules appear deeply basophilic because of the dense packing of the nuclei.

- Epithelial cells are arranged in intertwining cords, cords enclose small irregularly shaped islands of edematous connective tissue.
- Malignancy in the lesion shows glandular formation, squamous differentiation and sarcomatous change with high mitotic rate.

Differential Diagnosis
- Cutaneous lymphadenoma
- Cylindroma
- Metastatic carcinoma.

Case History: A 38-year-old male with papular lesion on the face.

Diagnosis: Cryptococcus

Clinical Features
- Solitary lesion
- Lesions on uncovered parts
- History of trauma and direct inoculation
- Most often occurs in immunosuppressed patients but may occur in nonimmunosuppressed patients.
- Single lesion develops at the site of infection
- Solitary nodules that may ulcerate
- Cellulitis
- Ulcers
- Abscesses
- Panniculitis.

Microscopy

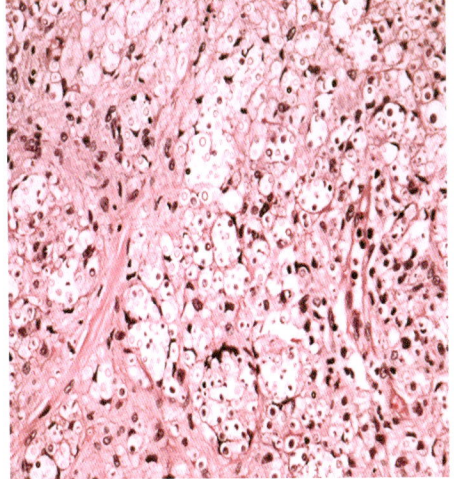

Fig. 17.19

- It is an oval, thick-walled spherule surrounded by a polysaccharide capsule.
- Two patterns of involvement can be seen.
  - The *first* is the gelatinous type, which shows numerous budding yeasts in a foamy stroma with a little or no inflammation.
  - The *second* is the granulomatous type, which shows fewer, smaller organisms and a granulomatous inflammatory infiltrate.

Special Stains
Methylene blue, alcian blue, or mucicarmine.

Case History: A 70-year-old male with large tense bullae over the trunk.

Diagnosis: Bullous pemphigoid

Clinical Features
Subepidermal blistering which can persist for weeks to months.

Microscopy

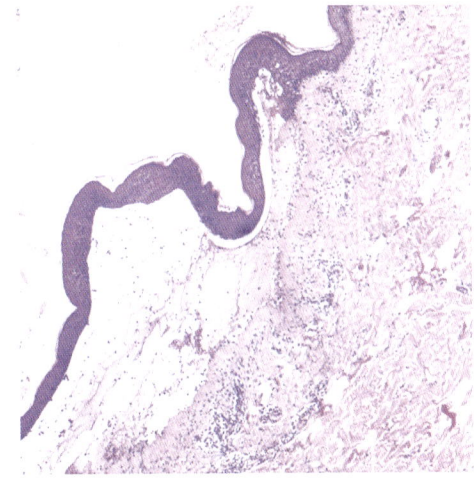

Fig. 17.20

- Subepidermal non-acantholytic unilocular blisters with festooning of dermal papillae, perivascular lymphohistiocytic infiltrate, eosinophilic microabscess, mild interface changes.
- NaCl split skin test: Antibody binds to epidermal side.

Immunohistochemistry

Linear IgG and C3 antibodies to hemidesmosomes at the lamina lucida of the basement membrane.

Differential Diagnosis

- **Dermatitis herpetiformis:** Papillary neutrophilic microabscesses, basal cell vacuoles, granular IgA pattern in dermal papillae by direct immunofluorescence, no circulating antibodies
- **Epidermolysis bullosa acquisita:** Reactivity on dermal side in salt split skin, fluorescence on the floor of the blister, while BP fluorescence is on the roof of the blister
- **Bullous lupus erythematosus:** Fulfills the criteria for SLE, including positive lupus serology (antinuclear antibodies); reactivity will be seen on dermal side in salt split skin

Case History: A 55-year-old female with large and flaccid bullae in oral cavity and scalp.

Diagnosis: Pemphigus vulgaris

Clinical Features

- Direct pressure to the center of the lesion is followed by lateral extension, Asboe-Hansen sign.
- Healing is accompanied by post-inflammatory hyperpigmentation but no scarring.

Microscopy

- Numerous, small, suprabasilar bullae with single row of keratinocytes attached to basement membrane.
- Prominent extension of acantholysis into the follicular infundibula.
- Minimal dermal infiltrate.

Differential Diagnosis

- Darier's disease
- Familial benign pemphigus
- Actinic keratosis.

Case History: A 50-year-old male with slowly enlarging erythematous patch.

Diagnosis: Bowen's disease

Clinical Features

Solitary slowly enlarging erythematous lesion common in sun unexposed areas.

Microscopy

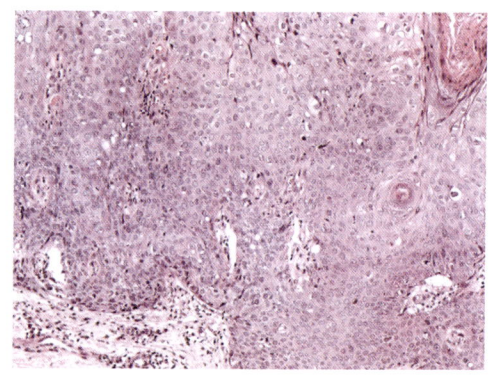

Fig. 17.22

- Wind-blown appearance of the epidermis.
- Atypia prominent throughout epidermis, includes hyperchromasia, multinucleation, individual cell dyskeratosis, increased mitotic figures of the nucleus.
- Surface keratinization and cytoplasmic vacuoles are present.

Immunohistochemistry

p53, high molecular weight CK.

Differential Diagnosis

- Bowenoid actinic keratosis
- Chronic arsenic ingestion.

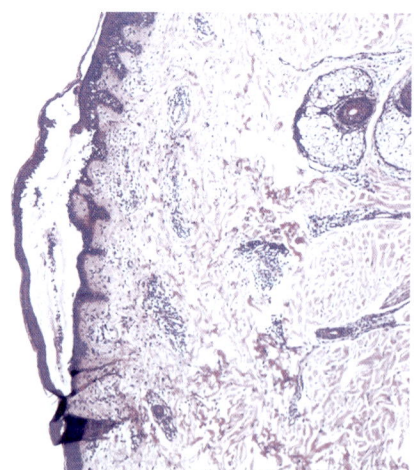

Fig. 17.21

Case History: A 65-year-old female with plum-colored nodule on trunk.

Diagnosis: Cutaneous lymphoma

Clinical Features

Subtypes include:
- Primary cutaneous follicle center lymphoma
- Primary cutaneous marginal zone lymphoma
- Intravascular large B cell lymphoma, diffuse large B cell lymphoma, leg type
- Diffuse large B cell lymphoma—other.

Microscopy

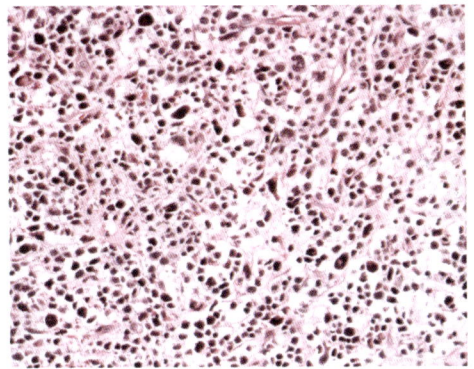

Fig. 17.23

Sheets of monoclonal population of lymphocytes showing atypia and mitosis.

Immunohistochemistry

Primary Cutaneous Follicle Center Lymphoma

- Positive for CD20 and CD79a with follicular pattern.
- Follicular and diffuse patterns of PCFCL typically BCL-6 positive.
- CD10 expressed in follicular pattern and typically negative in diffuse pattern.
- BCL-2, CD5, and CD43 negative.
- BCL-2 positivity suggests nodal origin with skin involvement.

Primary Cutaneous Marginal Zone Lymphoma

Positive for CD20, CD79a, and BCL-2.

Diffuse Large B Cell Lymphoma, Leg-type

BCL-2 positive. Positive for CD20, CD79a, MUM-1/IRF4 and usually BCL-6 or CD10.

Case History: An 18-year-old girl with round flesh colored papules.

Diagnosis: Lichen nitidus

Clinical Features

Round flat topped, flesh colored 2–3 mm papule predominantly in arm, trunk or penis.

Microscopy

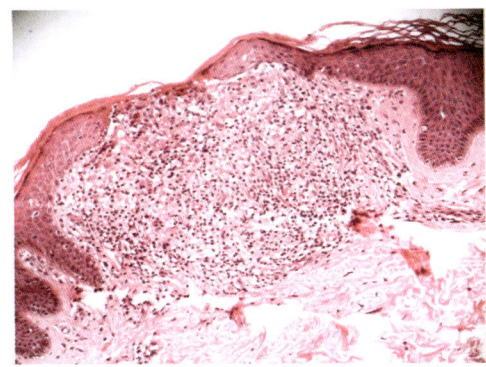

Fig. 17.24

- Well circumscribed mixed cell granulomatous infiltrate attached closely to the lower surface of the epidermis and confined to the widened dermal papillae.
- Rete ridges bend downward and inward, seem to clutch the infiltrate "claw clutching the ball" appearance.
- Thin suprapapillary epidermis with the vacuolar alterations of the basal layer and focal parakeratosis.

Case History: A 40-year-old male with brown red papules with scaling in legs.

Diagnosis: Amyloidosis

Clinical Issues

- *Lichenoid:* Seen at the age of 50–60 years. Intensely itchy rash that is scaly red brown in color on the shins, thighs, feet and forearm.
- *Macular:* Common in women lesions appear as flat dusky brown or grayish colored spot distributed symmetrically over the upper back and the shoulder blades, usually presenting in the early adult life. Itchiness is mild to severe.

- *Nodular:* Very rare present as a single or multiple firm pinkish brown nodules in the trunk, limbs or extremities and face, usually symptomless.

Microscopy

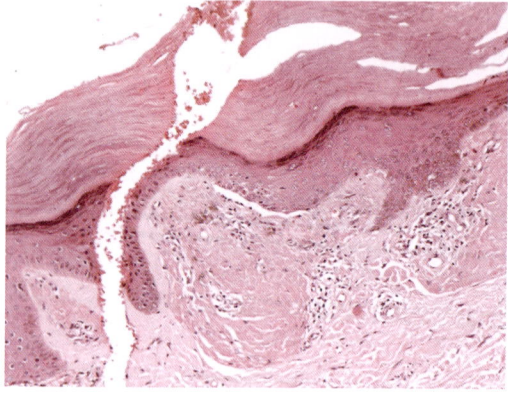

Fig. 17.25

- *Lichenoid:* Hyperkeratosis, acanthosis and basal hydropic degeneration. Small eosinophilic globules in the papillary dermis.
- *Macular:* Focal/small amount of eosinophilic faceted deposit in the papillary dermis also pigment incontinence.
- *Nodular:* Amyloid is not limited to the papillary dermis but is present in the entire dermis and can extend into the subcutaneous fat. Deposits are prominently seen even in the walls of small blood vessel and individual lipocytes with adjacent inflammatory tissue showing predominantly plasma cell.

Special Stain

Congo red stain.

Differential Diagnosis

Cutaneous pseudolymphoma.

CHAPTER 18
Non-Neoplastic Lesions of the Lymph Node

P Shanthi, S Gayathri

Case History: A 31-year-old female with fever for one week. Biopsy right cervical lymph node.

Diagnosis: Kikuchi lymphadenopathy.

Clinical Features
- The patients are young adults, predominantly women.
- More than 85% of the patients present with swollen cervical lymph nodes.

Microscopy

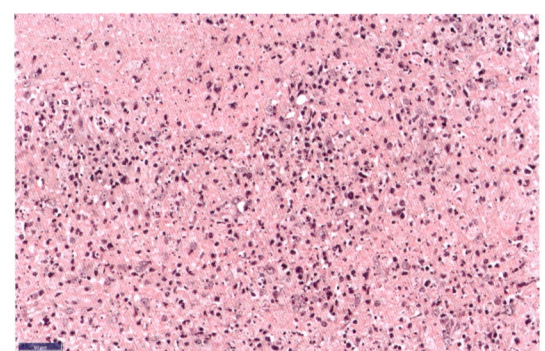

Fig. 18.1

- The lymph node architecture is partially maintained and residual follicles have reactive germinal centers.
- Patchy areas of necrosis and brightly eosinophilic fibrinoid deposits including nuclear fragments.
- Cells with abundant cytoplasm and peripheral compressed, crescentic nuclei resembling signet ring cells.
- Neutrophils and eosinophils are consistently absent, constituting a distinctive feature of this lesion.
- There is usually a degree of perilymphadenitis.

Histologically they may be classified into:
- Lymphohistiocytic type
- Phagocytic type
- Necrotic type
- Foamy cell type

Differential Diagnosis
- **Lymph node infarction:** It shows ischemic necrosis without nuclear debris involving the entire lymph node and sparing only a narrow subcapsular rim.
- **Systemic lupus lymphadenitis:** The foci of fibrinoid necrosis with nuclear debris may be similar; however, also present are hematoxylin bodies, neutrophils, numerous plasma cells and lesions of vasculitis including deposits of nuclear DNA (Azzopardi effect).
- **Necrotizing granulomatous lesions of tuberculosis.**
- **Non-Hodgkin lymphoma:** May be confused with Kikuchi-Fujimoto lymphadenopathy, because of obliterated sinuses and

the proliferation of plasmacytoid monocytes and immunoblasts, which may be misdiagnosed as lymphoma cells. However, in Kikuchi-Fujimoto lymphadenopathy, the reactive follicles, and the mixture of lymphocytes and histiocytes exhibit nonmalignant morphologic features.

Case History: A 20-year-old female with mass on left side of the neck for 2 months.

Diagnosis: Castleman lymphadenopathy.

Clinical Syndrome

Cases of localized CD demonstrate two major histologic variants—HV and PC. The HV variant, by far, is more common.

Hyaline Vascular Variant

- The variant occurs over a broad age range and, in most studies, males and females are equally affected.
- If patients with HIV infection are excluded, HV-CD occurs in younger patients than does plasma cell variant CD.
- Hyaline vascular CD usually presents as a large mass involving a lymph node (or group of lymph nodes).

Plasma Cell Variant

- The PC variant of CD accounts for 10 to 20% of localized or unicentric cases of CD.
- The PC-CD occurs over a broad age range, but patients tend to be older than those with HV-CD.

Microscopy

Hyaline Vascular Variant

- The histologic findings in HV-CD can be divided into two broad groups—follicular changes and changes in the interfollicular region.
- The proportions of the follicular and interfollicular abnormalities can be variable, comprising a spectrum—from cases characterized mostly by abnormal follicles, to cases with an equivalent degree of changes in the follicles and interfolicular region

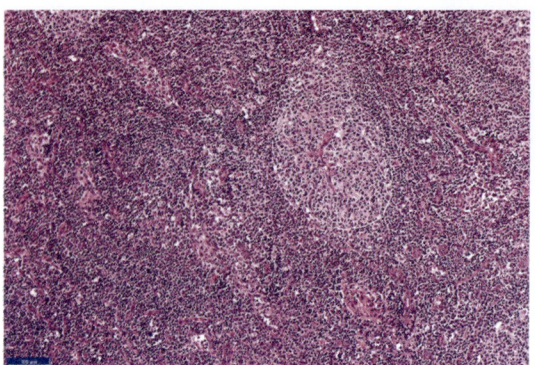

Fig. 18.2

(so-called classical HV-CD), to cases characterized mostly by changes in the interfollicular region (so-called stroma-rich CD).

- In classical HV-CD, the overall lymph node is preserved but distorted. Lymphoid follicles are increased, scattered throughout the cortex and medulla, and often contain two or more small germinal centers (so-called "twinning").
- The germinal centers are depleted of small lymphocytes and are composed of numerous follicular dendritic cells.
- Hyaline deposits, highlighted by the periodic acid–Schiff reaction, can be prominent within germinal centers.
- Sclerotic blood vessels radially penetrate the germinal centers, forming HV lesions (also known as "lollipop lesion").
- The mantle zones of the follicles are broad.
- In a subset of cases, the mantle zones are composed of concentric rings of small lymphocytes (onion skin pattern).
- The interfollicular regions are composed of numerous high endothelial venules with plump endothelial cells, and the vessels often have sclerotic walls.

Plasma Cell Variant

- In HHV-8 negative cases of PC-CD, the interfollicular areas and medulla are occupied by large sheets of mature plasma cells.
- Vascular proliferation in the interfollicular areas is variable. Follicles in PC-CD are

widely scattered, and may be large and hyperplastic or of normal size. The follicles contain germinal centers with polarization, mitoses, and histiocytes with nuclear debris.

Immunophenotype

- In both types of CD, B cells and plasma cells are polyclonal, and T cells show no evidence of an aberrant immunophenotype.
- In HV-CD, the HV follicles show numerous concentric rings of follicular dendritic cells that can be highlighted with markers (CD21, CD23, and CD35).
- In HHV-8 positive PC-CD, presence of HHV-8 can be shown using monoclonal antibodies specific for components of the virus.

Differential Diagnosis

Hyaline Vascular Variant

- In **Toxoplasma lymphadenitis,** the reactive follicles are large with well-developed germinal center.
- In burnt-out **HIV lymphadenitis,** pattern C, involuted follicles with hyalinized germinal centers and interfollicular vascular proliferation can be present and closely mimic HV-CD.
- In **follicular hyperplasia** of any cause (as seen in reactive lymphadenopathies), reactive follicles are large, often potingible-body macrophages.
- In **follicular lymphoma,** the neoplastic follicles are composed of a monotonous population of closely packed germinal center lymphocytes (centrocytes and centroblast) in variable proportions.

Plasma Cell Variant

- In the lymph nodes of untreated patients with **rheumatoid arthritis,** marked interfollicular plasmacytosis and reactive follicular hyperplasia may be present, similar to PC-CD.
- In lymph nodes involved by **lymphoplasmacytic lymphoma/Waldenstrom macroglobulinemia or marginal B cell** lymphomas, numerous plasmacytoid lymphocytes and plasma cells can be present.
- In **plasmacytoma,** sheets of atypical monoclonal plasma cells replace lymph node architecture without preservation of lymphoid follicles or sinuses.
- In some peripheral T cell lymphomas, particularly **angioimmunoblastic T cell lymphoma (AILT),** numerous plasma cells are present throughout the interfollicular regions of the lymph node.

Case History: A 20-year-old male with cervical lymphadenopathy since 2 weeks.

Diagnosis: Reactive lymphoid hyperplasia—follicular.

Microscopy

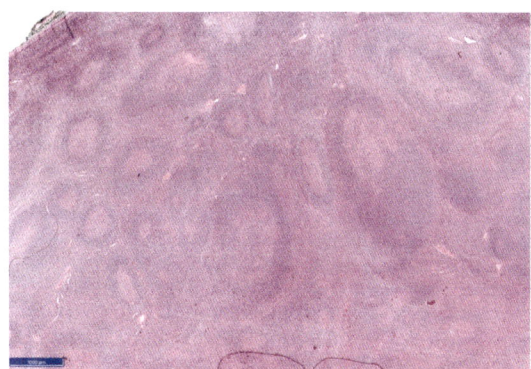

Fig. 18.3

- Follicles of varying sizes, mainly in the cortex.
- Shapes can be varying, often coalescing.
- Perinodal tissue does not show follicles.
- Rimmed by mantle cells. Exhibit polarity.
- Variation in cell types, centrocytes, centroblasts, tingible body macrophages. High mitosis.

Ancillary Tests

- **Special stains:** Reticulin stain shows poor reticulin fibers, no condensation.
- **Immunohistochemistry**: BCL-2 negative.

Differential Diagnosis

Florid follicular hyperplasia needs to be differentiated from follicular lymphoma.

Reactive Lymphoid Hyperplasia—Paracortical/Mixed

Gross
May have blackish appearance.

Microscopy
Paracortex expanded with high endothelial venules, lymphocytes, activated T cells, histiocytes, plasma cells, immunoblasts.

Immunohistochemistry
T cell markers, CD1a, EBV (if needed).

Differential Diagnosis
- Dermatopathic lymphadenitis
- Interfollicular Hodgkin lymphoma
- Peripheral T cell lymphoma.

Reactive Lymphoid Hyperplasia—Sinus Histiocytosis

Microscopy
Sinuses distended with lymphocytes, macrophages.

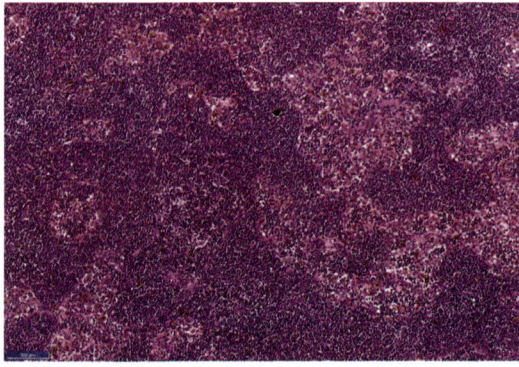

Fig. 18.4

Immunohistochemistry
T cell markers, CD1a and EBV.

Differential Diagnosis
- Metastasis
- Sinus histiocytosis with massive lymphadenopathy
- Intravascular DLBCL
- ALCL

Case History: A 10-year-old male with history of lump in the right axilla of axillary lymph nodes—firm, discrete.

Diagnosis: Sinus histiocytosis with massive lymphadenopathy (Syn: Rosai-Dorfman disease).

Clinical Features
- The age of patients ranged from newborn to 74 years (mean, 20.6 years).
- In addition to involving lymph nodes, still the principal site, in approximately one-third of patients, SHML, in the form of pseudotumors, can occur in a variety of extranodal sites.

Microscopy
- Involved lymph nodes are large and matted and exhibit fibrosis of the capsule and pericapsular fibro-fatty tissues.
- The architecture is altered by marked dilatation of the sinuses.
- The sinuses are obstructed by static lymph and contain a mixed population of cells, including lymphocytes, plasma cells, and histiocytes.
- The most characteristic cells in the sinuses are histiocytes that have marked phagocytic properties.
- The intracytoplasmic vacuoles contain engulfed cells, usually lymphocytes, plasma cells, or erythrocytes.
- Some cells, particularly lymphocytes in the vacuoles, are viable, reproducing the phenomenon of emperipolesis.

Immunohistochemistry
- SHML cells are positive for the monocyte/macrophage-associated antigens CD14, CD68 (KP-1), CD163, Ki-M1P, EBM 11 (Dako), HAM56 (Enzo), and MAC 387.
- In most cases, they also stain with antibodies to α_1-antichymotrypsin and α_1-antitrypsin, which suggest lysosomal activity, although lysozyme is weakly expressed, or is negative.

Differential Diagnosis

- **Sinus histiocytosis** is a nonspecific reaction of lymph nodes to infections and neoplasia. Lymphophagocytosis not present. Result of staining for S100 protein shows that only a few isolated cells are positive.
- **Granulomatous lesions** show epithelioid histiocytes arranged in typical patterns, multinucleated giant cells, and occasional necrosis. The individual epithelioid histiocytes do not resemble SHML cells, and are rarely positive for S100 protein.
- **Langerhans cell histiocytosis:** The histiocytes in these lesions have characteristic cytologic features with twisted nuclei and nuclear grooves. Eosinophils are frequent.

Case History: A 50-year-old female with axillary lymph node enlargement.

Diagnosis: Sinus histiocytosis (Syn: Sinus hyperplasia).

Site

Rarely occurs in pelvic nodes of prostate cancer and axillary nodes of breast cancer patients.

Microscopy

Dilated and prominent sinuses, often containing increased macrophages or sinus lining cells and polygonal histiocytes with rounded nuclei.

Differential Diagnosis

Signet ring cell carcinoma: May resemble signet ring carcinoma cells, but lack atypia and are mucin negative.

Case History: A 25-year-old male with matted lymph nodes in cervical region.

Diagnosis: Tuberculous lymphadenitis.

Microscopy

- Coalescing granulomas, often with central caseation. Langhans giant cells, rimming of lymphocytes, periadenitis common, AFB +, in immunosuppressed may show necrosis

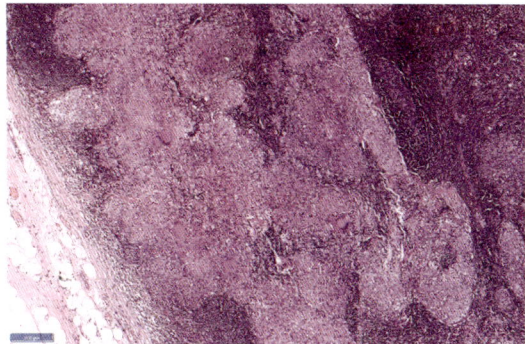

Fig. 18.5

with suppuration, teaming with acid-fast bacilli.
- Mycobacterial pseudotumor shows sheets of histiocytes often with elliptical shape with intracytoplasmic acid-fast bacilli.
- Atypical mycobacteria like MAC complex causes that.

Special Stains

Ziehl-Neelsen stain.

Differential Diagnosis

Other granulomatous diseases.

Case History: A 40-year-old female with history of fever and cough for 2 weeks. On examination, generalized lymphadenopathy—biopsy cervical lymph node.

Diagnosis: Cryptococcus lymphadenitis.

Microscopy and Special Stain

- In lymph nodes, the lesions consist of scattered or confluent noncaseous granulomas.
- These are in the forms of yeasts that may be barely visible as unstained circular forms with hematoxylin and eosin stain but are stained brilliant red with PAS or mucicarmine stain.
- Large numbers of degenerating yeasts release abundant gelatinous fluid that accumulates and forms cystic spaces surrounded by collagenous tissue.

- India ink can detect them in smears of sputum of cerebrospinal fluid or in touch preparations.
- An interesting albeit unexplained feature is the occasional association of cryptococcosis with sarcoidosis.

Differential Diagnosis

Histoplasma lymphadenitis, the yeasts are slightly smaller, although they show similar budding. Granulomas and yeasts containing giant cells are also present; however, the yeasts have no capsules and do not stain with mucicarmine.

Case History: A 3-year-old girl baby with fever and skin rashes since 1 week, biopsy cervical lymph node.

Diagnosis: Measles lymphadenitis

Clinical Features

- In primitive communities, measles affect children <2 years old, whereas in the United States, older children and teenagers may acquire the infection, which in such cases tends to be more severe.
- Pharyngitis, conjunctivitis, otitis, pneumonia, and in severe cases even encephalomyelitis may occur.
- Measles lymphadenitis may occur in the course of measles infection or days to weeks after vaccination with live-attenuated virus.
- The axillary, cervical, and inguinal lymph nodes are most commonly involved.

Microscopy

- The lymph node architecture displays the pattern of diffuse paracortical immunoblastic hyperplasia common to most viral lymphadenitides.
- This is characterized by the diffuse proliferation of immunoblasts and the relative depletion of small lymphocytes, which result in a mottled (moth-eaten) pattern.
- Multinucleated giant cells, independently described by Warthin and Finkeldey, usually appear in the prodromal phase of measles in various hyperplastic lymphoid tissues, including tonsils, adenoids, lymph nodes, spleen, appendix, and thymus.
- They tend to disappear with the rise in antibody titers or when the cutaneous eruption is established.

Immunohistochemistry

Reaction of these polykaryocytes with antibodies directed against CD3, CD4, and CD43 (Leu-22) indicated them to be of helper T cell origin.

Differential Diagnosis

- Viral lymphadenitides of various kinds (Epstein-Barr virus, cytomegalovirus, herpes simplex virus) exhibit the mottled pattern of diffuse paracortical immunoblastic hyperplasia, but do not usually the Warthin-Finkeldey giant cells.
- HIV lymphadenitis in the acute phase includes giant cells resembling the Warthin-Finkeldey cells of measles; however, they are accompanied by follicular lysis and patches of monocytoid cells.
- **Drug-induced lymphadenopathies** (particularly dilantin and other anticonvulsants) display atypical paracortical immunoblastic hyperplasia and disruption of germinal centers. A clinical history of hypersensitivity and long-term drug treatment may be revealing.

Case History: A 20-year-old male with history of painless mass in the submandibular region.

Diagnosis: Kimura disease

Clinical Features

Often subcutaneous mass of head and neck (including salivary glands), associated with regional lymphadenopathy but normal overlying skin.

Laboratory

Increased serum IgE, peripheral eosinophilia.

Microscopy

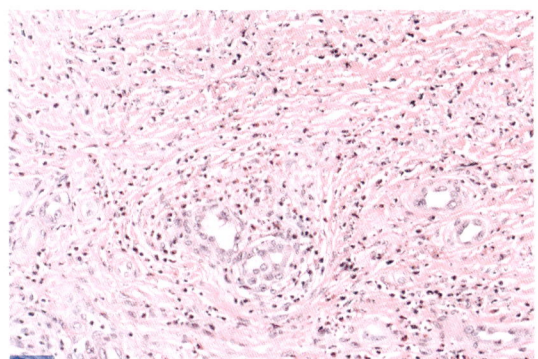

Fig. 18.6

- Germinal center hyperplasia with polykaryocytes, fibrosis and proteinaceous material in germinal centers.
- Folliculolysis, interfollicular eosinophils and eosinophilic abscesses.
- Increased paracortical plasma cells.
- Variable hyalinized vessels.
- Soft tissue lesions show proliferation of thin-walled vessels with eosinophilia.

Molecular Description

May be clonal rearrangement of T cell receptor delta gene.

Differential Diagnosis

Progressive transformation of lymph nodes.

Case History: A 28-year-old male with a single asymptomatic enlarged cervical lymph node.

Diagnosis: Progressive transformation of germinal center.

Clinical Features

- Usually presents with solitary asymptomatic lymphadenopathy of head and neck.
- Either self-limited or associated with lymphocyte predominant Hodgkin lymphoma.

Microscopy

- Germinal centers are markedly larger than normal, with indistinct margins; are

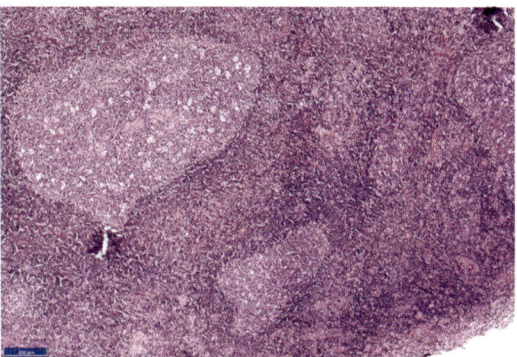

Fig. 18.7

composed of follicular mantle lymphocytes and extensive follicular dendritic cells.
- Tingible body macrophages are also present. Associated with more typical germinal centers. A large number of T cells are present. May have a few small hyaline vascular type germinal centers. Rarely have T cell rosettes.

Immunohistochemistry

May have BCL-2 expression in mantle B cells. CD20, CD45RA positive.

Differential Diagnosis

- Follicular lymphoma
- Hyaline vascular Castleman disease
- Nodular lymphocyte predominant Hodgkin lymphoma.

Case History: A 50-year-old male with a single swelling in the left inguinal region—inguinal node biopsy.

Diagnosis: Intranodal palisading myofibroblastoma

Clinical Features

Painless, slow-growing lymph nodes, usually inguinal.

Gross

Well circumscribed, gray-white with hemorrhage and peripheral nodal tissue.

Microscopy

- Spindle cell proliferation surrounded by hemorrhage and collagenous pseudo-

capsule; growing nodule compresses remaining nodal tissue.
- Bland spindle cells with areas of nuclear palisading, intraparenchymal hemorrhage and red blood cell extravasation, so-called amianthoid fibers. Extra- and intracellular fuchsinophilic bodies (best seen with SMA stain) are also seen.

Ancillary Stains

- **Spindle cells:** Smooth muscle actin, vimentin, cyclin D1.
- **So-called amianthoid fibers:** Elastic stains, trichrome, smooth muscle actin, collagen.

Differential Diagnosis

- Benign metastasizing leiomyoma
- Follicular dendritic cell sarcoma
- Kaposi sarcoma
- Schwannoma.

References

1. Iochim's Lymph Node Pathology, 4th edition.
2. Graham W. Slack. The pathology of reactive lymphadenopathies: A discussion of common reactive patterns and their malignant mimics. Arch Pathol Lab Med, Vol 140, September 2016; 881–93.

CHAPTER 19

Diagnostic Approach to Lymphoma

Marie Therese Manipadam

A precise diagnosis of lymphoma is important because
- Each type of lymphoma has distinctive pathogenesis, clinical manifestations and evolution.
- They are potentially curable neoplasms.
- The therapeutic strategies vary widely—ranging from wait and watch to very aggressive therapies with high risks of iatrogenic complications.
- The diagnosis of lymphoma is an integrated process and encompasses
  1. Clinical information
  2. H and E morphology
  3. Immunophenotyping
  4. Cytogenetics
  5. Molecular studies.

One needs to use a multiparametric approach to distinguish lymphoma from reactive lymphadenopathy.

Tissue sample sent to the laboratory for a suspected case of lymphoma can be sent for the following tests:
- Microscopy on appropriately fixed and stained tissue samples.
- Immunohistochemistry and/or flow cytometry.
- Cytogenetic analysis by Giemsa banding.
- FISH on cell suspensions, films, imprints or paraffin sections.
- Molecular genetic analysis by RT-PCR or gene sequencing.

Well-fixed lymph node tissue cut at 3 microns and stained with H and E is the cornerstone for the diagnosis of lymphoma regardless of the number of advanced ancillary tests available at hand.

Morphological Analysis of Lymph Nodes

Points to Note Under Low Power

Architectural patterns in lymph node
- Diffuse
- Nodular/follicular
- Mantle zone
- Marginal
- Interfollicular
- Sinusoidal
- Heterogenous

Points to Note Under High Power
- Cell size
- Monotonous/heterogenous
- Chromatin pattern
- Nucleoli
- Nuclear shape
- Cytoplasm

Cell size is a good guide to the grade of many types of NHL. In poorly fixed tissue or thick sections, cells assume shrunken appearance. Excess intense nuclear staining may mask subtle nuclear details. Hence, utmost importance has to be given to adequate fixation of lymph node tissues.

Assessing the Size of a Lymphoid Cell

Nucleus of a histiocyte is used for comparison. Large lymphoid cells have nuclei larger than that of a histiocyte nucleus. Medium-sized cell is comparable/slightly smaller than that of a histiocyte nucleus. Small lymphoid cells have nuclei much smaller than that of a histiocyte.

Lymphoid Neoplasms with Small Cells

- Follicular lymphoma grade 1–2
- Mantle cell lymphoma
- Marginal zone lymphoma
- CLL/SLL
- LPL

Lymphoid Neoplasms with Medium-sized Cells

- Burkitt's lymphoma
- Lymphoblastic
- Blastoid variant of MCL
- DLBL (rare variants composed of medium-sized cells)
- PTCL-NOS (variants composed of medium-sized monomorphic cells)
- NMZL

Lymphoid Neoplasms with Large Cells

- DLBL and variants and subtypes
- PTCL
- ALCL
- Follicular lymphoma grade 3B.

Features Favoring a Diagnosis of Lymphoma over Lymphoid Hyperplasia

- Abnormal architecture
- Invasive/destructive features
- Cytologic atypia.

Case History: A 70-year-old male, generalized lymphadenopathy and hepatosplenomegaly.

Diagnosis: Chronic lymphocytic leukemia/small lymphocytic lymphoma (CLL/SLL).

Clinical Features

- Usually older patients (median age 60 yrs) with disease in bone marrow, lymph nodes, spleen, liver
- Often presents with leukemia.
- CLL is the most common adult leukemia in Western countries.
- Usually associated with lymphadenopathy or hepatosplenomegaly.

Microscopy

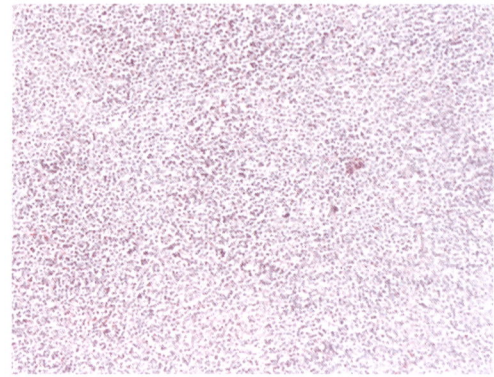

Fig. 19.1

- Effacement of nodal architecture by an infiltrate of small cells with round nuclei, clumped chromatin and prachromatin clearing.
- There is a pseudofollicular pattern with interspersed pale staining pseudofollicles or proliferation centers with ill-defined borders, enriched in larger cells—prolymphocytes and paraimmunoblasts.
- In the peripheral smear, CLL cells are small lymphoid cells with clumped chromatin and scanty cytoplasm.
- Smudge cells are typically seen.
- Prolymphocytes are usually <2% in peripheral blood films.
- CLL cases with marrow involvement usually have interstitial, interstitial/focal or diffuse patterns; paratrabecular pattern is not seen.

Ancillary Studies

Immunohistochemistry

- CD5, CD19, CD23; weak (low density) CD20 staining
- Light chain restriction
- Variable CD38, surface immunoglobulin, FMC7
- Some cases may have an atypical phenotype (CD5 negative or CD23 negative, FMC7+ or strong sIg.

Molecular
- 17p– (poor survival)
- 17p13 and 11q22–23 (associated with advanced disease)
- 12q trisomy, 13q14, 13q– (longest survival)

Transformation of SLL/CLL
- CLL can transform to a high grade neoplasm. Progression of CLL to B-PLL is extremely rare.
- Richter syndrome is transformation from B-CLL/SLL or other low grade B cell lymphoproliferative disorder to a pleomorphic lymphoma, such as diffuse large cell lymphoma.

Differential Diagnosis
Other low grade lymphomas with leukemic phase:
- Mantle cell lymphoma
- Follicular lymphoma
- Persistent polyclonal B cell lymphocytosis.

Case History: A 65-year-old male with low grade fever, generalised lymphadenopathy.

Diagnosis: Follicular lymphoma

Clinical Features
- Follicular lymphoma tends to present with painless, generalized lymphadenopathy.
- Involvement of extranodal sites, such as the gastrointestinal tract, central nervous system, or testis, is relatively uncommon.

Microscopy

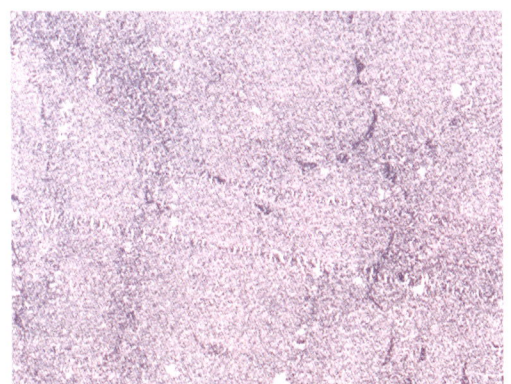

Fig. 19.2

- In most cases, at low magnification, a predominantly nodular or nodular and diffuse growth pattern is observed in involved lymph nodes.
- Two principal cell types are present in varying proportions: (1) Small cell with irregular or cleaved nuclear contours and scant cytoplasm, referred to as centrocytes (small cleaved cells); and (2) larger cells with open nuclear chromatin, several nucleoli, and modest amounts of cytoplasm, referred to as centroblasts.
- In most follicular lymphomas, small cleaved cells are in the majority.
- Follicular lymphomas are graded according to the proportion of centroblasts present.
- *Grade 1:* 0–5 centroblasts per high power field (HPF).
- *Grade 2:* 6–15 centroblasts per HPF.
- *Grade 3:* >15 centroblasts per HPF.

Ancillary Tests
Immunohistochemistry
- The neoplastic cells closely resemble normal germinal center B cells, expressing CD19, CD20, CD10, surface Ig, and BCL-6.
- Unlike CLL/SLL and mantle cell lymphoma, CD5 is not expressed.
- BCL-2 is expressed in more that 90% of cases, in distinction of normal follicular center B cells, which are BCL-2 negative.
- The nuclear protein BCL-6 is expressed in a majority of cases.

Molecular Cytogenetics
- The hallmark of follicular lymphoma is a (14;18) translocation that juxtaposes the IgH locus on chromosome 14 and the BCL-2 locus on chromosome 18.
- The t(14;18) is seen up to 90% of follicular lymphomas, and leads to overexpression of BCL-2.

Differential Diagnosis
- Reactive follicular hyperplasia
- Progressive transformation of germinal centers

- Nodular lymphocyte predominance—Hodgkin's disease
- Mantle cell lymphoma (nodular pattern)
- Pseudofollicular pattern in SLL/CLL.

Case History: A 71-year-old male with weight loss and fatigue for 3 months. He has generalised lymphadenopathy and splenomegaly. Biopsy of left axillary lymph node.

Diagnosis: NHL Mantle cell lymphoma.

Clinical Features

- Mantle cell lymphoma (MCL) is uncommon under the age of 40 occurs mostly in the sixth or seventh decade of life.
- Most patients present with stage III or IV disease with lymphadenopathy, hepatosplenomegaly, frequently with massive splenomegaly and marrow involvement (>50%).

Microscopy

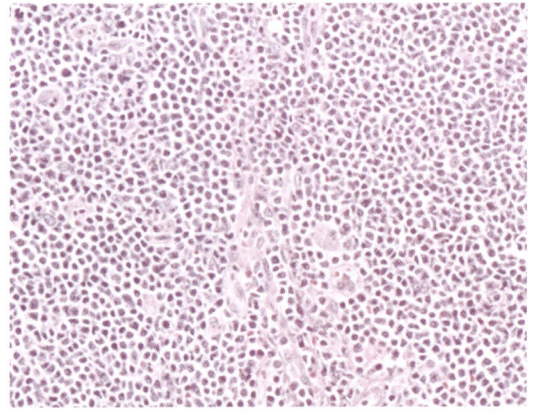

Fig. 19.3

- MCL demonstrates architectural destruction by a monomorphic lymphoid proliferation with a vaguely nodular, diffuse or mantle zone growth pattern.
- Most cases are composed of small to medium-sized lymphoid cells with slightly too markedly irregular nuclear contours, most closely resembling centrocytes.
- The nuclei have moderately dispersed chromatin but inconspicuous nucleoli.
- Neoplastic transformed cells resembling centroblasts, immunoblasts or paraimmunoblasts and pseudofollicles are absent.

Ancillary Tests
Immunohistochemistry

- The neoplastic cells are monoclonal B cells with relatively intense surface IgM ± IgD.
- They are typically CD5 positive, usually CD10 negative, BCL-6 negative, CD23 negative.
- All the cases are BCL-2 protein positive and virtually all expresses cyclin D1.

Molecular Genetics

- *Antigen receptor genes:* Immunoglobulin heavy and light chain genes are rearranged.
- *Cytogenetic abnormalities and oncogenes:* Almost all cases show t(11;14)(q13;q32) translocation between the immunoglobulin heavy chain and the cyclin D1 (CCND1, PRAD1, BCL-1) genes.

Differential Diagnosis

- Follicular lymphoma grade 1 can mimic nodular pattern of MCL.
- Blastoid or pleomorphic variants can often be misdiagnosed as DLBL. Immunohistochemistry for Cyclin D1 or fluorescent in situ hybridization for CCND1 translocation helps in the differential diagnosis.
- Lymphoblastic lymphoma is a differential diagnosis for blastoid variant MCL.

Case History: A 3-year-old boy baby with abdominal pain and fever—mesenteric lymph node biopsy.

Diagnosis: Burkitt's lymphoma

Clinical Feature

The abdomen is the most common anatomic location of disease in patients with sBL.

Microscopy

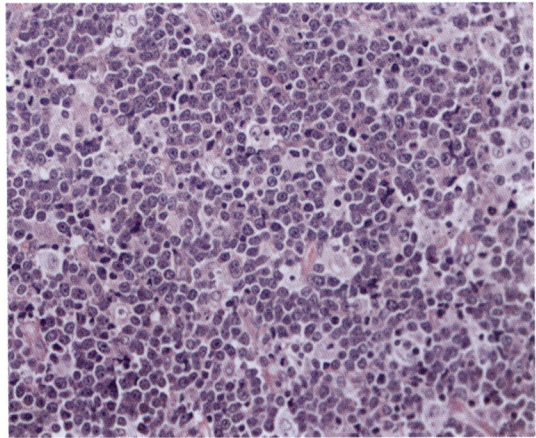

Fig. 19.4

- At low-power magnification, normal structures are replaced by lymphoma with a diffuse pattern.
- Large areas of coagulative necrosis or hemorrhage are common.
- There is also an usually high rate of individual cell apoptosis with numerous pyknotic nuclei and nuclear fragments that may lie free or are engulfed by phagocytic histiocytes.
- The characteristic finding is a "starry sky" pattern, although this is not specific and can be seen in any high grade non-Hodgkin lymphoma with a high cell turnover.
- This pattern is the result of scattered, relatively evenly dispersed histiocytes within a background of sheets of basophilic neoplastic lymphoid cells.
- The neoplastic lymphoid cells are remarkably uniform in size and shape.

Ancillary Tests

Immunophenotype

- Monotypic Ig + (usually IgM, '>'), pan-B cell antigens +, CD10+, BCL-6+, MUM1 −/+, EBV + (endemic) or −/+ (sporadic)
- CD43+/−, Ki-67+ (virtually all cells brightly)
- BCL-2−, TdT−, pan-T cell antigens negative
- CD23 −, CD138 −

Molecular Genetics

- Chromosomal translocations involving myc are the key molecular events involved in the pathogenesis of all types of BL.
- The most common translocation, occurring in 80% of cases, is the t(8;14) (q24;q32) in which myc is translocated to the derivative chromosome 14.

Differential Diagnosis

Classical BL has to be distinguished from DLBCL. This differential diagnosis is of utmost importance.

- **Precursor T- or B-cell lymphoblastic lymphoma/leukemia (T- or B-LBL)** also occurs in children and adolescents; however, T-LBL usually involves the mediastinum and lymph nodes above the diaphragm, whereas BL commonly affects abdominal organs. B-LBL in children usually presents as acute lymphoblastic leukemia.
- **Myeloid sarcoma** can involve orbital bones or the ovaries, similar to BL. Myeloid sarcoma also can exhibit a starry-sky pattern. However, cytologically the neoplastic cells of myeloid sarcoma have immature chromatin and thin nuclear membranes. Myeloid sarcomas express a variety of myeloid-associated antigens and lack Ig and most B-cell antigens.
- A starry-sky pattern is not present **Ewing sarcoma/peripheral neuroectodermal tumor (ES/PNET)**. These tumors often contain abundant intracytoplasmic glycogen, express CD99 in most cases, keratin in a subset, and lack B-cell antigens.
- A starry-sky pattern is absent in **neuroblastoma**. Deposits of hematoxyphilic DNA material, rosettes, intracytoplasmic neurosecretory granules shown by electron microscopy, and the absence of B-cell antigens also distinguish neuroblastoma from BL.

- **Embryonal Rhabdomyosarcoma** can occur in the jaws and orbit similar to BL. However, a starry-sky pattern is absent, the nuclei are spindle-shaped, and intracytoplasmic striations are sometimes visible. Immunophenotyping is very helpful as embryonal rhabdomyosarcoma expresses a number of muscle-associated markers and lacks B-cell antigens.

Case History: A 6-year-old male with fever and petechial rash since 3 weeks. Supraclavicular and cervical lymph nodes enlarged.

Diagnosis: T-lymphoblastic lymphoma

Clinical Features

- Patients who present with the clinical picture of pre-T LBL tend to be adolescents and relatively young adults.
- These patients present with widespread lymphadenopathy that is usually preferentially located above the diaphragm.
- A mediastinal mass is common, presents in 50 to 75% of patients.
- The clinical course of patients with pre-T ALL/LBL is very aggressive.

Microscopy

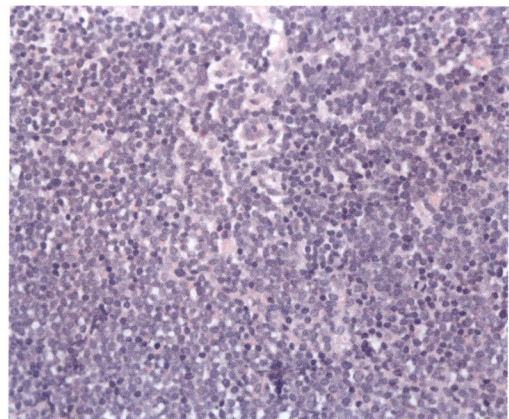

Fig. 19.5

- T-LBL replaces lymph nodes in a diffuse pattern. In most cases, the lymph node architecture is completely replaced.
- A starry-sky pattern can be present and most often is a focal finding.
- Cytologically, in routinely stained tissue section, lymphoblasts are usually smaller than the nuclei of benign histiocytes and have a high nucleus-to-cytoplasm ratio with minimal cytoplasm.
- Mitotic figures are often numerous.
- The chromatin of the neoplastic cells is fine and has been referred to as "dusty".
- Nucleoli are either absent or inconspicuous.
- The nuclear contours can be either highly irregular or round, referred to as convoluted or nonconvoluted respectively.

Ancillary Tests

- Focal PAS+ (block-like)
- TdT +, CD7+, CD2+, CD5+ (except pro-T stage), CD1a+/– (cortical)
- Cytoplasmic CD3+, surface CD3+/–, CD4+/CD8+ or CD4–/CD8– or CD4+/CD8– or CD4–/CD8+
- CD43+, CD52+, CD99+, CD10+/– CD34+/–

Case History: A 30-year-old male, presenting with a progressively increasing swelling in the left side of neck. Loss of weight present.

Diagnosis: Diffuse large B cell lymphoma.

Clinical Features

- Patients typically present with a rapidly enlarging, often symptomatic mass at a single nodal or extranodal site.
- Patients may present with nodal or extranodal disease.

Microscopy

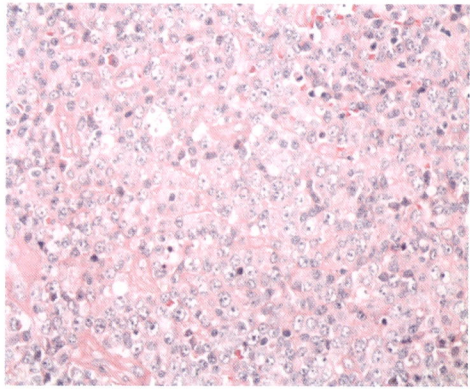

Fig. 19.6

- Diffuse large B cell lymphoma typically replaces the normal architecture of the underlying lymph node or extranodal tissue in a diffuse pattern.
- The perinodal soft tissue is often infiltrated; broad or fine bands of sclerosis may be observed.
- Cytologically, they are diverse and can be divided into morphologic variants.

Morphologic Variants
- Centroblastic
- Immunoblastic
- Anaplastic.

Differential Diagnosis
- DLBCL may form cohesive sheets or involve sinusoids, mimicking **carcinoma, melanoma** etc. In particular, nasopharyngeal carcinomas, neuroendocrine carcinomas, germ cell tumors (seminomas) and granulocytic sarcomas (chloromas) can be mistaken for DLBCL and should be considered in the differential diagnosis.
- In some cases, there may be aberrant phenotypic characteristics that make DLBCL difficult to identify [for example, **plasmablastic lymphoma** (PBL) may lack CD20, as may ALK+ DLBCL].
- **Burkitt's lymphoma** is a differential when DLBL has a predominant population of medium-sized cells, which can rarely occur.
- **Anaplastic large cell lymphoma** is a differential for anaplastic variant of DLBL. CD20 immunostaining will clinch the diagnosis.

Case History: A 40-year-old female, cervical and axillary lymphadenopathy

Diagnosis: Classical Hodgkin lymphoma and nodular sclerosis

Classification—WHO
- Lymphocyte predominant, nodular
- Classical Hodgkin lymphoma
- Nodular sclerosis
- Lymphocyte-rich
- Mixed cellularity
- Lymphocyte depleted

Clinical Features
- The mediastinal lymph nodes were commonly involved in up to 80% of cases with lesions of NS, whereas abdominal lymph nodes are affected by lesions of MC.
- Bulky lesions were seen in 54% of cases. The cervical and supraclavicular lymph nodes are most commonly involved in all forms of HL particularly NS.

Microscopy

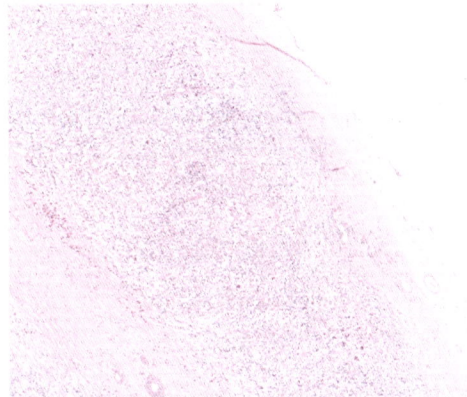

Fig. 19.7

- The cells of HL are heterogeneous, including neoplastic and non-neoplastic reactive cells give rise to multiple histologic pattern.
- Varying proportions of neoplastic and non-neoplastic cells give rise to multiple histological forms.

Cell Types of Classic Hodgkin Lymphoma
- *Non-neoplastic cells:* These are considered to represent an immune cellular reaction to the neoplastic cell component of HL.
- *Neoplastic cells*
    1. Reed-Sternberg cells
    2. Hodgkin cells
    3. Lacunar cell variant
    4. Mummified cell variant
    5. Anaplastic variant.

Histologic Patterns of Classic Hodgkin Lymphoma

- Nodular sclerosis
- Lymphocyte-rich
- Mixed cellularity
- Lymphocyte depleted

Immunohistochemistry

- Diffuse large B cell lymphomas express various pan-B markers such as CD19, CD20, CD22, and CD79a, but may lack one or more of these. Surface and/or cytoplasmic immunoglobulin (IgM > IgG > IgA) can be demonstrated in 50–75%.
- While the vast majority of anaplastic large B cell lymphomas express CD30, non-anaplastic cases may occasionally stain for CD30.

Molecular Genetics

Most cases have rearranged immunoglobulin heavy and light chain genes and show somatic mutation in the variable regions.

Differential Diagnosis

- **Nodular sclerosis**
  1. Infectious mononucleosis (IM).
  2. Diffuse large B cell lymphoma.
  3. Immunoblastic peripheral T cell NHL.
  4. Anaplastic large cell lymphoma.
- **Lymphocyte-rich classic type:** Lymphocyte predominant diffuse type is similar in that a large number of small lymphocytes comprise the tumor mass. However, in the classical type, R-S cells and their variants are scattered throughout the lymphocytes, whereas L&H (popcorn) cells are seen in the LP type.
- **Mixed cellularity:** Because of the characteristic cellularity of this type of HL, fewer problems of differential diagnosis arise.
- **Lymphocyte depletion:** Non-Hodgkin lymphoma large cell polymorphic tumors of B or T cell type may closely resemble the reticular subtype of LD. The criteria for differential diagnosis are based on immunohistochemistry. Malignant fibrous histiocytoma may be considered in the differential diagnosis of the diffuse fibrosis subtype of LD.

Case History: A 39-year-old male with isolated left upper deep cervical lymphadenopathy.

Diagnosis: Nodular lymphocyte predominant Hodgkin lymphoma.

Clinical Features

- Patients with NLPHL most often present with lymph node enlargement and have localized disease.
- Peripheral lymph nodes are most frequently involved by NLPHL, most often in the cervical, axillary or inguinal region.

Microscopy

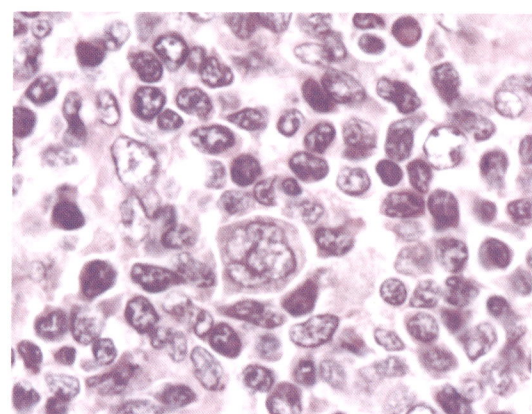

Fig. 19.8

- The classical pattern of NLPHL is that of large, expansile nodules that partially or totally replace the lymph node architecture.
- These nodules also displace and compress uninvolved lymphoid tissue at the periphery of the neoplasm.
- The neoplastic nodules vary in size, but most of them are larger than reactive lymphoid follicles and they usually have vaguer outlines than do reactive follicles.
- The neoplastic nodules are arranged closely, often in back-to-back fashion. The neoplastic nodules are composed of numerous, small, round lymphocytes; typical and epithelioid histiocytes; follicular dendrtic cells; and neoplastic LP cells, with the latter representing 1% or less of all the cells in the nodules.

Ancillary Tests

The large cells are CD20+, CD22, CD79a+, OCT2+, BOB1+, CD45+ (LCA), CD15−, CD30−/+

Differential Diagnosis

- **The Nodular variant of lymphocyte-rich classical HL** can resemble NLPHL. The absence of CD20 and presence of CD15, CD30, and EBV favour classical HL over NLPHL.
- **Follicular lymphoma:** Histologically, follicular lymphoma (FL) nodules are generally smaller; FL nodules are composed of a relatively monotonous population of centrocytes and cenroblasts in varying proportions. LP cells are absent. Immunopheno-typing can be helpful in this differential diagnosis.

Case History: A 60-year-old male with pancytopenia and splenomegaly.

Diagnosis: Hairy cell leukemia.

Clinical Presentation

- The most common presenting symptoms include weakness and fatigue, left upper abdominal pain, fever and bleeding.
- Most patients present with splenomegaly and pancytopenia with a few circulating neoplastic cells.
- Monocytopenia is characteristic.

Microscopy

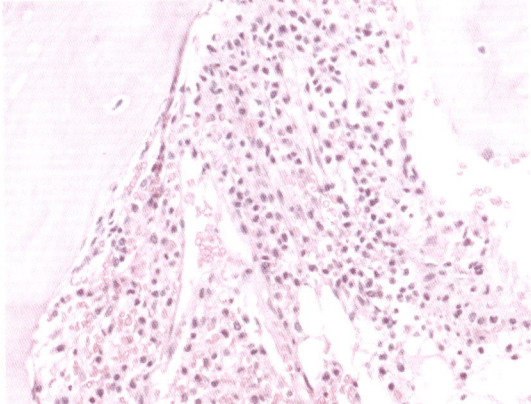

Fig. 19.9

- Bone marrow is often the first sample to be reach the lab because the patients present with pancytopenia.
- The aspirate often yields a dry tap.
- The bone marrow shows a patchy interstitial infiltrate of cells which appear spaced apart due to the presence of abundant clear cytoplasm.
- The cell borders in tissue sections are well defined. The nuclei are round or bean shaped.
- There may be some preservation of fat and hemopoietic marrow in early stages.
- The areas infiltrated by hairy cells are associated with increased reticulin deposition, often in a pericellular distribution which results in dry aspirate taps in many cases.
- The peripheral blood contains a variable number of cells with irregular hairy cytoplasmic projections.
- There is invariably monocytopenia.
- Lymph node involvement is rare.
- In the spleen, there is usually heavy infiltration of the red pulp with filling of the cords. Blood lakes (areas of hemorrhage) surrounded by hairy cells are typically present.

Ancillary Tests

- **Immunohistochemistry:** Hairy cell leukemia cells express pan-B cell antigens and are positive for Annexin A1, DBA44 (CD76), CD25 and with antibodies to TRAP. The cells express CD11c and CD123 and in frozen tissue or by flow cytometry can be shown to express CD103. The cells are positive for cyclin D1 in a significant proportion of cases but usually CD5 negative.
- **Molecular genetics:** BRAF V600E mutation to be present in all cases of HCl and rare in other splenic B cell lymphomas.

Differential Diagnosis

Other low grade B cell non-Hodgkin lymphoma of marrow.

Points to differentiate:
- Spaced infiltrate
- Pericellular increase in reticulin
- Annexin A1 positivity.

Case History: An 8-year-old boy with cervical and axillary lymphadenopathy and splenomegaly.

Diagnosis: ALK+ anaplastic large cell lymphoma (ALCL).

Clinical Features

- ALCL, ALK positive, is most common in children and young adults, with a marked male predominance.
- Although most patients present with nodal disease, a high incidence of extranodal involvement has been reported (involving skin, bone, and soft tissue).
- Approximately 75% of patients present with advanced-stage and systemic symptoms.

Microscopy

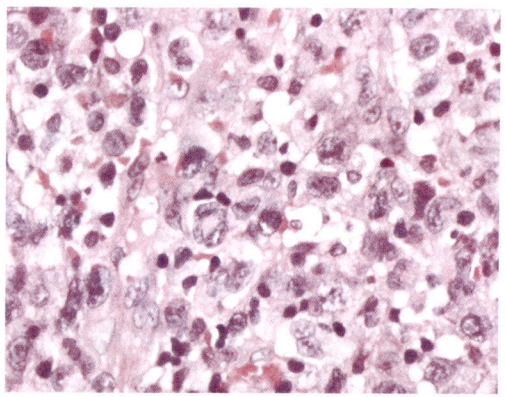

Fig. 19.10

- ALCL, ALK positive, is characterized by pleomorphic or monomorphic cells, which have a propensity to invade lymphoid sinuses.
- Classical ALCL usually displays a cohesive growth pattern.
- The cells have large, often lobulated nuclei with small basophilic nucleoli, so-called hallmark cells.
- The cytoplasm is usually abundant, amphophilic. A prominent Golgi region is generally visible.
- Small cell and lymphohistiocytic variants have a more aggressive clinical course.
- A consistent feature is the strong expression of CD30 antigen, a diagnostic hallmark.
- However, CD30 expression is not specific and can be seen in a variety of conditions, of course, including classical Hodgkin's lymphoma.

Ancillary Tests

- **Immunophenotype:** The cells exhibit an aberrant phenotype with loss of the T cell-associated antigens. Both CD3 and CD5 are negative in >50% of cases. CD2 and CD4 are positive in the majority of cases; CD8 is usually negative. The cells exhibit positivity for the cytotoxic-associated antigens TIA-1, granzyme B, and perforin. In addition, clusterin is generally present and represents another potentially useful diagnostic marker.
- **Molecular genetics:** The disease is associated with a characteristic chromosomal translocation, t(2;5)(p23;q35) involving NPM/ALK genes, respectively. A number of variant translocations has been identified that involve partners other than NPM. All lead to overexpression of ALK, although the cellular distribution of ALK varies according to the gene partners. In most of the cases, a clonal T cell receptor rearrangement is found, confirming a T cell origin.

Differential Diagnosis

- **Classical HL (CD15 negative):** PAX-5 is the best marker to use for this differential. CHL is PAX-5 positive and ALCL is negative. ALK IHC helps if ALCL is ALK+.
- **Anaplastic variant of DLBL** which has large, anaplastic tumor cells which can display a sinusoidal pattern and CD30 positivity. Positive staining for CD20 differentiates this entity from ALCL.

Table 19.1: Burkitt lymphoma versus lymphoblastic lymphoma

Burkitt lymphoma	Lymphoblastic lymphoma
Round nuclei	Round or convoluted
2–5 distinct nucleoli	Inconspicuous
Coarsely granular/clumped chromatin	Fine, dusty chromatin
Definite rim of cytoplasm-squaring	Scant cytoplasm
TdT negative, MIB-1 >95–100%	Tdt+, MIB-1 ~ 80–90%

Table 19.2: DLBL versus Burkitt lymphoma

DLBL	Burkitt lymphoma
Large- to-intermediate-sized cells	Intermediate sized
Varying size and shape	Uniform
Round to irregular vesicular nuclei, 1–3 membrane bound nucleoli	Round nuclei, clumped chromatin and small 2–5 nucleoli
Moderate cytoplasm DLBL	Scant, basophilic-squaring BL
Reactive lymphocytes present	Paucity of reactive lymphocytes in the background
MIB-1 can vary	95–100% MIB-1
Complex cytogenetics, t(8; 14) in 10%	Isolated t(8;14)

Table 19.3: Immunohistochemical markers for CHL versus NLPHL

CHL	NLPHL
CD 45 –	CD45+
CD30+	CD30–/+ (weak, focal)
CD15+	CD15–
CD20–/+ weak	CD20+ uniform, strong
PAX-5 weak	PAX-5 strong
CD79a–, OCT2/BOB-1–/+	CD79a+, OCT2 +, BOB1+
BCL-6–	BCL-6+
MUM-1+	MUM-1–
EMA–	EMA+

APPROACHES TO LYMPH NODE ARCHITECTURE

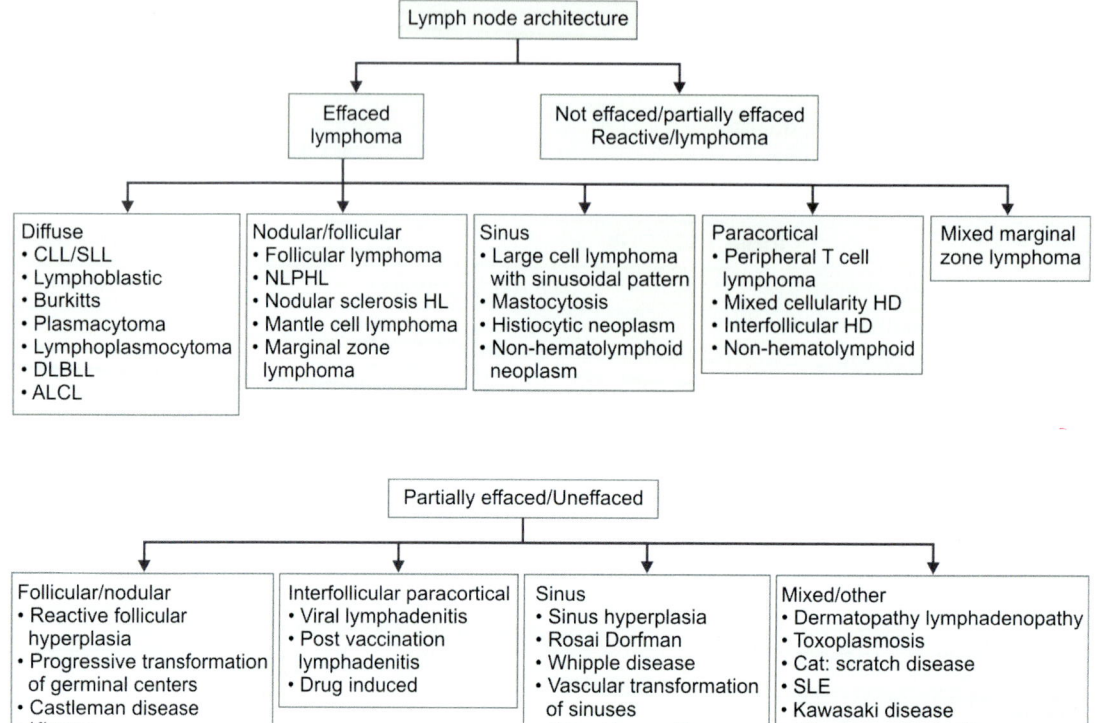

Contributed by Dr. G.A. Vasugi

IHC Profile

1. HD-Classical–CD45-Negative; CD15, CD30, PAX5- positive

   NCPHL-CD45, CD20-positive; CD15, CD30-Negative

   All B cell lymphoma – CD45, CD20, CD79a, PAX5- positive

2. SLL-CD5-Positive; CD23-Positive
3. MLL- Cyclin D1-positive; CD5-Positive
4. Follicular lymphoma–CD10-Positive, BCl2-positive, Ki67 low
5. Burkitts–Ki67 >90%, CD10, BCl2, MVC
6. B Lymphoblastic-Tdt–positive, CD10, CD34
7. Plasma cell neoplasm-CD20-negative, CD138- positive, CD19-Positive, Kappa and lambda

   T cell- CD3-positive, CD5, CD7-positive

   NK cell-CD56, CD3

   ALCL-CD3 positive, ALK-positive/negative, CD30-positive

   T lymphoblastic lymphoma–CD19, Tdt, CD3

Reference: Iochim-4th edition, Ackerman – 10th edition, Fletcher – 4th edition

Contributed by N. Priyathersini

CHAPTER 20

Endocrine Pathology

Rani Kanthan

Case History: A 60-year-old male with cavitron specimen sella turcica region.

Diagnosis: Pituitary adenoma (null cell)

Gross

Pituitary adenomas are soft lesions with a tan-brown discoloration.

Microscopy

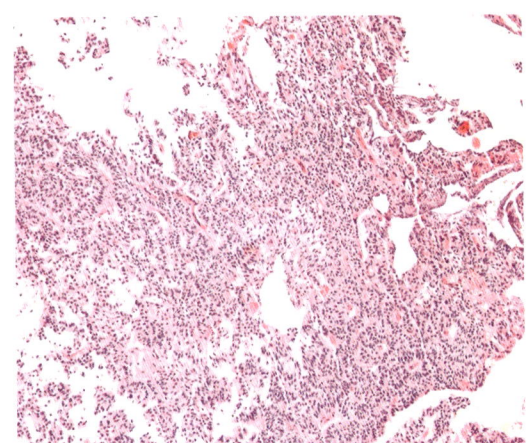

Fig. 20.1

- Variety of histologic patterns, including diffuse, papillary, and trabecular arrangements similar to those of other neuroendocrine tumors.
- Cytologically, tumor cells may be acidophilic, basophilic, or chromophobic.

Differential Diagnosis
- Rathke's cleft cyst
- Pituitary hyperplasia
- Germinoma
- Vascular aneurysm
- Sarcoidosis
- Infection
- Metastatic lesion

Case History: (a) A 62-year-old female with a right lobe thyroidectomy.

Diagnosis: Papillary carcinoma, cystic arising in a background of Hashimoto's thyroiditis

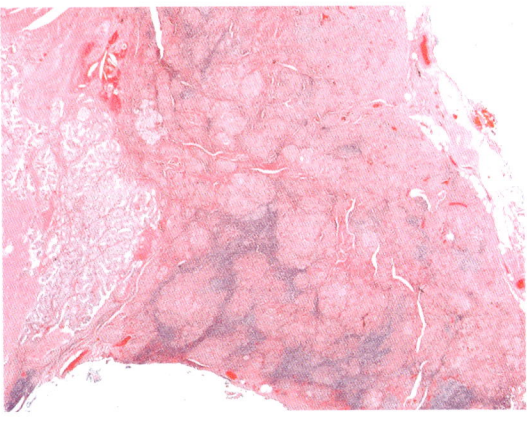

Fig. 20.2a

Case History: (b) A 26-year-old female with a right lobe thyroidectomy.

Diagnosis: Papillary carcinoma thyroid, classical type

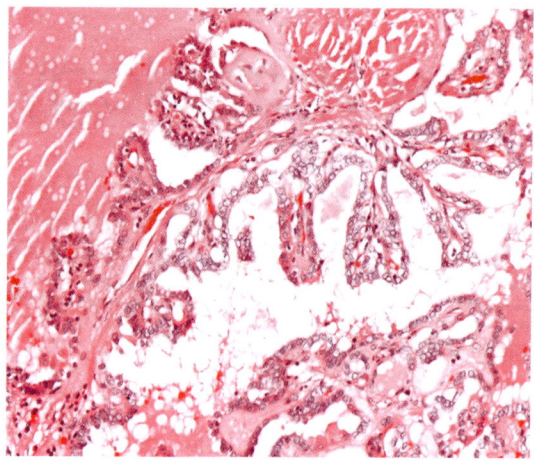

Fig. 20.2b

Case History: A 38-year-old male with total thyroidectomy.

Diagnosis: Papillary carcinoma, follicular variant

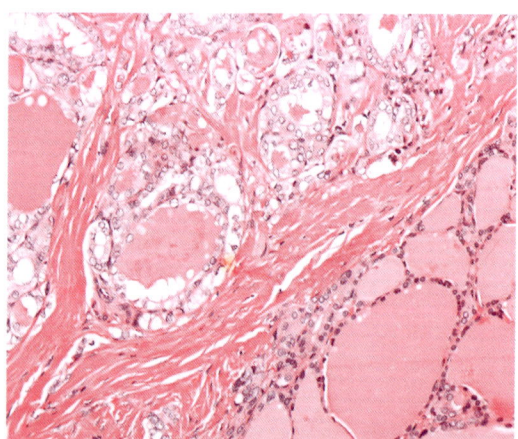

Fig. 20.2c

Case History: A 28-year-old female with a left hemithyroidectomy.

Diagnosis: Papillary carcinoma, multifocal arising in the background of a follicular adenoma, microfollicular pattern dominant

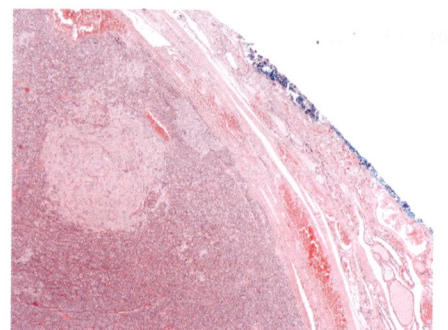

Fig. 20.2d

Case History: A 36-year-old female with Graves' disease—near total thyroidectomy.

Diagnosis: Papillary carcinoma—diffuse sclerosing

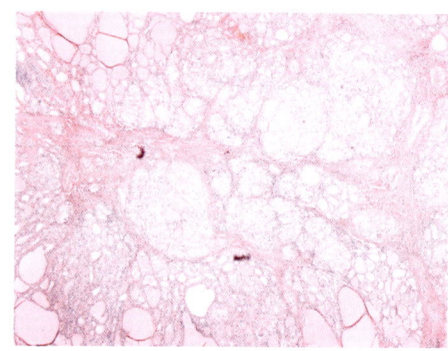

Fig. 20.2e

Case History: A 64-year-old female with a neck mass.

Diagnosis: Papillary carcinoma, thyroid involving parathyroid

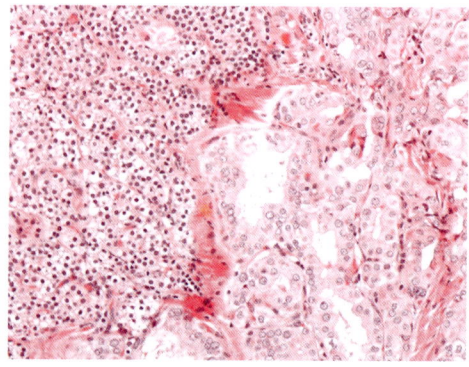

Fig. 20.2f

Clinical Features
- Usually presents as painless nodule or mass in neck or cervical node; usually cold on scan.
- Usually diagnosed by FNA.
- At presentation, 67% in thyroid only, 13% in thyroid and cervical nodes, 20% in nodes only.

Gross
- Can present as a yellow-white infiltrative mass with evidence of fibrous strands.
- The lesion can also be associated with cystic lymph node metastases, which could be the first presenting sign of tumor.

Microscopy
- The neoplastic papillae contain a central core of fibrovascular tissue lined by one layer, or occasionally, several layers of cells with crowded oval nuclei.
- Psammoma bodies that represent the "ghosts" of dead papillae within the cores of papillae or in the tumor stroma, but not within the neoplastic follicles.
- Characteristic nuclear feature of papillary carcinoma is the nuclear enlargement, overlapping, nuclear grooving, chromatin clearing, intranuclear cytoplasmic intrusion (pseudo-inclusion).
- *Immunohistochemistry:* Positive for cytokeratin-19, HBME-1, and galectin 3.

Types
- Columnar cell variant
- Cribiform morular variant
- Encapsulated follicular variant
- Encapsulated variant
- Follicular variant
- Macrofollicular variant
- Microcarcinoma variant
- Nodular fasciitis like stroma variant
- Oncocytic variant
- Solid variant
- Tall cell variant
- Warthin-like variant

Differential Diagnosis
- Dyshormonogenetic goiter
- Lymphocytic thyroiditis
- Papillary foci of Graves' disease
- Papillary thymic carcinoma
- Papillary variant of medullary carcinoma.

Case History: A 27-year-old female with a dominant right thyroid nodule.

Diagnosis: Follicular adenoma, oncocytic variant (Hürthle cell adenoma)

Clinical Features
- Presents with long-standing solitary thyroid nodule, almost always solitary.
- If multiple, diagnose as multinodular goiter with adenomatous change.

Laboratory Investigation
Patient is usually euthyroid.

Imaging
Usually "cold" nodule, may be "warm", but rarely "hot".

Gross
- Solitary, encapsulated, variable size (1–10 cm).
- Solid, fleshy, tan to light brown.
- Bulges when fresh, compresses adjacent thyroid.

Microscopy

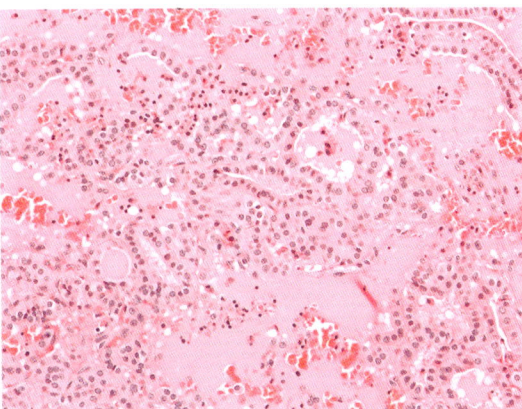

Fig. 20.3

- Completely enveloped by thin fibrous capsule.
- Architecturally and cytologically different from surrounding gland; surrounding thyroid tissue shows signs of compression.
- Closely packed follicles, trabeculae or solid sheets.
- Commonly secondary changes of hemorrhage, hemosiderin deposition, sclerosis, edema, necrosis, and cystic changes.
- No capsular or vascular invasion after thorough sampling (at least 10 blocks), no/rare mitotic figures, no papillary nuclear features.

Patterns
- Normofollicular
- Macrofollicular
- Microfollicular
- Trabecular/solid
- Cords/trabeculae with a few follicles.

Ancillary Tests
- *Immunohistochemistry:* Positive for thyroglobulin, low molecular weight cytokeratin. Negative for CK19.
- *Electron microscopy:* Abundant dilated endoplasmic reticulum; microvilli project into well developed lumina.
- *Molecular genetics:* Clonal; RAS (20 to 40%), PAX8-PPAR (5 to 20%), TSH-R and GNAS 1.

Differential Diagnosis
Follicular variant of papillary carcinoma.

Case History: (a) A 25-year-old female with a left thyroid mass.
(b) A 71-year-old male with a neck mass.

Diagnosis: (a) Follicular carcinoma, minimally invasive with capsular invasion

(b) Follicular carcinoma, widely invasive with capsular and vascular invasion

Clinical Features
- 75% women, older age than papillary carcinoma.
- Clinically solitary but not occult.

Metastases
- Does not invade lymphatics but does spread to lungs, liver, bone, brain via veins.
- Distant metastases common in grossly invasive disease:
  - 50% if vascular and capsular invasion
  - 75% if local invasion and vascular or capsular invasion.
- Metastases may pulsate because of their vascularity.

Imaging
- Usually "cold" on radionuclide scan.

Gross
- Gray-tan-pink.
- Usually single encapsulated nodule, focally hemorrhagic.
- Variable fibrosis and calcification.
- Large lesions may often be infiltrative.

Microscopy

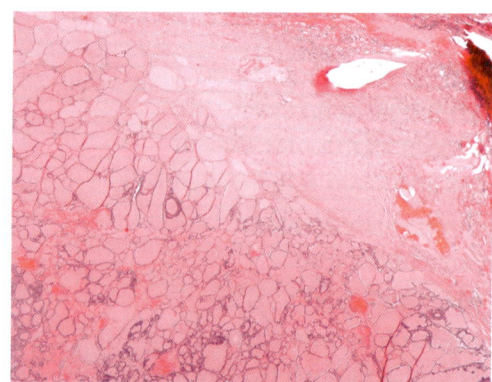

Fig. 20.4a

Endocrine Pathology

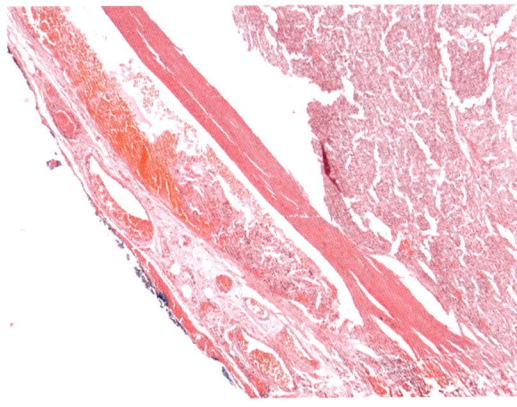

Fig. 20.4b

- Need convincing evidence of invasion of adjacent thyroid parenchyma, capsule (complete penetration) or blood vessels (medium-sized veins or larger vessels or beyond the capsule).
- Capsule is typically thick with calcification.
- Common architectural patterns are follicular or solid.
- Usually no squamous metaplasia, no nuclear features of papillary carcinoma, no psammoma bodies, no/rare lymphatic invasion.

Ancillary Tests

- *Immunohistochemistry:* Positive for thyroglobulin, low molecular weight cytokeratin, EMA, TTF1.
- *Electron microscopy:* Follicular cells converge towards central lumen.
- *Molecular genetics:* RAS mutations in 49%. PAX8-PPAR gamma rearrangement in 36%.

Differential Diagnosis

Atypical follicular adenoma.

Case History: A 69-year-old female with a left thyroid nodule.

Diagnosis: Poorly differentiated thyroid carcinoma

Clinical Features

- 50% have prior multinodular goiter
- 20% have prior differentiated carcinoma
- 20% have concurrent differentiated carcinoma.

Gross

Large solid tumor with necrosis and hemorrhage that invades adjacent structures.

Microscopy

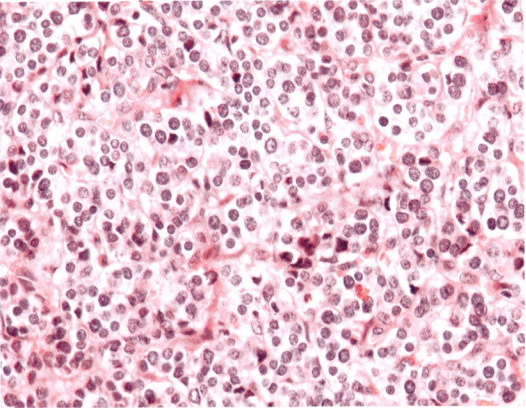

Fig. 20.5

Three Patterns

1. Large, pleomorphic giant cells resembling osteoclasts with cellular connective tissue septae, may have cavernous blood filled sinuses resembling aneurysmal bone cyst.
2. Spindle cells resembling sarcoma.
3. Squamoid cells that are relatively undifferentiated but also appear epithelial with occasional focal keratinization.

Ancillary Tests

- *Immunohistochemistry:* Positive for keratin, vimentin; p53 (well-differentiated tumor usually p53 negative); CD68 (osteoclast-like cells). Increased Ki-67 and PCNA PAX8 (79%). Negative for thyroglobulin, TTF1, BCL-2, calcitonin, desmin, muscle specific actin.
- *Molecular genetics:* BRAF mutations in 50%.

Case History: A 37-year-old male with a neck mass.

Diagnosis: Medullary carcinoma thyroid

Clinical Features
Invades locally, metastases to cervical and mediastinal nodes, lung, liver and bone; metastases may be initial presentation of disease and usually contain amyloid.

Laboratory Investigations
High serum calcitonin and chromogranin A levels.

Gross
- Single or multiple.
- Typically nonencapsulated, solid, gray-tan-yellow, firm, may be infiltrative.
- Larger lesions have hemorrhage and necrosis, tumor usually in mid or upper portion of gland.

Microscopy

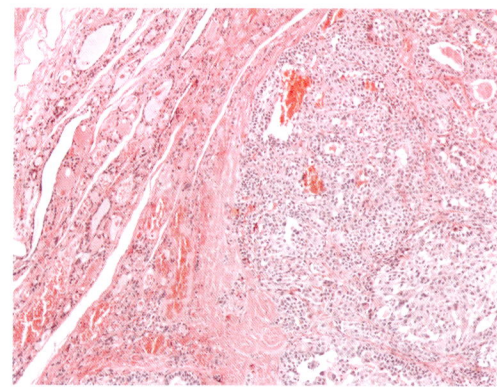

Fig. 20.6

- Round, polygonal or spindle cells in nests, cords or follicles, defined by sharply outlined fibrous bands.
- Tumor cells have granular cytoplasm and uniform round/oval nuclei with punctate chromatin.
- Stroma has amyloid deposits from calcitonin, prominent vascularity with glomeruloid configuration or long cords of vessels, coarse calcifications. Often angiolymphatic invasion.
- C cell hyperplasia presents in familial but not in sporadic cases.

Ancillary Tests
- *Special stain:* Congo red for amyloid.
- *Immunohistochemistry:* Calcitonin, CEA, low molecular weight keratin, chromogranin A and B, synaptophysin, neuron-specific enolase, TTF1, progesterone receptors.
- *Molecular genetics:* Activating mutations of RET different from those in papillary carcinoma.

Differential Diagnosis
- **Hürthle cell carcinoma**: Eosinophilic not amphophilic cytoplasm, no fibrous bands dividing cells into nests.
- **Insular carcinoma**: Thyroglobulin positive, calcitonin negative, no amyloid.
- **Metastatic neuroendocrine carcinoma**: Primary often discovered only on follow-up; primarily interstitial spread, multiple tumour foci, folliculotropism and rosettes, negative for calcitonin, focal/negative for CEA.

Case History: (a) A 37-year-old female with mediastinal mass.
(b) A 59-year-old female with myasthenia gravis.

Diagnosis: (a) Thymoma (lymphocytic predominant)
(b) Thymoma, predominantly epithelial type

Clinical Features
Associated with:
- Myasthenia gravis.
- Acquired hypogammaglobulinemia.
- Other immune-mediated disorders.

Gross
- Mostly encapsulated, 20% infiltrative into surrounding structures.
- Usually large (15–20 cm), yellow-gray with sharp lobulations.
- Cystic degeneration and calcification common.

Microscopy

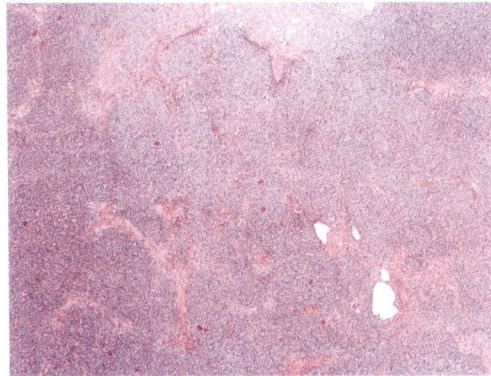

Fig. 20.7a

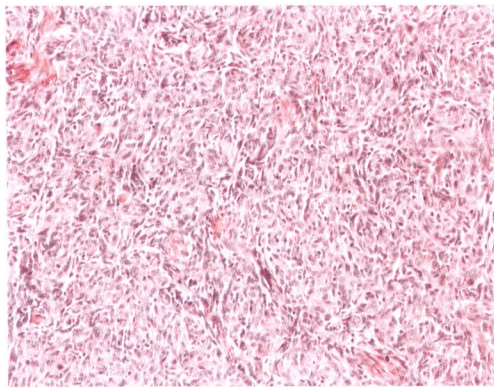

Fig. 20.7b

- *Non-invasive thymoma:* Medullary-type (spindle shaped) epithelial cells, with sparse infiltrate of thymocytes.
- *Mixed thymoma:* Mixture of medullary-type and cortical-type (polygonal) epithelial cells, with denser infiltrate of thymocytes. Capsule may be thick and calcified in both.
- *Invasive thymoma (cortical thymomas):* Cytologically bland cortical-type epithelial cells (abundant cytoplasm, vesicular nucleus) admixed with numerous thymocytes with infiltration of capsule. May have prominent vasculature, microcystic and pseudopapillary patterns, extensive sclerosis. Usually no well formed Hassall's corpuscles.
- *Thymoma with pseudosarcomatous stroma:* Highly cellular spindle cell proliferation without nuclear atypia.

Ancillary Tests

- *Immunohistochemistry*: Positive stains—CEA, CD3, EMA, keratin, Ki-67, S-100, CD205, Foxn1, PAX8, XIAP. Negative stain: CD70
- *Electron microscopy*: Branching tonofilaments, complex desmosomes, elongated cell processes, basal lamina.

Differential Diagnosis

- Thymic cyst
- Thymic carcinoid—well formed rosettes
- Lymphoma
- Seminoma
- Solitary fibrous tumor.

Case History: A 48-year-old man with myasthenia gravis.

Diagnosis: Malignant thymoma (invasive)

Clinical Features

- Aggressive
- Patients usually present with mass related symptoms.
- Always exclude other primaries, which are much more common (lung, trachea, bronchi, esophagus).
- Associated with hypercalcemia, elevated parathyroid hormone levels, pulmonary sarcoidosis.

Proposed Staging System

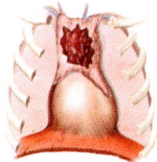 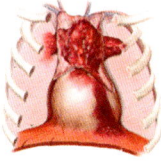 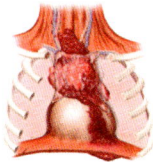

Proposed stage T1, tumor limited to thymic gland   Proposed stage T2, tumor invades nearby structures   Proposed stage T3, direct (continuous) extrathoracic beyond thoracic inlet or below diaphragm

Fig. 20.8a

Gross
- Fleshy, infiltrating, firm to hard, gritty with gray-white.
- Cut surface, no internal fibrous septation, necrosis and hemorrhage.

Microscopy

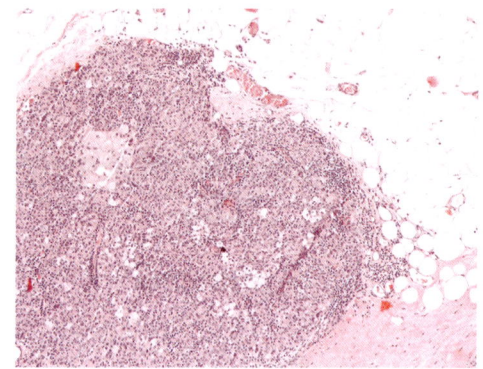

Fig. 20.8

- Mostly squamous cell carcinomas.
- Next most common variant is lymphoepithelioma-like carcinoma (sheets of cells with indistinct borders).
- Usually cohesive cellular growth, regularly round/oval nuclear outlines, eosinophilic nucleoli, geographic necrosis.
- Usually foci of medullary differentiation, abortive Hassall's corpuscles, rosettes, gland-like spaces, T-lymphocytes; no perivascular spaces.

Ancillary Tests
- *Immunohistochemistry*: Positive stains—keratin, CD5, CD70, often EMA, variable CEA, c-kit, GLUT1. Negative stains—proteasome beta subunit.
- *Electron microscopy*: Well-formed desmosome-like intercellular junctions, cytoplasmic tonofilaments that may insert into junctional complexes.

Differential Diagnosis
- Metastatic carcinoma
- Thymoma type B3: GLUT1 usually negative.

Case History: A 59-year-old man with a left adrenal mass.

Diagnosis: Adrenal myelolipoma with adrenal carcinoma

Clinical Features
- Incidental findings, either an autopsy or CT scanning for other reasons.
- Occasionally may attain a large size to become clinically apparent.
- Tumors are inactive hormonally.

Gross
- Soft, fleshy, well-circumscribed tumor with pushing border.
- Yellow areas with the appearance of adipose tissue alternate with hemorrhagic foci composed of bone marrow tissue.

Microscopy

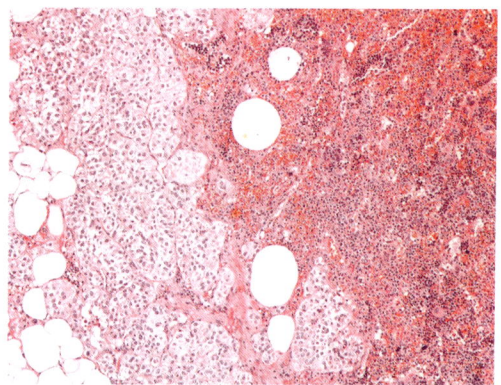

Fig. 20.9

- Composed of normal-appearing hematopoietic elements with all three cell lines typically represented.
- Variable amount of mature adipose tissue is seen.
- Compression of normal appearing adrenal cortex is seen at periphery.

Differential Diagnosis
Lipoma: Is rarely found in adrenal gland and is composed solely of mature adipose tissue. Lacks bone marrow elements.

Case History: A 59-year-old man with a left adrenal mass.

Diagnosis: Adrenocortical carcinoma

Clinical Features
- Sporadic adrenal cortical carcinoma is most common; however, it also occurs in hereditary syndromes:
  1. Li-Fraumeni
  2. Beckwith-Wiedemann
  3. MEN 1
  4. Carney complex
  5. Hereditary isolated glucocorticoid deficiency syndrome.
- Hormonal dysfunction or mass effect.
- Highly necrotic carcinomas may result in fever and thus simulate an infectious disease clinically.
- Palpable adrenocortical neoplasms are malignant in practically every instance.

Imaging
CT scan-central tumor necrosis, calcifications, more heterogeneous tumor.

Gross
- Usually large tumors weighing between 100 and 1000 gm; may measure more than 20 cm.
- Irregular, variegated, tan-yellow mass with infiltrative borders.
- Extension into adjacent soft tissue or surrounding organ is common.
- Cut surface often shows extensive hemorrhage and necrosis.

Microscopy

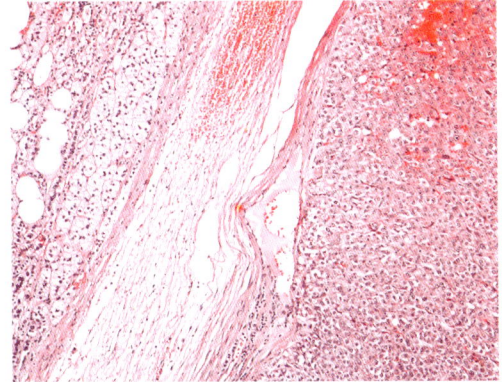

Fig. 20.10

- Characteristic pattern is that of broad trabeculae with anastomosing architecture. Other common patterns include solid or alveolar architecture.
- Infiltrative growth pattern: Tumor cells may resemble normal adrenal cortical cells; however, there is marked nuclear atypia, atypical and frequent mitoses (more than 5/50 high power fields), vascular and extra-adrenal invasion, and necrosis.
- Diagnostic features of malignancy include size (weight, >100 gm), vascular invasion, and metastasis.

Ancillary Tests
- *Immunohistochemistry*: Vimentin, inhibin-, steroidogenic factor-1 (SF-1), and melan-A positive. Cytokeratin may be negative or weakly positive. Synaptophysin may be positive. Chromogranin—negative. Ki-67 labeling index may be helpful to separate adenomas from carcinomas and has prognostic relevance. Cyclin E—positive staining correlates with advanced stage.
- *Electron microscopy:* Prominent rough and smooth endoplasmic reticulum; mitochondria with spherulated cristae; intracellular lipid droplets may be seen. These features are useful to characterize metastatic lesions as derived from adrenal cortex.

Differential Diagnosis
- **Adrenal cortical adenoma:** Is usually much smaller and lacks prominent hemorrhage or necrosis, pleomorphism, atypical mitotic figures, and vascular invasion. Adrenocortical adenomas show a greater expression of low molecular weight keratins and a lesser expression of vimentin than adrenocortical carcinomas.
- **Renal cell carcinoma:** Two features favoring the diagnosis of renal cell carcinoma are the presence of glands (particularly if they contain numerous red blood cells) and abundant cytoplasmic glycogen, but neither is pathognomonic. Immunohisto-

chemically strong positivity for cytokeratin, EMA, CD10, and Lewis blood group isoantigen favors renal cell carcinoma, whereas positivity for inhibin, Melan-A (Mart-1, A103), and synaptophysin favors adrenocortical carcinoma. Adrenomedullary tumors is more likely if chromogranin reactivity is present; synaptophysin is of no help since it stains both tumor types.
- **Pheochromocytoma:** Typically has solid nesting architecture (Zellballen) with indiscreet cell borders, abundant intracytoplasmic hyaline globules, strong synaptophysin and chromogranin positivity, and S-100 protein highlighting sustentacular cells.

Case History: A 55-year-old man with hypertension.

Diagnosis: Pheochromocytoma

Gross

- Varies from small, circumscribed to large, hemorrhagic and necrotic.
- Lobulated, yellow-red-brown.
- Chromaffin reaction: Fresh tumor turns dark brown if added potassium dichromate at pH 5–6.

Microscopy

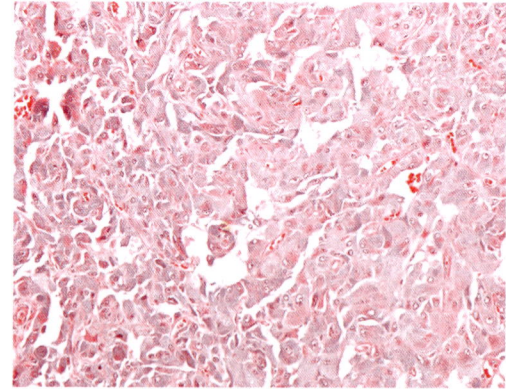

Fig. 20.11

- Zellballen, trabecular or solid patterns of polygonal/spindle-shaped cells in rich vascular network.
- Cells have finely granular basophilic or amphophilic cytoplasm.
- Intracytoplasmic hyaline globules.
- Round/oval nuclei with prominent nucleolus and variable inclusion-like structures.

Ancillary Stains

Chromogranin, synaptophysin, S-100 (sustentacular cells), PAS + diastase resistant hyaline globules and tenascin (strong in clinically malignant tumors).

Differential Diagnosis

Adrenocortical Carcinoma: Inhibin +, Melan A + and calretinin +.

Small Blue Cell Tumors

- Carcinoid
- Ewing/PNET
- Lymphoma
- Monomorphic Wilms' tumor
- Neuroblastoma
- Medulloblastoma
- Rhabdomyosarcoma
- Small cell carcinoma—neuroendocrine
- Carcinoma
- Small cell osteosarcoma

Case History: A 50-year-old male with exploration neck for hypercalcemia.

Diagnosis: Parathyroid adenoma

Gross

- Solitary.
- Well circumscribed tan nodule with delicate capsule.
- May undergo cystic change or hemorrhage.
- May have rim of normal tissue.

Microscopy

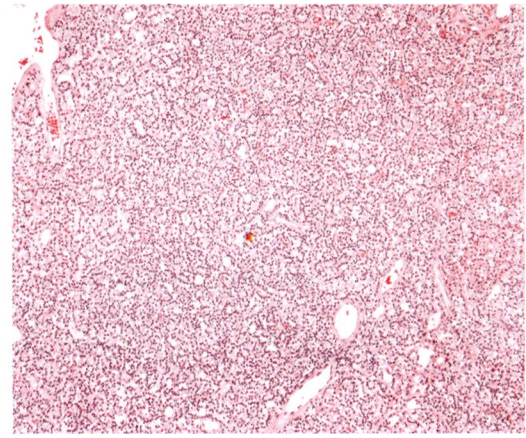

Fig. 20.12

- Encapsulated, cellular, homogenous lesions, rarely papillary, composed of chief cells with some oxyphil cells in delicate capillary network.
- Microfollicles resembling those in thyroid are common.
- Adipose tissue is rare.
- Minimal mitotic activity.
- May see clusters of bizarre nuclei.
- Usually no capsular invasion, no vascular invasion, no invasion of adjacent tissue.

Ancillary Tests

- *Immunohistochemistry*: Positive stains: Parathyroid hormone, glycogen, keratin, cyclin D1, neurofilament, renal cell carcinoma marker. Negative stains: TTF1
- *Molecular genetics*: Loss of heterozygosity in 1p.

Differential Diagnosis

Papillary adenomas resemble papillary carcinoma of thyroid.

Case History: A 60-year-old female with a hard palpable right-sided 2 cm neck mass.

Diagnosis: Parathyroid carcinoma

Clinical Features

- Usually detected because of palpable neck mass.
- Excessive PTH secretion, high serum calcium (>14 mg/dl, may recur after surgery).
- Clinical effects of hypercalcemia (skeletal disease 73%, renal disease 26%), vocal cord paralysis.
- Present in 15% with hyperparathyroidism-jaw tumor (HPT-JT) syndrome, a rare autosomal disorder.

Types

- Chief cell
- Oxyphil

Gross

May be circumscribed, gray-white, firm, irregular, may exceed 10 gm and adhere to adjacent structures.

Microscopy

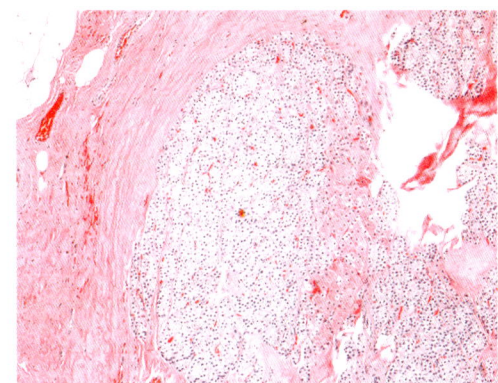

Fig. 20.13

- Uniform cells with minimal atypia in nodular or trabecular patterns with dense fibrous bands.
- Tumor cells are spindled, mitotic figures are frequent, atypical mitotic figures relatively specific, capsular invasion present.
- Vascular invasion, perineural invasion and soft tissue invasion usually reliable indicators of malignancy.

Ancillary Tests

- *Immunohistochemistry:* Positive stains—higher Ki-67 (4–6% or more), lower p27kip1 than adenomas/hyperplasia, cyclin D1, PAS (intracellular glycogen), PTH.
- *Molecular genetics:* Recently described in multiple endocrine neoplasia type 1 (MEN 1), although not a classic finding. One case of parathyroid carcinoma has been reported in MEN 2A syndrome.

Differential Diagnosis

Follicular thyroid carcinoma—PTH negative.

Case History: (a) A 48-year-old female patient with an incidental finding of a mass in the tail of the pancreas.

(b) A 51-year-old man with hypoglycemic episodes.

Diagnosis: (a) Pancreatic neuroendocrine tumor, well differentiated
(b) Pancreatic neuroendocrine tumor—insulinoma

Clinical Features

- Can occur as a part of 4 inherited disorders, including multiple endocrine neoplasia type 1 (MEN 1). von Hippel-Lindau disease (VHL), neurofibromatosis 1 (NF-1) (von Recklinghausen disease), tuberous sclerosis complex (TSC).
- Most secrete multiple hormones, but produce no symptoms that are non-syndromic.

Classification of Neuroendocrine Neoplasms

- Pancreatic neuroendocrine microadenoma
- Neuroendocrine tumor G1 (NET G1)/carcinoid
- Neuroendocrine tumor G2 (NET G2)
- Neuroendocrine carcinoma, NOS
- Large cell neuroendocrine carcinoma, small cell neuroendocrine carcinoma
- Enterochromaffin cell (EC), serotonin-producing neuroendocrine tumor (NET)
- Gastrinoma, malignant
- Glucagonoma, malignant
- Insulin producing carcinoma (insulinoma)
- Somatostatinoma, malignant
- VIPoma, malignant

Note: All considered malignant except microadenomas (less than 5 mm, usually incidental at autopsy), because no histologic criteria differentiate benign and malignant (except metastases).

Imaging

Tumors are hypervascular and circumscribed with octreotide scan.

Gross

- Pink (resembles spleen, lymph node)
- No well defined capsule, variable fibrous tissue, calcium, bone, and cysts.

Microscopy

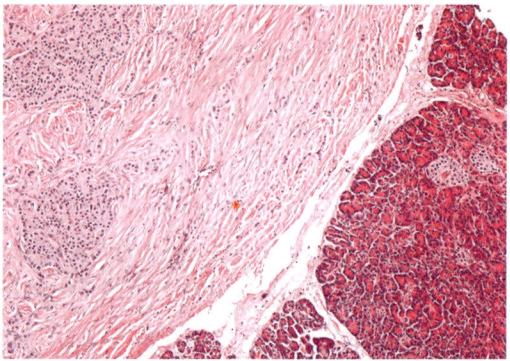

Fig. 20.13a

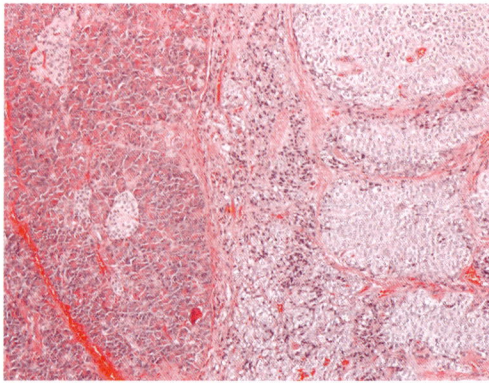

Fig. 20.13b

- Nests of polygonal cells with moderate to abundant eosinophilic cytoplasm resembling carcinoid tumors due to delicate vasculature, salt and pepper chromatin.
- Solid, gyriform, trabecular and glandular patterns with minimal to moderate fibrosis but NO desmoplasia.
- Amyloid is produced by insulin-secreting tumors.
- Cells are less polarized than acinar cell carcinoma. Rarely exhibits true glandular formations, hyaline globules in 5%.

Immunohistochemistry

- Chromogranin, synaptophysin, CEA; also, various hormones including insulin, glucagon, somatostatin, pancreatic polypeptide, gastrin, vasoactive intestinal polypeptide.
- Useful panel for determining pancreatic origin is islet1 +, PAX8 +, CDX2 +, TTF1 – PDX1 +, CDX2 +, TTF1 – and CK7 – may also be useful panel.

Differential Diagnosis

- **Chronic pancreatitis:** Cases with islet cell hyperplasia resemble pancreatic endocrine neoplasms.
- **IPMN:** Small, incidentally identified pancreatic endocrine tumors compress main pancreatic duct and present clinically, radiologically, and grossly as intraductal papillary mucinous neoplasm.
- **Pseudoneoplastic islet cell lesions:** Islets aggregate while rest of pancreas atrophies; islets at tail are compact, islets in head are diffuse and may appear infiltrative, usually have trabecular pattern and are pancreatic polypeptide positive; usually no perineurial invasion.
- **Solid pseudopapillary neoplasm:** Clear cytoplasmic vacuoles on cytology, alpha1-antitrypsin+, vimentin+, CD10+, PR+, nuclear staining for beta-catenin.
- **Usual ductal adenocarcinoma:** Marked nuclear atypia.

Case History: (a) A 50-year-old woman with a suprasellar mass.

(b) A 21-year-old woman with bitemporal hemianopia.

Diagnosis: (a) Craniopharyngioma, papillary variant, who grade 1.

(b) Craniopharyngioma, adamantinomatous type, WHO grade 1.

Clinical Features

- Grows slowly and damages hypothalamus compresses optic chiasm (causing bitemporal hemianopia).
- Blocks third ventricle (causing hydrocephalus).

Imaging

- Cysts typically large and a dominant feature.
- Solid component has soft tissue density of 90% enhancement.
- Calcification seen in 90% typically stippled and often peripheral in location.

Types

- *Adamantinomatous subtype:* Usually children (age 5–14 years); associated with catenin mutation.
- *Papillary subtype:* Usually older adults (age 50 +).

Gross

- Solid and cystic.
- Contents of adamantinomatous tumors resemble motor oil (color due to blood proteins, protein and cholesterol crystals secondary to hemorrhage).

Microscopy

Either adamantinomatous (pediatric type), papillary (adult type) or mixed.

Adamantinomatous

- Relatively poorly circumscribed, nests and trabeculae of epithelium in fibrocollagenous stroma.

- Peripheral cells show nuclear palisading. Central cells are loose and termed "stellate reticulum".
- Often shows abundant keratin with "wet" appearance.

Papillary

Well circumscribed, composed of cores of fibrovascular stroma lined by well differentiated squamous epithelium that may separate to form pseudopapillae.

Immunohistochemistry

Negative for CK8 and CK20.

Differential Diagnosis

- **Metastatic carcinoma**: Usually no calcifications, no squamous epithelium
- **Pilocystic astrocytoma**: Resembles if only gliosis is sampled; but is more cellular, has microcysts
- **Rathke cleft cysts**: CK8+, CK20+; both negative in craniopharyngioma.

APPROACHES TO ENDOCRINE

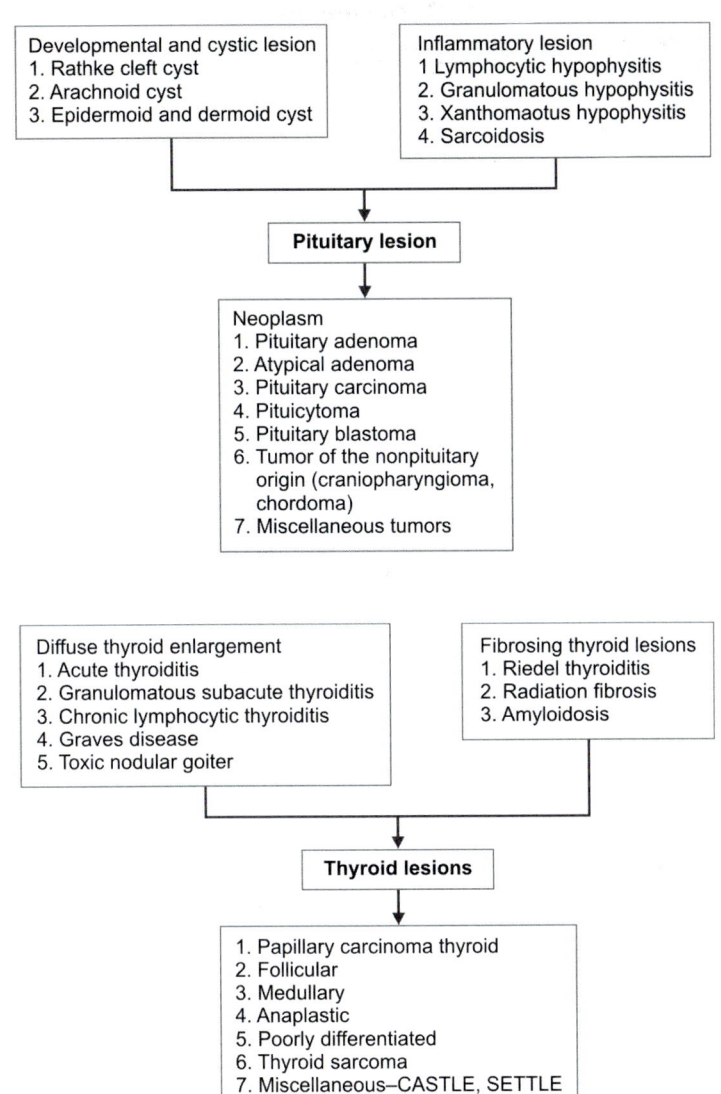

PARATHYROID

1. Parathyroid hyperplasia
2. Parathyroid adenoma
3. Atypical parathyroid adenoma
4. Parathyroid carcinoma
5. MEN syndromes
6. Miscellaneous lesions

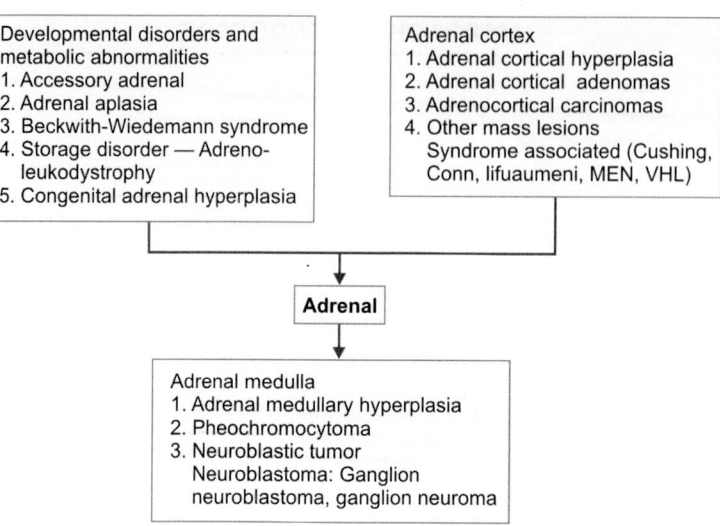

Contributed by Dr G.A. Vasugi

CHAPTER 21

Pap Smear—Gynecological Cytology

Swaminathan Rajendiran

PAP SMEAR

Game Plan

1. Objectives
2. Introduction
3. Sampling and preparation methods
4. Pap stain: Basic aspects
5. a. General approach to cytology
   b. Normal cells in a Pap smear
6. The 2014 Bethesda system (TBS)
   a. Specimen type
   b. Specimen adequacy
   c. General categorization (optional)
   d. Interpretation/results
      i. Negative for intraepithelial lesions/malignancy
      ii. Epithelial cell abnormalities
      iii. Others (endometrial cells in ≥45 yrs)
   e. Adjunctive testing
   f. Computer assisted interpretation
   g. Educational notes and suggestion (optional)
7. Quality control in cytology
8. Conclusion
9. References

Objectives

At the end of this presentation the participants should be:

1. Able to understand the importance of Pap stain.
2. Able to know the steps in Pap staining.
3. Able to apply the TBS criteria in the interpretation of the Pap smears.
4. Able to know the advances made in this field of gynecological cytology.

Introduction

George Papanicolaou 1883–1962: Pap stain is a multicolored staining technique, developed by George Papanicolaou, the father of cytopathology. He was born in Greece (1883) and in 1904, received his MD from University of Athens. He then served in Greek army. He got his PhD in Zoology, University of Munich in 1910. In 1913, he moved over to USA and was working as a research biologist at Cornell Medical College, New York. To start with, he was correlating the cytological changes in vaginal discharge of guinea pig in correlation with the ovarian and uterine cycle. He then applied the same theory to humans.

In 1923, he found abnormal cells from women with cervical cancer: Nobody acknowledged his theory at that time. In 1939, he joined with Dr Herbert F. Traut, a Gynecologist and worked to prove his idea. In 1943, they both published their findings as "Diagnosis of uterine cancer by the vaginal smear". The academic and clinical world started believing his work and he became very well known, occupied many positions and finally retired as Director, Papanicolaou Cancer Institute, Miami in 1961.

On 19th of Feb 1962, he died of heart attack at age 79. He rose to great heights by his hard work but was very humble and used to tell his admirers "I often feel that whatever I have accomplished has been largely a matter of good luck". US government honored him by releasing a stamp on 18th May 1978.

Till today Pap test is the most simple, painless and cost effective screening tool that has reduced the cervical cancer mortality (pre-Pap: 14 per 100,000, post-Pap: 4 per 100,000).

Sampling and Preparation Methods

Patient Instructions

- Pap smear should be taken 2 weeks after LMP.
- No vaginal medications, douches for 48 hours before the sampling.
- Intercourse is not recommended for 24 hours before the sampling.

Instructions for the Sampling Person

- Specimen obtained after insertion of non-lubricated speculum (can be moistened with warm water if necessary).
- Excess mucus or other discharges should be gently removed.
- Sample obtained before applying acetic acid or Lugol iodine.
- Optimal sample should include ecto- and endocervical components.

Conventional Smears

- Spatula or brush is used. In cases of spatula, a plastic rather than wooden one is recommended as the diagnostic material may get trapped between wooden fibers.
- After proper sampling, smears are made in an area that can be covered nicely by the cover slip.
- Immediate fixation is very critical either in 95% ethanol or spray fixation.

Liquid-based Preparation

- After collecting the material (often brush), it was placed in a liquid fixative (ethanol or methanol based) and transported to lab.
- Smears are made with the use of sophisticated instruments.

Advantages of liquid-based technologies	Disadvantages of liquid-based technologies
Immediate fixation, better cytology	Cost (conventional: ₹ 150, liquid based: ₹ 900 in India)
Lesser obscuring material like blood or mucus	Personal to prepare the slides
Improved diagnostic yield and specimen adequacy	Disposable accessories
Decreased rate of atypical smears	Training
Increased rate of dysplastic smears	Changes in the criteria
Availability of material for additional slides	Learning curve
Ancillary testing—HPV, Chlamydia, Gonorrhea, etc.	

Pap Stain: Basic Aspects

Nowadays, Pap staining is used to differentiate cells in smear preparations of various bodily secretions; the specimens can be gynecological smears (Pap smears), sputum, brushings, washings, urine, cerebrospinal fluid, abdominal fluid, pleural fluid, synovial fluid, seminal fluid, fine needle aspiration material, tumor touch samples, or other materials containing cells.

Pap staining is a very reliable technique. As such, it is used for cervical cancer screening in gynecology. The entire procedure is known as Pap smear.

The classic form of Pap stain involves 5 dyes in three solutions:

1. A nuclear stain, hematoxylin, is used to stain cell nuclei.
2. OG-6 counterstain (denotes the used concentration of phosphotungstic acid; other variants are OG-5 and OG-8). It stains keratin. Its original role was to stain the small cells of keratinizing squamous cell carcinoma present in sputum.

3. EA (eosin azure) counterstain, comprising three dyes; the number denotes the proportion of the dyes, e.g. EA-36, EA-50, EA-65.
   - Eosin Y stains the superficial epithelial squamous cells, nucleoli, cilia, and red blood cells. Light green SF yellow stains the cytoplasm of other cells, including non-keratinized squamous cells. This dye is now quite expensive and difficult to obtain, therefore, some manufacturers are switching to fast green FCF, however, it produces visually different results and is not considered satisfactory by some.
   - Bismarck brown Y stains nothing and in contemporary formulations it is often omitted.

On a well-prepared specimen, the cell nuclei are crisp blue to black. Cells with high content of keratin are yellow, glycogen stains yellow as well. Superficial cells are orange to pink, and intermediate and parabasal cells are turquoise green to blue. Metaplastic cells often stain both green and pink at once.

Pap stain comes in several versions, subtly differing in the exact dyes used, their ratios, and timing of the process. The difference between regressive and progressive staining will be dealt in the "Special stains" session (a favorite and useful question often asked in the practical examination).

General Approach to Cytology

A. Quantity

a. Number of normal and abnormal cells present plays a vital role in the diagnosis and in the differentiation of borderline lesions like ASC-US and dysplastic lesions like LSIL.
b. Specimen adequacy should always be kept in mind in negative cases (when there is no epithelial abnormality, if the specimen is inadequate, it has to be repeated).
c. At the same time, the specimen should be reported as adequate even if a small cluster (1–2 cells) of definitive atypical cells are seen (in other words, in the presence of epithelial abnormality… quantity does not matter … hope it is not confusing ….!!)

B. Quality

a. *Cell border:* Distinct or indistinct
b. *Amount of cytoplasm and its nature:* Scant or abundant with mucin.
c. *Number of nuclei:* Binucleation and multinucleation is common in epithelial lesions.
d. *Nuclear cytoplasmic ratio:* The most important in cytology:
   i. <1/3: Normal or ASC-US, AGC (Vide infra)
   ii. 1/3 to 2/3: Low grade epithelial lesion
   iii. >2/3: High grade epithelial lesion (this is good in almost all the organs)
e. The size, shape, distribution:
   i. Uniform size, shape distribution—normal
   ii. Variation in size, shape, distribution—abnormal (ASC-US, LSIL, HSIL)
f. Nuclear membrane regularity and chromatin content are also very important. The chromatin content is assessed by dividing

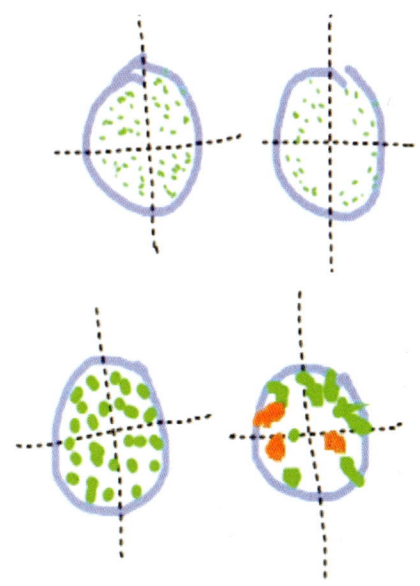

Fig. 21.1: Nuclear chromatin

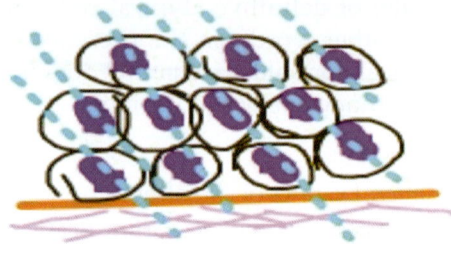

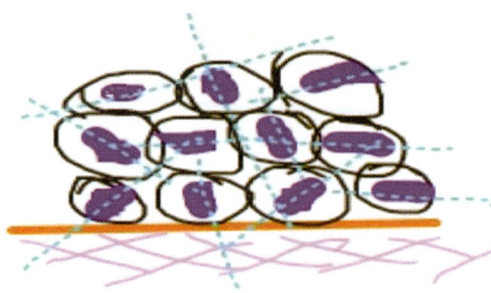

Fig. 21.2: Polarity

the nucleus into 4 quadrants (drawing a line along the long and short axis of the nucleus) and looking at the nature of chromatin and its distribution (Fig. 21.1)
  i. Fine, even (upper, left) : Normal
  ii. Fine, uneven (upper, right) : ASC-US
  iii. Coarse, even (lower, left) : Low grade lesions
  iv. Coarse, uneven (lower, right) : High grade lesions
g. Nucleoli size, shape and distribution also should be noted
  i. No or micronucleoli : Normal, ASC-US, SIL
  ii. Macronucleoli : Carcinoma
h. Polarity is determined by lines drawn along the long axis of the nuclei and it should run parallel to each other rather than crossing, to call it as polarity is maintained (Fig. 21.2)
  i. Polarity maintained (upper) : Normal, ASC-US, LSIL
  ii. Polarity lost (lower) : HSIL, carcinoma
i. Number of mitosis, normal or abnormal also forms part of cytological evaluation.

In a nutshell, with above features, nuclei will fall under 3 categories:
1. *Normal:* Uniform, evenly sized, shaped and distributed nuclei with fine-even chromatin.
2. *Low grade:* Slightly enlarged, overlapping, unevenly distributed mild to moderately pleomorphic nuclei with fine-uneven or coarse-even chromatin. Mitoses increased in number on careful analysis (you look for mitosis) but are of normal form. Polarity is maintained.
3. *High grade:* Markedly enlarged nuclei (more than 3 times the size of normal nuclei), pleomorphic nuclei with coarse-uneven chromatin. Mitoses increased in number (it will look at you ...!!) and abnormal forms seen. Polarity is lost.

Normal Cell Seen in a Pap Smear

A. Squamous Cells

- *Superficial cells:* Large polygonal cells with abundant pink/eosinophilic cytoplasm and pyknotic 5–6 micron nuclei (smaller than a RBC). Keratohyaline granules may be present in the cytoplasm. Estrogen is the hormone controlling these cells and hence increased in the states of estrogenic/hyperestrogenic conditions (follicular phase of the cycle, estrogen producing tumors).
- *Intermediate cells:* Large polygonal cells with abundant greenish cytoplasm with vesicular 8–10 micron nuclei (similar to or slightly larger than a RBC) with fine, evenly distributed chromatin. These cells are under the control of progesterone and hence predominant in luteal phase of the cycle and in hyper-progesterogenic states like pregnancy. (This forms the basis of hormonal evaluation and presence of more superficial cells in cases of pregnancy indicates hypoprogesterone and threatened abortion that can be treated by progesterone injections.)
- *Parabasal/basal cells:* As sampling is taken mainly from exfoliated cells and superficial layer of cervix, these deeper cells are seen

less in normal Pap smears. These cells are small round to oval cells with moderate amount of cytoplasm that is less in basal when compared to parabasal cells. The nucleus is slightly larger than intermediate cells (9–11 micron, slightly larger than a RBC). It is also vesicular with fine, evenly dispersed chromatin. Increased number of these cells can be seen in:
  - Cervical ulcers/erosions
  - Low estrogenic/androgenic phases, menarche, postpartum/postmenopause, Turner syndrome, status post-bilateral oophorectomy.
- *Metaplastic squamous cells:* Parabasal/basal like cells with rigid cytoplasm and arranged in a pavement like or "Cookie cutting" pattern.

B. Endocervical Cells

- Mucin producing cells with eccentrically placed round to oval vesicular nuclei and abundant vacuolated cytoplasm.
- End on view gives a "Honeycomb" appearance with uniformly sized, shaped and distributed cells. On lateral view, it appears as strips of columnar cells as seen in histology.
- Mitosis is not present.

C. Endometrial Cells

1. *Epithelial cells*
   - Balls of small cells with scant cytoplasm and dark nuclei
   - Nuclear molding is present
   - Chromatin is coarse granular in character (endocervical cells are referred as "grapes" and endometrial cells as "raisins")
   - Some time seen as straight or branched tubular structures
   - Often confused with HSIL, AIS and small cell carcinoma.
2. *Stromal cells*
   - Two types of cells: Dense spindle cells (deep) or loose "histiocyte" like cells (superficial). The nuclei are uniform with fine granular chromatin.
   - Capillaries can be seen passing through larger fragments.

D. Trophoblastic and Decidual Cells

- Syncytiotrophoblasts can be rarely seen in smears from pregnant woman.
- Large cells with abundant blue/pink cytoplasm with multiple round to oval dark nuclei.
- Not a reliable predictor of impending abortion.
- Decidual cells appear as isolated cells with abundant granular eosinophilic cytoplasm with a large vesicular nuclei and a prominent nucleoli.
- When you see these cells, a call to the clinician is warranted.

E. Inflammatory Cells

- Neutrophils are always seen and do not represent inflammation. You should see cellular changes such as perinuclear halo and pseudo-orangophilic cytoplasm before calling a smear as inflammatory changes.
- Lymphocytes and plasma cells can also be present, scattered in the background.
- Histiocytes are noted in cases of menstruation, pregnancy, postmenopause, foreign body, radiotherapy, endometrial hyperplasia and carcinoma.

F. Lactobacilli

- Gram-positive rods seen as blue rods in Pap stain.
- It is seen more in luteal phase, causing cytolysis (by metabolizing the glycogen of the squamous cells).

G. Artifacts and Contaminants

- *Corn flaking:* Refractile brown artifact due to air bubble trapped over superficial cells. Restaining and recover slipping may reverse this

- *Cockle burrs:* Club-shaped orange bodies arranged in a radial pattern. Composed of lipid, glycoprotein and calcium surrounded by histiocytes. Seen in pregnant patients and carry no clinical significance.
- *Trichome:* Pale yellow, large, star shaped, 3 to 8 legged structures. Produced by different plants and vary in color, size and shape.
- *Carpet beetle:* Arrow-shaped structures that are contaminant from tampons or gauze pads.

The Bethesda System 2014 (TBS)

It is a system used for reporting Pap smear results. It was introduced in 1988 and revised in 1991 and 2014. The name comes from the location (Bethesda, Maryland) of the conference that established the system. Clearly defined criteria are used for all the terminologies and the best of this system is, openly obtaining the opinion of the practising pathologists through the web portal. All possibilities are carefully considered, well debated and conclusions are drawn based on scientific evidences. The abridged Bethesda system is as follows:

A. Specimen type conventional or liquid based or others
B. Specimen adequacy
C. General categorization (optional)
  i. Negative for intraepithelial lesions/malignancy
  ii. Epithelial cell abnormality
  iii. Others
D. Interpretation/results
  i. Negative for intraepithelial lesions/malignancy
    1. Organisms
       a. *Trichomonas vaginalis*
       b. Candida
       c. Bacterial vaginosis
       d. Actinomyces
       e. Herpes simplex virus
       f. CMV
    2. Other non-neoplastic findings (optional, list not comprehensive)
       a. Reactive cellular changes (inflammation, repair, radiation, IUD)
       b. Glandular cells—status posthysterectomy
       c. Atrophy
       d. Endometrial cells (≥ 45 yrs)
  ii. Epithelial cell abnormalities
    1. Squamous cells
       a. Atypical squamous cells (ASC)
          i. Of undetermined significance (ASC-US)
          ii. Cannot exclude HSIL (ASC-H)
       b. Low grade squamous intraepithelial lesion (LSIL) includes HPV and CIN 1
       c. High grade squamous intraepithelial lesion (HSIL) includes CIN 2 and 3
       d. Squamous cell carcinoma
    2. Glandular cells
       a. Atypical glandular cells (specify endocervical, endometrial, NOS)
       b. Atypical glandular cells—favor neoplastic (specify as above)
       c. Endocervical adenocarcinoma *in situ*
       d. Adenocarcinoma (specify as above)
    3. Other malignancies
E. Adjunctive testing
F. Computer assisted interpretation
G. Educational notes and suggestion (optional)

A. **Specimen adequacy**
- Satisfactory
  a. Well preserved and visualized cells should be:
     i. 5000—for liquid-based preparation
     ii. 8000–12000—for conventional smears (reference images for conventional and spot counting for liquid-based preparations available in the web)
  b. Note the presence of transformation zone/endocervical cells (10 or more squamous metaplastic or endocervical cells). It is a "quality indicator" and the

clinicians have to take a call if there is no T zone/endocervical cell in a smear.
c. Obscuring elements (inflammation, blood, drying artifact, others) should be mentioned if it obscures 50–75% of cells.
- Unsatisfactory
  a. Specimen rejected
     i. Lack of or mismatched patient information
     ii. Slide broken beyond repair (unacceptable specimen due to other causes)
  b. Specimen processed
     i. Insufficient squamous cells
     ii. Obscuring elements more than 75% of epithelial cells

B. **General categorization (optional)**
   i. Negative for intraepithelial lesions/malignancy
   ii. Epithelial cell abnormality
   iii. Others

C. **Interpretation/results**
Negative for intraepithelial lesions/malignancy
1. *Organisms*
   a. *Trichomonas vaginalis*
      - 15 to 30 micron
      - Pear shaped
      - Pale, eccentrically placed nucleus
      - Red cytoplasmic granules (endoplasmic reticulum)
      - Often accompanied by leptothrix: Pathogenic long filamentous bacterium
   b. Candida
      - Pink yeast form, 3 to 7 micron in diameter, budding also may be present
      - Long pseudohyphae may be seen
      - Tangles of squamous cells around pseudohyphae (shish kebabs)
   c. Bacterial vaginosis
      - Curved bacilli or coccobacilli or mixed bacteria
      - "Filmy" appearance of the slide
      - Clue cells
   d. Actinomyces
      - Tangled clumps of Gram-positive bacteria (cotton balls)
      - Often associated with intrauterine devices (IUD)
   e. Herpes simplex virus
      - 3M: Multinucleation, molding of nuclei and margination of chromatin.
2. *Other non-neoplastic findings (optional, list not comprehensive)*
   a. Reactive cellular changes (inflammation, repair, radiation, IUD)
      - Enlarged nuclei with bi- or multinucleation
      - Prominent nucleoli
      - Cells running in one direction (school of fish) or being pulled out (like taffy)
      - In inflammation, perinuclear halo and pseudo-orangeophilia of the squamous epithelium noted (mere neutrophils are not enough for the diagnosis of inflammation).
      - *Radiation:* Large polychromatic, bizarre cells with enlarged nucleus, multinucleation and cytoplasmic/nuclear vacuolations. Nuclear cytoplasmic ratio is maintained.
      - *IUD:* Single or clusters of cells with cytoplasmic vacuolations (may resemble signet cell). The differential is adenocarcinoma and HSIL and be cautious in diagnosing these in the presence of IUD. Please ask for a repeat Pap after removing the IUD.
   b. Glandular cells—status posthysterectomy
      - Wrong history/patient
      - Partial hysterectomy
      - Rarely from bartholin/other para vaginal glands
      - Atrophic cells
      - Therapy-induced metaplasia of squamous cells
      - Fallopian tube prolapse
      - Vaginal adenosis/endometriosis
      - Rectovaginal/vesicovaginal fistula
      - Recurrent adenocarcinoma
   c. Atrophy

- Increased number of parabasal cells and basal cells in sheets and syncytial-like aggregates or hyperchromatic crowded groups.
- Naked nuclei (small cells) may be seen
- Cells have high nuclear cytoplasmic ratio but uniform chromatin.
- Pseudokeratinized cells (pink to orangeophilic cytoplasm) are due to degeneration.
- Severe atrophy can show dirty background with inflammation, debris, old blood, blue blobs (represent condensed mucus, degenerated bare nuclei or precipitating hematoxylin) and giant cells.
- In liquid based cytology, background of atrophic smear is cleaner.
- May resemble urothelial metaplasia, but cells have prominent intercellular bridges.
- Nuclei are uniform, evenly spaced, often elongated with grooves.

d. Others
- *Tubal metaplasia:* Strips of crowded, stratified columnar and goblet cells with terminal bar and cilia. The nuclei can be enlarged, pleomorphic and hyperchromatic, mistaken for AGC. The cilia and the terminal bar are diagnostic of tubal metaplasia.
- Keratotic cellular changes:
  - *Hyperkeratosis:* Anucleated, mature, polygonal squamous cells (prolapsed uterus). Can be a contaminant from vulvar area.
  - *Parakeratosis:* Small, heavily keratinized squamous cells with dense orangeophilic cytoplasm and small pyknotic nuclei. When these show nuclear atypia, should be called dyskeratosis and categorized as epithelial cell abnormality. History of previous epithelial cell abnormality with/without treatment should be obtained.
  - *Follicular cervicitis:* Commonly associated with Chlamydia infection. Heterogenous population of lymphoid cells with scattered tingible body macrophages. Some time clusters of follicular center cells are misinterpreted as HSIL. Most of the time the lymphoid cells are arranged as trails seen in a bone marrow aspirate, rather than clusters of HSIL cells.

Epithelial cell abnormalities
1. *Squamous cells* (Table 21.1)
   a. Atypical squamous cells (ASC)
      i. Of undetermined significance (ASC-US)
      ii. Cannot exclude HSIL (ASC-H)

		Table 21.1			
Character	ASC-US	ASC-H	LSIL	HSIL	Squamous cell carcinoma
1. Abnormal cells	Few		Many		
2. Classic koilocytes	Nil		Many	Few	
3. N:C ratio	<1/3	>2/3	1/3 to 2/3	>2/3	Varies
4. Nuclear membrane	Regular		Irregular		
5. Chromatin	Uniform, fine granular		Uniform, coarse	Clumped, adherent to nuclear membrane	
6. Nucleoli	Absent	Present	Absent	Absent	Present
7. Tadpole cells	Absent	Absent	Absent	Absent	Present
8. Tumor diathesis	Absent	Absent	Absent	Absent	Present
9. HPV typing	No/low risk		Low risk	High risk	High risk

b. Low grade squamous intraepithelial lesion (LSIL) includes HPV and CIN 1.
c. High grade squamous intraepithelial lesion (HSIL) includes CIN 2 and 3.
d. Squamous cell carcinoma

Koilocytes: Mono or binuclear cells with enlarge nuclei with fine granular chromatin with mild nuclear membrane irregularity and nuclear groove (resemble coffee bean). Cytoplasm shows a large cavitation with a sharp inner edge. Indicates HPV infection and qualifies for LSIL by itself.

2. *Glandular cells* (Table 21.2)
   a. Atypical glandular cells—AGC (specify endocervical, endometrial, NOS)
   b. Atypical glandular cells—favor neoplastic (specify as above)
   c. Endocervical adenocarcinoma *in situ*—AIS
   d. Adenocarcinoma (specify as above)

Atypical glandular cells—favor neoplastic

No defined criteria. It should be more than ASC and less than AIS. It is very easy to mention theoretically, but very difficult to apply practically. Hope they will remove this terminology in the future update ....!!!

Many times, glandular lesions may coexist squamous abnormality and we have to document both. Sometimes, it is very difficult to differentiate both, especially HSIL and AIS. The following findings favor AIS:

1. Strips of columnar cells
2. Feathering
3. Gland formation, rosettes
4. Absence of koilocytes
5. Clean background

Likewise, endocervical lesions and endometrial lesions are also difficulty to differen-

Table 21.2

Character	Normal	AGC	AIS	Adenocarcinoma
1. Abnormal cells	Nil	Few	Many	
2. Cell border	Distinct		Indistinct	
3. Pseudostratification	Nil	Present		
4. Feathering	Nil		Present	
5. Disorganization	No (honeycomb)	Yes (drunken honeycomb)		
6. Nuclear enlargement/ overlapping	No	Yes		
7. Chromatin	Fine, even	Coarse, even	Coarse, uneven	
8. Nucleoli	Nil	Micronucleoli		Macronucleoli
9. Mitosis	Nil	Nil/rare	Few	Many
10. Tumor diathesis	Nil			Present

Table 21.3

Character	Endocervical lesion	Endometrial lesion
1. Age of the patient	Young (reproductive age group)	Elderly (mostly postmenopausal)
2. Cell border	Distinct (grapes)	Indistinct (raisins)
3. Cytoplasm	More, mucin +	Less, foamy
4. Overcrowding of nuclei	Less	More (morphology not clear)
5. Feathering	Present	Absent
6. Associated histiocytes	Less	More
7. Tumor diathesis	Hemorrhagic	Watery
8. Associated HPV/HSIL	Present	Absent

tiate at times. The following tables may be useful (Table 21.3).

Other Tumors
Rare gynecological tumors: Small cell carcinoma, sarcomatoid carcinoma, MMMT, sarcoma, lymphoma, melanoma.
Metastasis: Common from ovary, fallopian tube, colon, stomach and breast.

3. Others (list not comprehensive)
   Endometrial cells in women ≥45 years:
   - Should be reported as "Negative for squamous intraepithelial lesion" with a note indicating:
     – Endometrial cells after the age 45, particularly out of phase or after menopause may be associated with benign endometrium, hormonal alteration and less commonly endometrial hyperplasia (12%) or carcinoma (6%).
     – Pap test with only histiocytes/superficial stromal cells should be reported as "Negative for intraepithelial lesion or malignancy". Histiocytes/superficial stromal cells alone do not have independent diagnostic significance and should not be reported in the same context as exfoliated glandular cells.
   e. Adjunctive testing
      i. Molecular testing for HPV, Chlamydia, Gonorrhea and others like p16
      ii. Indicate the test method
      iii. Result should be interpreted and understandable for the clinician
      iv. Result should be correlated with the cytological features.
   f. Computer assisted interpretation
      i. Type of instrument used for screening and interpretation
      ii. Screening by automation or manual and automated
         1. Correlation of automated and manual results
         2. Name of the technologist verifying the automated data
   g. Educational notes and suggestion (optional)
      i. Concise and consistent with the guidelines of professional organizations
      ii. Should be rendered in cases of:
         1. Unsatisfactory specimen (to improve the quality of repeat sample)
         2. Further triage and management
         3. Morphological features are ambiguous
         4. Complex cases

Quality Control in Cytology

It will be dealt in detail in another presentation, but for the completion sake, the following are included:
a. Errors have to be reduced
b. Ratio of ASC-US and AGC has to be within allowed percentage

Table 21.4: Measures to reduce the errors

Task	Error	Remedy
• Preparation	Douching/menses	Patient education
• Sampling	Lack of endocervix	Clinician education/samplers
	Inflammation/blood	Liquid-based preparation
• Fixation/staining	Air-drying/poor staining	Liquid-based preparation
• Locating cells	Incomplete scanning	Stage controllers
	Cells obscured	Liquid-based preparation
	Too few cells	Liquid-based preparation
		Computer screening
• Identifying cells	Significance not apparent	Computer screening
	Missing the cells	New regulations (CLIA 88)

c. Correlation of cytology with histology (biopsies, definitive surgery specimens)
d. External and internal quality control
e. In case of an error, do a RCA (root cause analysis) and CAPA (corrective and preventive action) (Table 21.4).

Conclusion

1. Pap smear remains one of the most successful cancer screening methods developed.
2. Criteria should be applied for the interpretation, starting from specimen adequacy.
3. The Bethesda system 2014 should be followed for consistency in the reporting.
4. Frequent updating regarding the diagnostic criteria and newer technologies available to use is a must.
5. Clinical correlation and follow-up is essential.

References

1. http://nih.techriver.net/index.php (.... images)
2. http://www.asccp.org/Link Click. aspx? fileticket=uUGOqspsCBU%3d&tabid= 5964

CHAPTER
22A
Cytology Slide Case Discussion Part I

K Swaminathan

Case Number 1: Pleural Fluid Cytology

History: A 59-year-old female patient presented with breathlessness, hemoptysis for one week. She had similar complaints for the past 2 months for which she received local medical aid. As the condition worsened she presented to the hospital for admission. X ray—massive pleural effusion. CT chest-Massive pleural effusion. Pleural fluid—hemorrhagic 900 ml tapped with rapid filling. Pleural fluid cytology.

Diagnosis: Smear positive for malignancy—metastatic adenocarcinoma deposits

Microscopy

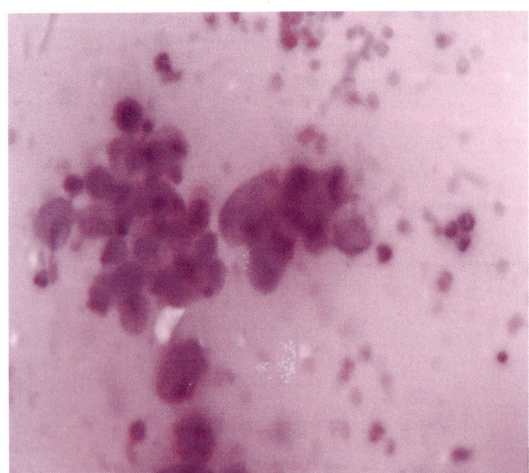

Fig. 22A.1a

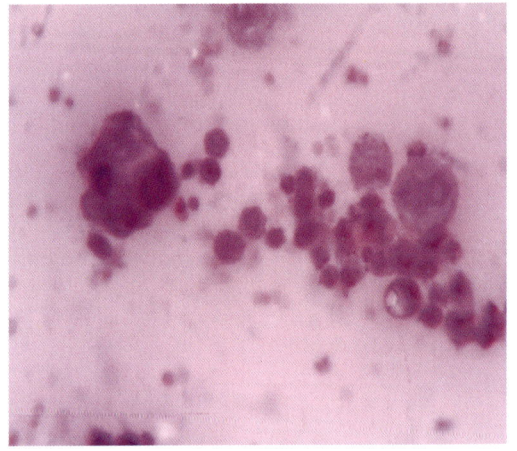

Fig. 22A.1b

Smear studied shows cohesive clusters of medium to large cells, arranged in cell balls in many areas with few cells with abundant mucinous cytoplasm with scattered reactive mesothelial cells, degenerated cells and lymphocytes in a hemorrhagic background.

Case Number 2: Pleural Fluid Cytology

History: A 32-year-old male person presented with difficulty in breathing for one month. H/O irregular fever, cough with expectoration. Diagnosed as tuberculosis and put on ATT. Defaulted with ATT. No lymphadenopathy and hepatosplenomegaly. X ray—massive pleural effussion. CT chest—massive pleural effusion. Pleural fluid-hemorrhagic 1200 ml tapped with rapid filling.

Diagnosis: Lymphocytic effusion of pleural fluid—possibily primary effussion lymphoma.

Microscopy

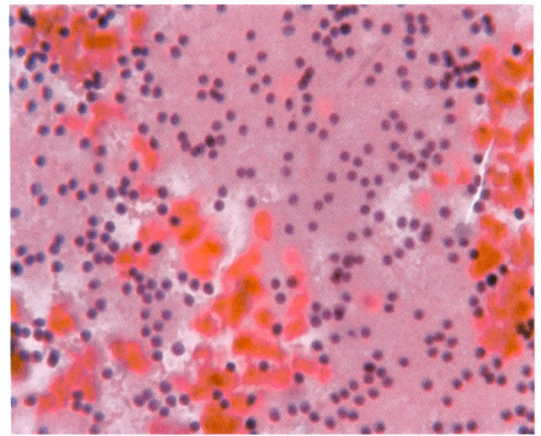

Fig. 22A.2

Markedly cellular smear in a hemorrhagic background composed of monotonous population of small lymphoid cells with scant rim of cytoplasm and round nuclei with coarse chromatin. Few bare nuclei and smudge cells seen.

Effusions with a lymphocyte differential of more than 50% are defined as lymphocytic effusion. They may be either exudative or transudative. Lymphomatous and leukemia pleural effusions are classically exudative. Similarly transudative effusions are seen in patients with renal failure and heart failure.

Case Number 3: Peritoneal Wash Cytology

History: A 68-year-old female patient presented with fullness of the abdomen for the past 3 months. She had a gradual increase in the fullness for the past 2 months with rapid increase in size since 3 weeks. Ultrasound examination revealed a complex mutiloculated cystic and solid mass of size 18 x 14cm in the right pelvis, ovaries could not be visualised separately with peritoneal fluid collection. She was taken up for a debulking surgery. Peritoneal wash sent for cytological analysis.

Diagnosis: Smears positive for malignancy—mucinous adenocarcinoma deposits

Microscopy

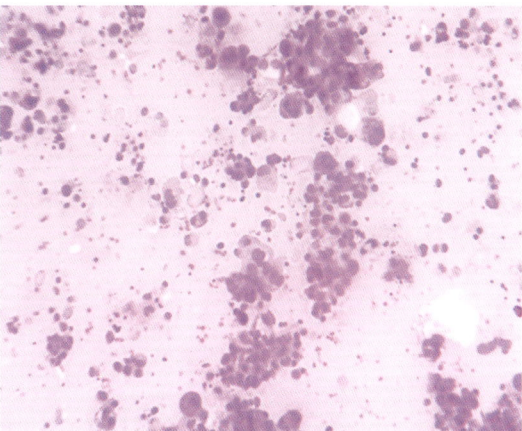

Fig. 22A.3

Smear studied shows cohesive clusters of large round to polygonal cells with abundant pale vacuolated cytoplasm with irregular nuclear outlines with abnormal chromatin clumping with few degenerated cells, few reactive mesothelial cells in a hemorrhagic background.

Malignant Effusions

Metastatic adenocarcinoma is the most common cause for malignant effusion and the most common primary site is the lung. Other sites include breast, ovary and GIT.

Table 22A.1: Segregation based on the cell size, pattern and cell type	
Cell size	Probable primary site of tumour
Small	Breast, stomach
Medium	Breast, stomach, lung, ovary
Large	Ovary, lung, breast
Cell pattern	Probable primary site of tumour
Papillae	GIT, ovary, breast, lung
Cell balls	Breast, ovary, lung
Indian file	Breast, stomach, pancreas
Single cells	Stomach, breast

Contd.

Table 22A.2: Segregation based on the cell size, pattern and cell type (Contd.)	
Cell type	Probable primary site of tumour
Signet ring cells	Stomach, intestine, ovary, lung
Clear cells	Ovary, kidney
Columnar cells	Colon
Bizarre cells	Lung, pancreas

Table 22A.3: Frequency of metastasis from different sites		
Gender	Pleural	Peritoneal
Female	Breast	Ovary
	Ovary	Breast
	Lung	GIT
	GIT	Endometrium
	Lymphoma	Lymphoma
Male	Lung	GIT
	GIT	Lymphoma
	Lymphoma	
Children	Lymphoma	
	Leukemia	
	Neuroblastoma	
	Rhabdomyosarcoma	
	Ewing's sarcoma	

Reactive Mesothelial Cell versus Adenocarcinoma Cells

Reactive mesothelial cells usually loose adhesions and appear as single cells. They may form small groups less than 10 cells. True acinus formation and three dimensional clusters are not the features of reactive mesothelial cells.

They have indistinct cytoplasmic membrane, dense greenish cytoplasm with pap or deep blue stain with MGG. They have a round nucleus and a central nucleoli. Small clusters of reactive mesothelial cells show "window" formation. Window formation is not seen in adenocarcinoma. Few mesothelial cells contain large vacuoles in their cytoplasm. These vacuoles are degenerative and contain neither glycogen, mucin nor lipid.

Cytomorphological Spectrum of Mesothelial cells

1. Uniform cell population
2. Oval to round nuclei
3. Centrally placed nuclei
4. Fine powdery chromatin
5. Inconspicuous nucleoli
6. Moderate translucent cytoplasm
7. Two zone cytoplasm
8. Peripheral vacuole with glycogen
9. Fuzzy cell borders due to microvilli
10. Mesothelial windows between the slides

Benign Conditions Simulating Malignancy

1. Chronic effusions of chronic renal failure
2. Congestive cardiac failure
3. Cirrhosis of liver
4. Long term peritoneal dialysis
5. Endometriosis/endosalpingiosis
6. Megakaryocytes in extramedullary hematopoiesis
7. Detached ciliated cell clusters in post-operative states

POINTS TO PONDER—CYTOLOGY OF EFFUSIONS

1. The three essential steps for an accurate diagnosis of effusions are:
   a. freshly tapped specimen
   b. immediate processing
   c. rapid fixation of the slide
2. **Gross Examination**

Table 22A.4	
Colour of the fluid	Probable diagnosis
Watery clear/pale yellow	Congestive cardiac failure, cirrhosis, Malnutrition
Cloudy, turbid,	Infections
Milky white, chylous	Thoracic duct obstruction, trauma, leukemia, lymphoma
Bloody, darck chocolate brown	Malignancy, Trauma, infarction,
Green	Biliary tract disease
Viscid	Pseudomyxoma peritonei, mesothelioma

3. **Fixatives:**
   a. Papanicolaou fixative—mixture of 95% alcohol and ether [1:1 ratio]
   b. 95% alcohol
   c. 100% methanol
   d. 80% isopropyl alcohol
   e. Carnoy's fixative (95% alcohol, chloroform and glacial acetic acid in ratio of 6:3:1) for hemorrhagic fluids.
   Minimum time for fixation is 10 to 15 minutes.
4. **Common stains:**
   Papanicolaou stain and MGG is recommended.
5. **Ancillary techniques:** The various ancillary techniques used are
   a. Immunocytochemistry
   b. Desorption technique
   c. Electron microscopy
   d. Image morphometry
   e. Flow cytometry
   f. AgNORs
   g. Telomerase activity
   h. Lectin binding assay
   i. PCR and FISH

Light's Criteria for Exudative Effusion

The pleural fluid is an exudate if one or more of the following criteria are met:
1. Ratio pleural fluid protein/serum protein >0.5
2. Ratio pleural fluid LDH/serum LDH >0.6
3. Pleural fluid LDH more than two-thirds the upper limit of normal serum LDH

Immunocytochemistry of Effusions

Categorisation of effusion immunomarkers:

Ideal Positive Mesothelial Markers

1. Calretinin—sensitive
2. D2–40 (Podoplanin)—sensitive
3. Cytokeratin 5/6
4. WT 1

Ideal Negative Mesothelial Markers

1. Ber-EP4
2. mCEA
3. MOC-31
4. BG-8
5. B72.3

Case Number 4: Bronchial Wash Cytology

History: A 64-year-old male patient presented with breathlessness for 2 weeks. H/o cough with expectoration, three episodes of hemoptysis and vague chest pain. Investigations revealed an irregular hilar mass 5.5 × 4.5 cm in the right lung. Patient subjected to flexible fibro-optic bronchoscopy and bronchial wash slides given for analysis.

Diagnosis: Smears positive for malignancy non-small cell carcinoma probably squamous cell carcinoma lung.

Microscopy

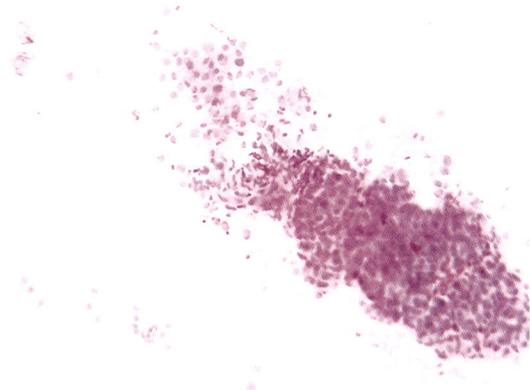

Fig. 22A.4

Smear studied shows exfoliated ciliated bronchial cells admixed with reserve cells, occasional muciphages and clusters of polygonal cells with dense eosinophilic cytoplasm and large irregular nuclei with occasional dyskeratotic cells. The background shows cell debris, acute and chronic inflammatory cells.

Table 22A.5: Cytologic mimics of pulmonary squamous cell carcinoma

Cytological features	Squamous cell carcinoma	Squamous metaplasia	Pulmonary infarction	Vegetable material
Cellularity	Hypercellular	Hypocellular	Hypocellular	Hypocellular
Background	Necrosis ++	No necrosis	Hemosiderin laden macrophages	No necrosis
Pattern	Sheets, single cells	Single cells	Single cells	Loose single cells
Cell type	Strap cell, tadpole cells, polygonal	Mature squamous	Cuboidal, columnar	Rectangular, thick refractile cell wall
Cytoplasm	Variable, dense	Dense, Basophilic	Variable	Basophilic
Nucleus	High N/C ratio	Round and central	Round to oval	Small
Nuclear membrane	Irregular	Smooth	Irregular	Smooth
Chromatin	Granular, irregular	Fine granular	Fine granular	Degenerated
Nucleoli	Prominent	Normal	Normal	Normal
Others	Keratin pearls			

Case Number 5: FNAC–Mass Lung

History: A 48-year-old male patient presented with breathlessness for 2 months. H/o cough with expectoration with one episodes of hemoptysis present. Treated as a case of tuberculosis of lung. Defaulted from treatment. Investigations revealed an irregular mass 2.5 × 2 cm in the peripheral region of lower lobe of right lung. Patient also had a tiny nodular lesion in the right adrenal gland. Patient subjected to CT guided fine needle aspiration cytology of the mass.

Diagnosis: Suggestive of adenocarcinoma right lung

Microscopy

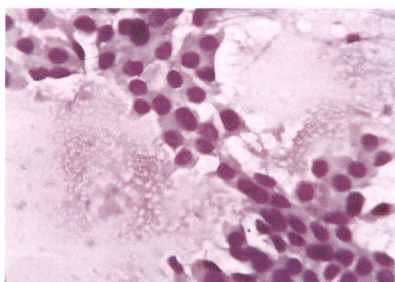

Fig. 22A.5a

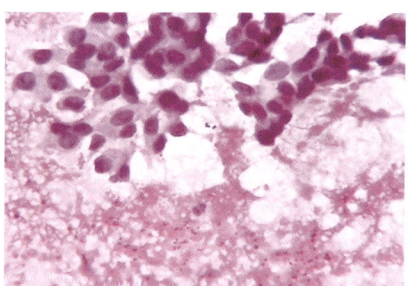

Fig. 22A.5b

Smear studied shows loose clusters of medium to large sized round to polygonal cells with variable cytoplasm and round to oval nuclei with moderate anisokaryosis. Few cells tend to form acinar pattern with isolated degenerated cells and mucin laden cells in a hemorrhagic background.

Common Differential Diagnosis

1. Metastatic adenocarcinoma
2. Large cell carcinoma
3. Atypical adenomatous hyperplasia
4. Reactive bronchiolar cells
5. Mesothelioma

Immunostaining with TTF-1 is the best single marker of primary origin.

- A basic panel with CK 5/6, CK7, p63 and TTF -1 will help in the process of diagnosis.
- Squamous cell carcinoma—positive for CK 5/6, p63
- Adenocarcinoma—positive for CK7, TTF-1
- Calretinin—positive for mesothelioma
- Synaptophysin, chromogranin and CD56—neuroendocrine tumours

Table 22A.6: Cytologic mimics of pulmonary adenocarcinoma

Cytological features	Adenocarcinoma	Clear cell	Hamartoma tumour	Granular cell tumour	Atypical pneumocytes	Reactive bronchial cells	Bronchial cell hyperplasia	Goblet cell hyperplasia	Therapy related
Cellularity	Hyper-cellular	Hypo-cellular	Hypo-cellular	Hyper-cellular	Hypo-cellular	Hypo-cellular	Hyper-cellular	Hyper-cellular	Hypo-cellular
Background	Necrosis ++	No necrosis	No necrosis	No necrosis	No necrosis	No necrosis	No necrosis	No necrosis	Necrosis ++
Pattern	Clusters, acini, single	Clusters, single	Sheets	Loose	Clusters with knobby borders	Cohesive	Papillary	Small	Cohesive/dyscohesive
Cell type	Cuboidal, columnar, polygonal	Polygonal	Epithelial	Polygonal	Cuboidal	Cuboidal columnar	Columnar	Columnar	Polygonal
Cytoplasm	Scant, moderate, mucoid	Vacuolated	Scant	Granular	Moderate vacuolated	Moderate	Moderate, mucin rich	Mucin rich	Vacuolated, variable, two toning
Nucleus	High N/C ratio, eccentric	Round to oval	Round to ovalc	Round to oval	Round to oval	Variable	Small	Small	Irregular enlargement
Nuclear membrane	Irregular	Smooth	Smooth	Smooth	Smooth	Smooth	Smooth	Smooth	Irregular
Chromatin	Granular, irregular	Fine granular	Fine granular	Fine granular	Fine granular	Fine granular	Fine granular	Fine granular	Irregular
Nucleoli	Prominent	Normal	Normal	Normal	Normal	Normal	Normal	Normal	Macronucleoli
Others	Intranuclear inclusions ++	HMB 45 positive	Ciliated cells +	S 100 positivity	—	—	—	Normal goblet to bronchial cell ratio 1:6	

Table 22A.7: Common pitfalls in pulmonary cytology

Pitfalls	Cause	Solution
Clinical presentation	Acutely Ill patient/ no mass	Bronchogenic carcinoma patients never present with acutely ill Be wary of a malignant diagnosis in the absence of a mass
Specimen cellularity	Low cellularity	Never report on malignancy if cellularity is inadequate Adhere to the cytomorphological criteria strictly
Cytological backgound	Clean background/ obscured by inflammation	Be wary of a malignant diagnosis in a clean background. Be wary of a malignant diagnosis in a background obscured by inflammation
Cytomorphology	Overlapping features	Make a diagnosis of malignancy after excluding the potential mimics.

Case Number 6: Fnac Mass Breast

History: A 59-year-old female patient presented with an irregular vague lump in the left breast for 6 months. No recent increase in size of the swelling noted. On examination the swelling was 3 × 2.5cm in the upper outer quadrant, mobile. No nipple discharge. Skin over the swelling normal. Mammogram was done which revealed an irregular mass with speculated margins with a diagnosis of suspicious of malignancy. FNAC was done for the mass.

Diagnosis: Suggestive of malignancy— lobular carcinoma of breast

Microscopy

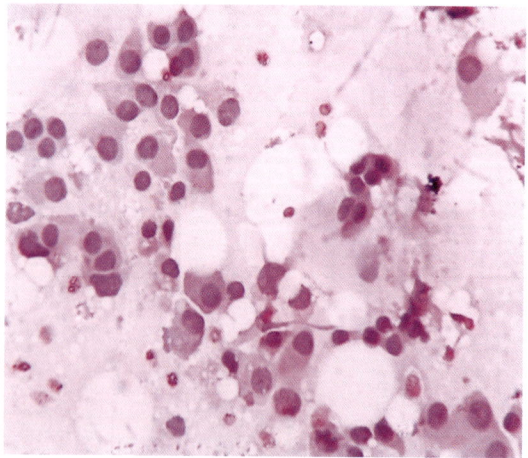

Fig. 22A.6a

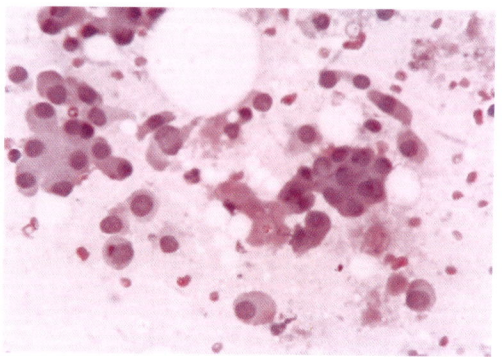

Fig. 22A.6b

Moderate cellularity with many isolated single cells with variable cytoplasm and eccentrically placed nuclei. Few of the clusters show intracytoplasmic vacuoles with a targetoid appearance sometimes compressed and indented the nucleus. The shape of the nucleus was irregular angular, triangular, indented, and occasionally budding. The background often was thick, eosinophilic, and sometimes had crushed material interspersed with fatty vacuoles.

In cases of sparse cellularity the diagnostic clues are
1. Irregular and abnormal nuclear outline
2. Eccentric location of nuclei
3. Dense cytoplasm
4. Intracytoplasmic lumina
5. Mucin droplets
6. Tendency to form small chains
7. Absence of bipolar stromal nuclei

Case Number 7: Nipple Discharge Cytology

History: A 32-year-old female presented to the surgical OPD with complaints of nipple discharge for the past 2 weeks. The discharge was thin and watery to begin with and now appears blood stained. On examination a small nodular mass felt in the subareolar region. Firm in consistency with vague tenderness. Smears prepared from nipple discharge cytology.

Diagnosis: Suggestive of a papillary neoplasm of breast—intraductal papilloma

Microscopy

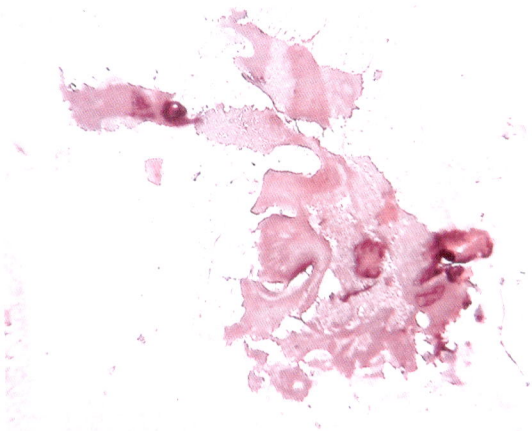

Fig 22A.7

Smear studied shows many complex folded branching epithelial sheets and finger like fragments. Few strands of dense fibrovascular stroma seen. The epithelial cells show isomorphic nuclei with occasional palisading of columnar cells. The background shows scattered hemosiderophages and cyst macrophages.

Common Differential Diagnosis

The conditions include:
1. **Low grade papillary carcinoma:** Presence of long slender papillae with ramifying edges and cellular atypia suggests a papillary carcinoma. Increased cellularity, nuclear crowding, loss of cell cohesion favor malignancy.
2. **Fibroadenoma:** Papillary like epithelial fragments may be seen in fibroadenoma. These papillae are usually finger shaped and lack the complex pattern of papillomas. A background with single bipolar nuclei and stromal fragments with myxoid material are in favor of fibroadenoma.

Case Number 8: FNAC Mass Breast

History: A 29-year-old female presented to the surgical OPD with a huge mass 8 × 8cm in the right breast.

There was a gradual increase in size with no pain/tenderness. No nipple discharge. The mass was mobile with pushing margins. Opposite breast normal. No lymphnodes palpable

Diagnosis: Phyllodes tumour of breast

Microscopy

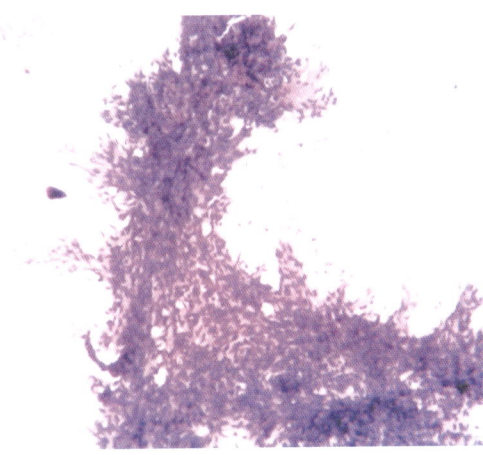

Fig. 22A.8

Cellular smear with large stromal fragments. The stromal cells have benign plump nuclei with retained cytoplasm with small clusters of benign epithelial cells with bland cytological features.

Common Differentials

Cellular fibroadenoma: Difficult to distinguish, clinical examination often gives us clue. Howeever presence of huge stromal fragments and stromal cells with minimal atypia helps in the diagnosis of phyllodes tumour of breast.

Case Number 9: FNAC Swelling Thyroid

History: A 27-year-old female presented to the surgical OPD with swelling in front of the neck. She had the swelling for the past 6 months and she had noticed recent increase in body weight. On examination there was diffuse enlargement of thyroid which was moving with deglutition. FNAC of the swelling thyroid was done.

Diagnosis: Hashimoto's thyroiditis

Microscopy

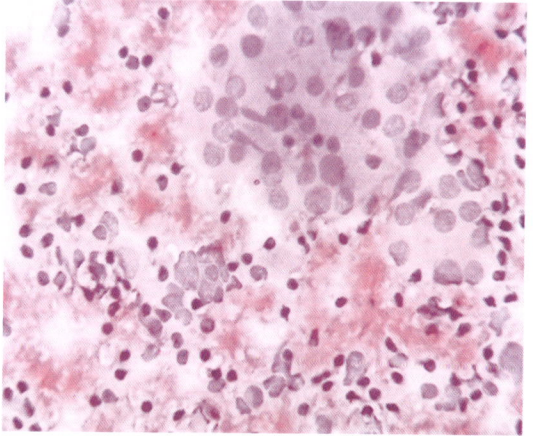

Fig. 22A.9a

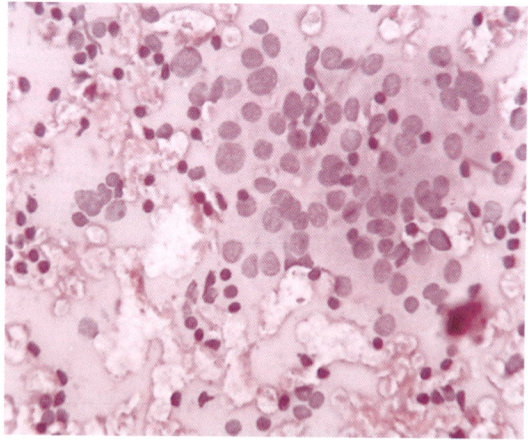

Fig. 22A.9b

Smear studied shows prominent clusters of Hurthle cells with abundant granular eosinophilic cytoplasm and round nuclei with dense lymphoplasmacytic infiltration and variable colloid. Occasional multinucleate giant cells are seen.

Discussion

The most common problem in the diagnosis of Hashimoto's thyroiditis is to differentiate between the bare thyroid nuclei and the lymphocytes. The follicular cells have more homogenous chromatin and dense nuclear rim than a lymphocyte.

Conditions with Increased Lymphocytes in Smears

Lymphoid cells can be seen in **the diffuse sclerosing variant and Warthin's like variant of papillary carcinoma** and in few cases of nodular goiter.

It is often difficult to distinguish low grade MALT lymphomas from Hashimoto's thyroiditis in few cases. If the lymphocytic infiltration is florid with very sparse epithelial cells care must be taken to exclude lymphoma.

Hashimoto's thyroiditis can also be mistaken for **granulomatous thyroiditis**. But the presence of uniform lymphocytic infiltration and prominent Hurthle cells help in the diagnosis. The granulomatous thyroiditis usually have a polymorphous infiltrate with giant cells and epitheloid cells.

Hurthle cells in groups may be confused with **papillary carcinoma**. The points in favor of the Hurthle cells are the granular quality of the cytoplasm. In papillary carcinoma the cell to cell boundary is very distinct.

Hurthle cell nodules of Hashimoto's may be confused with **Hurthle cell neoplasm**. This can be resolved by analyzing the nuclear polymorphism of the Hurthle cells. The extent of the nuclear variability is less in Hurthle cell neoplasm when compared with Hashimoto's thyroiditis.

Case Number 10: FNAC Diffuse Thyromegaly

History: A 32-year-old female presented to the ENT OPD with painful deglutition with fever and malaise. On examination there was diffuse enlargement of thyroid. Tenderness on palpation.

No evidence of hyper or hypothyroidism. FNAC of the swelling thyroid is done.

Diagnosis: Subacute granulomatous thyroiditis (dequervian's thyroiditis)

Microscopy

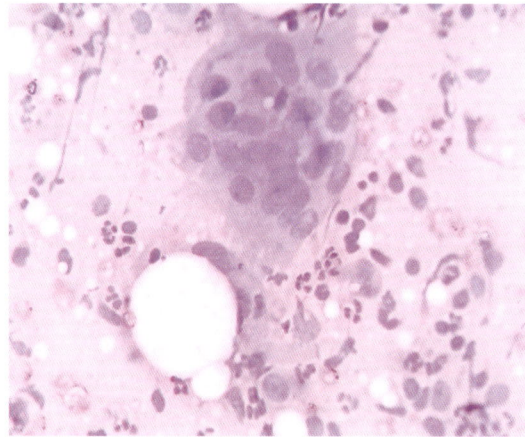

Fig. 22A.10a

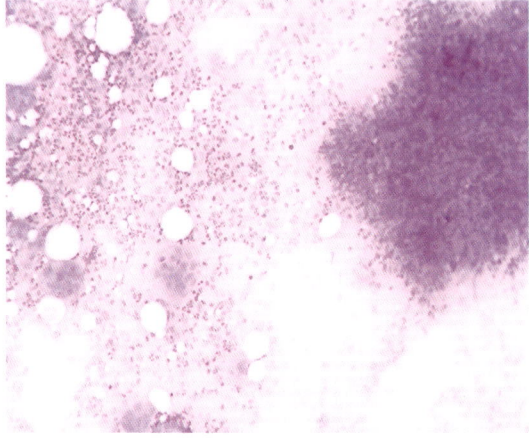

Fig. 22A.10b

Smear studied shows loose collection of epithelioid cells with many multinucleate giant cells and degenerated follicular epithelial cells. The background is dirty with cell debris, colloid, neutrophils, lymphocytes and macrophages.

Differential Diagnosis: Granulomatous changes in thyroid may also be seen as:

1. Histiocytic response to hemorrhage
2. Reaction to spilled colloid
3. Adjacent to a thyroid neoplasm
4. Following robust clinical examination (palpation thyroiditis)
5. Mycobacterial infection
6. Fungal infection
7. Sarcoidosis
8. Vasculitis
9. Foreign body reaction

Case Number 11: FNAC Mass Thyroid

History: A 70-year-old Male presented to the casualty with an irregular mass in front of neck. Recent increase in the size of the mass. H/O dysphagia present. Difficulty in breathing observed. Firm to hard in consistency. Partly moves with deglutition. FNAC of the swelling thyroid was done.

Diagnosis: Anaplastic carcinoma thyroid

Microscopy

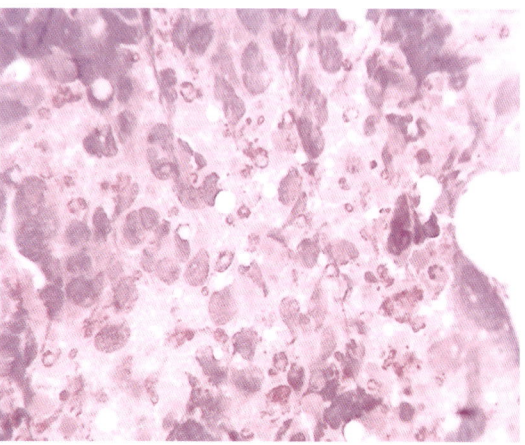

Fig. 22A.11a

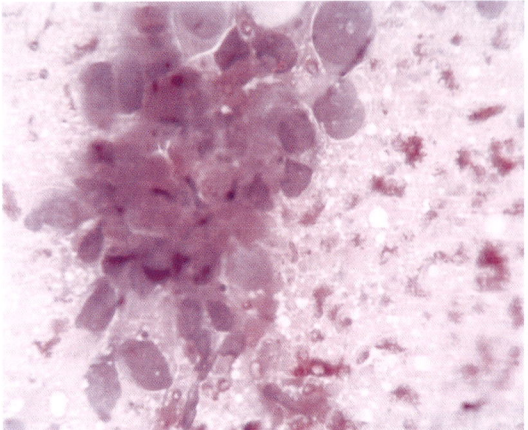

Fig. 22A.11b

Cellular smear with polymorphic population of cells, predominantly plump spindle cells, Large bizarre mononuclear cells, Multinucleated giant cells, cells with bizarre nuclei and prominent macronucleoli are seen. Occasional atypical mitotic figures are seen. Background with hemorrhage and necrosis.

Differential Diagnosis

1. Plemorphic variant of medullary carcinoma
2. Bizarre cells of a degenerating multinodular goiter.
3. Follicular neoplasms following radio-therapy/chemotherapy.
4. Metastatic carcinomatous deposits.

Case Number 12: CT Guided FNAC Osteolytic Lesion—Humerus

History: A 62-year-old female presented to the orthopaedic OPD with swelling in her left elbows for 2 weeks. She was a domestic helper and had a recent fall in her workplace. On examination there was an oblong swelling in the lower end of left humerus. Tenderness was present. X-ray revealed a pathological fracture of lower left humerus with an osteolytic lesion. CT guided FNAC was done.

Diagnosis: Metastatic deposits humerus—primary papillary carcinoma thyroid

Microscopy

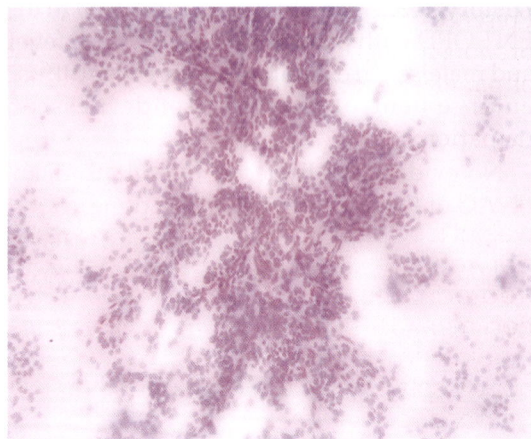

Fig. 22A.12a

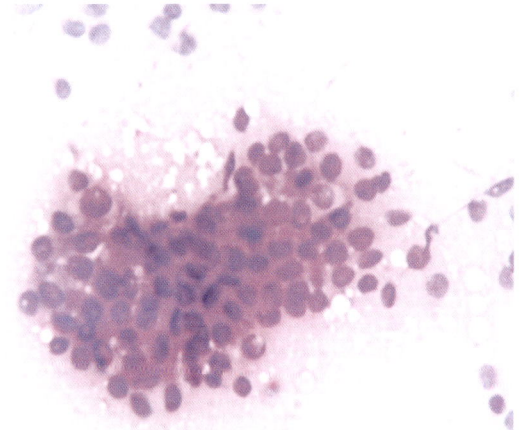

Fig. 22A.12b

Smear studied shows papillary clusters of round to polygonal cells with eosinophilic cytoplasm and round to oval nuclei with pale chromatin and prominent intracytoplasmic inclusions. Few of the cells show prominent grooves. The background shows cell debris and hemorrhage.

Criteria for Diagnosis of Papillary Carcinoma

1. Papillary structures without blood vessels
2. Fine granular chromatin
3. Intranuclear inclusions
4. Nuclear grooves
5. Psammoma bodies

Definite Criteria—More than 3

Presence of nucleomegaly, nuclear atypia and prominent nucleoli indicate metastatic lesions of papillary carcinoma.

Case Number 13: FNAC Cervical Lymphnode

History: A 42-year-old male person. H/O fever, weight loss and sweating. Multiple palpable cervical lymph nodes. Diagnosed and treated as tuberculosis. No response to treatment. USG—multiple Cervical, axillary, mediastinal, Mesenteric adenopathy with hepatosplenomegaly. FNAC of the cervical lymphnode was done.

Diagnosis: Hodgkin's lymphoma.

Microscopy

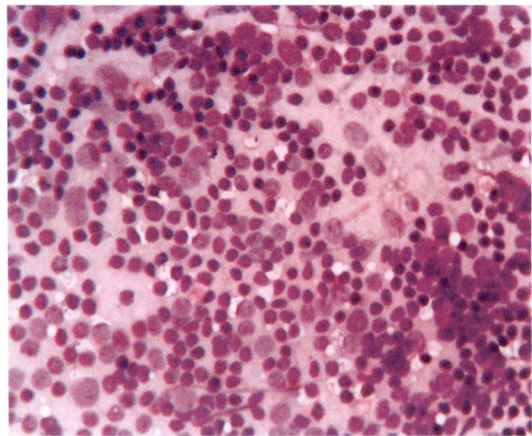

Fig. 22A.13

Smear studied shows a heterogeneous population of lymphoid cells, plasma cells, histiocytes, eosinophils. Prominent binucleate Reed Sternberg giant cells. Few scattered mononuclear Hodgkin's cells.

Conditions with Reed Sternberg Look Alike Cells

1. Infectious mononucleosis
2. Toxoplasma lymphadenitis
3. Angio-immunoblastic lymphadenopathy
4. Pleomorphic T cell lymphoma
5. Anaplastic large cell lymphoma
6. Metastatic nasopharyngeal carcinoma
7. Dendritic follicular cell sarcoma
8. Rheumatoid arthritis
9. Drug induced lymphadenopathy.

Case Number 14: FNAC Inguinal Lymphnode

History: A 48-year-old male patient presented to the surgical OPD with a swelling in the right inguinal region for the past one month. There was a gradual increase in the size of the swelling. No pain or tenderness. A provisional diagnosis of right inguinal adenopathy was made and the case was sent for FNAC. FNAC of the inguinal node done.

Diagnosis: Metastatic malignant melanoma deposits lymph node.

Microscopy

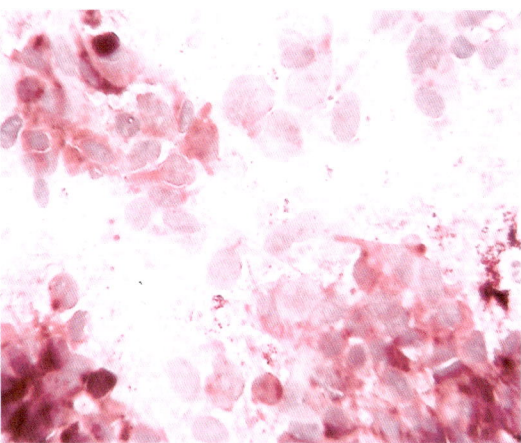

Fig. 22A.14

Smear studied shows many clusters of round to polygonal cells with abundant cytoplasm with eccentrically placed nuclei with variable anisokaryosis. Few cells show prominent intranuclear inclusions and occasional binucleate cells are seen. Many cells show intracytoplasmic melanin pigmentation.

Diagnostic Points

1. Polymorphic dissociated cells
2. Cytoplasm with pigment granules

3. Vacuolated cytoplasm (negative pigmentation)
4. Cells with large nucleoli
5. Cytoplasmic invaginations into the nucleus.

Appearance of Melanin Pigments with Various Stains

1. Brownish—Pap
2. Brown and dusty—HE
3. Bottle green/black–MGG
4. Fontana Masson—Positive
5. Perl's stain—Negative
6. PAS stain—Negative
7. Z-N stain—Negative

Case Number 15: CT Scan Guided FNAC Mediastinal Mass

History: A 30-year-old male presented with difficulty in breathing with chest pain. Investigations revealed a mass in the anterior mediastinum. CT scan guided FNAC of the mass was done.

Diagnosis: Metastatic malignant melanoma deposits lymphnode

Microscopy

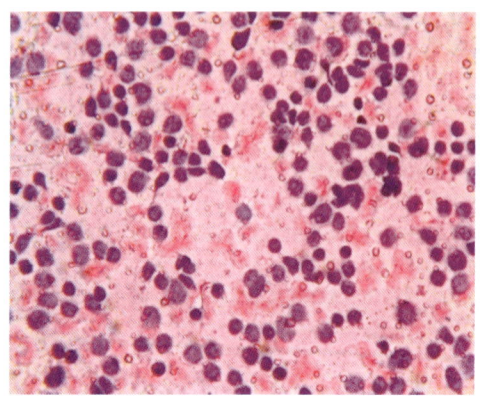

Fig. 22A.15

Smear studied shows clusters of oval to polygonal cells with round to oval nuclei admixed with lymphoid cells with scant rim of cytoplasm with few degenerated cells in the background.

Table 22.8: Differential Diagnosis for Mediastinal Lesions					
Features	Thymoma	Germinomas	Non-Hodgkin's lymphoma	Hodgkin's lymphoma	Metastatic small cell carcinoma
Mediastinal location	Anterior, superior	Anterior	Anterior, middle	Anterior, middle	Middle
Cell arrangement	Cohesive	Non-cohesive	Non-cohesive	Non-cohesive	Loose choesion, rows of cells
Tumor cells	Epithelial cells with mild to moderate cytoplasm	Cell with large nuclei and prominent nucleoli	Immature lymphoid cells	Classical Reed Sternberg's cell and its variants	Small cells large than mature lymphocytes, cell to cell moulding present
Lymphoid cell	Mature looking, small	Mature looking, small	Immature mono-morphic cells	Mature looking, small	Malignant cells are small but larger than mature lymphocytes
Background	Lymphoglandular bodies from lymphoid cells	Trigroid	Lymphoglandular bodies	Lympoglandular bodies	Chromatin threading
Ancillary tests	CK+	PLAP+	LCA+ Light chain B-NHL present	CD15+, CD30+	NSE+, chromogranin+

CK = cytokeration, PLAP = Placental leukocyte alkaline phosphatase, LCA = Leukocyte common antigen, NSE = Neurone specific enolase, NHL = Non-Hodgkin's lymphoma + = positive.

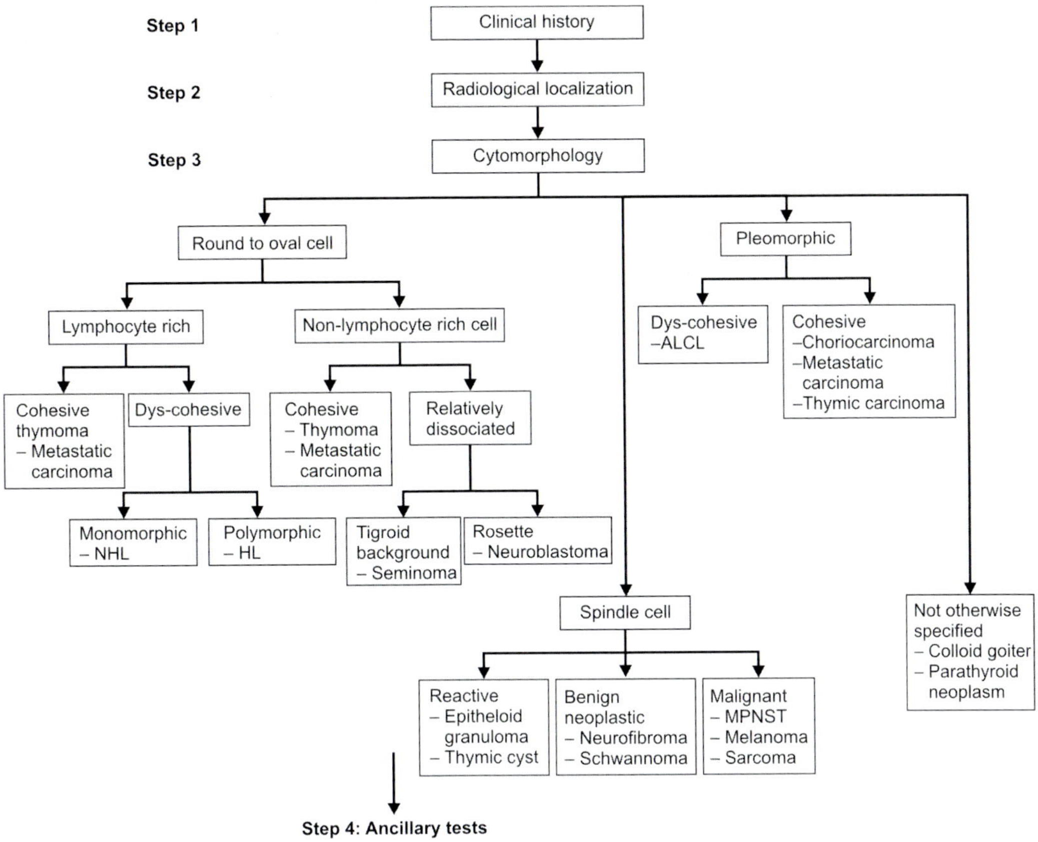

```
Step 1          Clinical history
                      ↓
Step 2          Radiological localization
                      ↓
Step 3          Cytomorphology
              ↙              ↘
     Round to oval cell      Pleomorphic
       ↙         ↘           ↙        ↘
  Lymphocyte   Non-lymphocyte  Dys-cohesive   Cohesive
    rich        rich cell      –ALCL          –Choriocarcinoma
                                              –Metastatic
                                               carcinoma
                                              –Thymic carcinoma

  Lymphocyte rich:
   Cohesive      Dys-cohesive
   thymoma
   – Metastatic
    carcinoma

   Monomorphic   Polymorphic
   – NHL         – HL

  Non-lymphocyte rich cell:
   Cohesive      Relatively
   – Thymoma     dissociated
   – Metastatic
    carcinoma

   Tigroid       Rosette
   background    – Neuroblastoma
   – Seminoma

                Spindle cell
         ↙         ↓         ↘
     Reactive    Benign       Malignant          Not otherwise
     – Epitheloid neoplastic  – MPNST            specified
      granuloma  – Neurofibroma – Melanoma       – Colloid goiter
     – Thymic cyst – Schwannoma – Sarcoma        – Parathyroid
                                                  neoplasm

Step 4: Ancillary tests
```

Abbreviation: NHL= Non hodgkin's lymphoma, HL= Hodgkin's lymphoma, Ca= Carcinoma, ALCL= Anaplastic large cell lymphoma, MPNST= Malignant peripheral nerve sheath tumor

Case Number 16: FNAC Submandibular Nodule

History: A 62-year-old female presented with an irregular swelling in the submandibular region for 6 months. There was a gradual increase in size with occasional pain over the swelling. Skin over the swelling normal. FNAC of the mass was done

Diagnosis: Mucoepidermoid carcinoma.

Microscopy

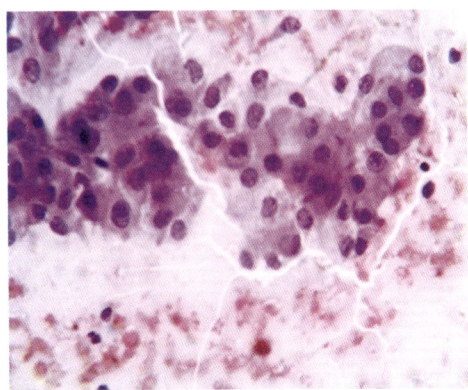

Fig. 22A.16

Smear studied shows small cohesive clusters of cells with well defined finely vacuolated cytoplasm and bland nuclei. The cells show prominent intracellular mucin with few cells with dense eosinophilic cytoplasm – squamoid cells. Background with mucus and cell debris.

Grading of Mucoepidermoid Carcinoma

Histopathologic feature	Point value
1. Cystic component <20%	2
2. Neural invasion	2
3. Necrosis	3
4. 4 or more mitoses/10 HPF	3
5. Anaplasia	4

Tumour Grade Point Score
- Low   0–4
- Intermediate 5–6
- High   7 or more

Case Number 17: FNAC Parotid Nodule

History: A 25-year-old female presented to the surgical OPD with a nodule in the right parotid. She has noticed the swelling for the past 3 months and there was a gradual increase in the size of the nodule. No history of pain or tenderness seen. FNAC of the nodule was done.

Diagnosis: Benign salivary gland neoplasm –pleomorphic adenoma parotid.

Microscopy

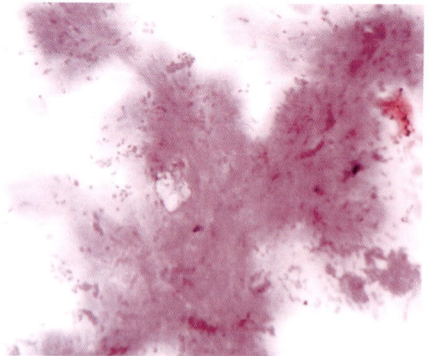

Fig. 22A.17a

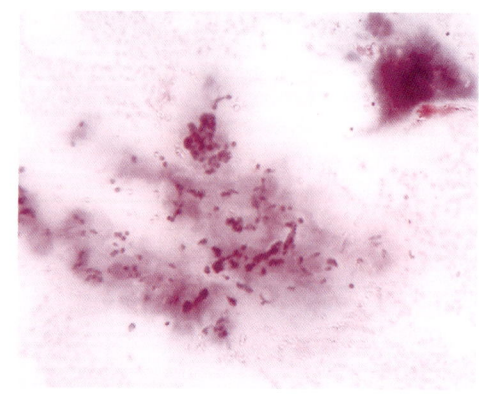

Fig. 22A.17b

Smear studied shows small nests and clusters of acinar epithelial cells with regular ovoid nuclei and bland nuclear chromatin with oval shaped myoepithelial cells in a fibrillary chondromyxoid ground substance in the stroma.

The common problem is to distinguish pleomorphic adenoma from adenoid cystic carcinoma. Presence of well defined cytoplasm, bland, finely granular nuclear chromatin favor pleomorphic adenoma whereas scanty cytoplasm, high nucleocytoplasmic ratio, nuclear molding and hyperchromasia favor adenoid cystic carcinoma.

Case Number 18: FNAC Nodule Hard Palate

History: A 46-year-old female presented with a nodular swelling in the oral cavity. On examination there was a nodular mass in the palate 2 × 2 cm. Skin over the nodule was normal. FNAC of the nodular mass done.

Diagnosis: Adenoid cystic carcinoma

Microscopy

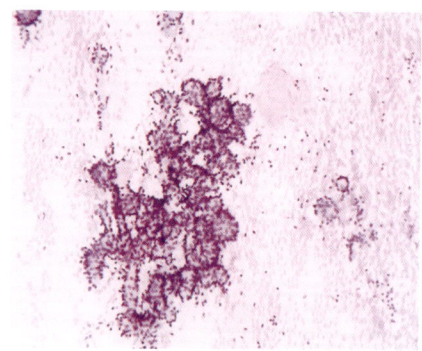

Fig. 22A.18a

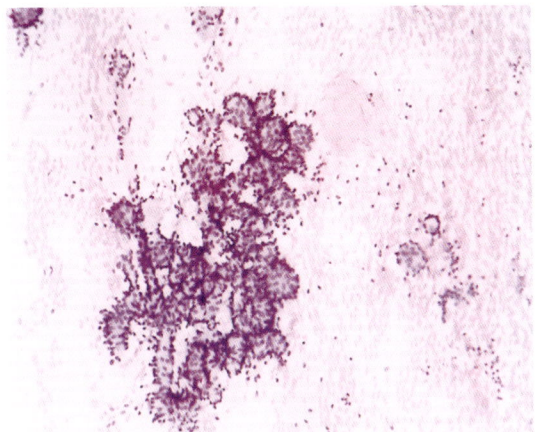

Fig. 22A.18b

Smear studied shows clusters of round to oval cells with scanty rim of cytoplasm and high nucleocytoplasmic ratio. Few naked nuclei seen. Prominent hyaline spherical globules are seen.

Conditions with Hyaline Stromal globules

1. Basal cell adenoma
2. Canalicular adenoma
3. Basal cell adenocarcinoma
4. Pleomorphic adenoma
5. Polymorphous low grade adenocarcinoma
6. Epithelial myoepithelial carcinoma.

The hyaline globules in pleomorphic adenoma tend to be smaller, fewer in number, with less define outlines. The pleomorphic adenoma contain myoepithelial cells with intact cytoplasm whereas the adenoid cystic carcinoma has many bare nuclei in the background.

Case Number 19: FNAC Nodule Parotid

History: A 49-year-old female presented with a nodular mass in the parotid area for 2 months. There is a rapid increase in size with pain and tenderness. Skin over the mass was normal. No facial nerve involvement. FNAC of the mass was done.

Diagnosis: Malignant myoepithelioma parotid gland

Microscopy

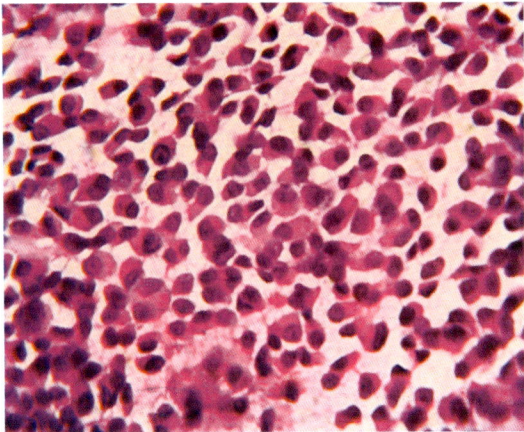

Fig. 22A.19

Cellular smear with sheets and clusters of plasmacytoid cells. Abundant eosinophilic granular cytoplasm and moderate cellular and nuclear atypia. Mitotic figures present. Background with cell debris and necrosis.

Criteria for Diagnosis

1. Composed of a single myoepithelial cells
2. Predominantly plasmacytoid
3. Significant nuclear pleomorphism
4. Coarse nuclear chromatin
5. Prominent nucleoli

Differential Diagnosis

The most common condition to be considered is metastatic melanoma deposits.

Case Number 20: USG Guided FNAC Mass Liver

History: A 48-year-old male presented with pain abdomen. On examination there was a mass palpable in the right hypochrondrium. Ultrasound revealed a mass in the left lobe of liver. USG guided FNAC of the mass was done.

Diagnosis: Hepatocellular carcinoma liver

Microscopy

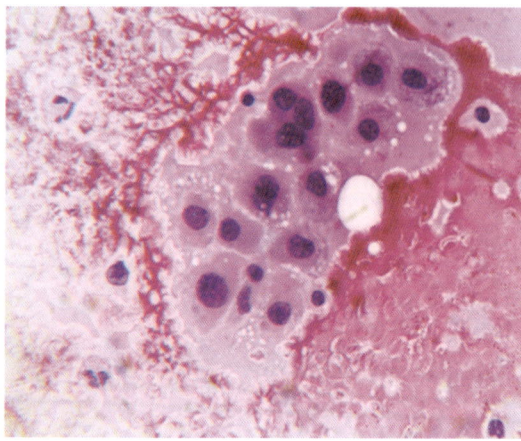

Fig. 22A.20

Smear studied shows many dyscohesive clusters of polygonal hepatocytes with variable cytoplasm and large nuclei with moderate anisokaryosis and prominent macronucleoli. Few cells show prominent intranuclear inclusions. Few degenerated cell debris are seen in the background.

Common Cytological Findings

1. Smooth-edged clusters with peripheral wrapping by the endothelial cells
2. Cohesive sheets of hepatocytes with transgressing vessels
3. Acinar formations
4. Increased N/C ratio
5. Macroeosinophilic nucleoli
6. Reduced number of binucleate cells
7. Background free of bile duct epithelial cells

Use of Immunomarkers to Differentiate Primary Versus Metastatic Tumour

- HepPar-1: Diffuse granular cytoplasmic positivity (favors HCC)
- Glypican-3: Positive in HCC
- CK 7, CK 10: Negative in HCC
- TTF-1: Cytoplasmic staining in HCC

Case Number: 21 CT scan Guided FNAC Mass Liver

History: A 2-year-old male child presented with pain abdomen with a mass abdomen for one month. There was a rapid increase in size. CT scan huge heterogeneous mass of the liver. CT scan guided FNAC of the mass done.

Diagnosis: Hepatoblastoma

Microscopy

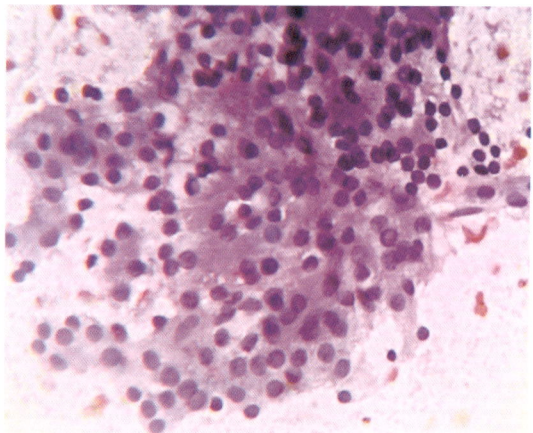

Fig. 22A.21

Highly cellular smear with clusters, acinar pattern and rosettes of round cells. The cells are small with high N C ratio, scant to moderate cytoplasm, round to oval nuclei with condensed chromatin. The cells resembling foetal hepatocytes. It is one of the most common primary hepatic malignancy in children. Usually occurs less than 5 years of age. Third common after NB and WT. Elevated serum AFP levels are seen in few cases. Presence of extrahepatic tumour, multifocal location, vascular invasion and distant metastasis indicate poor prognosis.

Differential Diagnosis

- Foetal type hepatoblastoma vs hepatocellular carcinoma.
- Embryonal type hepatoblastoma vs pediatric small round blue cell tumours.

Case Number 22: USG Guided FNAC Testicular Mass

History: A 34-year-old individual presented with a swelling on testis with gradual increase in size. No pain/tenderness. Oval mass firm in consistency. USG—mass confined to right testis. No significant abdominal lymphadenopathy. USG guided FNAC done.

Diagnosis: Mixed germ cell tumour of testis consistent with teratocarcinoma

Microscopy

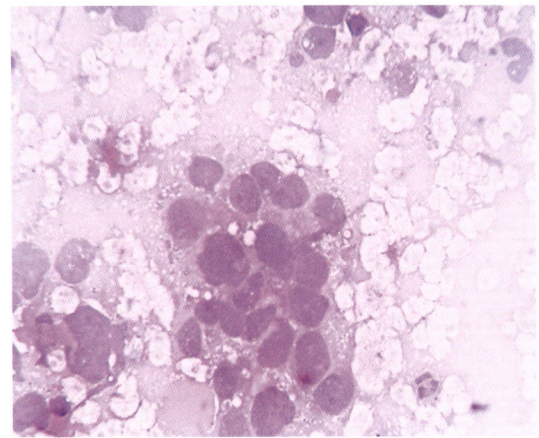

Fig. 22A.22

Cellular smear with acinar and glandular pattern of cells. The cells are large with vesicular nuclei and prominent nucleoli. Cell borders are indistinct. Few cells with vacuolated cytoplasm. Ocassional syncytiotrophoblastic giant cell. Background rich in hemorrhage and necrosis.

Case Number 23: Aspiration from Pouch of Douglas

History: A 64-year-old female presented with pain in abdomen. On examination she was diagnosed to have a right adnexal mass with fullness of the pouch of Douglas.

Aspiration of POD was done.

Diagnosis: Smear positive for malignancy consistent with papillary cystadenocarcinoma ovary

Microscopy

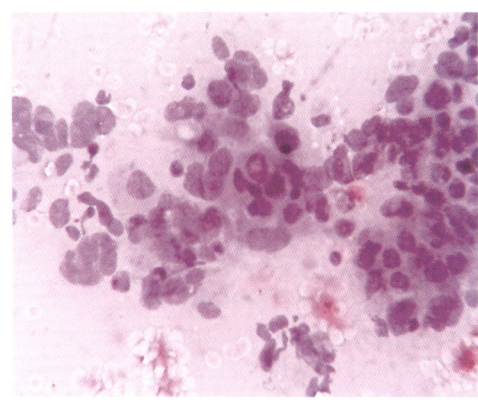

Fig. 22A.23

Smear studied shows round to oval cells arranged in papillary pattern with variable eosinophilic cytoplasm and nuclei with moderate anisokaryosis. Ocassional psammoma body like structures are seen. Few degenerated cells and few cyst macrophages are seen in the background.

Case Number 24: CT Guided FNAC of Mass Pancreas

History: A 54-year-old male patient presented with vague pain in the abdomen. CT scan revealed a mass like lesion in the junction of the body and tail of pancreas. CT guided FNAC of the mass was done.

Diagnosis: Suggestive of maliganncy—pancreatic endocrine tumour

Microscopy

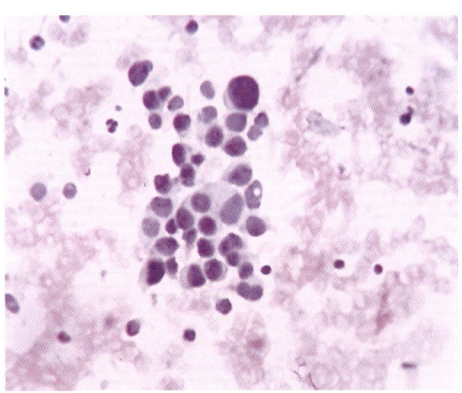

Fig. 22A.24

Smear studied shows clusters of large cells with large nuclei with stippled chromatin pattern and focal palisading of the nuclei with few fragmented cells in a hemorrhagic background.

Criteria for Diagnosis

1. Solid sheets of cells
2. Predominantly single cells with stripped nuclei
3. Rosette like structures
4. Plasmacytoid population of cells
5. Round nuclei with finely stippled chromatin
6. Ocassional binucleation
7. Scant to moderate delicate cytoplasm

Differential Diagnosis

- Acinar cell carcinoma
- Benign acinar cell clusters
- Solid pseudopapillary tumour
- Metastatic renal cell carcinoma

Case Number 25: USG Guided FNAC Nodule Duodenum

History: A 46-year-old male patient presented with vague pain in the abdomen. Ultrasound shows a diffuse thickening of the duodenal wall with apparent nodularity. FNAC of the nodule was done under USG guidance.

Diagnosis: Neuroendocrine tumour duodenum

Microscopy

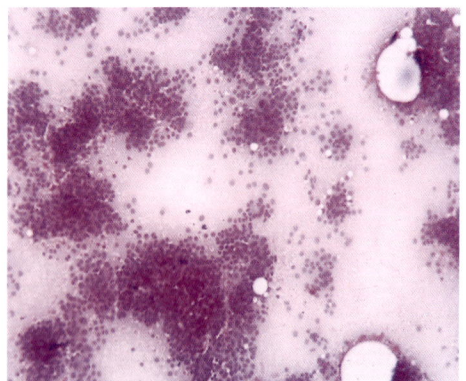

Fig. 22A.25a

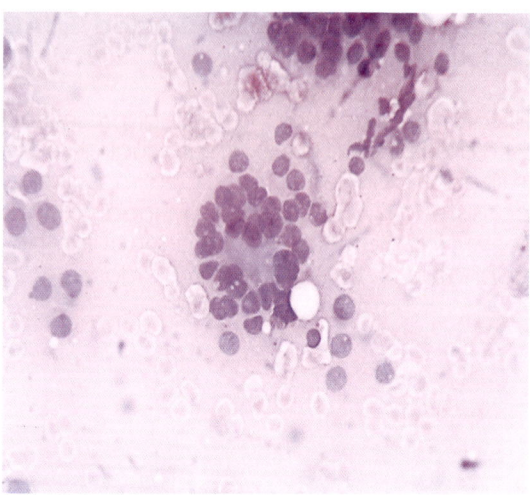

Fig. 22A.25b

Smear studied shows cohesive clusters and nests of round cells with scant rim of cytoplasm and round nuclei with stippled chromatin with few areas showing nuclear palisading within a hemorrhagic background.

WHO Classification of Neuroendocrine Tumours

- Well differentiated neuroendocrine tumour
- Well differentiated neuroendocrine carcinoma (Small/large)
  - Presence of metastases
  - Infiltration into the muscularis propria or angioinvasion
- Poorly differentiated neuroendocrine carcinoma
- Mixed adeno neuroendocrine carcinoma (MANEC)

Case Number 26: FNAC Lesion Rib

History: A 55-year-old female presented with a nodular swelling over the chest wall. Investigations shows an expansile lesion of the fourth rib on the right side. FNAC of the lesion was done.

Diagnosis: Suggestive of plasmacytoma rib

Microscopy

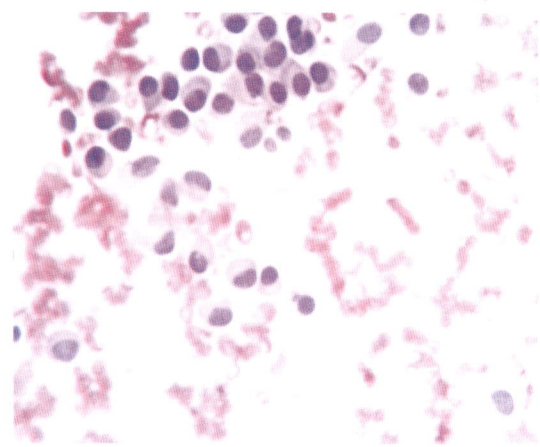

Fig. 22A.26

Smear studied shows many scattered plasma cells with abundant cytoplasm and eccentrically placed nuclei with many binucleate plasma cells in a hemorrhagic background.

Case Number 27: USG Guided FNAC Mass Kidney

History: A 65-year-old male presented with frequent abdominal pain. Ultrasound revealed a nodular mass 2 × 2cm in the right kidney. The mass was aspirated under ultrasound guidance.

Diagnosis: Oncocytoma kidney

Microscopy

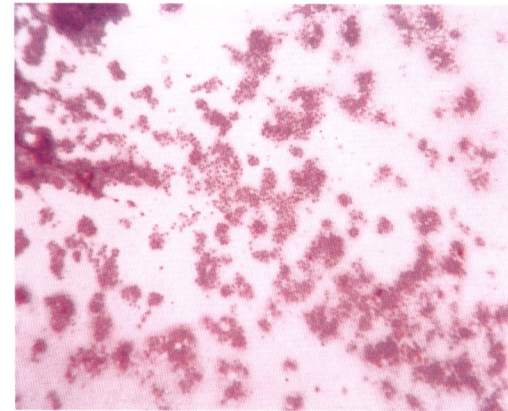

Fig. 22A.27a

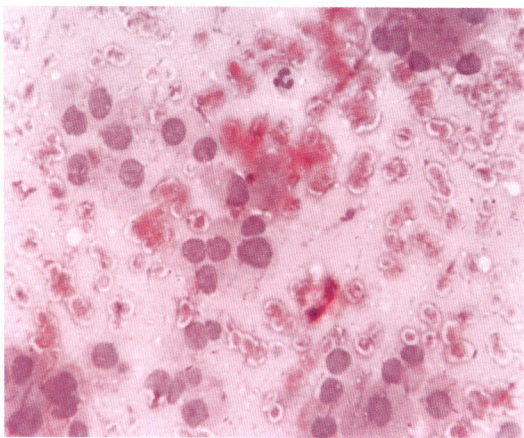

Fig. 22A.27b

Smear studied shows loose clusters of round to polygonal cells with abundant eosinophilic granular cytoplasm and clear cell borders. The nuclei was round to oval in a hemorrhagic background.

Criteria for Diagnosis

1. Numerous large single cells
2. Pale basophilic granular cytoplasm
3. Round regular nuclei
4. Binucleation/multinucleation
5. Prominent nucleoli
6. Minimal nuclear atypia

Differential Diagnosis

The common differentials include
- Clear cell renal cell carcinoma
- Chromophobe renal cell carcinoma.

Case Number 28: FNAC Soft Tissue Mass—Thigh

History: A 56-year-old male presented with a mass in the upper thigh. There was a recent increase in the size of the mass. Skin over the mass appears normal. FNAC of the mass was done.

Diagnosis: Suggestive of spindle cell sarcoma consistent with fibrosarcoma.

Microscopy

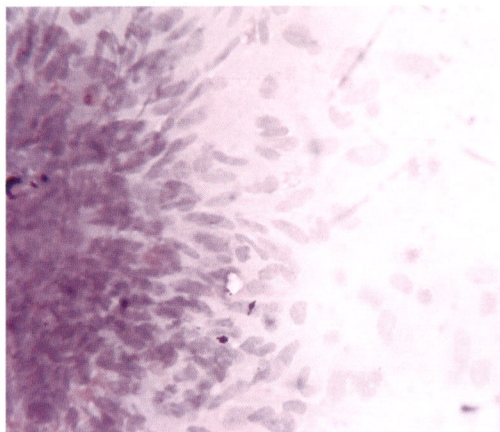

Fig. 22A.28a

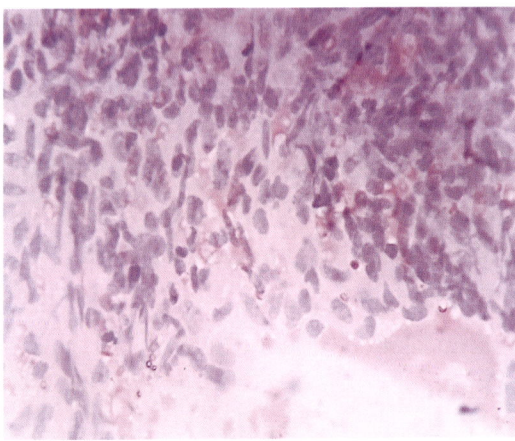

Fig. 22A.28b

Smear studied shows clusters of spindle cells with variable cytoplasm and elongated nuclei with mild to moderate anisokaryosis with coarse chromatin and degenerated cell debris in the background.

Generally Grouped into
- Spindle cell sarcoma
- Round cell sarcoma
- Myxoid sarcoma
- Pleomorphic sarcoma

Cytological features of common spindle cell sarcomas:

Fibrosarcoma
- Young adults
- Highly cellular
- Spindle cells
- Pale vesicular cytoplasm

Leiomyosarcoma
- Oval nuclei
- Adults
- Moderate/poor cellularity
- Spindle cells
- Abundnat acidophilic/cyanophilic cytoplasm
- Perinuclear vacuoles
- Cigar nuclei, pleomorphism +/−

Synovial Sarcoma
- Extremities
- Short spindle cells
- Uniform vesicular nuclei
- Micronucleoli
- Epithelial cells +

Malignant Peripheral Nerve Sheath Tumour
- Adults
- Cellular
- Spindle cells
- Fibrillary cytoplasm
- Wavy nuclei, pleomorphism ++

Case Number 29: FNAC Soft Tissue Mass Gluteal Region

History: A 55-year-old male patient presented with a swelling in the gluteal region for the past 6 months. The mass was 3.5 × 3cm, firm to hard in consistency with restricted mobility. The skin over the swelling was normal. A provisional diagnosis of a calcified epidermoid cyst was made. FNAC of the swelling was done.

Diagnosis: Calcinosis cutis

Microscopy

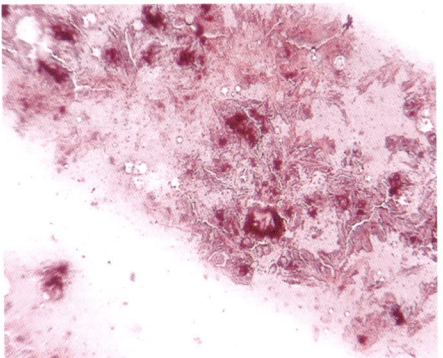

Fig. 22.29

Smear studied shows many scattered basophilic granular calcific material with few scattered lymphocytes and occasional plasma cells in the background.

Case Number 30: CT Guided FNAC of Lumbosacral Lesion

History: A 59-year-old male patient presented with complaints of low back ache for the past 3 months. He had taken native treatment for the pain. He reported to the ortho OPD for the complaints. Patient localised the pain to the L5 S1 region. No obvious swelling noted. X-ray of the lumbosacral spine showed an irregular lytic lesion of L5 and S1 with soft tissue shadow. CT scan also showed a destructive lesion of the vertebra with adjoining soft tissue lesion. CT guided FNAC of the mass done.

Diagnosis: Chordoma

Microscopy

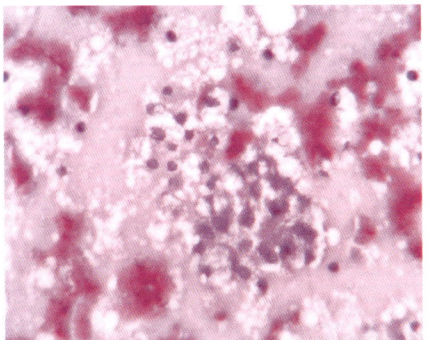

Fig. 22A.30

Highly cellular smear with many scattered large cells with vacuolated cytoplasm and round to oval nuclei with mild ansionucleosis with few oval to spindle cells in a hemorrhagic background.

Differential Diagnosis

- Chondrosarcoma
- Chordoid chondrosarcoma
- Metastatic clear cell carcinoma
- Myxofibrosarcoma

Case Number 31: Squash Cytology of Buccal Ulcer

History: A 68-year-old male patient presented with an ulceroproliferative lesion of the buccal mucosa. The lesion was ulcerated with exudates and indurated base. Scrape cytology of the lesion was done.

Diagnosis: Smear positive for malignancy – squamous cell carcinoma

Microscopy

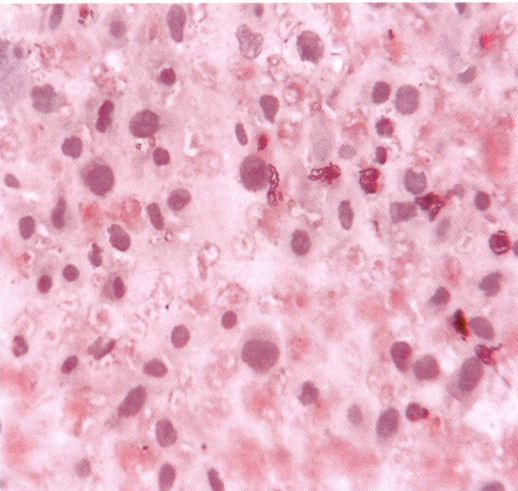

Fig. 22A.31

Smear studied shows clusters of round to polygonal cells with dense eosinophilic cytoplasm and large irregular nuclei with chromatin clumping with anucleate squames, acute and chronic inflammatory cells, degenerated cell debris in the background.

Cytological Criteria

1. Nuclear crowding
2. Nuclear hyperchromasia
3. Increased N/C ratio
4. Dyskeratotic cells
5. Tadpole/strap cells

Case Number 32: CT Guided FNAC Paraspinal Lesion

History: A 15-year-old boy presented with pain and swelling of the back for one month. He had low grade fever on and off. CT scan showed collapse of the D10 vertebra with paraspinal lesion. CT scan guided aspiration of the paraspinal region was done.

Diagnosis: Caseating granulomatous inflammatory pathology consistent with pott's spine

Microscopy

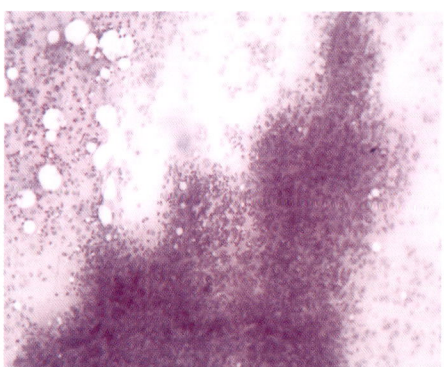

Fig. 22A.32a

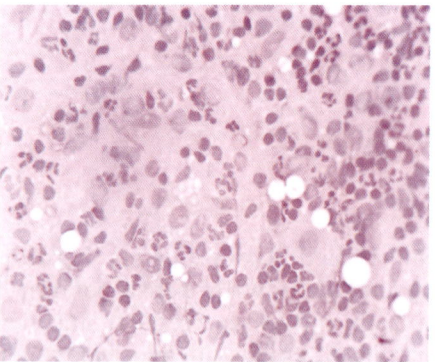

Fig. 22A.32b

Smear studied shows loose cohesive clusters of epithelioid cells with indistinct cytoplasm and oval nuclei with many reactive lymphocytes within a necrotic background.

Case Number 33: CT Scan Guided FNAC Nodule Liver

History: A 48-year-old male patient was referred to the medical gastroentrology for pain abdomen in the right hypochondrium. The patient was anaemic, not jaundiced. No ascitis was seen. Spleen was palpable. Ultrasound showed nodular mass lesion of the liver with provisional diagnosis of Regenerative nodule. FNAC of the nodule done.

Diagnosis: Extramedullary hematopoiesis liver

Microscopy

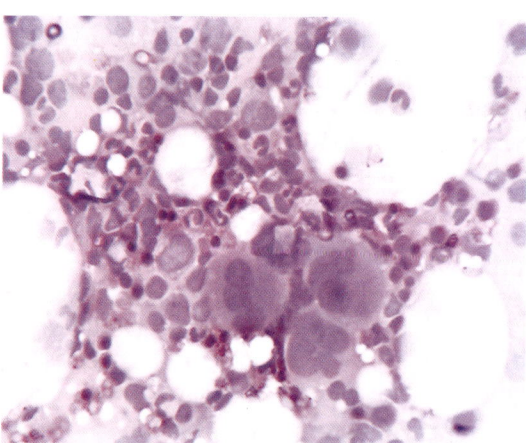

Fig. 22A.33

Smear studied shows scattered hematopoietic cells with many normoblasts, promyelocytes and prominent megakarycytes in a hemorrhagic background.

Case History: A 64-year-old male patient presented with breathlessness for 2 weeks. History of cough with expectoration, three episodes of hemoptysis and vague chest pain. Investigations revealed an irregular hilar mass 5.5 × 4.5 cm in the right lung with massive pleural effusion. Pleural fluid tapping done and smears for analysis.

Diagnosis: Smear positive for malignancy consistent with small cell carcinoma lung

Microscopy

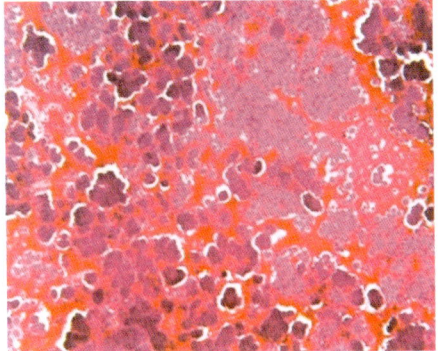

Fig. 22A.34

Smear studied shows sheets and clusters of small cells with scant rim of cytoplasm and round nuclei with coarse condense chromatin with many degenerated smudged cells and many nuclear fragments with occasional mesothelial cells seen.

Case History: A 60-year-old female presented with a lump in the left breast. There was a gradual increase in size. The mass was of variable consistency. Mobile. Nipple, skin over the mass normal. Opposite breast normal. No lymph nodes palpable. FNAC of the lump breast was done.

Diagnosis: Colloid carcinoma breast

Microscopy

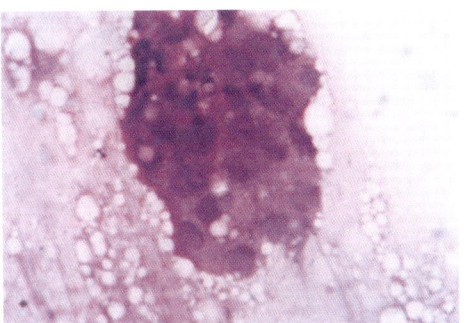

Fig. 22A.35

Smear studied shows small clumps of cells floating in pools of mucin in the background. The cells shows mild to moderate nuclear atypia with abundant cytoplasm and presence of intracytoplasmic mucin.

Case History: A 49-year-old male person case of pain in abdomen for one month. No specific location. CT scan—nodular lesion of the right adrenal gland. Incidental finding. CT scan guided FNAC of the adrenal lesion was done.

Diagnosis: Myelolipoma

Microscopy

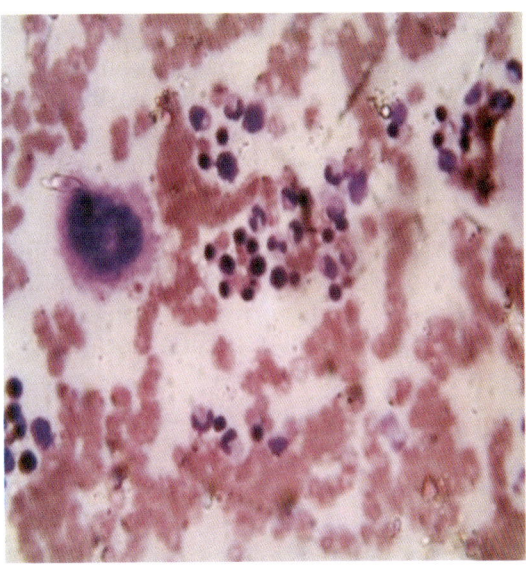

Fig. 22A.36

Smear studied shows bone marrow with hemopoietic cells comprising erythroblasts, myeloid cells and prominent megakaryocytes with fatty are as in the background.

Case History: A 60-year-old male presented with a nodular lesion in the left parotid with gradual increase in size. No pain and tenderness. On examination, the nodule 2 × 2 cm in the left parotid, mobile and cystic. No involvement of the facial nerve.

Diagnosis: Warthin's tumor—parotid

Microscopy

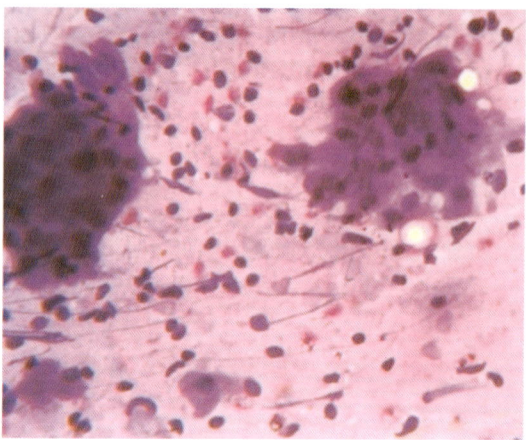

Fig. 22A.37

Smear studied shows cohesive clusters of round to polygonal cells with eosinophilic granular cytoplasm, uniform nuclei. Degenerated cell debris, many lymphocytes and mucin are seen in the background.

CaseHistory: A 24-year-old female presented with a nodular swelling in the forearm.The nodule was 1.5 x 1 cm, mobile. Skin over the swelling normal. FNAC of the nodule was done.

Diagnosis: Benign adnexal tumor of skin consistent with chondroid syringoma

Microscopy

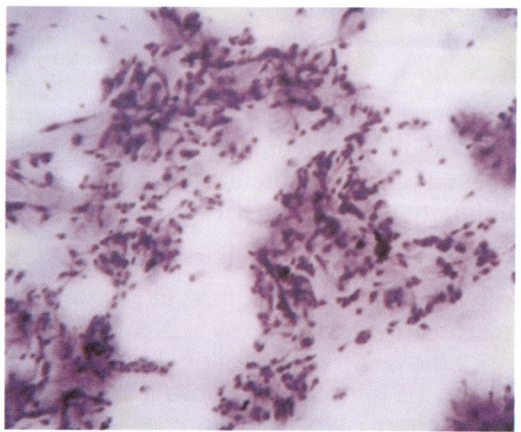

Fig. 22A.38

Smear studied shows clusters of round to oval cells with pale cytoplasm with oval to elongated nuclei with fine granular chromatin in a background with myxoid areas.

Case History: A 65-year-old female presented with a recent onset swelling of left parotid. She had underwent renal transplant surgery an year back. O/E the nodular mass was 3x3cm, soft and fluctuant. FNAC was done. 1.5 cc of pus-likematerial was aspirated.

Diagnosis: Organizing abscess parotid with non-tyrosine crystalloids

Microscopy

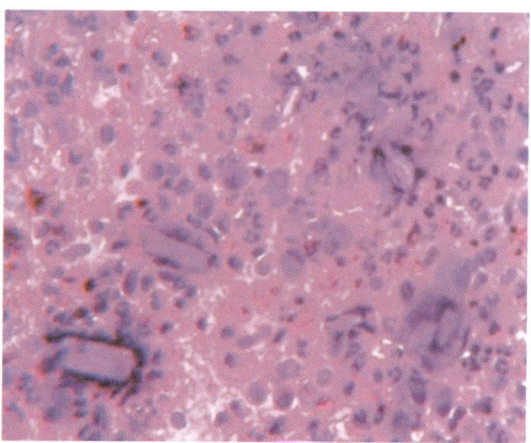

Fig. 22A.39

Smear studied shows many neutrophils, degranulated cells, cell debris, cyst macrophages and many scattered crystalloid substances in the background.

Case History: A15-year-old boy presented with pain and swelling of the back for one month. He had low grade fever on and off. CT scan showed collapse of the D10 vertebra with paraspinal lesion.CT scan guided aspiration of the paraspina lregion was done.

Diagnosis: Caseating granulomatous inflammatory pathology consistent with Pott's spine

Microscopy

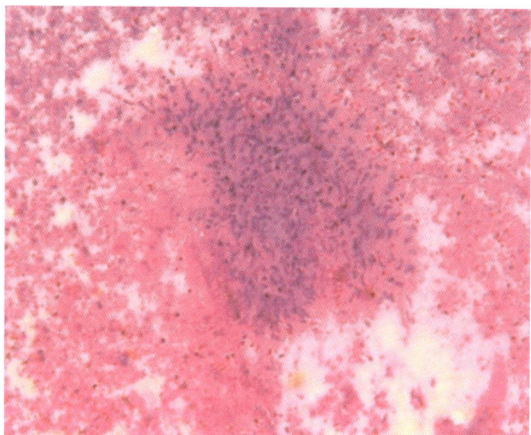

Fig. 22A.40

Smear studied shows loose cohesive clusters of epithelioid cells with indistinct cytoplasm and oval nuclei with many reactive lymphocytes within a necrotic background.

CHAPTER 22B

Cytology Slide Case Discussion Part II

N Siddaraju

Case History: Fine needle aspirate of liver in a 67-year-old male (1 Pap).

Diagnosis: Malignant endothelial neoplasm

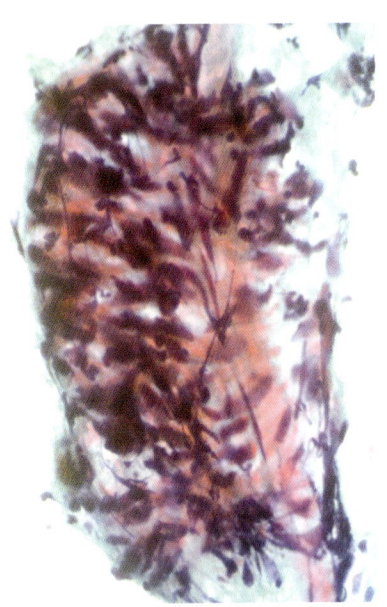

22B.1

Cytologic Picture
- Aspirate-frankly hemorrhagic.
- Rare fragments of atypical spindle cells lining the basement membrane-like material.
- Occasional spindle cell fascicles exhibiting nuclear palisading and wavy nuclei giving an impression of neurogenic tumor.
- ICC—strong CD31 expression of neoplastic cells and S-100 negativity.

Points Worth Remembering
- Hemangioma is the commonest vascular tumor of liver.
- Hemangioendothelioma and angiosarcoma are less common.
- Hemangioendothelioma and angiosarcoma are not always distinguishable on cytology due to overlapping cytomorphology.
- Necrosis and increased mitotic activity (indicative of angiosarcoma) are not always reflected in the cytologic material.
- Neoplastic endothelial tumors may have 'spindle cell' or 'epithelioid' morphology.

Morphologic 'Clues' of Malignant Endothelial Neoplasms

These include:
- Obvious hemorrhagic aspirate with variable cellularity (despite the ideal FNA technique).
- Acinar/rosettoid structures and cells and cell clusters seen in association with three dimensional elongated endothelium-lined vascular structures.
- Signet-ring like cells reminiscent of intra-cytoplasmic lumina and occasional such

lumen containing a single erythrocyte, suggestive of endothelial differentiation.
- Erythrophagocytosis and vacuolated cytoplasm.

Other Features Described in Literature
- Round to ovoid cells scattered throughout the smear, loose clusters and sheets of cells with moderate to abundant dense cyanophilic cytoplasm.
- Embracing cells or cell in cell pattern
- Tumor cells varying in size from 2–7 times the size of an RBC.
- Nuclear features described are coarse chromatin, rare intranuclear inclusions, prominent nuclear grooves and nuclear indentations causing an angulated or multilobated appearance.
- A few cells with dense cytoplasm having concentric lamination, and a few binucleated, multinucleated, spindle and bizarre cells, and scarce mitotic figures.

Case History: A 2-year-old boy baby presented with an abdominal mass (1 MGG).

Diagnosis: Wilms' tumor (WT) with predominant blastemal component

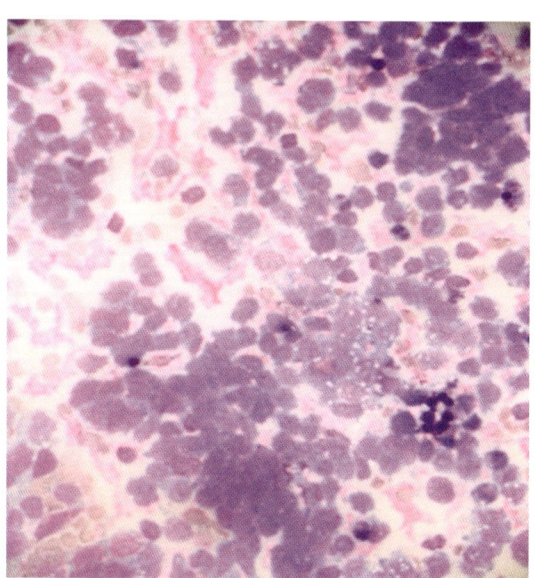

Fig. 22B.2a

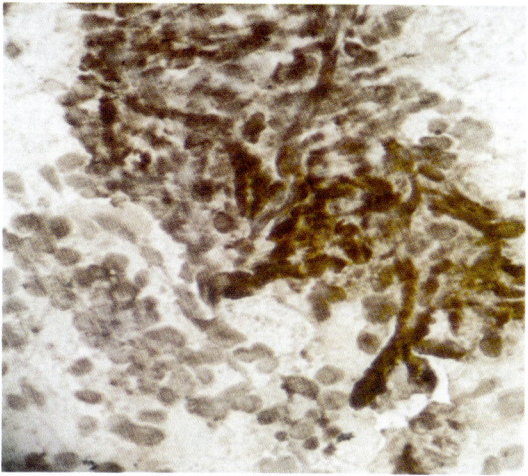

Fig. 22B.2b: Vimentin

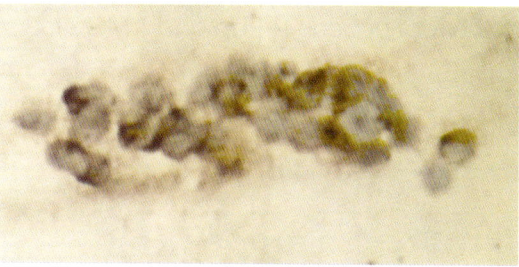

Fig. 22B.2c: Pan CK

Cytologic Picture of the Given Case
- High cellularity.
- Dominated by small, undifferentiated blastemal cells having a high nuclear cytoplasmic ratio and evenly dispersed coarse chromatin.
- Focally, blastemal cells are tightly packed.
- Abundant magenta granular matrix material. No obvious epithelial or mesenchymal cellular elements.

Points to be Remembered
- Blastemal cells in presence of recognizable epithelial and mesenchymal components (triphasic pattern) allow an easy diagnosis of WT.
- Microarchitectural patterns such as rosettes, tubules or cords in smears represent epithelial differentiation.

- Epithelial cells are larger with more cytoplasm and cellular cohesion than blastemal cells.
- Stromal cells are identified by their spindled nature and loose arrangement within a collagenous or myxoid matrix.
- Rarely, smooth muscle and skeletal muscle differentiation may be noted.
- Clinico-radiologic features should always be considered, when evaluating smears from a Wilms' tumor. The differential diagnoses include other small blue round cell tumors such as neuroblastoma, PNET/Ewing. Clear cell sarcoma of kidney.

Case History: An 88-year-old male with a hisotry of swelling in the left inguinal region and at the root of penis. FNA from the swelling at the root of penis (1 Pap and 1 MGG).

Diagnosis: Undifferentiated malignant tumor with an epithelioid morphology (immunohistochemically proven synovial sarcoma—poorly differentiated)

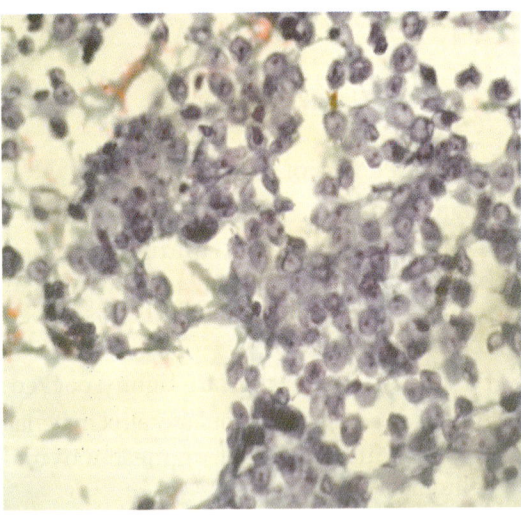

Fig. 22B.3

Cytologic Picture

Inguinal aspirate: Non-diagnostic
Aspirate from swelling at the root of penis:
- High cellularity.
- Monomorphic, undifferentiated malignant cells having plasmacytoid to polygonal morphology.
- Cells arranged in solid sheets, vague glandular and pseudo-alveolar pattern.
- Vesicular nuclei, prominent nucleoli.
- Increased mitotic activity.
- Distinct cell borders in MGG smears and wispy cytoplasmic borders in Pap-stained smears.
- No hemorrhagic or necrotic background.

Cytologic Differential Diagnosis

i. Clear cell sarcoma
ii. Epithelioid sarcoma
iii. Metastatic poorly differentiated carcinoma
iv. Metastatic melanoma
v. Epithelioid variant of malignant peripheral nerve sheath tumor
vi. Epithelioid angiosarcoma
vii. Epithelioid synovial sarcoma
viii. Non-Hodgkin lymphoma.

Subsequent Biopsy Findings

- Relatively vascular, solid tumor with focal areas of hemorrhage and necrosis.
- Fairly monomorphic tumor cells, with only a focal and mild pleomorphism.
- Striking increase in mitotic activity.
- Absence of distinct nodular pattern.

Differential Diagnosis

Similar to cytologic DD.
- *Proximal type of epithelioid sarcoma:* Excluded by the absence of distinct nodular pattern with central area of necrosis within the nodules a (nodular pattern with central area of necrosis is highly characteristic of epithelioid sarcoma). Moreover, it also lacked so-called 'rhabdoid features' described in the proximal type of epithelioid sarcoma. Tumor cells—positive for pan CK, CK-8, CK-5/6, EMA, vimentin, CD99 and S-100, while negative for desmin.
- *Synovial sarcoma:* Positivity for pan CK, CK-8, CK-5/6, EMA, vimentin, CD99 established the diagnosis.
- *Clear cell sarcoma:* Excluded by S-100 positivity but melan-A and HMB-45 negativity.

- *Metastatic melanoma:* Excluded by S-100 positivity but melan-A and HMB-45 negativity.
- *Poorly differentiated prostatic adenocarcinoma:* Excluded by PSA negativity.
- *Malignant endothelial neoplasm:* Excluded by CD31 and CD34 negativity.
- *Epithelioid MPNST:* Though S-100 positive, it is excluded by positive expression of pan CK, CK-8, CK-5/6, EMA, vimentin and CD99.

Final Diagnosis

Poorly differentiated synovial sarcoma.

Message from the Case

Pathologists should be aware of the sarcomas exhibiting an exclusive epithelioid morphology and their clinicopathologic/immunohistochemical differences.

Case History: A 3-year-old male presented with a history of recurrent scalp swelling (1 Pap and 1 MG).

Diagnosis: Langerhans cell histiocytosis (LCH)

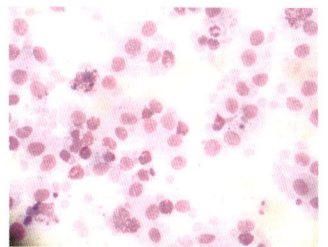
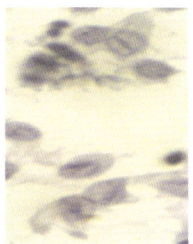

Fig. 22B.4a Fig. 22B.4b

Cytologic Picture

- Cellular with sheets of cells.
- Increased histiocytes showing delicate chromatin, inconspicuous nucleoli and indented/grooved (coffee bean) nuclei.
- Large numbers of eosinophils admixed with other inflammatory cells.
- A few mitotic figures and giant cells.

Points to Remember

- Immunocytochemically, LCH cells express CD1a antigen, fascin (both expressed only in LCH and not in normal histiocytes) and S-100 protein.
- Ultrastructurally, they display characteristic Birbeck's granules.
- Due to mixed inflammatory component, cytologically, it is likely to mimic an inflammatory lesion.
- Careful attention to nuclear morphology and ICC using CD1a resolves the diagnostic dilemma.

Case History: A 55-year-old male with a mass lesion in the left lobe of liver (1 Pap)

Diagnosis: Hepatocellular carcinoma (HCC)

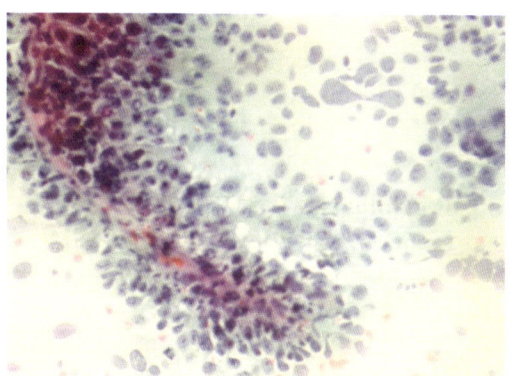

Fig. 22B.5a

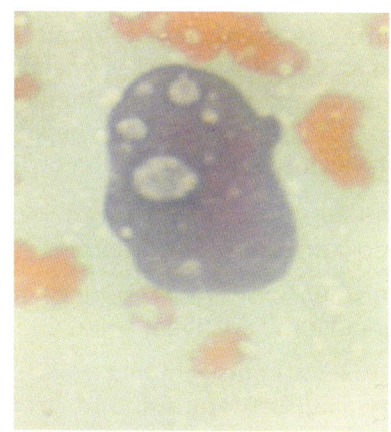

Fig. 22B.5b

Cytologic Picture

- Clusters of neoplastic hepatocytes forming trabeculae, acini or sheets.
- Hepatocytic clusters rimmed by endothelial cells.
- Blood vessels traversing hepatocytic clusters.
- Polygonal cells with abundant cytoplasm, central nuclei and prominent nucleoli.
- Many, large, stripped naked nuclei
- Intranuclear inclusions.
- Intracytoplasmic hyaline inclusions (not seen in the present case).
- Intracytoplasmic bile pigment.
- Absence of bile duct epithelium.
- However, features vary from case to case. FNAC plays a vital role in the diagnosis of malignancies involving the liver such as primary hepatocellular carcinoma (HCC), metastatic malignancies, in particular, metastatic carcinomas and cholangiocarcinomas.

Role of cytology and ICC in HCC

- Although, there are well established cytomorphologic criteria for diagnosing HCC, cytopathologists land up with frequent dilemma, particularly in distinguishing HCC from metastatic adenocarcinomas.
- Hep Par-1, glypican 3, arginase 1 are useful markers for diagnosing HCC and distinguishing it from metastatic adenocarcinomas. CK-19 is a marker of cholangiocarcinoma and useful in distinguishing it from HCC. Also, neoplastic hepatocytes display cytoplasmic expression of TTF-1.

Case History: Sputum sample from a 50-year-old female patient (1 Pap), and

Case History: Bronchial washings from a 55-year-old female patient (1 MGG).

Diagnosis: Adenocarcinoma cells in respiratory samples (sputum and bronchial washings)

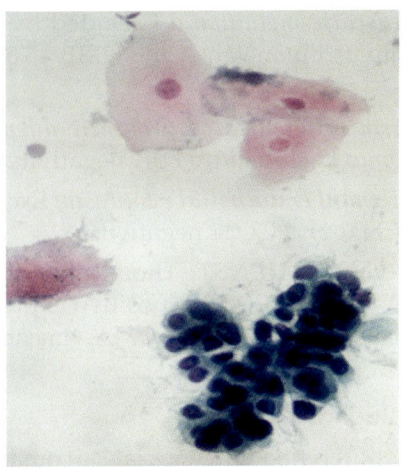

Fig. 22B.6a: Sputum

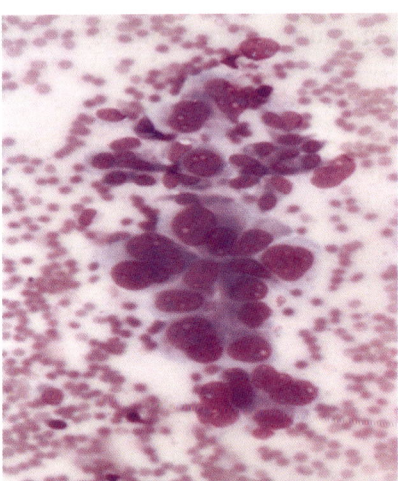

Fig. 22B.6b: Bronchial wash

General Cytologic Picture

- Most adenocarcinomas of acinar type show a mixture of cell clusters, tissue fragments and single cells.
- Tissue fragments show cells arranged in syncytial groupings, acini, tubules and papillary clusters.
- Nuclei are round to ovoid or lobulated with vesicular chromatin, prominent centrally located macronucleoli.

- Cytoplasm is granular to finely vacuolated or distended with large vacuoles.
- Mucinous type of bronchoalveolar carcinoma (BAC) shows ball-like clusters and papillary fronds. The cells may or may not display secretory vacuoles and the nuclei exhibit finely granular chromatin and inconspicuous nucleoli. The cytoplasmic microvilli may simulate cilia.
- Mucinous type of BAC shows more abundant cytoplasm.
- A minor proportion of BAC is poorly differentiated with marked nuclear atypia.
- The cases provided (sputum smear and bronchial brushings) are frankly positive for adenocarcinoma cells, exhibiting predominantly an acinar pattern.
- Sputum smear in addition to presence of adenocarcinoma cells, revealed numerous yeast and pseudohyphal forms of Candia species.

Case History: Synovial fluid sample for interpretation (1 MGG).

Diagnosis: Synovial effusion in gouty arthritis

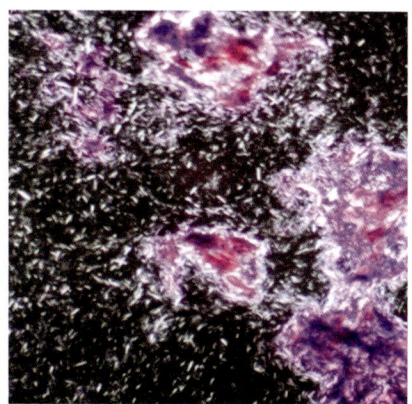

Fig. 22B.7b

Gross Nature of Synovial Fluid (Present Case)

Curdy white appearance (referred as 'urate milk').

Cytologic Picture

- Individual as well as clumps and bundles of slender or hair-like, needle shaped crystals.
- Seen in association with clumped fibrin, white cells and cell debris.
- Crystal size ranged from <1 to 20 μm
- Spherical aggregates of MSU crystals—referred to as 'beach balls' formation.
- In plain light-slender or hair-like
- In compensated polarized light—strongly negatively birefringent.

Points to Remember

- MSU crystals of gout should be differentiated from calcium pyrophosphate dehydrate crystals (CPPD) of pseudogout.
- CPPD crystals exhibit varied shapes (rhomboid, rod-like, ovoid or cuboid).
- CPPD crystals are weakly positively birefringent.
- Simplest method of identifying MSU crystals in synovial fluid—wet mount film examination.
- MSU crystals are identifiable in Pap-stained smears as well.

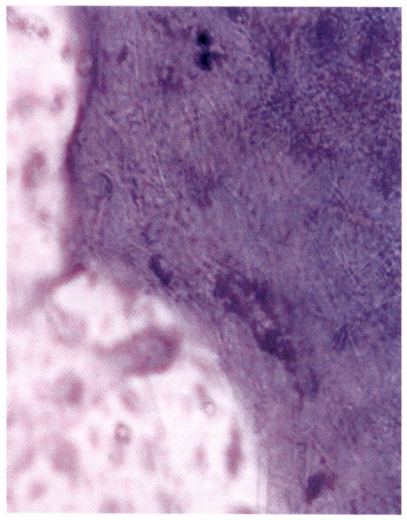

Fig. 22B.7a

- Accurate characterization of MSU crystals requires polarizing microscopy.
- Accuracy of polarizing microscopy depends on concentration of urate crystals in synovial fluid.
- A low concentration and smaller size of crystals may result in a false negative report.
- In cases with negative result on light microscopy—electron microscopy (EM) can be useful.
- Threshold level of crystals for reliable identification on light microscopy: 10–100 mg/ml.

Case History: Urine cytology for interpretation (1 MGG).

Diagnosis: Low grade papillary urothelial carcinoma (in voided urine)

- Very useful in follow-up of patients with known and treated cases of urothelial malignancy.
- High grade urothelial tumors are readily diagnosable, while low grade papillary urothelial neoplasms are not always easy to diagnose.
- Other sensitive (but not specific) techniques used for detection of urothelial malignancy in urine.
  i. Assessment of telomerase activity
  ii. Fluorescence *in situ* hybridization (FISH)
  iii. Flow cytometry (FCM)

It is essential to know if sample sent is voided or catheterized urine; because, unlike voided urine which contains the exfoliated cells, the catheterized sample is likely to contain mechanically disrupted papillary-like clusters (which are) normal) derived from urothelial mucosa. Such clusters in voided urine suggest possibility of a low grade papillary urothelial neoplasm (even in the absence of nuclear atypia), while the similar clusters in catheterized sample does not convey the same.

Case History: Pleural fluid from a 60-year-old male patient with suspected malignant effusion (1 MGG).

Diagnosis: Tuberculous pleural effusion with caseous necrotic material in pleural fluid

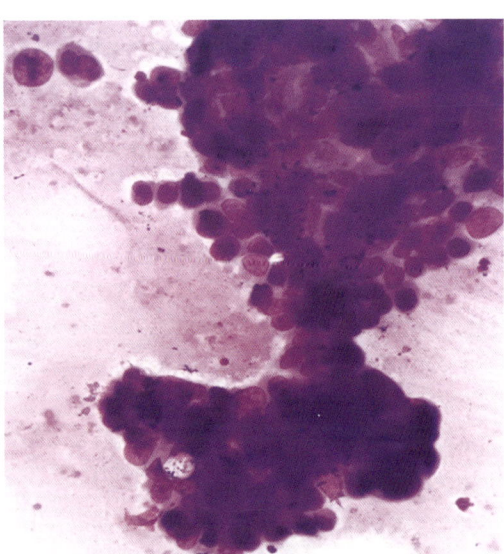

Fig. 22B.8

Cytologic Picture

A few papillary clusters of mild to moderately atypical urothelial cells.

Points to Remember

- Urine cytology is the first-line investigation for detection of clinically occult and *in situ* urothelial tumors.

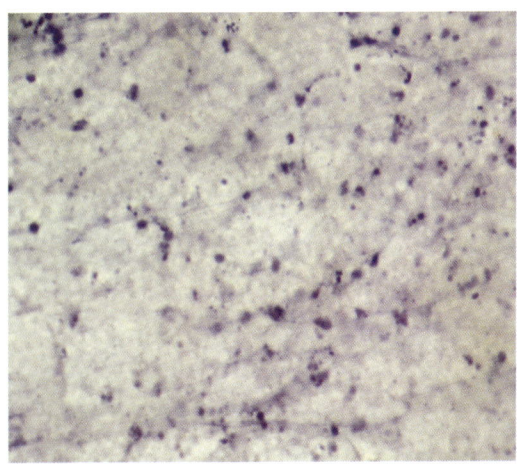

Fig. 22B.9

Cytologic Picture

Gross appearance: Turbid

Microscopic Picture

Caseous material (AFS positive).

Other Possible Cytologic Findings in Tuberculous Effusions

Marked increase in lymphocytes (80–100%) with very few or no mesothelial cells.

1. Tuberculous effusions of short duration may contain some neutrophils and mesothelial cells.
2. Paucity or absence of mesothelial cells in tuberculous pleural effusion is said to be due to deposition of fibrin on the pleural surface that either seals off or destroys the mesothelial cells.
3. Multinucleated giant macrophages, epithelioid cells and frank caseous necrotic material are a rare finding.

Case History: A 60-year-old male presented with intestinal obstruction and abdominal distension for 1 week duration (to emphasize role of ICC).

Diagnosis: Adenocarcinoma cells with varied cytomorphology in serous body fluids

Useful Points to Remember in Malignant Effusions

1. Positive malignant cytology of serous body fluids upstages the disease.
2. Serous body cavities can be involved virtually by any of the primary tumors.
3. The most common cause of malignant effusion in females—breast and ovarian carcinomas.
4. The most common cause of malignant effusion in men—bronchogenic and gastrointestinal adenocarcinomas.
5. Ancillary techniques used to distinguish mesothelial vs adenocarcinoma cells.
6. Use of proliferative markers argyrophilic nucleolar organizer region (Ag NOR) studies.
7. Ploidy analysis by DNA flow cytometry (FCM)
8. Cytogenetics
9. Telomerase assay
10. Electron microscopy (EM)
11. Immunocytochemistry (ICC)

Malignant Cells in Effusion

- *Large-sized malignant cells:* Common in squamous cell carcinoma (SCC), melanoma and some cases of adenocarcinomas.
- *Medium-sized malignant cells:* Common in gastric, pulmonary and pancreatic adenocarcinomas.
- *Small-sized malignant cells:* Common in small cell carcinoma of lung, Wilms' tumor and neuroblastoma.

General Features of Malignant Cells

- Pleomorphism with bizarre forms
- High nuclear to cytoplasmic (N : C) ratio
- Hyperchromasia
- Single or multiple, irregular, macronucleoli
- Abnormal mitoses.

Features of Adenocarcinoma

- Smoothly contoured cohesive clusters
- Eccentrically placed abnormal nuclei
- Vacuolated cytoplasm
- Papillary and glandular pattern or morula-like cell balls
- Cannibalism (a tumor cell phagocytozed by another tumor cell)
- Multiple Barr bodies.

Useful Morphologic Clues of Mesothelial Cells

- Small monolayers with narrow windows
- Clusters with knobby contour
- Dual cytoplasmic zones in individual cells (peripheral paler and central denser cytoplasm)
- Lacy skirt cell borders.

Useful Morphologic Clues of Adenocarcinoma Cells

- 3-D clusters with smooth contour
- Crowded nuclei within clusters
- Irregular nuclear/nucleolar membranes
- Absent windows, or presence of broader windows reminiscent of mucin vacuole
- Individual cells lacking pale ectocytoplasmic and denser endocytoplasmic zones.

Role of Cyto-/Histochemical Stains

- PAS with/without diastase is useful for demonstration of neutral mucin (sensitivity—37 to 62%)
- Pattern of PAS positivity—diffuse cytoplasmic in adenocarcinoma cells; while granular with peripheral localization in mesothelial cells.
- Mucicarmine—24 to 41% sensitive.
- Alcian blue with and without hyaluronidase—useful for differentiating adenocarcinoma *vs* mesothelioma.

Role of Immunocyto-/Histochemistry

1. *Useful epithelial markers:* Carcinoembryonic antigen (CEA), epithelial membrane antigen (EMA), E-cadherin (EC), B-72.3, Ber-Ep4, Leu-M1 and MOC-31.
2. *Useful mesothelial markers:* Calretinin, thrombomodulin, vimentin, desmin, fibronectin, CK-5/6, WT-1 and HBME-1.

Possible Clues for Identification of Primary Site in Malignant Effusions

- Proliferation spheres or morula-like clusters in pleural fluid-invasive ductal carcinoma.
- Discrete small, malignant cells with a high N : C ratio, nuclear irregularity, presence of Bull's eye inclusions (cell with tiny eosinophilic globule within the cytoplasmic vacuole), and cells exhibiting Indian-file arrangement—lobular carcinoma of breast.
- Discrete malignant signet ring cells entangled in a patchy mucoid background in ascitic fluid—diffuse type of gastric adenocarcinoma/colonic adenocarcinoma.
- Prominent papillary clusters in the ascitic fluid sample, in an elderly female manifesting with abdominal mass—papillary ovarian adenocarcinoma.
- Relatively bland-looking sparse adenocarcinoma cells in an abundant thick mucoid background showing chicken-wire capillary network is diagnostic of pseudomyxoma peritonei.
- Atypical keratinized squamous cells—SCC (rare).
- Clusters of small cells with stippled chromatin and nuclear molding—neuroendocrine carcinoma.
- Presence of architectural features reminiscent of adenocarcinoma, but with hypervacuolated cytoplasm and intracytoplasmic/extracellular hyaline globules—yolk sac tumor.

Case History: A 55-year-old female presented with a cutaneous nodule (1 MGG).

Diagnosis: Cutaneous metastasis from carcinoma breast

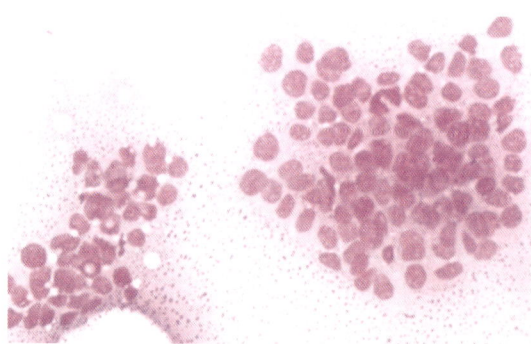

Fig. 22B.10

Cytologic Findings

Clusters of adenocarcinoma cells.

Note: Morphologic features of cutaneous metastatic deposits vary according to the primary site. In most cases, a previous history of primary malignancy assists in predicting the primary site of malignancy. In the present case, the patient had the history of primary breast carcinoma and hence the diagnosis was relatively straight forward.

Points to Remember

1. Most frequent sites of cutaneous metastasis—scalp, head and umbilicus (any site may be involved)
2. Common primary sites in females—breast, colon, lung and ovary
3. Common primary sites in males—lung, colon, oral cavity, kidney and stomach
4. Clinical presentation—papules or nodules of 1–3 cm size and rarely larger nodules
5. When solitary—its distinction from a primary carcinoma is difficult.
6. Examples of primary skin malignancies—cutaneous mucinous adenocarcinoma, adenocarcinoma of mammary-like glands of vulva, cutaneous signet ring cell carcinoma, cutaneous carcinoid and adnexal carcinomas.

Case History: 47-year-old female with a swelling in the neck (1 MGG).

Gross Nature of Aspirate
Blood mixed particulate.

Interpretation
Bethesda category IV; follicular neoplasm.

Cytologic Picture
- High cellularity.
- Monomorphic cells with repetitive follicular pattern.
- Both individual and clustered uniform microfollicles.
- Nuclear overlapping.

Differential Diagnosis
Adenomatous nodule and follicular variant of papillary carcinoma (FVPTC).

Points to Remember
- General features of a follicular neoplasm.
- High cellularity.
- Lack of colloid.
- Prominent follicular pattern with repetitive microfollicles.
- Uniform nucleomegaly.
- Significant overlapping of nuclei of follicular cells.
- Absence of atretic naked nuclei.

Possible Features of Hyperplastic/Adenomatous Nodule

1. High cellularity with prominent follicular pattern.
2. Presence of a significant amount of colloid
3. Features indicative of secondary changes in a nodular goiter such atretic naked nuclei, significant anisonucleosis of follicular cells, cyst macrophages and sometimes the presence of Hürthle cell change.

Features Favoring FVPTC
- Syncytial clusters
- Uniform nucleomegaly
- Nuclear crowding/overlapping
- Ovoid or pear-shaped nuclei
- Dusty chromatin
- Scanty gummy colloid.
- Though uncommon, other features indicative of conventional PTC such as the nuclear grooving, metaplastic change, cellular swirls, micropapillae and multinucleated giant cells also need to be looked for.

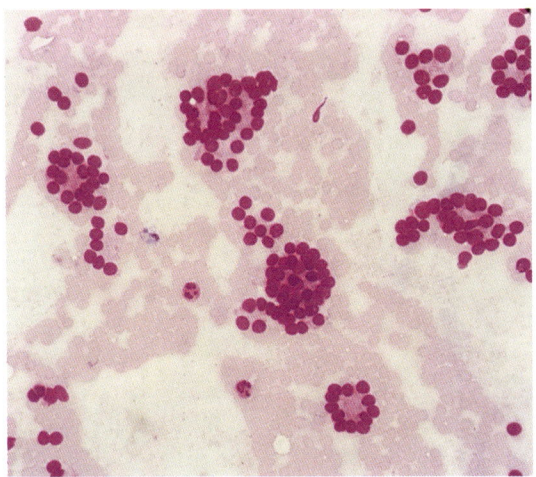

Fig. 22B.11

- Intranuclear cytoplasmic inclusions characteristic of conventional PTC and some of the PTC variants' are an extremely rare finding in an FVPTC.

Case History: A 47-year-old female with a swelling in the little finger (1 MGG).

Diagnosis: Giant cell tumor of tendon sheath (GCTS or nodular tenosynovitis)

Common age group: 30–50 years
Predilection: Slight female preponderance
Common sites: Fingers, wrist, ankle/foot and knee
Typical presentation: Long-standing painless swelling
X-ray: Soft tissue swelling sometimes eroding adjacent bone.
Gross nature of aspirate: Particulate.

Key Cytologic Features

- Presence of multinucleated osteoclastic type of giant cells.
- Dissociated cell pattern.
- Cell components: Mononucleated histiocyte/osteoblast-like cells and spindle cells.
- Atypia—uncommon.
- Mitotic figures—rare.
- Nuclear grooves and intranuclear inclusions —rarely described.

Note: Cytologically, GCTS is easily distinguished from a giant cell tumor of bone; GCT of bone exhibits a high cellularity with microbiopsy fragments composed of ovoid to spindle cells, having numerous osteoclastic type of giant cells adhering to the margins of the tissue fragments and cell clusters.

Case History 24: A 32-year-old female presented with swelling in the left submandibular region.

Diagnosis: Low grade mucoepidermoid carcinoma.

Age group: All age groups.
Sites: Both major and minor salivary glands.
Gross nature of aspirate: Mucoid.

Cytologic Picture

- Dirty background of mucus and debris that stain purplish blue.
- Cohesive clusters/sheets/small streams of cells within the mucus.
- A predominant population of mucus secreting cells with bland nuclear features.
- Less obvious intermediate and squamous cells.
- Neoplastic cells resembling macrophages.
- Sometimes, a few mast cells are also noticeable.
- Metachromatically stained intracytoplasmic mucin content in Romanowsky-stained smears.
- Squamous cells, when present resemble the metaplastic cells of a cervical smear.
- Frank keratinization is unusual.

Differential Diagnosis of a Low Grade MEC

- Papillary mucinous cystadenocarcinoma (rare)—papillary pattern and mucoid background.
- Mucus retention cyst—sparse cellularity abundant mucus.
- Rarely Warthin's tumor—oncocytes and lymphocytes in a proteinaceous fluidy background.

Case History: A 44-year-old male presented with right renal mass (1 MGG).

Diagnosis: Renal angiomyolipoma

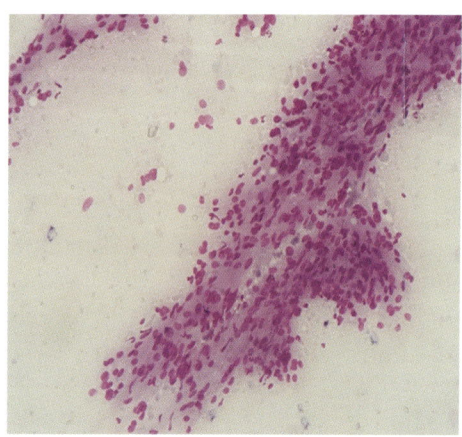

Fig. 22B.12

Approach to Diagnosis
Clinically: Renal mass
Imaging: Indicative of RCC/angiomyolipoma.
Gross nature of aspirate: Blood mixed particulate.

Cytologic Picture
- Prominent epithelioid morphology of neoplastic cells.
- Arborizing endothelial strands lined by epithelioid cells.
- Neoplastic cells—round to ovoid nuclei, bland chromatin and ill-defined cytoplasmic borders.
- Intranuclear cytoplasmic inclusions.

Points to Remember
- It is a benign tumor derived from the peri vascular epithelioid cells composed of an admixture of smooth muscle, fat and thick walled blood vessels.
- Around 50% of cases are associated with tuberous sclerosis.
- Remaining cases are sporadic.
- A few cases reported in association with von Recklinghausen's disease and autosomal dominant polycystic disease.
- Angiomyolipomas associated with tuberous sclerosis tend to be smaller, bilateral, multiple and asymptomatic with an early age (mean age: 25 years) of onset.
- Sporadic cases manifest at a later age (mean age: 25 years) with larger tumors flank pain and hematuria.
- Imaging studies (CT scan) can detect fat within the tumor and hence can diagnose/suspect angiomyolipoma.
- Though a benign tumor, histologically, atypical features such as nuclear pleomorphism, mitoses and necrosis can be seen in angiomyolipoma.
 Smooth muscle component often displays epithelioid morphology with abundant eosinophilic cytoplasm and eccentric nuclei having prominent nucleoli.
- Fine needle aspirates are usually hemorrhagic.
- Smears show cohesive tissue fragments as well as singly lying cells.
- Smooth muscle component displays highly varied morphology ranging from mildly atypical, spindle cells to round leiomyoblast-like round cells or pleomorphic cells. These cells amidst adipose tissue may raise a suspicion of liposarcoma.
- In absence of adipose tissue elements—mimic carcinoma, high grade sarcoma and sarcomatoid carcinoma.
- Cases of epithelioid angiomyolipomas presenting with prominent intranuclear inclusions are on record. Such cases are often misdiagnosed as renal cell carcinoma.
- Cases reported so far in the cytology literature have not shown consistent presence of thick-walled blood vessels. Blood vessels seen in a few documented cases are indistinguishable from those seen in the normal fat.
- However, thick-walled blood vessels are usually demonstrable in cell block sections of the aspirates. The smooth muscle cells are positive for vimentin, actin and desmin.
- In problematic cases melanocytic markers such as HMB-45 and melan-A are useful.
- A correct preoperative cytodiagnosis of angiomyolipoma can avoid unnecessary nephrectomy.

Case History: A 45-year-old male presented with swelling over the right shoulder.

Diagnosis: Myxoid liposarcoma
Gross nature of aspirate: Particulate.

Cytologic Picture
- High cellularity.
- Spindle cells admixed with prominent myxoid matrix.
- Focal arborizing capillaries.
- Occasional lipoblast.

Differential Diagnosis

- *Myxoid malignant fibrous histiocytoma (high grade myxofibrosarcoma):* Multinucleated giant cells.
- *Extraskeletal myxoid chondrosarcoma:* Intense metachromasia with dense appearance of the matrix material.

Myxoid Fibrosarcoma

- Benign myxoid neoplasms.
- Myxoid lipoma.
- Myxoma—sparse cellularity.
- Ganglion cyst—viscous fluid.
- Neurofibromas.
- Spindle cell lipoma.
- A few clusters of monomorphic basaloid cells.
- Peripheral palisading of basaloid cells.
- Presence of calcific material.
- Absence of nuclear atypia.
- Absence of ghost cells.

Differential Diagnosis

Varies depending on cytomorphologic variability; in the present case.

- Pilar cyst.
- Pilomatrixoma.
- Dermoid cyst.
- Calcified epidermal inclusion cyst.
- Additional cases as spotters.

Case History: A 42-year-old female with scalp swelling (1 MGG).

Diagnosis: Pilar cyst/pilomatrixoma

Cytologic Picture

- Cellular smear.
- Clumps of anucleate squames.
- A few clusters of monomorphic basaloid cells.
- Peripheral palisading of basaloid cells.
- Presence of calcific material.
- Absence of nuclear atypia.
- Absence of ghost cells.

Differential Diagnosis

Varies depending on cytomorphologic variability; in the present case.

- Pilar cyst.
- Pilomatrixoma.
- Dermoid cyst.
- Calcified epidermal inclusion cyst.

Case History: A 29-year-old male with inguinal swelling (1 MGG).

Diagnosis: Undifferentiated malignant tumor S/O metastatic amelanotic melanoma

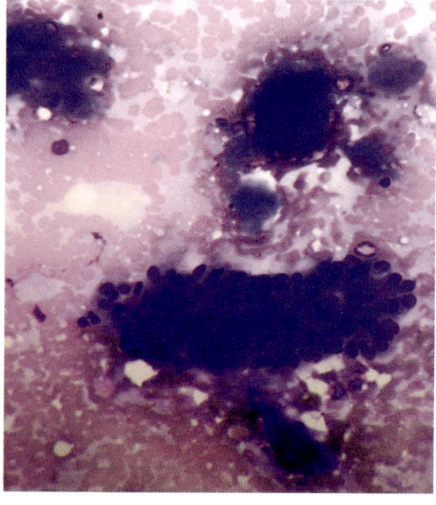

Fig. 22B.13

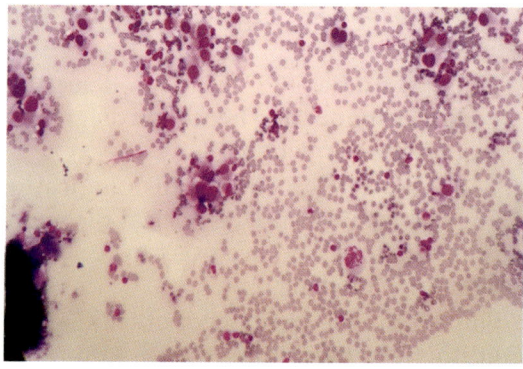

Fig. 22B.14

Cytologic Picture

- Moderate cellularity (high cellularity is a common finding).
- Discohesive cells and loose clusters.
- Marked pleomorphism (anaplasia).
- Abundant cytoplasm.
- Prominent nucleoli.
- Increased mitoses.

Differential Diagnosis

Depends on clinical presentation, morphologic variation.

Case History 29: A 30-year-old female with a solitary thyroid nodule (1 MGG).

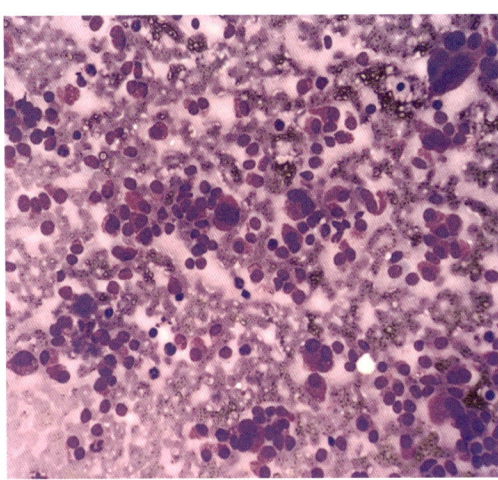

Fig. 22B.15

Interpretation

Bethesda category VI; malignant; medullary thyroid carcinoma.

Cytologic Picture

- Cellular smears
- Discrete/loose clusters of predominantly plasmacytoid cells.
- Rare follicle-like structures
- Bi- and tri-nucleate plasmacytoid cells.
- Prominent cytoplasmic red granularity.

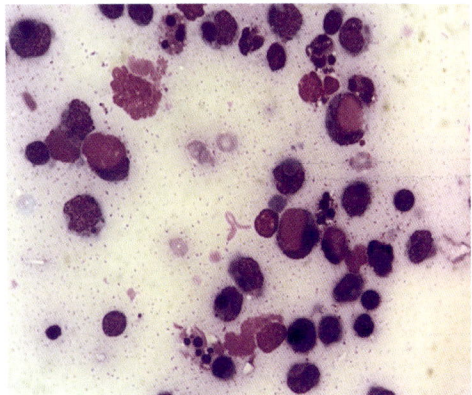

Fig. 22B.16a

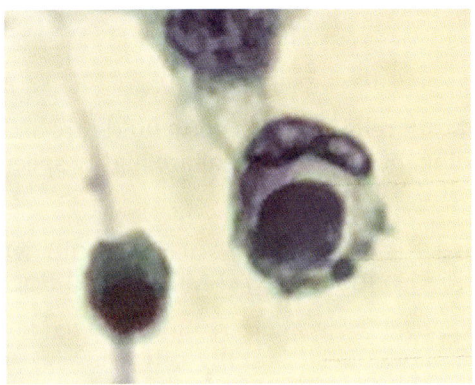

Fig. 22B.16b

Differential Diagnosis

- In the given case—none.
- Depending on morphologic features: paraganglioma, Hurthle cell neoplasm, anaplastic carcinoma.

Case History: Pericardial fluid sample from a 25-year-old female patient (1 MGG).

Diagnosis: LE cells in pericardial fluid

Cytologic Picture

- Cellular smears.
- Sheets of cells; predominantly of monocytic lineage.
- Admixed with many neutrophils.
- Many extracellular LE bodies.
- Several classic LE cells.
- Hemorrhagic background.

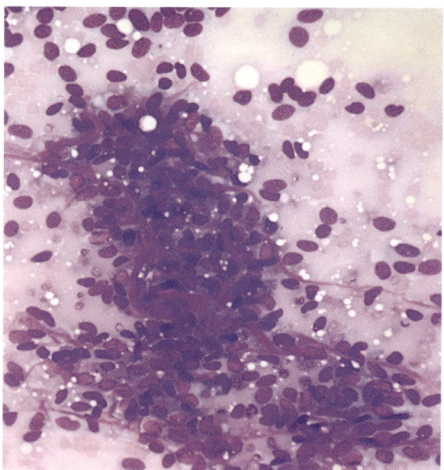 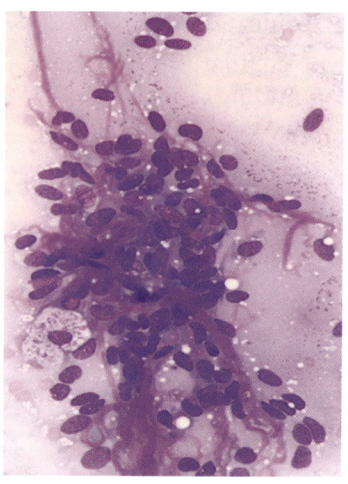

Fig. 22B.17a   Fig. 22B.17b

Note: LE cells in serous body fluids are a rare finding, but when present are highly specific for SLE.

Case History: A 40-year-old male with swelling in the left leg (1 MGG and 1 Pap).

Diagnosis: Low grade spindle cell sarcoma (S/O monophasic spindle cell synovial sarcoma/MPNST)

Cytologic Picture
- Highly cellular smears.
- Tight fascicles of monomorphic ovoid to spindle cells.
- Intervening collagenous matrix.
- Occasional loose clusters/fragments.
- Ovoid to spindly nuclei mostly with pointed ends.
- Scanty to moderate amount of tapering cytoplasm.
- No necrosis.
- No obvious mitoses.

Differential Diagnosis
Fibrosarcoma, monophasic spindle cell synovial sarcoma/MPNST.

CHAPTER 23

Hematology

Febe Renjitha Suman

NB
- PS—peripheral smear
- BMA—bone marrow aspirate
- BMB—bone marrow biopsy
- DD—differential diagnosis

Suggested Reading
Questions may be asked—refer to book.

APPROACH TO EXAMINATION OF PERIPHERAL BLOOD SMEAR

Macroscopy
Blue: Myeloma
Grainy: RBC agglutination
Blue specs at tail end: ↑WBC and ↑platelets
Holes: Lipemia

REPORTING FORMAT FOR PERIPHERAL SMEAR
Microscopy
RBC:
- Anisocytosis—Mention the types
- Poikilocytosis: Mention the types
- NN/MH/Microcytic/Macrocytic
- Schistocytes—% if MAHA, NRBC

WBC: ↑/↓ Neutrophil—left shift, toxic change, atypical cells, hypersegmentation
Lymphocyte—prolymphocyte, etc. Atypical cells
Others
Blasts: Uniform/Varying shape, size
Cytoplasm: Color, amount, granulation, vacuolation.
Nucleus: Shape, N : C ratio, chromatin, nucleolus
Background cells
Platelets: ↑/N/↓, morphology
Parasites: Species.
Any other cells in the background.

BONE MARROW ASPIRATE
Approach to Reporting a BMA
- *Low power:* Bony spicules
- *High power:* Particles, cell trails
- *Cellularity:* Proportion of cells to empty fat vacuoles in the vicinity of bone spicules
- *Adequacy:* Megakaryocytes
- *Abnormal clusters:* Metastatic tumor, lymphoid aggregates, granuloma
- Oil immersion
  1. To determine various types of cells of marrow
     i. Normal/hyperplasia/decrease
     ii. Maturation
     iii. Any dysplastic changes
     iv. Blasts, early precursors
     v. Any abnormal morphology of cells
  2. Any abnormal localization of cells
  3. Any clusters/granuloma—description
  4. Osteoblasts/osteoclasts
  5. Fat/endothelial cells/fibroblasts/fibrosis
  6. Iron and reticulin stain
  7. DC for 500 cells to be done (not in the examination).

BONE MARROW BIOPSY

Approach to Reporting a Bone Marrow Biopsy
1. Cellularity
2. Myeloid erythroid ratio
3. Maturation of myeloid series
4. Maturation of erythroid series
5. Eosinophils/basophils/mast cells
6. Megakaryocytes
7. Presence of other cells—lymphocytes, plasma cells, histiocytes, osteoblasts, fibroblasts.
8. Any proliferation/clusters/infiltrate
9. Stromal abnormalities—granuloma, fibrosis, necrosis, serous atrophy of fat
10. Hemosiderin
11. Vessel abnormality/amyloid deposits
12. Bone changes—Paget's cell, osteodystrophy, osteosclerosis.

Case History (1): A 46-year-old slender female feeling tired on climbing stairs. Routine investigations done. RBC count 3 million cells/cumm.

Impression: Microcytic hypochromic anemia. Probably iron deficiency anemia.

PS
- *RBC:* Anisopoikilocytosis, microcytic hypochromic, pencil cells, tear drop cells and occasional fragmented cells.

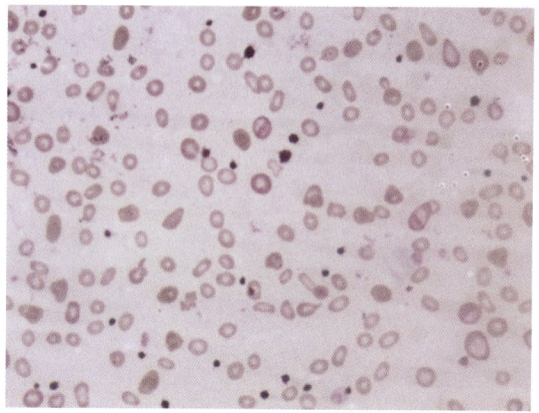

Fig. 23.1

- *WBC:* Normal in number and distribution.
- *Platelet:* Adequate and normal morphology.

Points to Remember
- Leucocytosis—chronic inflammation
- Thrombocytosis—iron deficiency due to chronic bleeding, anemia of chronic inflammation
- Basophilic stippling—lead poisoning
- Anemia in an adult male—mostly due to hidden bleeding.

Clues
Age/sex, symptoms, RBC count.

Table 23.1: Impression—microcytic hypochromic anemia, probably iron deficiency anemia					
DD	Iron deficiency	Thalassemia minor	Anemia of chronic inflammation	Sideroblastic anemia	Lead poisoning
Serum ferritin	↓	↑/N	↑/N	↑	N
Serum Fe	↓/N	↑/N	↓	↑	Variable
TIBC	↑	N	↓	↓/N	N
Transferrin saturation	↓	↑/N	↓	↑	↑
FEP/ZPP2	↑	N	↑	↑	↑
BM iron	Absent	↑/N	↑/N	↑	N
Sideroblasts	Absent	N	Absent/few	↑(ring)	N (ring)
RBC count	↓	N/↑	↑	N/↓	N/↓
RDW (anisocytosis)	↑↑	N/↑	↑	N	N
Mentzer index	>13	<13	NA	NA	NA
HPLC/HB electrophoresis	–	↑HbA2	–	–	↑
ALA and lead level	–	–	–	–	↑
Absolute reticulocyte count	↓	N/↑	N	N	↑

Suggested Reading
- Iron metabolism
- Biochemical biologic reference range.

Case Histroy (2): A 45-year-old man was admitted with chest pain and fever for 2 days. He complained of left hypochondrial pain for 2 years. Physical examination revealed mild jaundice, Hb 12 gm%.

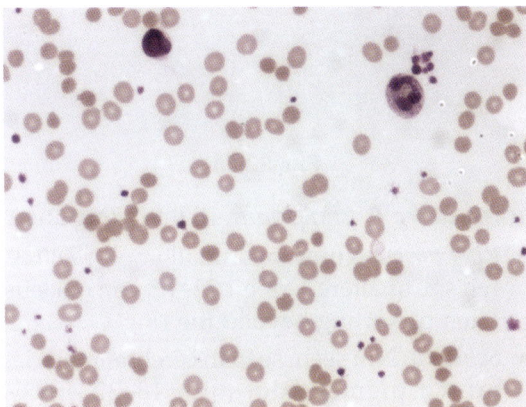

Fig. 23.2

PS
- *RBC:* Mild anisocytosis, polychromasia with microspherocytes.
- *WBC:* Normal in number and distribution
- *Platelet:* Adequate, normal morphology.

Impression: Hereditary spherocytosis

Invest
1. MCHC
2. Reticulocyte count
3. Serum bilirubin and LDH
4. Family history/testing
5. Osmotic fragility
6. Autohemolysis
7. Flow cytometric (dye-binding) test: EMA
8. Acidified glycerol lysis time
9. Cryohemolysis
10. Membrane protein electrophoresis

DD
1. Immune hemolytic anemia—DAT
2. Heinz body hemolytic anemia—bite cells, blister cells, Heinz body (methyl violet)
3. MAHA—schistocytes, helmet cells, thrombocytopenia
4. Burns—budding RBCs, triangular RBCs
5. SS disease—sickle cells, target cells
6. Water dilution hemolysis.

Points to Remember
- Age, Infancy, childhood, old age
- CBC—MCHC elevated
- History of jaundice, left hypochondrial pain
- Triad: Anemia, jaundice, splenomegaly—anyone may be given in history.

Suggested Reading
Inheritance, mutation, pathophysiology.

Case History (3): A 23-year-old female was admitted in ICU for seizure. Routine blood investigations led the patient to be shifted to hematology unit from neurology unit.

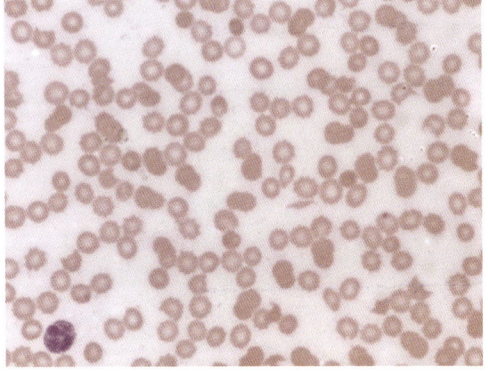

Fig. 23.3

PS
- *RBC:* Anisopoikilocytosis with NN RBC, microspherocytes, bizarre RBCs, helmet cells, schistocytes, polychromasia, NRBCs +, basophilic stippling +, diffusely basophilic RBC +.
- *WBC:* Leucocytosis with left shift.
- *Platelet:* Thrombocytopenia.

Imp: Microangiopathic Hemolytic Anemia
Probably thrombotic thrombocytopenic purpura.

DD
1. TTP—pentad

2. HUS—no neurological symptoms
3. DIC—coagulation parameters, D. dimer
4. Disseminated carcinomatosis
5. Post-transplant
6. Malignant hypertension
7. Venoms and toxins
8. Sepsis—toxic change in neutrophils
9. Antineoplastic drugs—history
10. *HELLP syndrome*—liver enzymes, pregnancy

Suggested Reading

- Pathophysiology of TTP/HUS.
- Therapeutic plasmapheresis.

Case History (4): Spot diagnosis

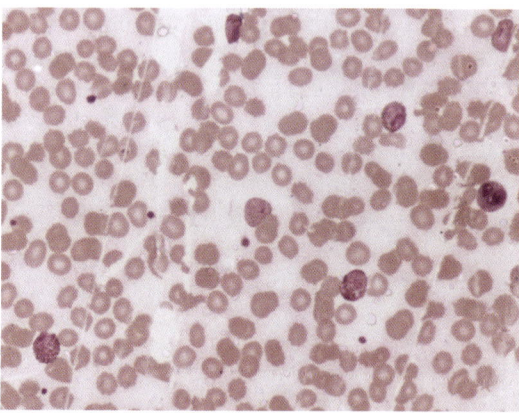

Fig. 23.4

Impression: *P. vivax* in Thin Film

- *Ring:* 2.5–3 µm, RBC enlarged and distorted, blue cytoplasmic ring, red nuclear mass, unstained area.
- *Schizont:* 9–10 µm contains 12–24 merozoites, rosette with yellow brown pigment at the centre.
- *Gametocyte:* Microgametocyte—cytoplasm light blue large diffuse nucleus.
- Macrogametocyte: Cytoplasm deep blue, small nucleus.

DD

- Ring form—platelet on RBC
- Trophozoite—stain artefact

Case History 5(a): Spot diagnosis.

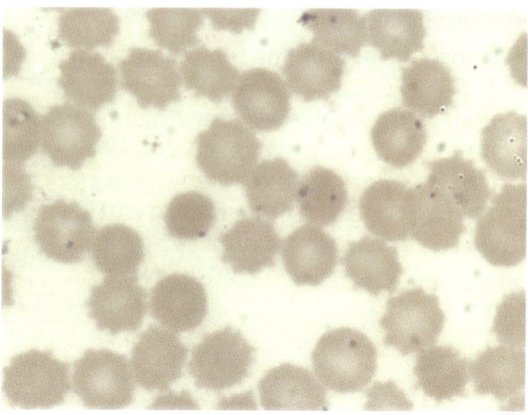

Fig. 23.5a

Impression: *P. falciparum* in Thin Film

- *Ring forms:* Numerous small, multiple, red cell size unaltered, ring 1.25–1.5 µm, nucleus often projecting beyond the ring
- *Schizont:* Not seen, seen in cerebral malaria, brown pigment dot with 18–32 merozotes
- *Gametocyte:* Crescentic, deep blue cytoplasm with pointed ends, brownish pigment near the centre (macrogametocyte), broader blunt end, light blue cytoplasm, nuclear granules scattered (microgametocytes)

DD

Ring forms: Babesia species

Case History 5(b): Spot diagnosis

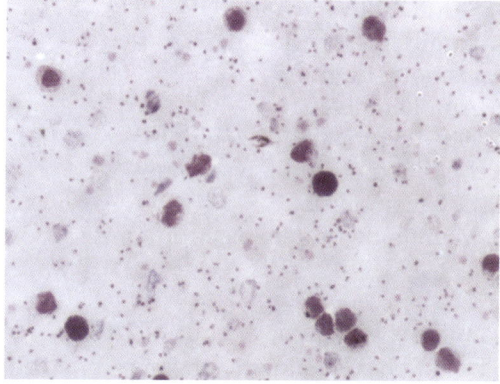

Fig. 23.5b

Impression: *P. falciparum* in Thick Film

Points

- If only ring forms are seen—suspect *P. falciparum*
- If all stages seen—suspect *P. vivax*
- Always look for both species—mixed infection
- Thick film—lysed RBCs, large volume, 0.25 µl blood/100 fields, blood elements concentrated
- Thin film—fixed RBC, single layer, smaller volume, 0.005 µl blood/100 fields
- Automation (hematology analyzer) based malaria detection?
- Please read up with different analyzer manuals.

Invest

1. QBC
2. Flourescent microscopy
3. Malarial antigen—chromatogram/ELISA.
4. Malaria serology—antibody
5. PCR

Case History (6): An 18-year-old Omani woman flown to India was seen in the emergency department for fever and abdominal pain.

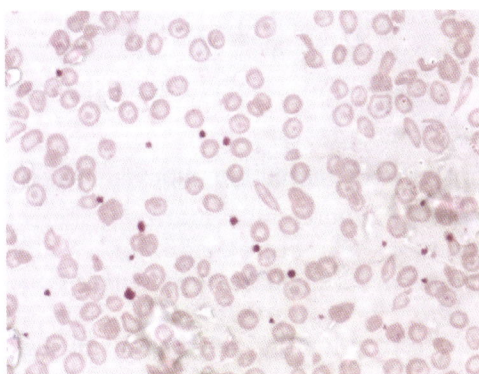

Fig. 23.6

PS

- *RBC:* Anisopoikilocytosis with microcytic hypochromic RBCs, sickle cells and target cells.
- *WBC:* Polymorphonuclear leucocytosis
- *Platelet:* Adequate with normal morphology

Impression: Hemolytic Anemia due to Hemoglobinopathy Probably HbS/Beta-thalassemia

DD: Sickle Cell Anemia

- Age—early, clinical—symptomatic HB 4–8 gm/dl
- Marked anisocytosis, plenty of sickle cells
- *Target cells rare:* Other RBCs usually normocytic normochromic.

Points

- HBS/β^0 *thalassemia:* Clinical course similar to homozygous sickle cell anemia.
- Hbs/β^+ *thalassemia:* Milder condition to be distinguished from sickle cell trait by microcytosis, hemolytic anemia, PS—sickle cell, target cells; splenomegaly.
- *Sickle cell trait:* Clinically normal except in hypoxic conditions.

Invest

1. Sickling test
2. HbS solubility test
3. Hb electrophoresis
4. HPLC
5. Globin chain electrophoresis
6. Isoelectric focussing
7. Mass spectrometry
8. Molecular study

Case History (7): A 24-year-old primigravida regularly attending antenatal clinic not responding to iron therapy.

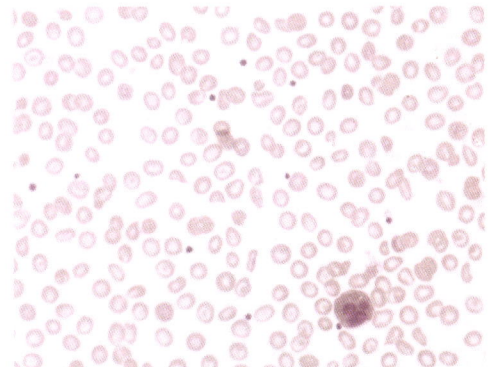

Fig. 23.7

PS

- *RBC:* Microcytic hypochromic
- *WBC:* Normal in number and distribution
- *Platelet:* Adequate, normal morphology
- *HP:* Absent

Impression: Microcytic Hypochromic Anemia

Probably hemoglobinopathy—beta-thalassemia trait

DD (Refer Case 1)

Investigations: Hb electrophoresis, HPLC, mutation studies, globin chain electrophoresis.

Case History (8): A 1-year-old boy baby with Hb 6 gm/dL.

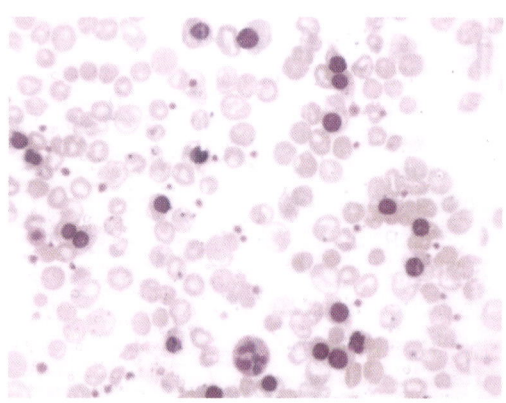

Fig. 23.8

PS

- *RBC:* Anisopoikilocytosis, microcytic hypochromic, polychromasia, nucleated RBCs, plenty of target cells noted.
- *WBC:* Normal in number and distribution
- *Platelet:* Adequate normal morphology
- *HP:* Absent

Imp: Thalassemia Major

Investigations: *Refer case 7*

Points

1. Age
2. By HPLC—thalassemia intermedia (not transfusion dependant)
3. Resistant to iron therapy

Suggested Reading

- Various hemoglobinopathies
- Mutations
- Chromatogram/electrophoresis.

Case History (9): A 67-year-old male patient with generalized lymphadenopathy and WBC count of 1,30,000/cumm.

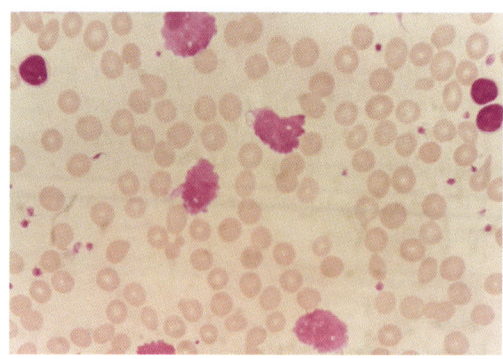

Fig. 23.9

PS

- *RBC:* Normocytic normochromic, some RBC agglutinates.
- *WBC:* Uniform population of mature small lymphocytes with round nuclei, clumped chromatin, scant cytoplasm. Broken cells (smear/smudge) seen.
- *Platelets:* Thrombocytopenia (advanced cases).

Impression: Chronic Lymphocytic Leukemia

- *BMA:* Hypercellular marrow—increased number of mature lymphocytes almost uniform. Normal hematopoiesis is reduced.
- *BMB:* Bone marrow diffusely infiltrated with small lymphocytes which are slightly larger than the average normal lymphocytes. Six histological patterns:
  1. Interstitial
  2. Nodular
  3. Diffuse packed
  4. Paratrabecular
  5. Random focal
  6. Intrasinusoidal

Points

Prolymphocytoid transformation:
1. Increased number of prolymphocytes—with prominent nucleolus and more abundant cytoplasm. > 55% PLL, < 55% atypical CLL
2. Co-existing AIHA—marrow shows erythroid hyperplasia.
3. Unusual pattern of infiltration—marked increase in reactive germinal centers (random/paratrabecular) in addition to diffuse infiltrate.
4. Diffuse pattern—poor prognosis; non-diffuse—good prognosis

DD

1. *Monoclonal B lymphocytosis:* circulating clonal cells are very less. Precursor of CLL.
2. *Polyclonal B cell lymphocytosis:* Binuclearity, deeply lobed nuclei, no clonality.
3. *Other Lymphoproliferative disorders:* Careful assessment of cytology and immunophenotype.
4. *DD in histology:* CLL non-para trabecular pattern.

Suggested Reading

1. Immunophenotyping, immunohistochemistry, cytogenetics and molecular genetics
2. Richter's transformation.

Case History (10): A 55-year-old male patient came with complaints of fatigue and dragging sensation in the abdomen. CBC showed increased WBC count, peripheral smear was performed.

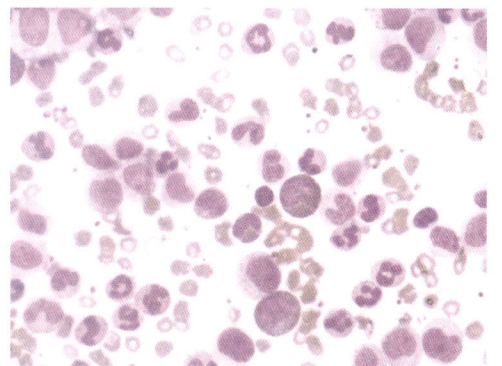

Fig. 23.10

PS

- *RBC:* Normocytic normochromic
- *WBC:* Leucocytosis with left shift and myelocyte bulge, basophilia and eosinophilia
- *Platelets:* Thrombocytosis/normal count
- *HP:* Absent

Impression

Chronic myeloid leukaemia—chronic phase

BMA and BMB

Increased cellularity and myeloid hyperplasia with normal/increased megakaryocytes. Small megakaryocytes increased, hypolobation present, macrophages increased, reticulin increased.

Invest

1. FISH/karyotyping
2. Quantitative RT-PCR for BCR-ABL
3. Serum uric acid + LDH
4. LAP score

DD

1. PS:
   a. *Leukemoid reaction:* History, splenomegaly not significant, more of neutrophils with left shift (remember CML neutrophilic variant), toxic granules, basophilia, eosinophilia not present.
   b. *Therapy with myeloid growth factors:* History, toxic granules type prominent granules. Counts may be less.
2. BMB—other MPN

   Refer case MF: Case no. 25

Points

1. Flow cytometry indicated only if CML-AP, CML-BP is suspected.
2. BM morphology at diagnosis essential to do quantitative bcr.abl
3. Monitoring response to therapy.
4. Criteria for CML-AP, BP.

Case History (11). A 29-year-old male with history of fever for 15 days and extreme fatigue.

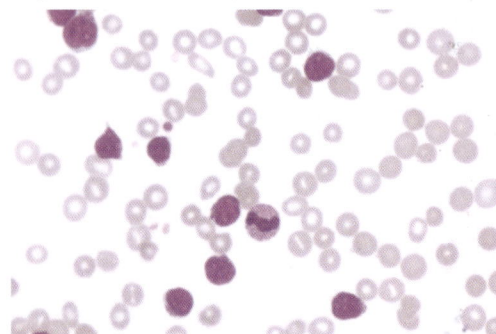

Fig. 23.11

PS
- *RBC:* Normocytic normochromic
- *WBC:* Leucocytosis with atypical cells resembling blasts; blasts are large, almost uniform, round with scanty cytoplasm which is granulated with high N : C ratio nucleus round to indented with fine chromatin and 2–3 prominent nucleoli. Background shows maturing myeloid cells. Platelets: Thrombocytopenia.
- *HP:* Absent

Impression: Acute Leukemia, Probably Myeloid in Origin—AML M2 (FAB)

DD, Invest, Learning Points

Refer AML.

Case History (12): A 2-year-old child presented with fever, failure to thrive.

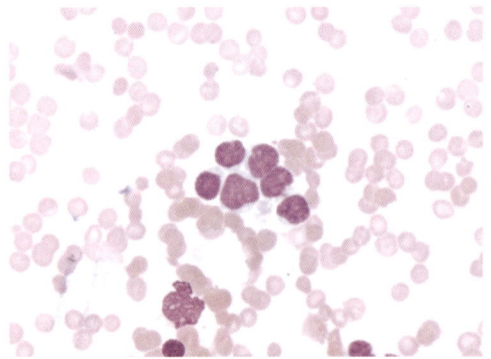

Fig. 23.12

PS
- *RBC:* Normocytic normochromic
- *WBC:* Atypical cells resembling blasts which show mild variation in size and shape with scanty agranular cytoplasm with large nucleus which shows indentation and clefting, chromatin is dense, with 1–2 nucleoli.
- *Platelets:* Thrombocytopenia
- *HP:* Absent.

Impression: Acute Lymphoblastic Leukemia

DD Invest, Learning Points

Refer ALL

Case History (13): A 50-year-old female with cervical lymphadenopathy

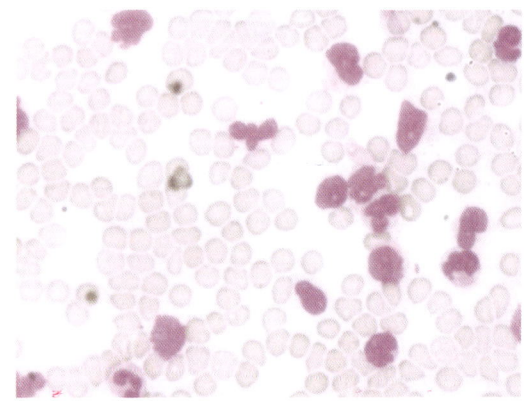

Fig. 23.13

PS
- *RBC:* Normocytic normochromic
- *WBC:* Leucocytosis with atypical cells having clover leaf-shaped nucleus.
- *Platelets:* Reduced
- *HP:* Absent

Impression: Acute Leukemia: Probably Lymphoid in Origin—T Cell Origin

Case History (14): An 11-year-old boy, exhausted while walking, not able to concentrate on studies. CBC and peripheral smear suggested bone marrow studies.

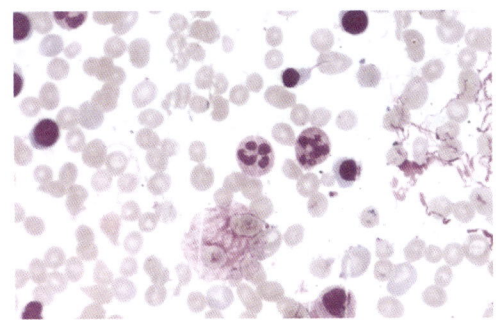

Fig. 23.14

BMA
- *Particles:* Present
- *Cellularity:* Hypercellular
- *Cell trails:* Present
- *Erythropoiesis:* Erythroid hyperplasia, megaloblastic maturation, nuclear—cytoplasmic asynchrony (look at—polychromatophilic normoblast)
- Granulopoiesis: All stages of maturation seen. Giant metamyelocytes and bands noted.
- *Megakaryocytes:* Increased/decreased/normal; hypolobation may be seen.

Impression: Megaloblastic Anemia

Differential Diagnosis
1. Congenital dyserythropoietic anemias. Age, biochemistry
2. Erythroleukemia—M6.

Invest
1. RBC histogram/MCV/pancytopenia/absolute reticulocyte count
2. Serum vitamin B_{12}/folic acid
3. Red cell folate
4. Methyl malonic acid assay—mass spectrometry
5. Serology—Ab to intrinsic factor (ELISA)/parietal cells (IIF)
6. Stool: Eggs/proglottids of *D. latum*.

Points
1. Biochemical investigations and serology for autoantibodies are available, which limited the bone marrow examination.

2. *Sequence of development:* Vitamin level ↓ → hypersegmented neutrophils → ovalomacrocytosis → definite megaloblastic BM → anemia.
3. *History of pancytopenia useful:* Pancytopenia with a hypercellular marrow.
4. *Age:* Any age.

Case History (15): A 60-year-old male with complaints of fatigue, DCT positive, peripheral smear showed indication for bone marrow study.

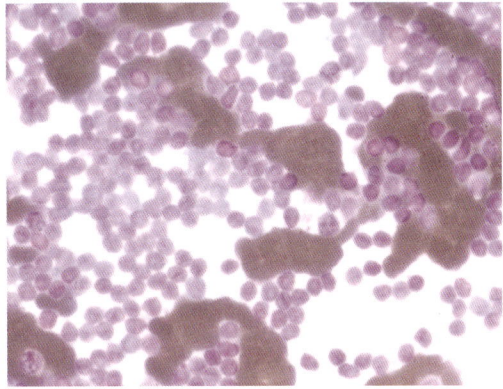

Fig. 23.15

Impression: BMA: Lymphoproliferative Disorder Probably Chronic Lymphocytic Leukemia

Description, DD, invest, learning points
Refer case 9:

Case History (16): A 4-year-old boy had lymph node biopsy, BM studies done for staging.

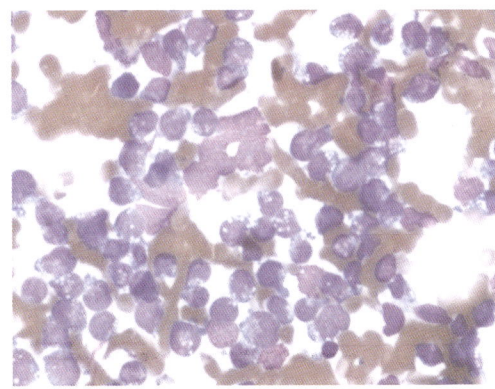

Fig. 23.16

BMA

- Particles—present
- Cell trails—present
- Erythropoiesis—suppressed
- Myelopoiesis—suppressed, with all stages seen
- Marrow heavily infiltrated with diffuse proliferation of large cells with basophilic and vacuolated cytoplasm and large nucleus which is indented with dense chromatin and occasional nucleoli, many degenerated cells and macrophages notes
- Megakaryocytes very occasional and smaller in size.

Points

1. Peripheral blood—N/circulating lymphoma cells (50% of cases).
2. Leukemic phase—not seen in endemic, common in AIDS.
3. Cell of origin—EBV related post-germinal center memory B cell. EBV negative cases, germinal center B cell.
4. BMA 5–20% of cases heavily infiltrated/decreased % of cells/increase in non-neoplastic cells.

BMB

Hypocellular marrow replaced by monotonous population of round to oval cells with scant vacuolated cytoplasm, large nucleus with prominent nucleoli and increased mitosis.

Impression: Lymphoproliferative Disorder—Burkitt Lymphoma

DD

- BMA: Usually straightforward
- BMB
  1. Blastoid variant of mantle cell lymphoma (spectrum of neoplastic cells small lymphocytes to medium-sized cells with a nuclear chromatin similar to lymphoblast: CD10 – CD5 +, cyclin D1 + vs BL -CD10 +, CD5 –, cyclin D1–)
  2. Grey zone lymphoma, B cell lymphoma unclassifiable—features intermediate between DLBCL and BL.
  3. Alveolar rhabdomyosarcoma—vacuolated cells.

Case History (17): A 62-year-old male with extreme tiredness, admitted with a Hb of 7 gm%. His serum iron, vitamin B_{12} are elevated.

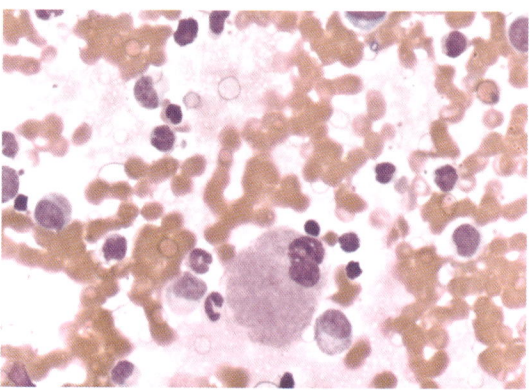

Fig. 23.17

BMA

- Particles—present
- Cell trails—present
- Cellularity—hypercellular
- Erythropoiesis—markedly suppressed, a few cells appear to be of normoblastic maturation
- Granulopoiesis—myeloid hyperplasia with increase in myelocytes, agranular myelocytes and metamyelocytes seen. Eosinophils and basophils show dysplastic changes.
- Megakaryocytes—present, hypolobated forms seen.
- Lymphocytes and plasma cells—present.

Imp: Myelodysplastic Syndrome (MDS/MPN)

Features of MDS

DYSERYTHROPOIESIS

PS

- Oval macrocytes (normal B_{12}/folate)

- Hypochromic microcytes (normal iron studies)
- Dimorphic RBCs

BM
- RBC precursors with more than one nucleus or abnormal nuclear shapes.
- Round nucleus with lobes or buds, nuclear fragments, internuclear bridging, basophilic stippling and ring sideroblast.

DYSMYELOPOIESIS
PS
- Persistence of basophilia in the mature WBC
- NC asynchrony
- Abnormal granulation of the cytoplasm (agranular bands—misinterpreted as monocytes)
- Abnormal nuclear feature—hyposegmentation, hypersegmentation, nuclear rings.

BM
- Nuclear cytoplasmic asynchrony (persistent basophilic cytoplasm)
- Cytoplasmic changes—uneven staining, basophilia as a dense ring. Abnormal granulation (agranular promyelocytes may be mistaken for blasts) abnormal nuclear shapes. Granulocytic hypoplasia/hyperplasia.

DYSMEGAKARYOPOIESIS
PS

Giant platelets/abnormal granulation, circulating micromegakaryocytes.

BM

Large megakaryocytes, micromegakaryocytes, micromegakaryoblast, multiple separated nuclei. Reticulin increased.

DD
1. Megaloblastic anemia
2. Copper deficiency
3. CDA
4. Drugs/Parvovirus B19/HIV
5. PNH.

Suggested Reading

WHO classification, cytogenetics.

Case History (18): A 38-year-old female patient presented with swollen and bleeding gums.

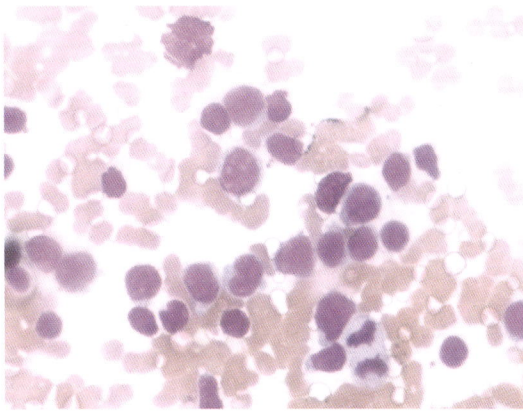

Fig. 23.18

BMA
- Particles—present
- Cell trails—present
- Cellularity—hypercellular
- Erythropoiesis—markedly suppressed
- Granulopoiesis—myeloid hyperplasia with increase in blasts, 2 population of blasts seen.
- Myeloblasts—large with scanty granulated cytoplasm with large nucleus and fine chromatin and 2–3 nucleoli; also seen are monoblasts which are very large with moderate amount of cytoplasm with nucleus appearing folded, having fine chromatin.
- Megakaryocytes—very occasional.

Imp: Acute Leukemia Probably of Myeloid Origin—AML-M4 (FAB)

DD, Invest, Suggested Reading

Refer acute myeloid leukemia.

Case History (19): A 4-year-old child presented with fever, peripheral smear showed atypical lymphocytes.

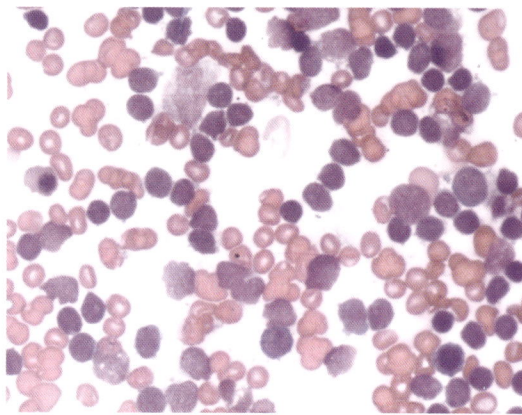

Fig. 23.19

BMA

- Particles—present
- Cell trails—present
- Cellularity—hypercellular
- Erythropoiesis—suppressed
- Granulopoiesis—suppressed, all stages of maturation seen
- Megakaryocytes—present
- Lymphoid cells—there is diffuse proliferation of atypical lymphoid cells with scanty blue cytoplasm and high N : C ratio, round to slightly indented nucleus, with dense chromatin.

Impression: Acute Leukemia—Probably Lymphoid in Origin (ALL)

DD, Invest, Suggested Reading

Refer ALL

Case History (20): A 60-year-old male patient presented with backache, proteinuria ++.

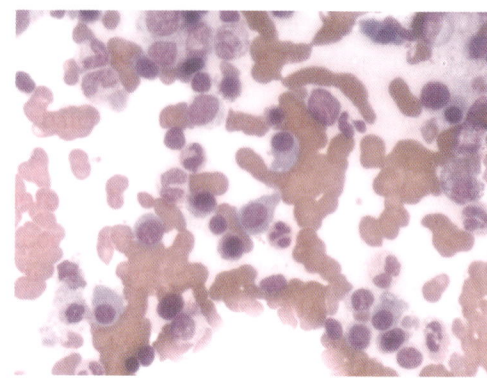

Fig. 23.20

BMA

- Particles—present
- Cell trails—present
- Cellularity—hypercellular
- Erythropoiesis—suppressed
- Granulopoiesis—suppressed, all stages of maturation seen
- Megakaryocytes—present
- Plasma cells—increased, with more than 30% of nucleated cells.

BMB

Sections show hypercellular marrow with diffuse infiltration by plasma cells and plasma blasts. Trilineage hematopoiesis seen but suppressed.

Impression: Features are Suggestive of Myeloma

To be confirmed by > 10% clonal plasma cells with CRAB features as 60% clonal plasma cells with SLIM features.

Invest

1. Protein electrophoresis
2. Immunofixation
3. Free light chain assay (serum/urine)
4. Renal function tests
5. Bence Jones proteins.
6. Immunohistochemistry—monoclonality—kappa/lambda.
7. Serum calcium
8. Hb
9. CT/PET/MRI/X-ray

DD

1. Reactive plasmacytosis—history and light chain assay
2. Lymphoplasmacytoid lymphocytes
3. Large cell lymphoma/carcinoma *vs* plasmablastic myeloma
4. Other plasma cell neoplasms.

Learning Points

Trephine biopsy 3 types:
1. Homogenous nodules of plasma cells occupying half of high power field.
2. Mononuclear cells as aggregates occupying the space between the fat cells.
3. Diffuse plasmacytosis with monotypic light chain expression.
4. If a few plasma cells are present in BM with a strong clinical suspicion M band/free light chain. CD138 and monoclonality to be done.

Suggested Reading

Criteria for all plasma cell dyscrasias, amyloidosis, cytogenetics.

Case History (21): A 37-year-old lady noted increasing fatigue and scattered purpura. She had non-steroidal anti-inflammatory agent for her wrist pain 3 months prior.

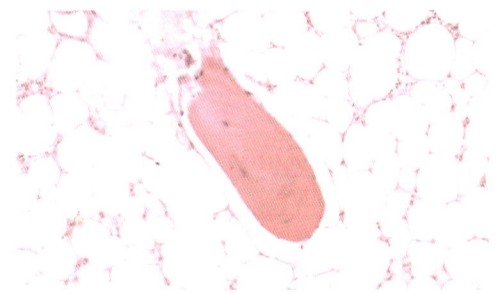

Fig. 23.21

BMB

Section shows bony trabeculae enclosing marrow particles showing only fatty marrow. Scanty population of plasma cells and lymphocytes seen.

Impression: Aplastic Anemia

- *Peripheral smear:* Pancytopenia
- Normocytic normochromic anemia, macrocytes present/absent, reticulocyte count reduced
- *BMA:* Aplastic/hypocellular/hypo- and normocellular-hyper/dry tap
- Dyserythropoiesis may be seen. But no dysplasia of granulocyte or platelet cell lines
- *BMB:* <25% cellularity, decrease of hematopoietic cells
- Cellular areas contain lymphocytes, plasma cells, macrophages, mast cells and eosinophils
- Reactive lymphoid aggregates
- Iron increased, reticulin normal
- Bone osteoporosis/increased osteoblastic and osteoclastic activity.

DD

1. Hypoplastic MDS (15%)
   - Look for cluster of blasts
   - Dyspoiesis in 1 or more cell lines, megakaryocyte clusters, reticulin fibrosis, megaloblastosis. Ringed sideroblasts. CD34 cell count increased.
2. Hypoplastic AML
   - Look for blasts
3. PNH
   - History of hemolysis, increased reticulocyte count. Look for areas of erythroid hyperplasia; always rule out PNH by investigations
4. Aplastic ALL (children)—increased lymphocytes, blasts

Points to Remember

Splenomegaly absent in AA

Table 23.2: Grading			
	NSAA	SAA	VSAA
Cellularity	<25%	<25%	<25%
Absolute neutrophil count	>500/mm^3	<500/mm^3	<200/mm^3
Platelet count	>20,000/mm^3	<20,000/mm^3	<20,000/mm^3
Reticulocyte count	>1%	<1%	<1%

Learning Points
1. Acquired causes most common especially in adults.
2. Inherited causes present usually before 10 years.
3. HbF increased in Fanconi anemia, normal/increased in DKC.
4. Chromosomal fragility increased
5. Genetics—trisomy 6, trisomy 8, abnormalities of chromosome 5/7.
6. Mutation—TERC in autosomal dominant DKC, DKC1 in X-linked DKC.

Case History (22): A 6-year-old male with proptosis, BMB done.

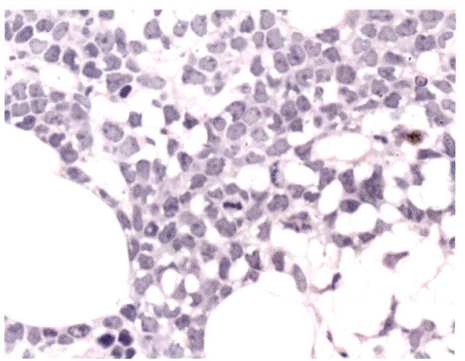

Fig. 23.22

Impression: Burkitt's Lymphoma

Description of the slide, DD, investigations, learning points: *Refer* to case 16.

Case History (23): A 60-year-old male patient presented with backache, proteinuria ++.

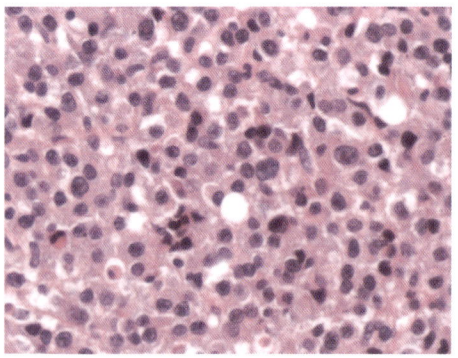

Fig. 23.23

Impression: Plasma Cells Myeloma

Description of the slide, DD, invest, learning points: *Refer* to case 20.

Case History (24): A 70-year-old male presented with splenomegaly. Peripheral smear showed leukoerythroblastic picture.

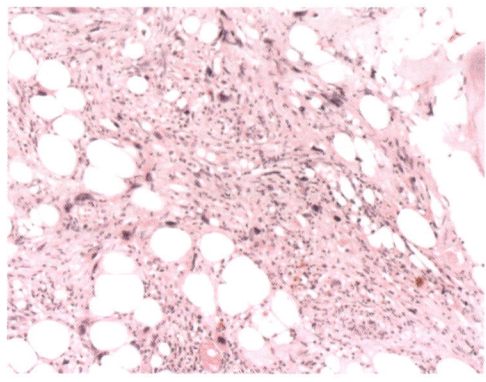

Fig. 23.24

BMB
Section shows bony trabeculae enclosing a cellular marrow with suppression of myeloid and erythroid series, there is increase and streaming of megakaryocytes in a background of abundant fibrosis.

Impression: Myelofibrosis—Fibrotic Phase

Description
- *Peripheral smear:* Leucoerythroblastic picture/pancytopenia with increase in eosinophil, basophil. Sometimes leucocytosis with blasts may be seen.
- *BMA:* Dry tap.
- *BMB:* May be edematous. Contains sparse dysplastic megakaryocytes with diffuse fibrosis. Scattered granulocyte precursors may be seen. Streaming of hematopoietic cells noted. Reactive lymphoid nodules may be present. Sinusoids obliterated. Thickening of bone trabeculae seen.

DD
Lymphoma/infiltration by carcinoma—when there is dense fibrosis, it is necessary to look for malignant cells. IHC may help.

- Points—reactive lymphoid nodules, amyloidosis seen sometimes
- Peripheral blood—CD34+ cells increased.

Suggested Reading

MF—reticulin grading, cytogenetics, WHO criteria

Case History (25): A 65-year-old male patient came with complaint of dragging sensation in the abdomen.

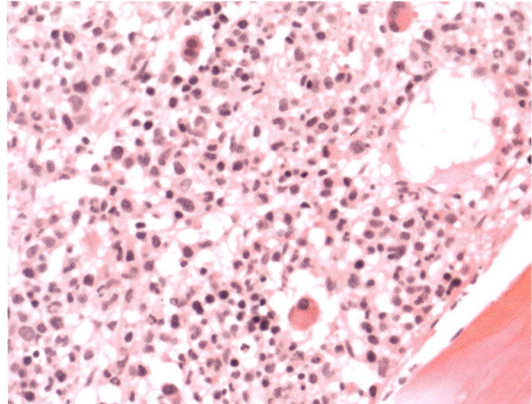

Fig. 23.25

BMB

Bony trabeculae enclosing a hypercellular marrow showing trilineage hematopoiesis, erythroid is markedly suppressed, there is myeloid hyperplasia with all stages of maturation seen with the precursors predominating. There is megakaryocyte hyperplasia, clustering and dysplastic changes.

Impression: Myelofibrosis—Prefibrotic Phase

Points

- *BMB:* Diffusely hypercellular with increase in all hematopoietic cell lineages with relatively normal maturation. Granulocytic precursors show an abnormal clustering in the intertrabecular spaces.
- Megakaryocytes are increased and varying in size with hypolobation. Some of them have hyperchromatic and hyperlobated nuclei. Clustering of megakaryocytes seen abnormally close to the endosteum.

Sinusoids are increased and distended, may have hematopoietic cells.
- *Peripheral blood:* Leukoerythroblastic blood film with tear drop cells. Dysplastic changes in the granulocytes and platelets. Circulating micromegakaryocytes.
- *BMA:* May be difficult, shows hypercellular fragments with increase in cells of all lineages and dysplastic megakaryocytosis.

DD

1. *Acute myelofibrosis:* Splenomegaly, tear drop cells, leukoerythroblastic picture, circulating blast cells, pancytopenia present.
2. *Other MPN:* Cytogenetics
   - PV—increased erythropoiesis
   - CML—increased myelopoiesis
   - ET—megakaryocytes in loose clusters or scattered, large deeply lobated, with staghorn like nuclei, less pleomorphic than MF.

Case History (26): A 59-year-old female patient presented with generalized lymphadenopathy, BMB done.

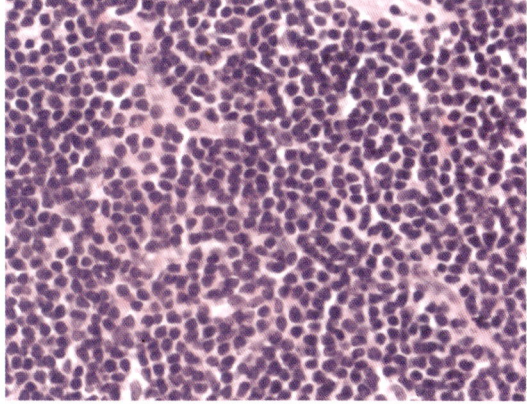

Fig. 23.26

BMB

Section shows bony trabeculae enclosing hypercellular marrow showing diffuse infiltrate of lymphoid cells. Normal trilineage hematopoiesis suppressed.

Impression: Chronic Lymphocytic Leukemia

Refer case 9.

Case History (27): A 9-year-old male presented with history of skin rashes, CBC showed WBC count 90,000/cumm.

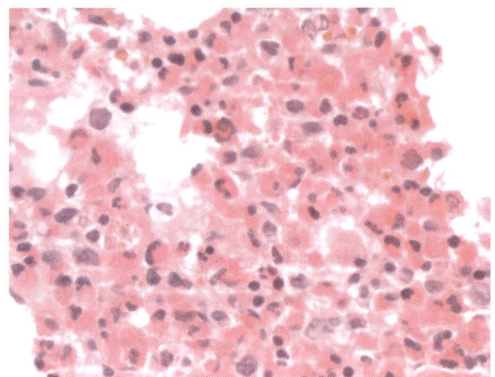

Fig. 23.27

BMB

Section shows bony trabeculae enclosing a cellular marrow with suppression of erythroid and megakaryocyte series. There is diffuse proliferation of eosinophils and precursors, few large cells resembling blasts are scattered.

Imp: Features are that of Acute Myeloid Leukemia—Probably M4-Eo

- DD, invest—refer to acute leukemia
- Points—inv (16) (p13.1q22) or t(16;16) (p13; q22); CBFB-MYH11

Case History (28): A 2-year-old male came with complaints of fever and sore throat.

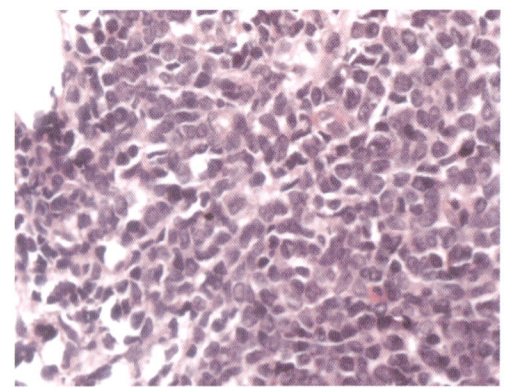

Fig. 23.28

BMB

Section shows bony trabeculae enclosing a cellular marrow composed of atypical cells that are round to irregular in shape, scant cytoplasm, increased NC ratio, hyperchromatic nucleus.

Impression: Acute Leukemia, Probably Acute Lymphoblastic Leukemia

DD, investigations, points—*refer* acute leukemia.

Case History (29): A 35-year-old male with known history of tuberculosis presented with symptoms of anemia.

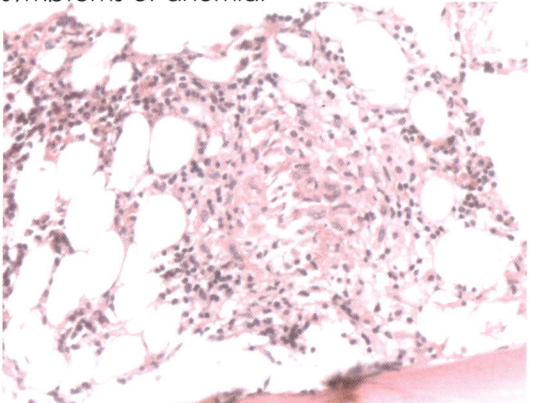

Fig. 23.29

BMB

Section shows bony trabeculae enclosing a hypocellular marrow. Erythropoiesis suppressed, granulopoiesis shows all stages of maturation, megakaryocytes seen. Multiple epithelioid granulomas with Langhans type giant cells seen.

Impression: Chronic Granulomatous Inflammation of Tuberculous Origin

Special Stains

AFB, PAS, PAS-D, Giemsa.

Case History (30): A 3-year-old male with a retroperitoneal mass, BM was done for staging.

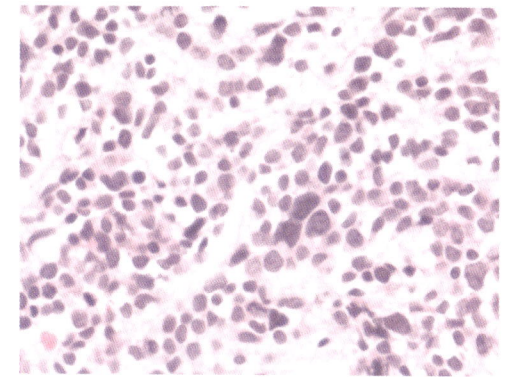

Fig. 23.30

BMB

Section shows bony trabeculae enclosing cellular marrow with foci of trilineage hematopoiesis. The marrow is infiltrated by monotonous sheets of atypical cells that are small round blue cells with scant cytoplasm and hyperchromatic nucleus.

Impression: Metastatic Deposit—Small Round Cell Tumor, Probably Neuroblastoma

DD

Any small blue cell tumor. IHC, clinical features, site, cytogenetics, molecular testing to differentiate.

IHC

Vimentin, synaptophysin, chromogranin positive. CD45, CD99, myogenin negative.

Case History (31): A 63-year-old male with multiple bony metastasis.

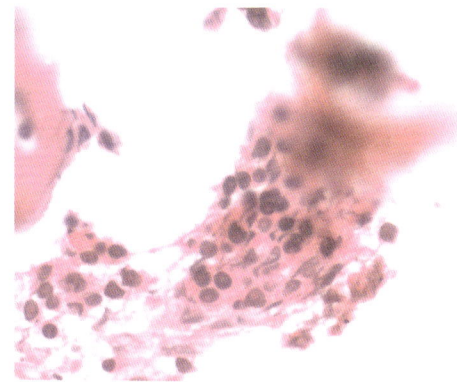

Fig. 23.31

BMB

Section shows bony trabeculae enclosing a scanty marrow, marrow shows clusters of large atypical cells with necrosis admixed with marrow cells. There is mild increase in plasma cells.

Impression: Metastatic Carcinoma

IHC

- Positive for vimentin, cytokeratin
- Negative for CD45, CD138, CK7, CK20.

Case History (32): A 5-month-old girl baby presented with symptoms of anemia with RBC count 1 million/mm^3. WBC, platelets normal.

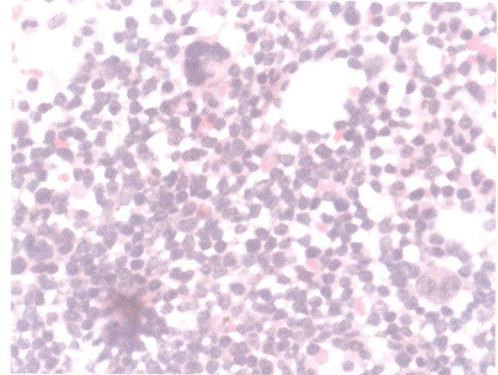

Fig. 23.32

BMB

Section shows cartilage and bony trabeculae enclosing marrow particles, marrow cellular erythroid is markedly suppressed, early precursors of erythroid series are noted. All stages of myeloid series noted. Megakaryocytes seen scattered in between.

Impression: Pure Red Cell Aplasia

IHC

CD45 positive in 80% of the cells, MPO positive in 60% of CD45 + cells.

PS

- *RBC:* Normocytic normochromic/macrocytic (Blackfan-Diamond syndrome)
- *BMA:* Cellularity—normal/reduced, striking reduction of maturing erythroid cells.

Proerythroblasts are usually present in normal numbers. Other lineages normal, hematogones and mature lymphocytes may be increased.
- *BMB:* Bone marrow cellularity reduced, lack of erythroid islands and maturing erythroblasts, large proerythroblasts with strongly basophilic cytoplasm are seen. Non-specific inflammatory changes may be seen.

Points

1. Blackfan-Diamond syndrome—first year of life
2. Transient erythroblastopenia of childhood—neutropenia moderately severe.
3. Older children, adults—Parvovirus B19 infection, HIV, drugs, transplant chemotherapy.

DD

1. Hematological neoplasm—increase in proerythroblast, increase of hematogones (look for maturing cells which are absent)
2. MDS—other lineage dysplasia.

ACUTE LEUKEMIA

Acute Myeloid Leukemia

Criteria: >20% blasts
- *Peripheral blood:* Counts usually less than 1,00,000/hyperleukocytosis/normal
- *BMA:* Hypercellular marrow, erythroid and megakaryocyte suppression, myeloid hyperplasia, morphology depends on the subtype.
- Hypocellular in case of early AML developing from AA, PNH, hMDS

Morphology
- FAB classification
- *Cytogenetics:* WHO classification.

AML-M0

- *PS:* Agranular blasts, large with high NC ratio, fine chromatin, nucleus round to indented. No myeloid differentiation. Presence of occasional hypogranular neutrophils provide a clue to myeloid nature.
- *BMA:* Medium-sized blasts with fine chromatin in the nucleus and 1–2 faint nucleoli, matured cells +/–.

AML-M1

- *PS:* More than 90% myeloblasts without evidence of maturation (<10% promyelocytes to neutrophils), Auer rod variable.
- *BM:* Medium-sized blasts with eosinophilic cytoplasm and nucleus with fine chromatin and 2–3 nucleoli, maturing cells—a few/absent.

AML-M2

- Myeloblasts <90%
- *PS:* Cytoplasmic globules and vacuoles, prominent Auer rods present, granules +, maturing cells +; mostly associated with t(8; 21)—10% of AML, 30–40% cytogenetic abnormality.
- *BM:* Blasts with eosinophilia and large nucleus with prominent 2–3 nucleoli with maturing cells of neutrophil and eosinophil lineage.

AML-M3

- *Promyelocytes and blasts:* Hypergranular (classic M3)—cytoplasm shows prominent azurophilic granules, Auer rods frequent with faggot cells. Nucleus folded, granulated, granules obscure the borders.
- *Microgranular (M3v):* Cytoplasm shows fine small granules, Auer rods rare, nucleus irregular and folded.
- *PML hyperbasophilic:* Granules sparse, strongly basophilic, high NC ratio, cytoplasmic budding +, Auer rods absent.
- *BM:* Infiltrate of abnormal promyelocytes—large cells with plenty of granulated cytoplasm, nucleus—oval or bilobed with single prominent nucleolus.

AML-M4

PS: Hyperleukocytosis usually, the cells have monocytic characters as well as myeloblastic characters are seen. Promonocytes and monoblasts noted.

AML-M4 Eo

- Immature eosinophils with eosinophilic or basophilic granules with monocytoid nucleus.
- *BM:* Shows a mixture of cells of monocyte and granulocyte lineage, predominantly eosinophils, basophils may also be present. Some eosinophils have basophilic granules. Blast—cells are usually around 20%.
- Criteria for AML—M4 blasts >20% of NEC, granulocytic component >20% of NEC, monocytic component >20% of NEC.
- And PS monocytes >5 × 10^9/L
- And cytochemical proof of monocytic differentiation.

AML-M5

- *PS:* Monoblasts are large cells with round or oval nucleus, a delicate chromatin pattern and plentiful cytoplasm, promonocytes are similar cells with nuclear irregularity or lobated with single nucleolus (WHO classification regards these as blast equivalent)
- *M5a:* Poorly differentiated—predominantly monocytic component, monoblasts are more.
- *M5b:* Predominantly monocytic component, monoblasts less.
- *BM: M5a*—BM monocytic component >80% of NEC, monoblasts >80% of BM monocytic component.
- *M5b:* BM monocytic component >80% of NEC, monoblasts <80% of BM monocytic component.

AML-M6

- *PS:* RBC—macrocytes, schistocytes, tear drop forms, pincered cells, basophilic stippling, and circulating erythroblasts may be seen. Occasional dysplastic erythroids noted.
- *BMA:* Hypercellular with megaloblastic change, erythroid cell abnormalities—multinuclearity, cytoplasmic vacuoles, karyorrhexis. Myeloblasts ++.
- *BMB:* Erythroid hyperplasia with sheet-like arrangement. Precursors vary in size with megaloblasts/bizarre forms. Nuclear lobulation and fragmentation noted. Myeloblasts are also noted.

AML-M7

- *PS:* Pancytopenia, a few micromegakaryocytes and megakaryoblasts seen. (They are similar in size to myeloblasts, high NC ratio and agranular, basophilic cytoplasm, peripheral cytoplasmic blebs may be seen.) Giant and hypogranular platelets may be seen.
- *BMA:* Myeloblasts and megakaryoblasts are seen, micromegakaryocytes and dysplastic megakaryocytes seen. 50% are megakaryoblasts, Often BMA is dry tap due to fibrosis.
- *BMB:* Above changes with fibrosis.

Points

1. Report to be written as acute leukemia probably myeloid in origin and FAB category to be mentioned to be confirmed and categorized by immunophenotyping and cytogenetics.
2. Clues in the history—anemia, low RBC count, thrombocytopenia, fever.
3. Bleeding gums, gum hypertrophy, skin lesions favor M4, M5.
4. History of extramedullary disease favor M5.
5. DIC—APML
6. Children—M5a
7. Down's syndrome—M7.

DD

1. ALL-M0 and ALL-M0-M1 very difficult to distinguish. ALL—effacement of bone marrow, cells with less cytoplasm, condensed chromatin. AML—residual

myeloid cells with dysplastic features seen. M6 and M7—cytoplasm more.
2. Aplastic anemia/hypocellular *vs* hypocellular AML (*see* aplastic anemia).
3. Large cell NHL *vs* M5a—lymphadenopathy *vs* gum infiltration and fine chromatin in M5a.
4. Leukemoid reaction—history of infection and alcohol abuse, sometimes hypocellular marrow with increased blasts can occur in the above conditions. Look for toxic granules, criteria of blast %.
5. APML:
   a. Therapy with myeloid growth factors—maturation preserved, Auer rods not found.
   b. CML: All stages of maturation present, increased eosinophils, basophils.
   c. AML-M2: not many promyelocytes, faggot cells absent
   d. AML-M5, M3v hyperbasophilic
   e. Mast cell leukemia/basophilic leukemia.
6. M6:
   a. AML-M6 *vs* megaloblastic anemia: Pancytopenia, macrocytes, no circulating nRBCs, hypersegmented neutrophils, biochemistry.
   b. Myelodysplasia: Dysplasia in myeloid; megakaryocyte abnormality, blasts % <20%.
7. M7:
   a. Primary myelofibrosis
   b. AML in a hypocellular marrow
   c. Metastasis
   See myelofibrosis
8. Blast crisis of CML—eosinophilia, basophilia helps in identification of CML.

Learning Points

Cytochemistry, immunophenotyping characteristics, cytogenetics and molecular characteristics.

Acute Lymphoblastic Leukemia

- PS-RBC—low count
- WBC—low/normal/increased

Peripheral lymphoblasts seen, sometimes absent.
- FAB L1 ALL—small uniform cells with regular cell outlines, high NC ratio, round nucleus, homogenous chromatin, inconspicuous nucleoli.
- L2—blasts large, pleomorphic, cytoplasm plentiful, nuclei vary in shape, nucleoli prominent.
- L3—Burkitt lymphoma like cells.
- Platelets—thrombocytopenia.

BMA

Marrow is markedly hypercellular heavily infiltrated by leukemic blasts, normal hematopoiesis is suppressed. Blast cells appearance—*refer* to PS.

BMB

Infiltrated with lymphoblasts which replace most of the hematopoietic and fat cells. Infiltrating cells vary in size, are about twice the diameter of RBC, large nucleus and minimal cytoplasm, chromatin is finely stippled with one or two medium-sized nucleoli.

Points

1. >25% lymphoblasts infiltration into the BM—ALL; <25% lymphoma.
2. Immunophenotyping is done for categorization of ALL.
3. Immunohistochemistry can be done on biopsy.
4. Cytogenetic and molecular genetic analysis to be done.
5. Prognosis depends on immunophenotype, epidemiology, clinical variables and genetic characters.
6. Preleukemic episode of marrow aplasia presenting with pancytopenia may cause difficulty in diagnosis. Neutropenia is more marked than thrombocytopenia. In BMB small hypercellular areas with lymphoid infiltrate are noted.
7. Bone marrow necrosis may complicate ALL—aspirate contains only necrotic cells.

DD

1. Reactive lymphocytosis—atypical cells can be seen in viral infections—cytoplasm blue and moderate—plenty. Clinical history is important.
2. AML—cytoplasm more than ALL, nucleus irregular, granules, maturing cells, dysplastic features in background cells.
3. Small cell tumors of childhood (remember leukemic lymphoblasts may fail to express CD45) differentiate by IHC.
4. Lymphoid blast crisis of CML—known case of CML with basophilia.

Case History (33): Middle aged man came with history of fever 3 weeks and extreme fatigue.

PS

- *RBC:* Normocytic normochromic.
- *WBC:* Leukocytosis with blasts which vary in size and shape, large, scanty cytoplasm a few having granules. Nucleus large with some of them, having indentation, dense chromatin and occasional ones showing inconspicuous nucleolus.
- *Platelet:* Marked thrombocyotopenia.
- *Impression:* Acute leukemia probably acute myeloid leukemia—M0.

Case History (34): A 35-year-old female admitted with history of fever since a month and bony pain.

PS

- *RBC:* Normocytic normochromic
- *WBC:* Leukocytosis with blasts which vary in shape and size with scanty cytoplasm and large round nucleus with fine chromatin which is indented in some and prominent 2–3 nucleoli. Background cells are a few lymphocytes and occasional neutrophils.
- *Platelets:* Thrombocytopenia.
- *Impression:* Acute leukemia probably acute myeloid leukemia—M1.

Case History (35): Middle-aged man admitted with history of fever since 2 weeks and bony pain and tenderness.

PS

- *RBC:* Normocytic normochromic
- *WBC:* Leukocytosis with blasts which vary in size and shape; cytoplasm scanty, granulated in some with Auer rods. Background neutrophils and eosinophils seen.
- *Platelets:* Thrombocytopenia.
- *Impression:* Acute myeloid leukemia—M2.

Case History (36): A 29-year-old male IT professional, developed purpuric spots and bleeding gums. He had on and off fever earlier for about 3 weeks.

PS

- *RBC:* Microcytic hypochromic
- *WBC:* Leukocytosis with atypical promyelocytes, some of them granulated, other showing deeply indented nuclei.
- *Platelets:* Thrombocytopenia.
- *BMA:* Particles with cell trails present, normoblastic hypercellular marrow with suppressed erythropoiesis, myeloid hyperplasia with increase in atypical promyelocytes, occasional megakaryocyte noted.
- *BMB:* Bony trabeculae enclosing a cellular marrow. Erythropoiesis suppressed. Myeloid hyperplasia with increase in blasts and atypical cells resembling promyelocytes. Megakaryocytes adequate.
- *Impression:* Acute myeloid leukemia—M3: Acute promyelocytic leukemia.

Case History (37): A 50-year-old man with pharyngitis, O/E gum hyperplasia observed.

- *Peripheral smear: RBC:* Normocytic normochromic.
- *WBC:* Leukocytosis with increase in number of blasts. Blasts are of two types—myeloblasts and monoblasts. Maturing of cells with myeloid and monocytic differentiation noted.

- *Platelets:* Thrombocytopenia.
- *Impression:* Acute myeloid leukemia-M4.

Case History (38): A 36-year-old male with fever and massive splenomegaly.

PS

- *RBC:* Normocytic normochromic.
- *WBC:* Leukocytosis with left shift, basophilia, eosinophilia and increased blasts.
- *Platelets:* Adequate.
- *Impression:* Chronic myeloid leukemia—accelerated phase.

BMA

Particles with cell trails present. Erythropoiesis suppressed, myeloid hyperplasia with increase in blasts noted. Eosinophilia, basophilia present. Megakaryocytes seen.

Case History (39): Known case of CML, on treatment, increasing anemia at review.

PS

- *RBC:* Normocytic normochromic.
- *WBC:* Leukocytosis with left shift, basophilia and increased blasts noted.
- *Platelets:* Thrombocytopenia.
- *Impression:* Chronic myeloid leukemia—blast phase.

Case History (40): A 32-year-old female with anemia and hepatosplenomegaly.

PS

- *RBC:* Normocytic normochromic.
- *WBC:* Eosinophilic leukocytosis with atypical eosinophils.
- *Platelets:* Adequate.
- *Impression:* Eosinophilia—probably chronic eosinophilic leukemia (CEL) or hypereosinophlic syndrome (HES).

BMA and BMB

↑ eosinophils and precursors
Blasts: <20%.

DD

1. CEL—criteria.
2. HES—no firm evidence of leukemia. No potential cause of reactive eosinophilia
3. Cytokine driven hypereosinophilia—look for a clone of T lymphocytes.
4. Reactive eosinophilia—look for all the causes.
5. Eosinophilic variant of CML—BCR-ABL
6. AML-M4 Eo.

Suggested Reading

1. Criteria
2. Flow chart for diagnostic pathway.

Case History (41): A 65-year-old man with splenomegaly, BCR-ABL positive.

PS

- *RBC:* Normocytic normochromic.
- *WBC:* Leukocytosis with left shift, predominantly neutrophils, eosinophila.
- *Platelets:* thrombocytosis.
- *HP:* Absent.
- *Impression:* Neutrophilic variant of CML.

Case History (42): A 45-year-old female with splenomegaly, BCR-ABL positive.

PS

- *RBC:* Normocytic normochromic, nRBCs present.
- *WBC:* Leukocytes with predominantly eosinophils and atypical eosinophils. Myelocytes and metamyelocytes are also increased.
- *Platelets:* Adequate.
- *Impression:* CML—eosinophilic variant.

Case History (43): A 55-year-old male splenomegaly WBC count > 30 x 10^9/L, BCR-ABL negative.

PS

- *RBC:* Microcytic hypochromic
- *WBC:* Neutrophilic leukocytosis

- *Platelets:* Adequate
- *HP:* Absent
- *Impression:* Chronic neutrophilic leukemia.

Case History (44): A 41-year-old female, mild splenomegaly low grade fever on and off, fatigue present.

BMA

- Particles—present
- Cellularity—hypercellular
- Erythropoiesis—suppressed
- Granulopoiesis—suppressed
- Megakaryocytes—occasional
- Lymphocytes, plasma cells—present
- There is increase in monocytoid cells with a few blasts.
- *Impression:* Chronic myelomonocytic leukemia.

Case History (45): A 3-month-old girl baby, with repeated episodes of infection.

BMA

- *Particles present:* Cell trails present
- *Cellularity:* Normocellular
- *Erythropoiesis:* Normoblastic maturation
- *Granulopoiesis:* Suppressed with precursors showing large granules and vacuolation
- *Megakaryocytes:* Present
- A few cells, resembling hemophagocytes seen
- *Impression:* Chédiak-Higashi syndrome, with hemophagocytosis.

Case History (46): Spot diagnosis.
- *RBC:* Anisopoikilocytosis with predominantly eliptocytes. The other cells being normochromic cells WBC: Normal in number and distribution.
- *Platelets:* Adequate with normal morphology
- *HP:* Absent
- *Impression:* Eliptocytosis.

Case History (47): Smear from newborn (day 2) with jaundice. Bilirubin 12 mg/dl.
- *RBC:* Normocytic normochromic with microspherocytes and # RBCs.
- *WBC:* Normal in number and distribution
- *Platelets:* Thrombocytosis
- *HP:* Absent
- *Impression:* ABO incompatibility

Case History (48): A 5-month-old-baby had jaundice and anemia at the onset of fever. Viral markers negative.

PS

- *RBC:* Microcytic, with bite cells
- *WBC:* Normal in morphology and distribution
- *Platelets:* Adequate
- *Impression:* G6PD deficiency.

Case History (49): Spot diagnosis: Impression: Mixed infection.

Case History (50): Spot diagnosis: Impression: Cold agglutination.

Case History (51): An 1-year-old boy failure to thrive with progressing hepatosplenomegaly.

BMB: Bony trabeculae enclosing marrow particles. Trilineage hematopoiesis suppressed. Megakaryocytes scattered. There is diffuse proliferation of enlarged macrophages with pale fibrillary cytoplasm and eccentric nucleus.

Impression: Storage Disorder—Gaucher's Disease

- *PS:* N/Pancytopenia/Gaucher's cells after splenectomy, monocytes + for TRAP.
- *BMA:* Large round to oval cells with voluminous faintly basophilic cytoplasm with wrinkled/fibrillar appearance and small eccentric nucleus. Erythrophagocytosis +/−. Foamy macrophages↑
- *BMB:* Isolated/clumps/sheets/replacing large areas of marrow.

- *Cells:* Abundant pale staining cytoplasm (watered silk/crumpled tissue paper), osteolysis ±/−.

DD

1. Pseudo-Gaucher cells
   Seen in CML and variants, AML, thalassemia major, CDA, lymphoma (rare)—negative for iron stain.
2. Multiple myeloma/lymphoplasmacytic lymphoma cells containing Ig.
3. AFB in immune suppressed—macrophages packed with AFB.

Points

- *Gaucher cells:* Sudan black B +, PAS +, NSE+, TRAP+, iron+.
- *Assay for β-glucocerebrosidase.*

Suggested Reading

Storage disorders.

Case History 52: A 52-year-old male with hepatosplenomegaly and pancytopenia.

BMB: Bony trabeculae enclosing marrow particles, trilineage hematopoiesis suppressed. There is diffuse proliferation of widely spaced cells which are large with faint basophilic cytoplasm and round to indented nucleus. Cells are surrounded by empty spaces.

Impression: Lymphoproliferative Disorder—Hairy Cell Leukemia

- *Peripheral smear:* Pancytopenia/neutropenia/monocytopenia
- *Hairy cells:* Larger than CLL with irregular cell border, abundant faint basophilic cytoplasm. Nucleus round/oval/indented/bilobed. Nucleolus: Not apparent.
- *BMA:* Dry tap/prominent mast cells amidst neoplastic cells.
- *BMB:* Focal extensive/diffuse/interstitial (hypocellular marrow)
- *Fried egg appearance:* Widely spaced mononuclear cells (10–25 μm).
- Pale clear cytoplasm and cytoplasmic retraction (reticulin increased, stippled chromatin). Mitosis ↓. Reactive plasma cells, lymphocytes and mast cells seen. Residual hematopoiesis—erythroid clusters and megakaryocytes seen. Reticulin fibrosis noted. Collagen absent.

CHAPTER 24

Approach to Bleeding Disorders

Febe Renjitha Suman, Rithika Rajendran

INVESTIGATING A CLINICALLY SUSPECTED BLEEDING TENDENCY

Comprehensive clinical evaluation	
Platelet/vascular	*Coagulation*
Female predominance	Male predominance
No family history	Positive family history
Mucocutaneous bleed	Deep hematomas

↓

Screening tests (vascular, platelet and coagulation)

↓

Confirmatory tests

Sample Collection

Venous samples, from relaxed patient in warm area (stress and exercise—↑ factor VIII, vWFag., fibrinolysis), no pressure cuff (to avoid hemoconcentration, platelet release, activation of clotting factors)

Order of blood—draw Second (blue top evacuated tube), process within 2 hours

Anticoagulation 32 g/L (0.109 M) solution of trisodium citrate, 9:1 ratio

↑ **HCT:** Citrate adjustment.

Tests for Vascular and Platelet Phases

Sample

Platelet rich plasma (centrifuge at 150–200 g for 5 min at room temperature. Platelet count ~2 lakhs/mm³)

1. **Bleeding time:** Ivy's method standard incision (2–3 mm long, 3 mm deep; 40 mm Hg) made on the volar surface of forearm. Measure time till bleeding stops. Normal range 2–7 min. Prolonged: Thrombocytopenia, platelet function disorders, vWD, vascular abnormalities, severe deficiency of factor V, XI, or afibrinogenemia.
2. **Platelet enumeration:** Automated cell counters/manual—verify by PS.
3. **Platelet volume measurements:** Automated cell counters. MPV normal range: 8.4–10.4 fl.
4. **Platelet morphology:** Peripheral smear.
5. **Platelet function assays:** Avoid drugs/beverages/foods that affect platelet function for 10 days. Fasting overnight is preferable.
   a. Adhesion tests
   b. Aggregation tests
   c. Investigation of granular content and release
   d. Flow cytometry: Glycoprotein surface expression, activation, P-selectin (CD62) surface expression, fibrinogen binding, annexin binding (to phosphatidyl serine), conformational changes in IIb, IIIa, platelet granule fluorescence.

Tests of Coagulation Phase

First-line coagulation tests: PT/APTT/Platelets/TT/fibrinogen.

Sample

Platelet poor plasma (PPP) (centrifuge at 1500–2000 g for 15 min at room temperature. Platelet count <10,000/mm³ QC: Run 1 sample through hematology analyser everyday)

PROTHROMBIN TIME

Used to assess extrinsic and common pathway. Time required for the clotting of citrated plasma in the presence of optimal concentration of tissue extract (thromboplastin) and calcium.

Principle

Tissue factor (thromboplastin) binds factor VII to initiate coagulation.

Reagents

1. PPP
2. Thromboplastin Commercial tissue factor obtained from rabbit brain/heart/lung or recombinant (*E. coli* produced human tissue factor + synthetic phospholipids)
3. Calcium chloride (0.025 mol/L)

Methods

1. Manual
2. Automated (semi/fully)

Procedure

Incubate at 37°C 0.1 ml plasma + 0.2 ml PT reagent (thromboplastin+ Ca^{2+}) → Mix and record endpoint (stopwatch). Duplicate + control.

Interpretation

Normal range: 11—16s
Critical value: 30s

International Normalized Ratio (INR)

$$\frac{Test\,PT^{ISI}}{MNPT}$$

Mathematical calculation that corrects for the variability in PT results caused by variable sensitivities (ISI) of the thromboplastin reagents used by the lab. Used for patients receiving stable orally administered anticoagulant therapy. Therapeutic range 2–3.

Control Plasma (MNPT)

20 healthy men and women (not pregnant, not taking OCP). Log geometric mean normal PT calculated.

International Sensitivity Index (ISI)

Measure of responsiveness of reagent relative to WHO international reference preparation. Mentioned by the manufacturer. ISI close to 1 is ideal.

ACTIVATED PARTIAL THROMBOPLASTIN TIME

Used to assess intrinsic and common pathway. Time required for the clotting of citrated plasma after the activation of contact factors and addition of phospholipid (partial thromboplastin) and calcium chloride.

Principle

Factors XII and XI are activated in the presence of cofactors prekallikrein and HMWK by kaolin, then FIXa/VIIIa activates FX.

Reagents

1. PPP
2. APTT reagent (kaolin + phospholipid)
3. Calcium chloride (0.025 mol/L)

Methods

1. Manual
2. Automated (semi/fully)

Procedure

Incubate at 37°C 0.1 ml plasma + 0.1 ml APTT reagent (kaolin + phospholipid) → Wait 1 min → Add 0.1 ml warmed $CaCl_2$ → Mix and record endpoint (stopwatch). Duplicate + control.

Interpretation of APTT

Normal range: 26–40 sec
Critical value: 70 sec

Prolonged PT

Congenital	Acquired
Deficiency of factors VII Deficiency of II, V or X	Warfarin Vitamin K deficiency Liver disease

Prolonged APTT

Congenital	Acquired
Deficiency of factors VIII, IX, XI Deficiency of factor XII, HMWK, PK (non-bleeders) von Willebrand disease	Heparin Lupus anticoagulant Factor VIII inhibitor Vitamin K deficiency Liver disease

Prolonged PT/APTT

Congenital	Acquired
Multiple factor deficiency Deficiency of factors V, X or II Combined V and VIII deficiency Afibrinogenemia/hypofibrinogenemia Dysfibrinogenemia	Vitamin K deficiency Liver disease Super therapeutic warfarin Super therapeutic heparin Direct thrombin inhibitors DIC

Approach to Prolongation

Rule out pre-analytical variables/acquired causes

Mixing Test

- **Principle:** Only 50% factor activity is needed for clotting.
- **Method:** Patient plasma 50% + Pooled normal plasma 50% → Incubate at 37°C for 1 to 2 hours (time, temp. dependant) → Perform test (PT/APTT)
- **Interpretation:** Corrected—factor deficiency

Not corrected—inhibitor (antibody/heparin/FDP/paraproteins).

CHAPTER 25

Automation in Hematology/Clinical Pathology

Febe Renjitha Suman, S Sri Gayathri

1. Complete blood count
2. ESR
3. Coagulation
4. Point of care testing
5. Urine analysis

ADVANTAGES

1. High level of precision and accuracy
2. Less labor
3. Rapid performance
4. Aberrant results are flagged for subsequent review
5. Embedded quality control programs

DISADVANTAGES

1. High capital.
2. Need calibration and maintenance.
3. Certain counts/flagging/results need manual checking.

Types

1. Semi-automated
   a. Requires some steps to be done manually
   b. Measures small number of variables
2. Fully automated
   a. Requires only sample presentation
   b. Measures 8–40 parameters
   c. Quality control analysis embedded
   d. Bar code reading
   e. Comprehensive information processing systems (interfacing)

Automated Hematology Analyzers (CBC—Counters)

The basic components are:
   i. Electrical system
   ii. Hydraulic system
   iii. Pneumatic system
   iv. Computer system.

Based on Coulter Principle (Fig. 25.1)

Blood sample is diluted in diluents which is a good conductor of electricity. The cells pass through the aperture by hydrodynamic

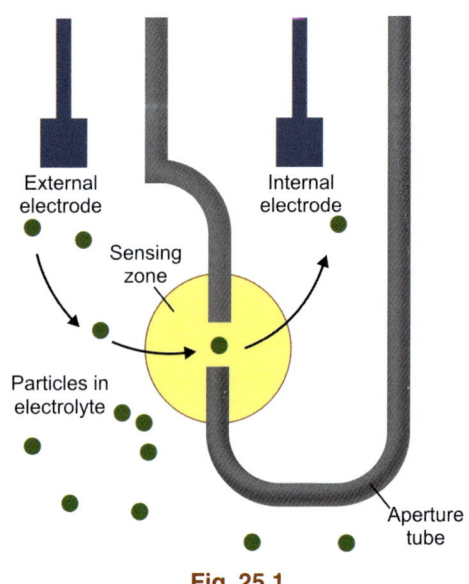

Fig. 25.1

focusing. As the cells pass through the aperture resistance/impedance is created causing change in voltage and pulse, the number of pulses in proportional to the number of cells. The size of the voltage pulse is proportional to the volume of cell. The RBCs and platelets are counted in the RBC chamber. Particles of 2–20 fl are counted as platelet and those above 35 fl as RBCs. Then WBC diluents with RBC lyse reagent releases Hb. WBC is then counted. Hemoglobinometer measures hemoglobin by photo calorimetry read at wavelength of 535 nm. The solutions are either cyanmethemoglobin or sodium lauryl sulfate. The pulses obtained are analysed for editing, coincidence correction and digitalization. The technology used for differential counts includes light scattering and absorbance when the cells pass through a laser beam. The light scattered 180°C to the light source is called *forward angle light scatter* (FALS) which determine cell volume. Light scattered 90°C to the light source is side scatter (SS) which is the function of the cell contents like complexity of the nucleus and granularity of the cells. The cell information seen on the screen is called a bitmap (Fig. 25.1).

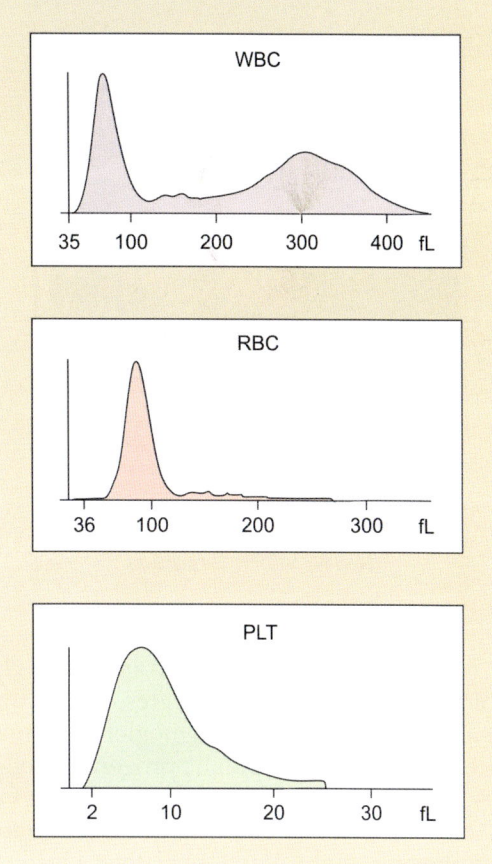

Fig. 25.2

Histogram (Fig. 25.2)

1. *RBC:* Symmetrical bell-shaped curve left shift—microcytic, right shift— macrocytic, camel humps—bimodal MCV is calculated from the area under the peak. RDW is measured at 20% level. Indices are calculated. In some machines MCV is measured and Hct is calculated.
2. *WBC:* Generated with size of cells (fl) in X-axis and number on the Y-axis. Three group of cells are seen in the histogram. Lymphocytes between 35–90 fl, mid and cell count (eosinophils, basophils, monocytes, blasts and promyeolocytes) between 90 and 160 fl and neutrophils between 160 and 300 fl. Counters can be 3 part, 5 part, 7 part differential.
3. *Platelets:* Counting and sizing lead to histogram at volume sizes 2–30 fl. MPV is calculated and PDW is width of the curve of distribution of platelets.

Scatterogram (Fig. 25.3)

Graph representing the distribution of two variables in the same population. The technologies used for scatter plot are volume, conductivity and scatters (VCS), peroxidase staining and fluorescence flow cytometry. The position that the dots appear on the cytogram screen are due to SS, the degree of FALS, absorption of light by each cell and dyes. Low FALS and SS—lymphocytes, increase FALS and SS is seen with monocyte, then neutrophils and highest with eosinophils. Basophil requires different windows. NRBCs are counted as WBCs.

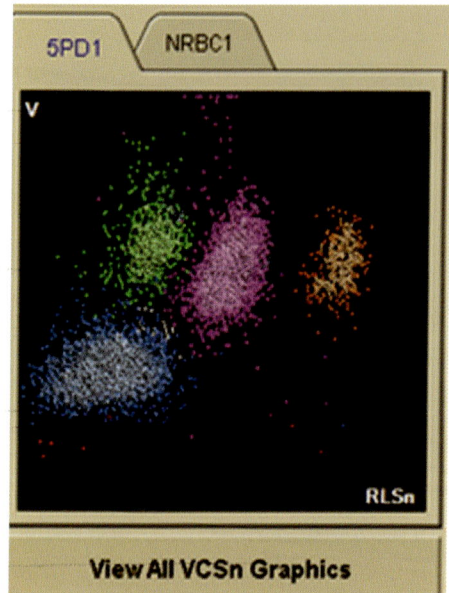

Fig. 25.3

Advanced parameters: Seen in high technology analysers. Reticulocytes, immature reticulocytes, reticulocyte hemoglobin, immature platelets, hematopoietic progenitor cells, absolute counts, NRBC correction, flagging for malarial parasites, blast, left shift, variant lymphocyte, giant platelet, platelet clumps, dimorphic reds, microcytes, macrocytes, hypochromasia. Flagging to review smear is also indicated.

Hb Estimation by HemoCue

Fingerprick blood drop is kept in a microcuvette in the strip which is coated with sodium deoxycholate (hemolyses the RBC), sodium nitrite (converts Hb to methemoglobin), sodium azide (converts methemoglobin to meth-hemoglobinizide). Absorbance of methemoglobinizide is measured at 570 nm. Results are displayed in 60 seconds in gm/dl on serum. Battery operated, portable, rapid and accurate method. Useful in acute clinical situations and blood camps.

ESR

The blood collected in the relative cuvettes (Na citrate/EDTA) is carefully mixed by the instrument. Then the samples are left to stand for a period in order for the sedimentation to take place. By means of a digital sensor (opto-electronic unit), the instrument automatically determines the sedimentation level of the erythrocytes following which the data is processed and then either automatically printed or shown on the display. Westergren method (1 hour) = Vesmatic method (25 minutes). Processing 20–80 samples at a time, external bar code reader, quality control set-up, temperature correction, display set-up, printer set-up available.

Coagulation

Coagulometers

Types (end point detection):
a. *Mechanical:* Magnetic steel ball (stationary/rotating) and viscometry
b. Optical:
   1. Turbidometry
   2. Chromogeneic
   3. Nephelometry
   4. Immunologic
c. Electrochemical

Mechanics of Coagulometers

Positive displacement pipetting, robotics for preparing and handling, computers for sample recognition data compilation and reporting of results, software to integrate results into HIS/LIS; some have centrifugation step. Contains monitoring devices and internal mechanism to maintain constant 37°C temperature throughout testing sequence.

Mechanical

In the stationary steel ball method sample cuvette rotates and steel ball remains stationery in a magnetic field. The formation of fibrin strands around the ball produces the movement. In the rotating steel ball method steel ball rotates under the influence of a magnet. The formation of fibrin strands around the ball stops it rotating which is detected by sensor.

Photo Optical

The formation of a fibrin clot in the plasma makes it denser optically. The light intensity is reduced when exposed to light at a wavelength of 660 nm. Chromogenic—color production and transmitted light detection.

Nephelometry

Quantifying plasma proteins based on the specific reaction of the protein being measured with highly specific antisera. Detects the amount of agglutination of particles by reading the increasing amount of light scattered at a 90° angle as agglutinates are formed.

Immunologic

The increase in light absorbance is proportional to the size of the agglutinates, which in turn, is proportional to the antigen level present in the sample, which is read from a standard curve.

Uses of Automated Coagulometers

Faster, visual errors in clot detection reduced, all the parameters of coagulation can be done including platelet function in advanced ones, clot waveform analysis can be done, sample rejection of inappropriate samples.

Electrochemical (IN Ratio Meter)

Uses single-use test strip is made of laminated layers of transparent plastic coated with tissue thromboplastin. Each test strip has a sample well where blood is applied. The device detects a change in electrical resistance when blood clots. Point of care testing device.

Platelet Aggregometer

The light transmittance of PPP is 100% and PRP plasma is 0%. The light transmittance is measured utilizing photometry and monitored on a chart recorder in waveform. When agonist is added PRP tends to aggregate and light transmittance increases. Five agonists, namely ADP, ristocetin, adrenaline, arachidonic acid, and collagen are added in different strengths. Variation in the characteristic wave with each agonist help in differentiating disorders affecting platelet aggregation and anti-platelet drug monitoring.

Platelet Function Analyser (PFA 100/200)

Simulator of platelet adhesion and aggregation in an environment that simulates an injured blood vessel. More sensitive screening test than the bleeding time. It is a non-specific test, not diagnoses any single disorder. The instrument has a bioactive membrane on which added citrated blood coated with collagen epinephrine/ADP. A pressure sensor detects the formation of a platelet plug which closes aperture in the membrane. Time is recorded. The result is a function of platelet count, platelet activity, von Willebrand factor activity.

Thromboelastography

Whole blood based analysis, monitors hemostasis in its entire process of clot initiation through clot lysis, measures the net effect of all hemostatic components interacting together during the clotting process. Demonstrates the hemostatic potential of a blood sample at a given point of time. Sample of whole blood is placed in a cup which has a pin carefully connected to a torsion wire. As the cup rotates in a back and forth movement, the aggregates formed within the cup cause the wire to become more rigidly placed and reflected via either an optical or magnetic detector.

The uses are:
  i. Illustrates function and dysfunction in the hemostatic system.
  ii. Allows physicians to give appropriate amount of FFP, cryo and platelets to control hemorrhage.
  iii. Reduces unnecessary use of blood products.
  iv. Allows effective management of hypercoagulability.
  v. Differentiates surgical from pathological bleeding.

Point of Care

The pieces of equipment used to test at bedside:
1. Electrochemcial (IN ratio meter)
2. Thromboelastography
3. Hemocue

Urine Analysis

Chemical analysis can be performed by using reagent strips. The strip reader is used to read the strips. The technically advanced urine analysers are able to read sediments by floweytometry (Sysmex UF systems) or digital imaging with (APR) auto particle recognition (Iris IQ system) or automated microscopy with digital imaging (sedi MAX). By flowcytometry the cells and casts in the uncentrifuged urine is categorised according to their fluorescence, size, impedance and forward scattered light. Digital imaging with APR classify and quantify urine particles in uncentrifuged urine based upon size and shape. The instrument which works on the principle of automated microscopy with digital imaging produces a monolayer of urine sediment by centrifugation in a special cuvette. The sediment is analysed by bright field microscope.

References

1. Dacie and Lewis Practical Hematology. 11th edn, 2011.
2. User manual Beckman Coulter, LH 780, 2011.
3. User manual Sysmex CS 2400, 2013.

CHAPTER 26
Component Preparation and Therapy

Vinod Panicker, R Krishnamoorthy

TRANSFUSION MEDICINE

Transfusion medicine is a multispeciality which includes blood banking, immunohematology, transfusion therapy, clinical practice, transplantation science and regenerative medicine.

Blood donors are the backbone of any blood transfusion service.

DONOR ELIGIBILITY CRITERIA

The prospective donor should appear to be in good health.
- **Age:** Donors should have completed 18 years of age and regular donors may continue to donate till the age of 65 if they are eligible otherwise.
- **Hemoglobin:** Hb should not be less than 12.5 gm/dl and the hematocrit should not be less than 38%.
- **Weight:** Donors weighing 45 to 55 kg can donate 350 ml and those weighing above 55 kg may donate 450 ml of blood.
- **Blood pressure:** BP should be in the range of 100/60 to 160/90 mm of mercury.
- **Temperature:** Temperature should not exceed 37.5°C/99.5°F.
  Pulse: Pulse should be between 60 and 100 per minute and regular.
- **Donor skin:** Skin at the venipuncture site should be free of any skin lesions.

There are specified periods of deferral for different medical conditions during which an individual is not eligible to donate either temporarily or permanently. In any case, the Medical Officer of the BTS takes the decision.

The interval between two consecutive whole blood donations should be minimum 3 months.

The Potential of Human Blood
Red Blood Cells
- To compensate the loss of blood after surgery, or
- To treat severe anemia.
  Storage: 42 days in the refrigerator (SAGM) 35 days (CPDA).

Fresh Frozen Plasma
- To correct a deficiency in coagulation factors, or
- To treat shock from burns or massive bleeding
  Storage: 1 year in the freezer.

Platelet Concentrates
- To treat or prevent bleeding due to low platelet levels.
- To correct functional platelet problems.
  Storage: 5 days at room temperature (20–24°C).

Cryoprecipitate

To correct fibrinogen deficiencies

Storage: 1 year in the freezer.

Component Preparation (for Safe and Adequate Therapy)

Components should be separated within 6–8 hours from the time of blood collection.

Component separation has to be done in a closed system of double/triple/quadruple bags under the laminar airflow bench.

If transfer bags are used, use a SCD (sterile connecting device).

Ensuring Sterility (for Safe Component Therapy)

- Sterile connecting device
- Laminar flow cabinet

Quality Control of Equipment (for Effective Component Therapy)

Each centrifuge should be calibrated for optimum speeds and times of spin for the preparation of each component.

A relative centrifugal force applicable for every component.

Relative centrifugal force formula:
Radius × (RPM) 2 × 1.118 1000

Storage (Proper Product Quality Maintenance)

Equipment used for storage should be monitored—must have

- Generator backup
- Alarms
- Thermograph charts

Storage Time (for Proper Product Quality Maintenance)

- Whole blood/PRBC in CPDA at 2–6°C in a BBR—35 days.
- Red cell suspension in additive (SAGM) — 42 days. Frozen red cells <–65°C in freezer for up to 10 years—cryopreservatives needed.
- Fresh frozen plasma, cryoprecipitate, cryo poor plasma <–30°C in a plasma freezer— 1 year from the date of collection.
- Platelet concentrate 20–24°C in a platelet agitator-cum-incubator 5 days.
- Peripheral blood stem cells—BBR (blood bank refrigerator), for up to 72 hours and freezer at <–80°C if used later than 3 days after cryopreservation.

Cellular Components (for Cellular Therapy)

- Red cell concentrate
- Red cells in additives
- Frozen red cells
- Rejuvenated red cells
- Platelet concentrate
- SDP (single donor platelets) prepared by apheresis
- Granulocytes by apheresis
- Leukoreduced components using leukocyte
- Filters

Plasma Components (Components Used for Therapy)

FFP (fresh frozen plasma)

Cryoprecipitate

Cryo poor plasma

Plasma Derivatives (Components Used for Therapy)

- Albumin 5% and 25%
- PPF (purified protein fraction)
- Factor concentrates
- Immunoglobulin obtained by fractionation.

BLOOD COMPONENT THERAPY

- *Red cells:* To restore tissue oxygenation.
- *Platelets:* To treat bleeding due to thrombocytopenia.
- *FFP:* Coagulation factor deficiencies
- *Cryoprecipitate:* As a source of fibrinogen.
- Factor VIII and von Willebrand factor.
- Specific factor concentrates.

Advances
- Leukoreduction
- Irradiation
- Peripheral blood stem cell collection
- Multiple component collection.

Leukoreduction (Done for RBC and Platelet Therapy): Methods of Leukoreduction
- Leukoreduced after collection using pre-storage filters.
- Blood is leukoreduced during collection by using in line filters.
- Leukoreduction done during transfusion using bedside filters.

Indications for Transfusion of Leukoreduced Blood Components
- To minimize febrile non-hemolytic transfusion reactions
- Neonatal transfusions
- Hemato-oncological malignancies
- Transplant recipients
- Prevention of HLA alloimmunization
- Platelet refractoriness in multitransfused patients
- Prevention of transmission of leukotropic viruses such as EBV (Epstein-Barr virus) and CMV (cytomegalovirus).

Blood Irradiation in Component Therapy
Indications
Prevention of transfusion associated graft versus-host disease (TA-GVHD) in cellular blood products given to:
- Patients receiving products from first-degree relatives or HLA-matched donors regardless of patient's immune status.
- Immunocompromised patients such as:
  - Infants (particularly premature) up to 4, 6, or 12 months depending on institutional policy.
- Intrauterine transfusion and/or neonatal exchange transfusion recipients.
- Congenital immunodeficiency, disorders of cellular immunity (i.e. SCID, DiGeorge)
- Hematopoietic progenitor cell transplant recipients.
- Hodgkin's disease, leukemia, or lymphoma patients.
- Patients treated with nucleoside analogs (i.e. fludarabine).
- Patients requiring granulocyte transfusions.*
- Solid organ tumor patients undergoing intense chemotherapy (controversial and not universal).
- Solid organ transplant recipient (controversial and not universal).
- Aplastic anemia with severe lymphocytopenia (controversial and not universal)
- Viral inactivation.

Blood Irradiation Process (Protocol for Effectiveness and Safety)
- Place the bag to be irradiated into the instrument.
- Move out of the room when the radiation process is on which lasts three minutes.
- The radiation dose applied is 25 Gy
- Personnel monitoring system (personnel safety monitor)
- Keep the room always under lock and key.

Apheresis Instrument (Uses in Component Therapy)
- *Single donor platelets (platelet apheresis):* One unit equivalent to 6 units of random donor platelets.
- *Red cell apheresis:* 1 or 2 units of packed red blood cells can be collected by this method.
- Granulocyte apheresis.
- *Peripheral blood stem cell collection:* Harvested
- Autologous and allogenic stem cells
- Therapeutic apheresis or therpeutic plasma exchange.

Apheresis Instrument (Use in Platelet Therapy)
- Indications for single donor platelets or platelet apheresis
- Mainly when platelet counts fall <20,000/µl

Common Indications
- Leukemias
- Myelodysplastic syndrome
- Aplastic anemia
- Chronic ITP
- Dengue

Red Cell Apheresis
Indications
- Polycythemia
- In hereditary hemochromatosis, red cell apheresis removes excess iron twice as fast as manual whole blood phlebotomy.
- Red cell exchange in sickle cell disease.

Granulocyte Apheresis
Indications
- Granulocyte therapy in severe leukopenia
- Granulocyte removal in leukemia with a very high count
- Granulocyte apheresis is undertaken in patients with ulcerative colitis.
- Granulocyte and monocyte apheresis suppresses symptoms of rheumatoid arthritis.
- Granulocyte and monocyte apheresis is also beneficial in patients with skin diseases like pustular psoriasis, allergic vasculitis and Behçet's disease.

Therapeutic Apheresis or Therapeutic Plasma Exchange
Definition: Therapeutic plasma exchange (TPE, plasmapheresis) is an extracorporeal blood purification technique designed for the removal of large molecular weight substances from the plasma.

Examples of these Substances
These include:
- Pathogenic autoantibodies
- Immune complexes
- Cryoglobulins
- Myeloma light chains
- Endotoxin
- Cholesterol containing lipoproteins.

Indications
Neurology
- Acute Guillain-Barré syndrome
- Chronic inflammatory demyelinating polyneuropathy
- Myasthenia gravis.

Hematology
- Hyperviscosity syndromes
- Thrombotic thrombocytopenic purpura (Exchange with plasma)
- Cryoglobulinemias
- Post-transfusion purpura.

Renal
- Goodpasture's syndrome
- ANCA (antineutrophil cytoplasmic antigen)
- Positive nephritis.

Metabolic
- Refsum's disease
- Hypercholesterolemia.

CHAPTER 27

Blood Bank—Laboratory Procedures

R Krishnamoorthy

There are different methods of doing blood grouping and cross matching. Blood grouping and Rh typing procedures using test tubes (tube method) are described below. Automated methods using the gel technology are also presently available.

Approximate speed of centrifugation using a laboratory (bench top) centrifuge.

Plasma/Serum

Separation in a test tube—3000 rpm × 10 minutes (from a sample of whole blood)
For cell washing—2000 rpm × 2 min (using normal saline)
For grading agglutination of 1000 rpm × 1 min

For performing immunohematology tests, a 3–5% red cell suspension in saline has to be prepared so that the red cell antigens would be present in optimal proportion to the antibody (present in commercial antisera or donor/patient serum) to be added subsequently. The serum: cell ratio normally used in immunohematology testing by the tube method is 2:1.

Preparation of 3–5% Red Cell Suspension

Wash the packed red cells at least once (with normal saline) and decant the entire supernatant after washing. Wash the red cells until the supernatant is clear and does not show hemolysis. To 5 ml of normal saline in a test tube, add 3–4 drops of the washed packed red cells using a Pasteur pipette. This will be a 3% RBC suspension (approximately).

Blood Grouping and Rh Typing

For ABO grouping, both "Forward" and "Reverse" grouping (back typing) should be carried out. There should be no discrepancy between the forward and reverse grouping results for a given blood sample. The principle of forward and reverse grouping is based on Landsteiner's law.

Forward grouping is done to look for unknown antigens on the red cells using known anisera. Reverse grouping is done to look for antibodies in serum.

ABO interpretation chart

Forward grouping				Reverse grouping			
Anti-A	Anti-B	Anti-AB	Anti-H	A cell	B cell	O cell	Blood group
+	0	+	+	0	+	0	A
0	+	+	+	+	0	0	B
+	+	+	+	0	0	0	AB
0	0	0	+	+	+	0	O
0	0	0	0	+	+	+	Bombay O

Rh Typing

Agglutination with anti-D is interpreted as Rh(D) positive and no agglutination with anti-D as Rh(D) negative. For all Rh(D) negative donor samples, weak D testing should be carried out.

CROSSMATCHING

Crossmatching is done to ensure compatibility between
a. The patient's serum and donor red cells (major crossmatch)
b. The donor plasma and patient's red cells (minor crossmatch)

Major crossmatch has to be carried out if donor packed red blood cells (PRBCs) are to be issued to a patient (recipient). Minor crossmatch has to be carried if plasma products like fresh frozen plasma (FFP) are to be issued.

Procedure

Take 2 test tubes and label them as 'major' and 'minor' appropriately.

Major crossmatch	Minor crossmatch
2 drops patient's plasma/serum + 1 drop of donor red cell suspension (3–5%)	2 drops donor's plasma/serum + 1 drop of patient's cell suspension (3–5%)
Mix	Mix

↓

Centrifuge at 1000 rpm × 1 min. Read result
(saline crossmatch)

↓

Incubate at 37°C for 30 min. Centrifuge and read.

↓

Wash 4 times with normal saline.

After the last wash, decant the supernatant entirely and add 1 drop of Coombs' serum **Coombs' crossmatch** to the dry cell button. Mix, centrifuge and read the results.

Interpretation

If agglutination is present at any stage, it is incompatible. If no agglutination, it is compatible. (Grade the agglutination as 4+, 3+, 2+, 1+, etc.) 0 denotes absence of agglutination.

Grading of Agglutination

4+—presence of one solid agglutinate
3+—several large agglutinates with a clear background
2+—medium-sized agglutinates with a clear background
1+—small agglutinates with turbid background.

COOMBS' TEST

Direct Coombs' Test (DCT)

- EDTA sample should be used.
- Prepare a 3–5% red cell suspension of the sample. Take 2 drops of the 3–5% red cell suspension in a test tube.
- Wash the red cells 3 to 4 times with normal saline. Decant the supernatant entirely after the last wash.
- Add 1 drop of polyspecific Coombs' serum to the dry cell button. Mix, centrifuge and read the results.
- If there is no agglutination, incubate the test tube at room temperature for 5 min. Centrifuge and read the results.

Interpretation

- If agglutination is present, DCT is positive.
- If no agglutination is seen, DCT is negative.

Positive Control

Positive controls (IgG sensitized "O" positive RBCs) and negative controls (known DCT negative RBCs) should be run in parallel when testing any sample to validate the test.

Applications of DCT: In investigation of suspected HDN, HTR, AIHA, DIHA.

Indirect Coombs' Test (ICT)

- Take 3 test tubes and label them as PC (for positive control), NC (for negative control) and 'test'.

- Add 2 drops of diluted (1:4) IgG anti-D to the tube labeled PC
- Add 2 drops of saline to the tube labeled NC
- Add 2 drops of patient's plasma/serum to the tube labeled 'test'
- Add 1 drop of pooled "O positive" red cells (3–5% suspension) to all 3 tubes
- Incubate all 3 tubes at 37°C for 45 min.

Wash the tubes 3–4 times with normal saline.

After the last wash, decant the supernatant entirely and add 1 drop of Coombs' serum to the dry cell button in all the 3 tubes. Mix, centrifuge and read the results.

Interpretation
- If agglutination is present, ICT is positive
- If no agglutination, ICT is negative.

Applications of ICT: The principle of ICT is applied in doing (a) antibody screening, (b) antibody identification, (c) compatibility testing, and (d) phenotyping for certain red cell antigens.

In both DCT and ICT, to all tubes that do not show agglutination, add 1 drop of IgG sensitized "O positive" red cells, mix, centrifuge and read. There should be agglutination.

Relevant Blood Bank Topics
- Blood donor selection
- Whole blood collection
- Blood components: Preparation, storage and uses
- TTI screening
- Forward grouping and reverse grouping
- Crossmatching
- Antibody screening and identification
- Coombs' test
- Transfusion reactions
- Autologous transfusion
- Apheresis
- Blood substitutes
- Stem cells

CHAPTER

28
Immunohistochemistry

S Rajendiran

GAME PLAN

1. Objectives
2. Introduction
3. Uses of IHC
4. Methodology
5. Quality control measures
6. Interpretation of results
7. Common IHC markers in use
8. Advances in IHC
9. Conclusion
10. References

Objectives

At the end of this presentation the participants should be:

1. Able to understand the principles of IHC
2. Able to perform IHC with a good control on quality
3. Able to interpret IHC stained slides
4. Able to use panels of IHC markers for diagnosis, prognosis and theranosis.

Introduction

IHC is identification of antigen located in a tissue by adding an antibody. This antigen antibody complex is made visible by a detection system with different color that can be seen by the light microscope. Clear idea of the terminologies is very essential for a clear understanding.

Polyclonal antibody production

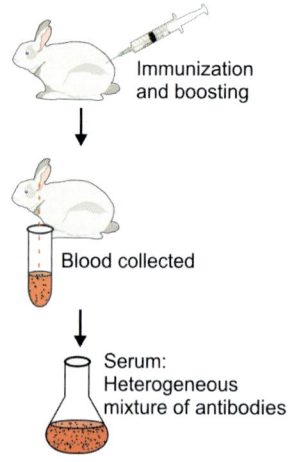

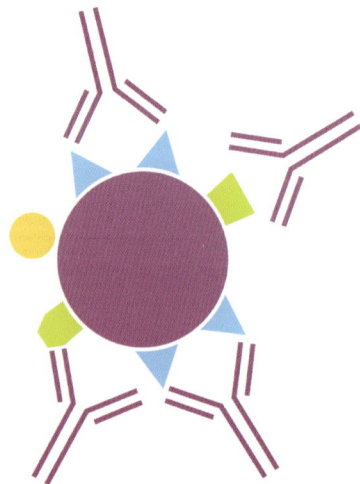

Fig. 28.1: Polyclonal Ab reacts with various epitopes of an antigen

Immunohistochemistry

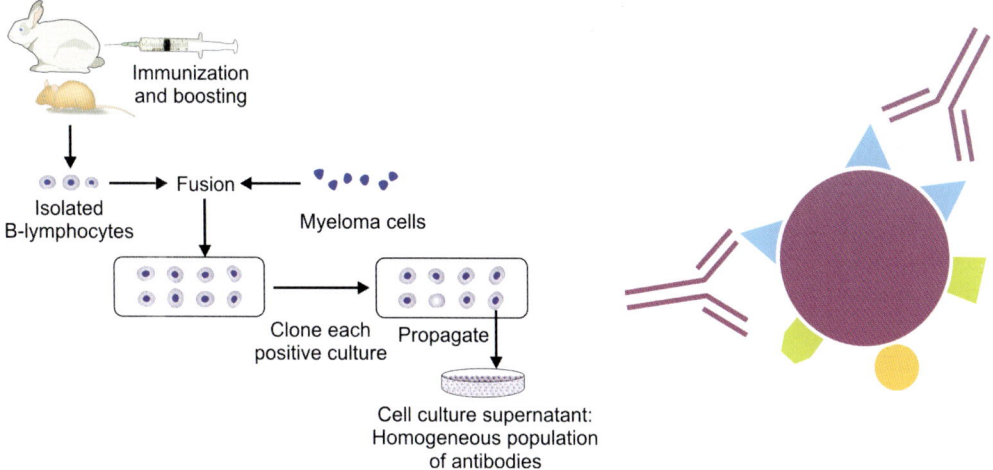

Fig. 28.2: Monoclonal Ab reacts with a particular epitope of an antigen

1. *Antigen:* What we are looking for in a tissue section. It can be a cellular substance (cytokeratin) or an organism (CMV).
2. *Antibody:* What was raised against an antigen. This can be monoclonal or polyclonal. It is usually IgG or IgM.
3. *Enzyme:* Attached to the antibody and act on the substrate to produce a colored end product (Horseradish peroxidase, calf intestine alkaline phosphatase).
4. *Substrate:* On which enzyme can act.

   DAB: Diaminobenzidine tetrahydrochloride: Brown color end product AEC—3-amino-9-ethyl carbazole—red color end product.

Uses of IHC

1. Diagnosis
   a. Cell of origin of primary tumors (carcinoma *vs* lymphoma)
   b. Organ of origin of secondary tumors (metastasis from lung or breast)
   c. *In situ* or invasive malignancy (basal cell markers—p63 in breast and prostate)
   d. Identification of infectious agents (CMV)
   e. Identification of extracellular material (amyloidosis due to β_2-microglobulin)
2. Prognosis
   a. Ki-67 in glial tumors, meningiomas and neuroendocrine tumors
   b. HER2/neu in breast carcinoma
3. Theranosis
   a. To guide specific therapy—c-kit in GIST, ER/PR/HER2/neu in breast carcinoma
4. Methodology

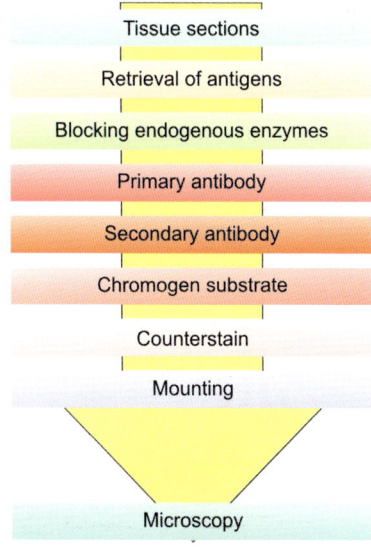

Fig. 28.3

Points to Pay Attention During the Procedure

1. Slides should be positively charged or coated with adhesive (albumin or lysine) to avoid dislodgement of the sections during the process.
2. Antigen retrieval enhances the sensitivity by unmasking antigen or its epitopes.
    a. Heat induced epitope retrieval (HIER): Pressure cooker, microwave (buffers used are sodium citrate, 1 mM EDTA or Tris EDTA)
    b. Enzymatic antigen retrieval (proteinase K, pepsin)
    c. Combined a and b
3. Antibody—pay attention to the storage temperature, dilution needed, incubation time and temperature.
4. Handle the chromogen carefully, especially DAB as it is a carcinogen.
5. Each test should be standardized in each lab as the working condition and other environmental factors are different.

Methods of Signal Amplifications

1. Direct method
2. Indirect method
3. PAP method
4. Avidin biotin complex (ABC)
5. Labeled streptavidin biotin (LSAB)
6. Polymeric method (dextran polymer)
7. Catalyzed signal amplification method (CSA)—amplification of tyramide
8. Rolling circle amplification (RCA)—amplification of oligonucleotide tail.

The newer technologies are increasing the sensitivity of antigen detection and the sensitivity chart as follows:
- *Standard:* ABC, PAP, LSAB
- *Moderate:* Polymeric method
- *Most:* CSA, RCA

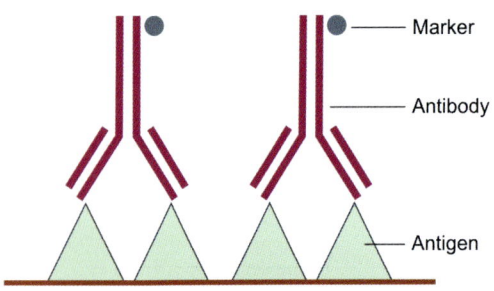

Fig. 28.4: Direct method

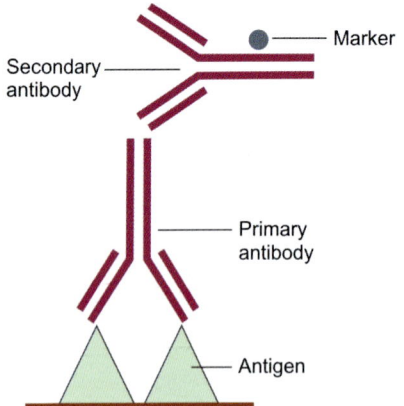

Fig. 28.5: Indirect method

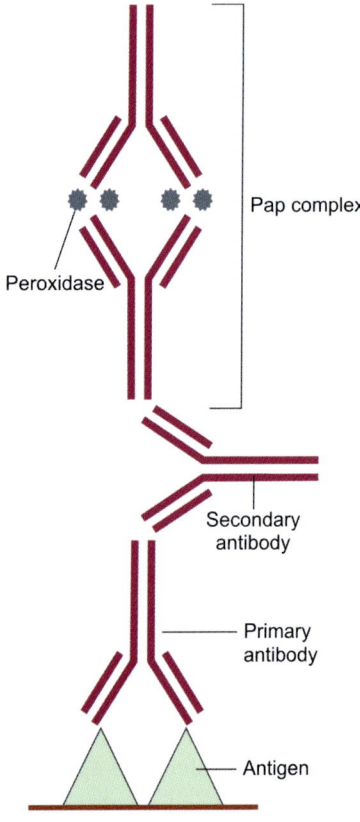

Fig. 28.6: PAP method

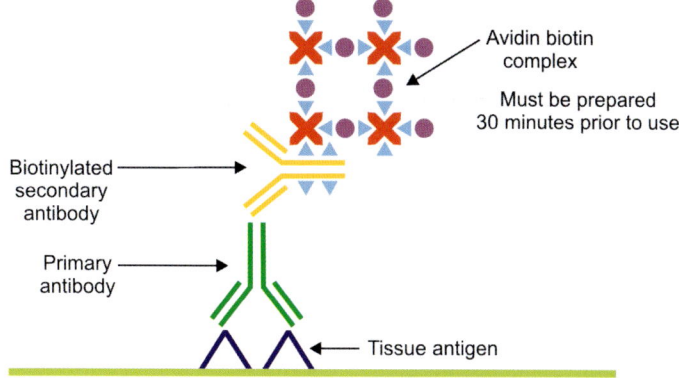

Fig. 28.7: Avidin biotin complex (ABC)

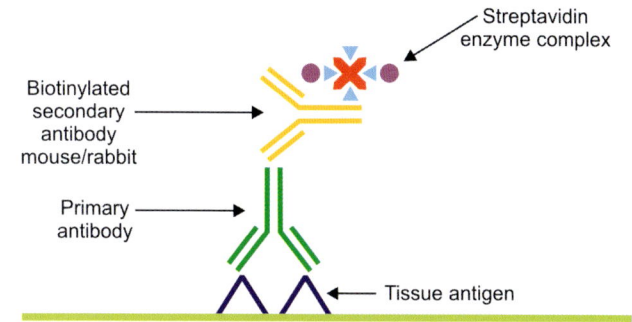

Fig. 28.8: Labeled streptavidin biotin (LSAB)

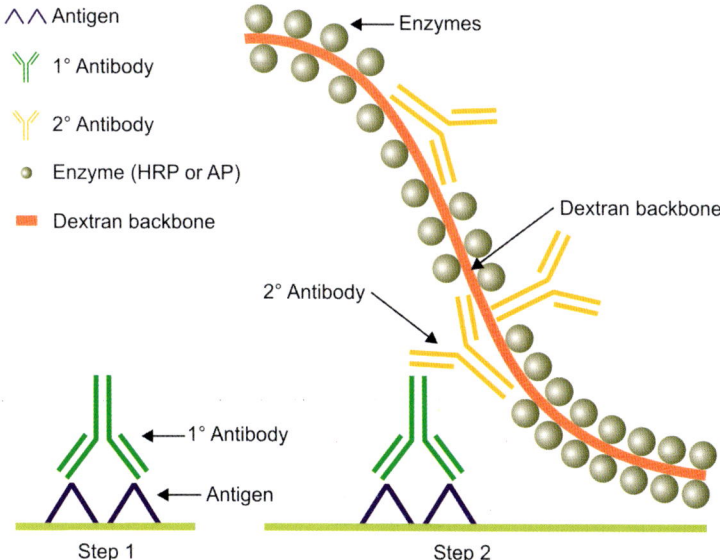

Fig. 28.9: Polymeric method (dextran polymer)

Quality Control Measures

The quality measures should be taken in the pre-, intra- and post-analytical phases. When interpreting the results, all the following factors should be kept in mind as each plays a vital role during the process.

Table 28.1
Pre-analytic
Test selection
Specimen type
Acquisition, pre-fixation/transport time
Fixation, type and total time
Processing, temperature
Analytic
Antigen retrieval procedure
Selection of 'primary' antibodies
Protocol; labeling reagents
Reagent validation
Control selection
Technician training/certification
Laboratory certification/QA programs
Post-analytic
Assessment of control performance
Description of results
Interpretation/reporting
Pathologist, experience and CME specific to IHC

A brief note on the control sections is important. They endure that each step of the complex IHC procedure has been performed carefully.

Positive Control

Running the test on a tissue known to be immunoreactive for a particular primary antibody. It should have positive staining. If it is negative, the result of the IHC on that batch would not be reliable. To verify the presence of antigenicity, vimentin should also be run as a control. This tests the presence of antigen, integrity of the antibody and validates the methodology.

Negative Control

Same section used for the positive control should be used but the primary antibody is replaced by non-immune antiserum in the same dilution as primary antibody. The slide should show a negative result and it validates the methodology. If a negative control is positive, no significance should be given to that batches IHC slides and the whole process should be repeated.

Interpretation of IHC

1. Location of the positivity
   a. Cellular
      i. *Cell membrane:* EMA, HER2/neu
      ii. *Cytoplasm:* Granular—organelles: HMB45, fibrillary actin, diffuse thyroglobulin
      iii. Nuclear: ER, PR, TTF1, p63
   b. Extracellular
      i. *Amyloid:* Calcitonin, light chains
2. Intensity
   a. Weak (mild)
   b. Intermediate (moderate)
   c. Strong
3. *Number of immunoreactive cells:* This depends upon the nature of antigen under investigation and the lesion. Usually a percentage of positive cells should be given in the interpretation. The terminology "focal" and "diffuse" can also be used.

Criteria for a Positive Result

This also varies from antigen looked for and the lesion under investigation. After a positive interpretation, all the three factors mentioned above should be included.

For example: In a case of rhabdomyosarcoma, the interpretation of IHC as follows:

Myogenin is positive. It shows nuclear positivity, moderate in intensity, in a diffuse pattern involving 90% of the tumor cells. Cytokeratin, LCA and chromogranin are negative.

Common IHC Markers in Use

Each cell lineage has its own markers. More than one marker can be there for one cell of origin. It is always better to use a panel having positive and negative markers rather than using a single marker.

The reason is although the markers are having a very good sensitivity and specificity none of them are 100% sensitive and specific.

And always remember that IHC is an ancillary study and its findings should be correlated with the H and E features and a good clinicopathological correlation should be present for a given final diagnosis.

Before going for the panel of markers, let us see the important markers indicating the lineage of the cells. Whenever more than one marker is available the most significant one are mentioned for teaching purpose and always keep it in mind that cross reaction can happen and nonspecific positivity can arise and hence H and E correlation is a must.

When you are encountering a marker for the first time, the cellular location of the marker is indicated by:

1. Nuclear and cytoplasmic
2. Nuclear
3. Membranous and others—cytoplasmic

Table 28.2

Cell lineage	Marker
Adipose tissue	S-100
All the cells	Vimentin
Chondrocyte	S-100
Epithelium	Pancytokeratin, EMA
Glial tissue	GFAP
Lymphoid cells	LCA (CD45)
Melanocyte	S-100, HMB45
Mesothelial cell	WT1, calretinin
Myeloid cells	MPO, c-kit
Myoepithelial cell	p63
Nerve	S-100
Skeletal muscle	Myogenin, desmin
Smooth muscle	Actin

Depending upon the H and E findings please use a panel of above said markers to narrow down the differential diagnosis. Then you can zero in the diagnosis by using another set of markers if it is clinically warranted.

Epithelial/Epithelioid Tumors

Once a tumor is positive for general epithelial markers, then they can be divided into 4 groups by performing CK7 and CK20. They are:
1. CK7+   CK20–
2. CK7–   CK20+
3. CK7+   CK20+
4. CK7–   CK20–

Table 28.3

CK7+ CK20– tumors	Other markers
Acinic cell carcinoma	34bE12, CAM 5.2, S-100
Adenoid cystic carcinoma	CEAm, p63, c-kit
Breast: Ductal carcinoma	GCDFP, ER, PR, E-cadherin
Breast: Lobular carcinoma	GCDFP, ER, PR (E-cadherin negative)
Cervical sq. cell ca.	HPV, p16
Choroid plexus tumors	GFAP, rare
Chordoma	EMA, S-100, brachyury
Craniopharyngioma	34bE1, CK5/6
Embryonal carcinoma	PLAP, CD30
Endometrial carcinoma	EMA, ER, PR
Lung: Adenocarcinoma	TTF1, surfactant protein, napsin
Meningioma: Secretory type	EMA, PR
Mesothelioma	WT1, calretinin
Ovary: Endometrioid ca.	EMA, WT1, ER
Ovary: Serous ca.	WT1, S-100, ER
Pleomorphic adenoma	P63, S-100, GFAP
RCC: Papillary and chromophobe	RCC marker, CD 10, PAX2, PAX8
Thyroid: Follicular	TTF1, p63, S-100, thyroglobulin
Thyroid: Papillary	TTF1, thyroglobulin
Thyroid: Medullary	TTF1, calcitonin, CEAm

Table 28.4

CK7– CK20+ tumors	Other markers
Colonic adenocarcinoma	CDX2
Merkel cell tumor	Chromogranin, synaptophysin

Table 28.5

CK7+ CK20+ tumors	Other markers
Cholangiocarcinoma	EMA, CEAp
Esophageal adenocarcinoma	–
Pancreatic ca.	DPC 4 lost in 55%
Ovarian mucinous	CDX2
Urothelial carcinoma	Uroplakin, thrombomodulin, p63

Table 28.6

CK7– CK20– tumors	Other markers
Adrenal cortical ca.	Inhibin, melan-A
Carcinoid	Chromogranin, synaptophysin
Epithelioid carcinoma	EMA
Esophageal, head and neck sq. cell ca.	p63
Seminoma	PLAP, CD117
Hepatocellular ca.	Hep Par-1, AFB, glypican
Lung: Sq. cell ca.	p63
Lung: Small cell ca.	TTF1, chromogranin, synaptophysin
Pheochromocytoma	Chromogranin, synaptophysin, S-100 (sustentacular cells)
Prostatic carcinoma	PSA
Renal cell carcinoma— clear cell type	RCC marker, CD10, PAX2, PAX8
Thymic carcinoma	CD5, p63, BCL-2
Thymoma	CD5, BCL-2 negative, p63 positive

Table 28.7 Small blue round cell tumors

Tumor	Markers
Melanoma	S-100, HMB 45, melan-A, microphthalmia TF2
Esthesioneuroblastoma	S-100, NSE
Neuroblastoma	NSE, NFP
Small cell carcinoma	Synaptophysin, chromogranin, TTF1
Merkel cell carcinoma	CK20 (dot-like +), synaptophysin, chromogranin
Desmo. small round cell tumor	Pan CK, EMA, desmin, WT1
Ewing/PNET	CD99, FLI-1
Medulloblastoma	NSE, synaptophysin
Rhabdomyosarcoma	Desmin, myogenin
AML	MPO, CD117
Lymphoma	LCA

Table 28.8: Spindle cell tumors

Tumor	Markers
Fascicular tumors	
DFSP	CD34
Endometrial stromal sarcoma	CD10, ER, PR

Contd.

Table 28.8: Spindle cell tumors (Contd.)

Tumor	Markers
Fibromatosis	β-catenin
GIST	DOG1, CD117, PDGFR-α
Leiomyosarcoma	Smooth muscle actin (SMA), caldesmon
Meningioma	EMA, PR
Mesothelioma Sarcomatoid type	WT1
MPNST	S-100, HNK1, PGP 9.5
Myofibroblastic tumors	Pan actin, smooth muscle actin
Perineuroma	S-100, EMA
Solitary fibrous tumor	CD34, CD99, MUC 4
Synovial sarcoma	EMA, CK, BCL-2, CD99, TLE1
Myxoid lesions	
Myxoid chondrosarcoma	S-100
Myxoid leiomyosarcoma	Actin
Myxoid liposarcoma	S-100
Epithelioid tumors	
Epithelioid leiomyosarcoma	SMA, caldesmon, CK
Epithelioid MPNST	S100, HNK1, PGP 9.5
Epithelioid sarcoma	EMA, CK, CD34
Granular cell tumor	Inhibin, S-100
PECOMA	HMB-45, melan A, SMA
Synovial sarcoma	EMA, CK, BCL-2, CD99, TLE1
Round cell tumors	
Desmo. small round cell tumor	Pan CK, EMA, desmin, WT1
Ewing/PNET	CD99, FLI-1
Glomus tumor	SMA, caldesmon
Neuroblastoma	NB84, NSE
Rhabdomyosarcoma	Desmin, myoglobin, myogenin
Pleomorphic tumors	
Leiomyosarcoma	SMA, caldesmon, CK
Liposarcoma	S-100
Rhabdomyosarcoma	Desmin, myoglobin, myogenin
Others	
Alveolar soft part sarcoma	TFE3
Angiosarcoma	CD31, CD34, FLI-1
Clear cell sarcoma	S-100, HMB45, melan-A
Kaposi sarcoma	HHV8, FLI1
Well and dedifferentiated liposarcoma	MDM2, CDK4

Table 28.9: Metastatic tumors of unknown origin

Type of tumor	Markers
Adrenal cortical tumor	Inhibin
Breast	GCDFP15, ER, PR
Carcinoid tumor, small cell carcinoma	Chromogranin, synaptophysin
Germ cell tumor	PLAP, OCT4, CD117
GIST	DOG1, CD117, PDGFR-α
Lung adenocarcinoma	TTF1
Lymphoma	LCA, CD3 (T cell), CD20 (B cell)
Prostate	PSA, PrAP, NKX 3.1
Sq. cell ca.	p63 (all SCC ... not specific for any site) p16/HPV (cervix, head and neck primary), CD5 (thymic sq. cell ca.)
Steroid tumors (ovarian stromal and hilar cell tr.)	Inhibin
Thyroid: Papillary and follicular	Thyroglobulin, TTF-1
Thyroid: Medullary carcinoma	Calcitonin, CEA
Trophoblastic tumors	Inhibin

Table 28.10: Specific differential diagnosis

Lung carcinoma

Small cell carcinoma	TTF1, chromogranin, synaptophysin
Adenocarcinoma	TTF1, ALK protein
Squamous cell carcinoma	p63
Epithelial mesothelioma	*Lung adenocarcinoma*
WT1, calretinin	TTF1, CEA
Signet cell carcinoma: Breast	*Signet cell carcinoma: Stomach*
ER, PR, GCDFP	CDX2, E-cadherin

Paget disease of skin and its differential

Mammary Paget	CK7, GCDFP15, HER2/neu
Extra-mammary Paget	CK20, GCDFP15
Sq. cell carcinoma *in situ*	p63
Melanoma *in situ*	S-100, HMB45
Hepatocellular carcinoma	*Cholangiocarcinoma*
HEP Par, CD10, CEAp, TTF1 (cyto), glypican	CEAm
Adrenal cortical carcinoma	*Pheochromocytoma*
Inhibin, MART1, synaptophysin	Synaptophysin, chromogranin, S-100 (sustentacular cell)

Contd...

Table 28.10: Specific differential diagnosis (Contd...)

Kidney tumors

Clear cell ca	RCC marker, CD10 +
Papillary ca	AMACR
Chromophobe	RCC maker +/−, CD10−
Oncocytoma	RCC marker, CD10−
Urothelial carcinoma	p63
Prostatic adenoca	PSA, PAP, AMACR, NAX 3.1
Endocervical ca.	Endometrial ca.
CEA, HPV, p16	Vim, ER, PR
Endometrial stromal sarcoma	Leiomyosarcoma
CD10	SMA, caldesmon

Germ cell tumors

Seminomatous seminoma	PLAP, CD117
Spermatocytic seminoma	CK, CD30 (Seminoma markers negative)
Embryonal carcinoma	SOX2, CD30
Yolk sac tumor	AFP, glypican-3
Choriocarcinoma	hCG, HPL, inhibin
Granulosa cell tumor	Inhibin, WT1
Sertoli cell tumor	Inhibin, EMA
Leydig cell tumor	Inhibin

Lymphomas

Table 28.11: NHL—B cell type

Tumor	Marker
Precursor lymphoblastic	CD19, CD79a, TdT, CD99
Small lymphocytic lymphoma	CD20, CD5, CD23, BCL-2
Mantle cell lymphoma	CD20, CD5, FMC, cyclin D1
Marginal cell lymphoma	No specific markers (exclusion diagnosis)
Follicular lymphoma	BCL-2, BCL-6, CD10
Burkitt lymphoma	CD10, BCL-6, EBER, Ki-67 (almost 100%)
Diffuse large cell lymphoma	CD20, BCL-6
Hairy cell leukemia/lymphoma	CD11c, CD25, CD103
Primary effusion lymphoma	HHV8, CD138
Plasmacytoma	CD138, CD56, EMA

Table 28.12: NHL—T cell type

Tumor	Marker
Precursor lymphoblastic	CD3, TdT, CD99
ALCL	Alk, CD30, EMA

Table 28.13: Hodgkin lymphoma (RS cells)

Tumor	Marker
Classic HL	CD15, CD30
Nodular LC predominant HL	CD45, OCT2

Table 28.14: Amyloidosis

Type	Marker
Primary AL	Kappa and lambda light chains
Secondary AA	Serum amyloid protein A (only IF now)
Dialysis associated	β_2-microglobulin
Tumor associated amyloid	Specific product (e.g. medullary carcinoma—calcitonin)
Alzheimer	β-amyloid
Other hereditary diseases	Transthyretin

Table 28.15: IHC for infectious agents					
Adenovirus	Aspergillus	B. henselae	BK virus	Candida	CMV
EBV (EBER, LMP1, EBNA2)		HBV	HSV1 and 2	HHV	HPV
H. pylori	Influenza A	JC virus	Leishmania	Listeria	Parvo B19
Pneumocystis	RSV	T. gondii	VZV	West Nile virus	
Prognostic markers	HER2/neu	Ki-67	p53	ER	PR

Table 28.16: Theranostic markers	
Tumor	Marker
GIST	CD117
Adenocarcinoma lung	EGFR, Alk
Breast carcinoma	ER, PR, HER2/neu, AR
B cell lymphoma	CD20

Advances in IHC

1. *IHC in tissue microarray:* Here, a recipient paraffin block is prepared by embedding multiple donor cores taken from different paraffin blocks.
   The main use is to perform IHC of multiple cases or multiple areas of same tumor in a single paraffin block. This helps not only in reducing the cost of IHC but also the time to do the IHC.
2. *IHC for dual markers:* This technique helps to view more than one marker (usually 2) in a given paraffin section. Different chromogens are used for different primary antibodies. Most commonly used in:
   a. B cell NHL to look for monoclonality of light chain (kappa and lambda expression)
   b. To differentiate *in situ* and invasive carcinoma (epithelial and myoepithelial markers in breast and prostate lesions).

Conclusion

IHC is a fabulous ancillary technique that helps the pathologists in many situations. But a few basic rules have to be remembered.
1. H and E is the gold standard and it cannot be replaced by IHC (IHC is a tool to be used cautiously… but remember "A fool with a tool is still a fool"…). A differential diagnosis should be formed before requesting the IHC by carefully reviewing the H and E features.
2. Never make a diagnosis based on IHC when the H and E findings are not supporting the IHC staining pattern.
3. Always call the clinician before ordering the IHC as some hidden history may help you to avoid doing IHC or to select the IHC markers.
4. At most caution is necessary during the interpretation. The markers may be positive in entrapped or surrounding benign cells in a lesion. The best example is TTF1 positivity in the benign alveolar epithelium in a biopsy showing pneumonia. Almost all the markers indicate the cell of origin and would not help in the differential diagnosis of benign or malignant condition (except a few like p53, AMACR).
5. Always use a panel, both positive and negative markers for a given lesion (for example, CK, TTF and LCA for a diagnosis of metastatic small cell carcinoma in a lymph node… as CK, TTF positivity and LCA negativity confirms the diagnosis and rules out lymphoma).

6. When all the markers are negative, make sure the antigenicity is preserved by demonstrating vimentin positivity. If it is also negative, you cannot rely upon the IHC findings.
7. Follow strict quality control measures. Pay attention when using new markers as aberrant expression may mean something that was not been reported/explained.
8. Keep updating your knowledge regularly as new markers are coming at astonishing speed.
9. Always get help from the seniors or experts in difficult cases.

References

1. www.google.com
2. http://www.dako.com/dist/08002_ihc_staining_methods_5ed.pdf
3. http://www.freefileforums.com/ebooks/3281926-manual_surgical_pathology_expert_consult_online_print.html

CHAPTER 29

Autopsy Highlights

G Barathi, Arthi M

ADULT AUTOPSY

After getting consent from the nearest relative, verify the name, IP number, age, sex and start the autopsy.

Instruments and Preparatory Equipment

- Cytology fixative
- Plain bulbs for blood and biochemical fluids
- Sterile tubes and swabs
- Syringe
- Spirit lamp
- Measuring cylinder
- Slide and smear
- Filter paper
- Microbiological broth
- Hack saw for cutting scalp
- Brain knife—10 inches for brain
- Enterotome
- Small scissor and long scissor, blunt end and pointed end
- Forceps—blunt/serrated scalpel, dissection knife
- Probes
- Bone cutting, knife
- Measuring tape, cartilage knife, chisel and hammer

External Examination

Head to Foot Examination

1. *Height to weight of the body:*
   – Height is measured using inch tape from head (crown) to heel.
   – Weight of the body is measured using digital weighing machine
2. *Head circumference:* Increased in hydrocephalus
3. *Chest circumference measured at the level of nipples:* Anteroposterior diameter is increased in emphysema and bronchitis
4. *Abdominal girth:* Abdominal distension due to gas/fluid.

General Examination

1. *Head:*
   – Scalp—look for injury, fracture of skull and texture of hair (in protein deficiency, decreased micronutrients like copper/selenium hair color changes)
   – Skull
2. *Mouth:* Open and look for gums and tongue
3. *Eyes:*
   – Conjunctiva: Jaundice/hemorrhage
   – Corneal opacity
   – Infections
4. *Nose and ear*
   – Discharge: Blood in injury to skull

5. *Neck:*
   - Palpate for any lymph node enlargement/carotids are examined for thrombus
   - Palpate for thyroid enlargement
6. *Examine the bony prominence:*
   - Shoulder—humerus
   - Neck—clavicle
   - Pelvis—iliac bone
7. *Thoracic cage:* Move the limbs to look for rigor mortis indicating the time of death
8. *Axilla:* Lymph nodes
9. *Breast:* Females particularly for any lump
10. *Ribs:* Any fracture and trauma
11. *Abdomen:* Organomegaly, ascites
12. *Umbilicus:* Position
13. *Abdominal skin:* Pinchability
14. *External genitalia:* Testis
15. *Inguinal region:* Lymph nodes
16. *Lower limbs:* Trauma
17. *Nails:* Color (pale/cyanosed) and clubbing
18. *Edema:* Pitting/nonpitting
19. *Femoral vein:* Collect blood for biochemical and microbiological culture
20. *Turn the body:* Look for congestion, trauma, abnormality.
    Sacral edema (dependent edema)—in bedridden patients.

Rigor Mortis

It is due to breakdown of ATP to ADP, thereby causing muscle fibers to contract. As ATP is resynthesized, rigor passes away. Muscular rigidity begins after 2–4 hours and disappears after 24–48 hours.

Livor Mortis (Postmortem Lividity/Postmortem Hypostasis/Postmortem Staining)

It is a consequence of the gravitational hypostasis of the blood in small superficial vessels in the dependent part of the body. First appears in the back of neck (most dependent part). Begins 30–45 min after death. Skin color is variable—commonly some shades of blue. Sometimes red if the body is kept in refrigerator.
- *Bright red:* Cyanide poisoning
- *Cherry red:* Carbon monoxide poisoning
- *Smoky grey:* Methemoglobinemia
- *Black:* Hydrogen sulfide poisoning.

Bony Deformities

- *Congenital deformity:* Achondroplasia/CTEV
- *Kyphosis:* Rickets/osteomalacia/fracture/collapse of vertebral bone
- *Lardosis:* Postural weakness/congenital
- *Scoliosis:* Poliomyelitis

Edema

Periorbital is the ideal place to check—due to loose connective, extracellular fluid collects fast in the loose areolar space.
- *Other areas:* Medial malleolus, sacral (bedridden patients), scrotal
- *Nonpitting edema:* Elephantiasis/hypothyroidism/Conn's syndrome
- *Pitting edema:* Nephrotic syndrome/acute nephritis/angioneuroticoedema/IVC obstruction/severe anemia.

Pigmentation

Generalized Pigmentation

1. Addison's disease
2. Hemochromatosis
3. Chronic malaria
4. Thyrotoxicosis
5. Cachexic patient

Localized Pigmentation

1. Pellagra
2. Neurofibromatosis
3. Chloasma
4. Chronic liver disease
5. Urticaria pigmentosa
6. Irradiation

Hypopigmentation

1. Leprosy
2. Leukoderma
3. Albinism
4. Fungal infections

Jaundice
- Yellowish discoloration of the sclera due to hyperbilirubinemia
- Jaundice with cyanosis—yellow blue or yellow green pigment
- Jaundice for long period in infancy—stain deciduous teeth green.

Hair
Distribution of hair on head, face, axilla, trunk, pubis and limbs are noted
- *Hair loss:* Debilitating illness or post-chemotherapy
- *Thick coarse hair:* Microcephalies
- *Thinning and drying of scalp hair*: Myxedema
- *In portal cirrhosis:* Loss of body hair in men or a change to female distribution of hair in late stages due to hyperestrogenism.

Face
To look for symmetry, cyanosis, fluid, froth from mouth, nose, ears
- Acromegaly
- Cretenism—widely spaced eyes
- Myxedema
- Mongolism—small skull with sloping forehead
- Down's syndrome.

Eyes
- Arcus senilis—ill-defined grey ring just inside the circumference of the cornea
- Kayser—Fleischer ring-greenish brown ring in the Descemet's membrane in Wilson disease
- Corneal opacity
- Cataract
- Exophthalmos—hyperthyroidism.

Nose
- Saddle nose—syphilis, leprosy and gargoylism
- Gangrene of the tip of the nose—bacterial endocarditis
- Large projecting friable polypoid mass—rhinosporidiosis
- Tumor

Ear
- *External ear:* Congenital abnormalities
- Hematoma
- *Bleeding from ear:* Internal (middle cranial fossa/head injury) hemorrhage
- *Gouty tophi:* Firm chalky nodules at the free border of the ear
- *Pinna damage:* TB, leprosy, syphilis, SLE
- *Pus discharge:* Otitis media

Mouth
- Oral candidiasis
- Condition of teeth (long standing tobacco—discoloration)
- Uremic frost—fine deposit of white crystals in severe azotemia.

Skull
- Palpation for fracture
- Local swelling
- Trauma

Cervical/Axillary/Inguinal Lymph Node
- Palpated and noted if enlarged
- Multiple/discrete/matted/size
- Soft/hard/mobility/location
- Warmth

Thyroid
- Size
- Nodularity
- Soft/firm/rubbery
- Adjacent lymph nodes

Neck Vessels
Engorgement

Thorax
- Look for symmetry
- Barrel-shaped chest seen in chronic respiratory disease.

Breast
- Size
- Mass lump—size, mobility, quadrant, consistency, number

- Nipple: Normal or retracted/puckered/fissure/inverted/Paget/discharge
- Areola: Normal or ulcerated/Paget
- Axillary nodes

Abdomen

- Presence or absence of protuberance or retraction
- Ascites
- Obesity
- Starvation
- Hernia
- Abdominal veins (cirrhosis)

External Genitalia

- General development
- Edema
- Local infection
- Positions of testis (if undescended search in inguinal canal)
- Scrotal skin
- Testis: Hydrocele/pyocele/hematocele/ulcer (STD)/torsion/tumor

Back

- Bedsores
- Spinal deformity (always turnover the body)
- Spina bifida, meningocele, meningomyelocele, cystic hygroma in pediatrics
- Adult: Pilonidal sinus
- Fistulous tract: TB/Crohn

General Condition of Skin

- Rash, petechiae, color, turgor.
- Dehydration.
- Edema, underlying infection/tumor.
- Pregnancy, ascites, obesity.
- Loss of elasticity of skin.
- Tightening of skin.
- Striae.
- *Spider angioma:* 2–5 mm, flat, red blue complexes seen on face, neck, thorax and arms in portal cirrhosis due to vasodilation due to hormonal changes.

Differential Diagnosis

Hereditary hemorrhagic telangiectasia/Osler-Weber-Rendu syndrome

- Wounds—swab for culture.
- Skin can be noted for petechiae, ecchymoses, purpuras, bullous lesions, etc.

Petechiae

- Pinpoint tiny hemorrhages less than 1 mm (<1 mm) in diameter.
- Hypoxia: Multiple organ failure m/s brain petechiae (red neurons are affected).
- Meningococcal meningitis.
- Subacute bacterial endocarditis.
- HIV, dengue fever (hemorrhagic viral diseases, Ebola and yellow fever).
- Vitamin C deficiency.
- Hematological complications due to thrombocytopenia as in acute leukemia, chronic lymphatic leukemia (CLL), CML (blast crisis).
- Platelet functional disorders.
- Aplastic anemia.
- Toxic shock syndrome (*Staphylococcus aureus*), fever + rashes.
- Asphyxia.
- Purpura (2–5 mm)—hemorrhage 2–5 mm in diameter.
- Ecchymoses (>5 cm)—hemorrhage >5 cm in diameter.
- Most common in coagulation factor deficiency like hemophilia A and B, factor 10 deficiency, etc.
- Hematoma—hemorrhage large enough to produce elevation of skin.

Purpura

- Hemolytic uremic syndrome.
- Microscopic angiopathies (red cell fragmentation syndrome) like TTP, ITP, DIC, HUS, liver failure (decrease of factors).
- Prosthetic valves, cerebral malaria, etc.

Definition of Macroscopic Terms

- *Macule:* Circumscribed flat lesion up to 5 mm distinguished from surrounding skin by its coloration.

- *Patch:* Circumscribed flat lesion >5 mm in diameter.
- *Papule:* Elevated dome shaped (or) flat topped lesion 5 mm and less.
- *Nodule:* Elevated dome shaped (or) flat topped lesion of spherical contour >5 mm across
- *Plaque:* Elevated lesion flat topped >5 mm, i.e. coalescent papules.
- *Vesicle:* Fluid filled raised lesion 5 mm or less.
- *Bulla:* Fluid filled raised >5 mm.
- *Blister:* Common lesion used to denote fluid filled lesion can be a vesicle or a bulla.
- *Pustule:* Discrete, pus filled raised lesion.
- *Wheal:* Itchy, transient, elevated lesion with variable blanching and erythema formed as a result of dermal edema.
- *Scale:* Dry, horny, plate-like excrescence.
- *Lichenification:* Thickening and rough skin.
- *Excoriation:* Breakage of epidermis.
- *Onycholysis:* Separation of nail plate.

Definition of Microscopic Terms

- *Hyperkeratosis:* Thickening of the stratum corneum.
- *Parakeratosis:* Retention of nuclei in the stratum corneum (on mucous membranes parakeratosis is normal)
- *Hypergranulosis:* Hyperplasia of the stratum granulosum.
- *Acanthosis:* Diffuse epidermal hyperplasia.
- Papillamatosis: Surface elevation caused by hyperplasia and enlargement of contagious dermal papillae.
- *Dyskeratosis:* Abnormal keratinization occurring prematurely within individual cells or groups of cells below the stratum granulosum.
- *Acantholysis:* Loss of intercellular connections resulting in loss of cohesion between keratocytes.
- *Spongiosis:* Intercellular edema of the epidermis.
- *Hydropic degeneration (swelling) ballooning:* Intracellular edema of keratocytes, often seen in viral infections.

- Exocytosis: Infiltration of the epidermis by inflammatory (or) circulating blood cells.
  Erosion: Discontinuity of the skin exhibiting incomplete loss of the epidermis.
- Ulceration: Complete loss of epidermis.
  Vacuolization: Formation of vacuoles within or adjacent to cells.
- Lentiginous: Linear patterns of melanocyte proliferation within the epidermal basal cell layer.

Conditions

- Macules:
  - <5 mm flat not raised
  - Typhoid, syphilis, focal (roseolar).
- Papules:
  - Elevated dome shaped <5 mm.
  - Measles, chickenpox, smallpox, drug eruptions like sulphonamides.
- Pustules: Staphylococcal
- Nodules:
  - Leprosy
  - Erythema nodosum
  - Tuberculosis (lupus vulgaris apple jelly nodules)
  - Secondary syphilis.
- Vesicles: Herpes, chickenpox.
- Café au lait patches: Dark brown patches, >5 in number is significant.
  a. Neurofibromatosis.
  b. Albright's syndrome

Where will you look for anemia?

- Lower palpebral conjunctiva.
- Tongue.
- Soft palate.
- Palm and nails.

Clubbing

Clubbing is bulbous enlargement of soft parts of the terminal phalanges with both transverse and longitudinal curving of the nails. It occurs due to interstitial edema and dilation of the arterioles and capillaries.

1. *Pulmonary:*
   - Bronchogenic carcinoma
   - Lung abscess

- Bronchiectasis
- TB with secondary infection
- Diffuse fibrosing alveolitis.

2. *Cardiac:*
   - Infective endocarditis
   - Cyanotic congenital heart diseases.

3. *Alimentary:*
   - Ulcerative colitis
   - Crohn's disease
   - Cholangitic cirrhosis

4. *Endocrine:*
   - Iatrogenic myxedema
   - Exophthalmic ophthalmoplegia
   - Acromegaly.

5. *Miscellaneous:*
   - Hereditary
   - Idiopathic
   - Unilateral—Pancoast tumor, subclavian and innominate artery aneurysm.
   - Unidigital—traumatic, tophi deposit in gout.
   - Only in upper limbs—in heroin addicts due to chronic obstructive phlebitis.

Pseudoclubbing

In hyperparathyroidism excessive bone resorption may result in disappearance of terminal phalanges with telescoping of soft tissues and a drumstick appearance of the fingers resembling clubbing. However, the curvature of the nail is not present.

Cyanosis

Cyanosis is bluish discoloration of the nails due to increased amount of reduced hemoglobin (more than 5 mg%) in capillary blood.

Types

1. *Central:* Skin, mucous membranes of tongue, palate, inner lip and conjunctiva.
2. *Peripheral:* Tip of nose, ear lobule, tip of finger, nailbed, cheek.
3. Mixed.

Central Cyanosis

It is due to increased circulation in warm areas like tongue, palate and inner lip.
- Cardiac—congenital cyanotic heart disease.
- TOF.
- Eisenmenger's complex
- Congestive cardiac failure.
- Pulmonary—chronic obstructive lung disease.
- Collapse and fibrosis of lung.
- Marked pulmonary destruction due to any cause.
- High altitude—due to low partial pressure of oxygen.

Peripheral

Occurs due to slowing of blood which allows more time for removal of oxygen by tissue.
- Cold (vasoconstriction).
- Increased viscosity of blood.
- Shock (cardiogenic).
- MI.
- Raynaud's disease.
- Polycythemia.

Mixed

- Acute left ventricular failure.
- Mitral stenosis.

Types of Incision

3 types (FM); some books 4 types.

A. Y-shaped Incision

Most commonly used:
- Begins at a point close to the acromian process.
- Extends down the breast across to xiphoid process
- From xiphoid process carried down to symphysis pubis.
- Umbilicus is usually avoided, so a slight curve to the left at umbilicus is taken. There are two reasons:
  1. To avoid cutting the ligament teres (umbilical remnant).

2. The fibrotic tissue below the umbilical skin is very difficult to suture after postmortem, it may not close to apposition giving way, which may be embarrassing.

B. Midline Incision (T-shaped)
Incision from suprasternal notch to symphysis pubis.

Then extends from suprasternal notch to over the clavicle to its center on both sides and then passes upwards over the neck behind the ear.

or

I-shaped incision: Just from the symphysis menti to symphysis pubis.

C. Inverted Y-shaped
In some cases before starting the autopsy a wooden block is placed under the back of the shoulder so that the neck is extended fully and the shoulder is flat for incision. The upper limbs of the Y shape is just beneath the breast to the xiphoid process of the sternum and extended down the midline up to the symphysis pubis, passing to the left of the umbilicus.

Why only from xiphoid process and neck incisions avoided?
To avoid disfigurement, body may be viewed before cremation.

In DIC, site of the suture has to be examined because there will be definite oozing of blood from the suture site.

What is morticea?
Reconstruction of the body after autopsy. After the incisions the skin along with the subcutaneous tissue is dissected laterally. A skin flap is dissected from the thorax to the abdomen muscle and ribs are exposed. Go as far lateral as possible.

Now do the test for pneumothorax (both sides have to be tested).
1. Make a pocket (pleural window) using the skin flap and thorax cage (chest wall), pour water into this pocket. Make a small knick into the intercostal space, if air is present in the pleural space it comes out as bubbles.
2. Another way is using a syringe without piston containing water and inject the needle into intercostal space, if pneumothorax is present air comes out of it.
3. In a case of tension pneumothorax the gas will escape with a definite hiss when the intercostal space is punctured.
4. Chest X-ray can be taken/CT scan.
5. Under seal water from the long tube.

PYROGALLOL TEST
It is usually done for air embolism in the right atrium. But can also be used for checking pneumothorax. 2% pyrogallol solution (4 ml) +4 drops (0.5 M) of sodium hydroxide. This is a yellow color solution which in presence of air turns brown.

If air is due to bacterial organism producing gas, there will not be color change to brown. It remains clear.

What is pneumothorax?
Air in the pleural cavity.

What are the types of pneumothorax?
1. Closed.
2. Open.
3. Tension.

What are the causes of pneumothorax?
1. *Traumatic:*
   a. Penetrating wounds—stab wound, fracture ribs, crush injury, lung biopsy, faulty tracheostomy.
   b. Nonpenetrating wounds—steering wheel impact against driver's chest.
   c. Following cardiothoracic surgery.
2. *Artificial:* For severe TB in older days.
3. *Spontaneous:*
   a. Ruptured emphysematous bullae.
   b. Ruptured congenital bullae.
   c. Pulmonary tuberculosis.
   d. COPD/suppurative lung disease like bronchiectasis, lung abscess, pneumonia, asthma.

e. Diffuse fibrosing pulmonary disease: Sarcoidosis, pneumoconiosis, interstitial fibrosis.
f. Pulmonary infarction.
g. Pleural neoplasm.
h. Miscellaneous—rupture of esophagus, Caisson's disease.

Differential Diagnosis

- *Large pulmonary cavity:* Hydropneumothorax.
- *Congenital large cyst:* Pyopneumothrax.
- *Eventration of diaphragm:* Hemopneumothorax.

Pyothorax

Pus in the pleural cavity. Example: Gangrene of lung, rupture of esophagus.

Most common bacterial organism: Klebsiella pneuomoniae, H. influenzae

Pus in the pleural cavity encapsulated by dense adhesions is termed empyema.

Lung abscess and pneumonia are common causes.

Hydrothorax (Effusion)

1. Myocardial failure
2. Chronic kidney/liver disease.

Hemothorax

Blood in the pleural cavity.
- Trauma.
- Most common due to tumor (malignant effusion).
- Tuberculosis.
- Disease of hemorrhagic diasthesis.
- Ruptured aneurysms.

After testing for pneumothorax, the dissection of rib cage is done. Sternoclavicular joint is dissected using bone saw or rib knife and the cut is extended down through the costochondral junction to the entire rib cage on either side and the bone is cut using bone nibbler or hammer chisel or rib rongeur. In children, the cartilage is easy to cut. Now the cut portion of the rib (anterior chest wall) along with sternum is reflected up the releasing any adhesions from beneath and removed. Marrow slides can be prepared using the sternum and fixed for examination.

Now the tongue is released from its posterior attachments, cutting through the soft palate and the inferior ramus of the mandible by releasing (cutting) the muscular attachments. The posterior (larynx) pharyngeal wall along with the epiglottis and tongue is now pulled forward. Care should be taken not to injure the neck vessels and thyroid. Examine all the neck structures for thrombus or emboli and then is pulled further down.

Examination of Pericardium

When the anterior chest wall is removed, look for all the thoracic organs *in situ*. Examine if dextrocardia is present, look for any herniation (diaphragmatic/hiatus hernia) or other congenital anamolies like number of lobes in the lung. Pathological conditions like adhesions, petechiae and hemorrhage on the organs.

Now that the pericardium is identified by the pulmonary conus that is present. A small nick is made on the fibrous pericardium and tested for air embolism from major vessels. The serous pericardium is also stripped and heart is delivered. If the blood culture is required it is ideal to take from the right atrium directly by using a syringe. The area is made sterile by using a heated spatula and right atrium is seared using hot spatula.

Dissection of the Abdominal

Abdominal incision is extended by cutting the peritoneum using a scissor and all the bowel loops are examined. Spleen and liver are examined. Look for emphysematous, volvulus, intussusceptions, adhesions or any other gross pathology. Right iliac fossa is looked carefully and appendix is examined. Bowel loops are retracted and reflected. Identify the duodenojejunal junction and tie two ligature 1 inch apart and cut in between the ligatures to avoid soiling. Similar ligatures are tied at the lower most portion of the rectum and cut it. Mesenteric fat is cut as close as to the bowel loop. Cut the bowel open at the anti-mesenteric end and pin it to a large board and examine the mucosal surface.

Tongue is pulled forward and along with epiglottis it is separated from the vertebral column. Neck vessels on both sides are severed at neck and sternoclavicular junction. Adhesions of lung to the back is released and enter block is pulled down, cut through the diaphragm and pull the bloc towards the prosector and removed 'en bloc'.

Bladder is removed along with prostate and urethra. Prostate is hard to feel. In the superior part of urinary bladder a cord-like structure, ductus deferens leads to inguinal canal. Muscle above is cut, ductus deferens is continued with spermatic cord and gently push the testis into the inguinal canal and to pelvis and delivered out.

Identify both the ureters. Bladder is released from the pelvic floor along with prostate, prostatic urethra and rectum. Thoracic and abdominal blocs together is removed (en bloc)

It is placed with the posterior part facing up. Always start dissection of the adrenals first, otherwise it may be lost. Left adrenal is semilunar shape, right adrenal is triangular in shape. Adrenals are golden yellow in color on cut surface. Start opening the aorta from descending aorta. Note renal ostia (press kidney to identify the renal artery—blood oozes out indicating the patency). Celiac, superior mesentery, renal and inferior mesentery ostia noted.

Kidneys are released. Open the aorta further, separate from lower IVC come all the way to the diaphragm where the aorta pierces the diaphragm and dissected.

Posterior to trachea esophagus is cut at the level of oropharynx from the neck structures. Cut through the diaphragm and kept along the abdominal cavity.

Thoracic Bloc

- Thyroid is first cut.
- Heart and lung fixed by perfusion technique.
- Larynx is cut through posterior aspect along with trachea. All are examined.
- Separate the heart from lung at the hilum along with great vessels.
- Pericardium is opened using inverted Y-shaped incision. Look for any fluid (normally 20–50 ml is present)
- Examining the great vessels are important—look for transposition and other congenital anomalies.
- Pulmonary artery bifurcation is examined for emboli.
- *Inflow–outflow method of dissecting heart:* Right atrium is opened by cutting the IVC and SVC. The foramen ovale is examined for any patency with the probe. The auricle is examined for clot. The right ventricle is opened by cutting through the tricuspid valve. The valves are carefully inspected and their lengths are measured. The pulmonary outflow tract is cut in the anterior wall of the right ventricle and continues up through the pulmonary valve and artery. The left atrium is opened by joining the right and left pulmonary veins. The left ventricle is cut down the left border of the heart. The outflow tract is opened from the apex along the anterior wall and then through the aortic valve and aorta. The aorta is examined for atheroma and fibrosis. The coronary vessels are opened along their length.

Identification Parts in Heart

- Heart along with great vessels.
- Right atrial appendage is triangular.
- Left atrial appendage long, narrow neck and multiple hooklets.
- Aorta is situated posteriorly and to the right.
- Pulmonary artery is anteriorly and to the left.
- Right atrial appendage is cut in front of IVC.
- Orifice is examined for tricuspid valve (3 fingers allowed).

- Cut through the right border of the heart into the right ventricle extending up to the right ventricular apex.
- Right atrium—sinus venereum, tricuspid annulus, right ventricular cavity.
- Pectinate muscle—rough internal structure.
- From right ventricular apex cut through the right ventricle parallel to the anterior ventricular septum and through the pulmonary artery.
- Feel through the pulmonary orifice (valve) cut extends into left pulmonary artery, 3 cusps examined, right pulmonary artery is also cut.
- Posteriorly, the pulmonary vein is connected and cut.
- Left border of heart.
- Left atrium and left ventricle and mitral valve examined.
- Put a probe into aorta and cut parallel to posterior interventricular septum extend into aorta arch and thoracic and abdominal aorta.

Right Atrium

- Pectinate muscle
- Smooth portion (trabeculae).
- Fossa ovalis—rimmed by limbus ovalis.
- IVC opening.
- Beneath the fossa ovalis is the opening (ostia) of the coronary sinus guarded by a valve.
- Tricuspid annulus—posterior tricuspid leaflet, septal, posterior.

Right Ventricle

Papillary muscles—anterior, medial (for surgeons).

Triangle of Koch

- It is to identify the AV node.
- Draw a line from the superior margin of the coronary sinus, goes down to meet the tricuspid annulus called central fibrous body which forms the apex. AV node pierces the central fibrous body and divides as right and left bundle branches.

Right Ventricle

- Rough ventricular trabeculae.
- Wall thin.
- Inlet portion and outlet portion.

Left Ventricle

- Smooth trabeculae.
- Wall thick.

Pulmonary Valves

- 3 cusps.
- Left, right (ligamentum arteriosus, a dimple in the pulmonary artery).

Left Atrium

Smooth portion

Mitral Valve

Anterior—broad; posterior—narrow.

Papillary Muscle

Chordae/commissural muscle.

Aortic valve

3 cusps

Coronary Artery Dissection

Identify right atrioventricular groove where right coronary artery is situated. Cut at 0.2–0.5 cm interval. Transversely cut through to look for thrombus. Calcification is seen in elderly people.

Posterior right atrioventricular groove—to trace right coronary artery.

Left coronary artery from ostia traced and cut—divides into left anterior descending (left IV groove) and left circumflex (left AV groove).

Myocardial infarction—cut longitudinal towards the myocardium to look for infarct (fresh or healed).

Pericardial Effusion

- Normally 5–50 ml fluid present, clear yellow to straw colored
- Can accumulate 500 ml–1 litre

- Pericardium is examined for effusion, pericarditis (bread butter in rheumatic fever), cardiac tamponade (cardiac filling is restricted) brown atrophy of heart, cardiomegaly, petechial hemorrhage.
- Dry pericardium—extreme dehydration as in cholera
- Transudate—hydropericardium
- Exudate—serous pericarditis
- Pus—purulent pericarditis
- Blood—hemopericardium

White spots called milky spots or soldier spots are seen as a result of old healed pericarditis.

Serofibrinous Pericarditis
- Rheumatic fever
- Recent MI.
- Uremia.
- Viral

Serofibrinous Pleural Effusion
- Early bronchopneumonia
- Pulmonary infarct
- Early TB

Fibrinopurulent
- Trauma
- Adjacent organ involvement
- TB pericarditis

Pleural Effusion
- Bronchopneumonia
- Lung abscess
- Trauma
- Putrid gangrene of lung
- Rupture of esophagus

Hemorrhagic
- Tumors
- Rupture of heart
- Aneurysm aortic/pulmonary artery
- Tuberculosis
- Malignant tumors
- Hemorrhagic diathesis
- Ruptured aneurysm

Terminologies
- *Mediastinopericarditis:* Heart is attached to adjacent structures by fibrous tissue
- *Constrictive pericarditis:* Adhesion that limits the diastolic expansion of heart. Most commonly seen in tuberculous pericarditis
- *Levicardia:* Apex pointing to left
- *Mesocardia:* Apex pointing to midline
- *Dextrocardia:* Apex pointing to right

Normal measurements of heart—measures 12 × 9 cm.

Weighs 300 gm in males and 250 gm in females

Valve	Diameter of the orifice
Pulmonary	– 2.5 cm
Aortic	– 2.5 cm
Mitral	– 3 cm
Tricuspid	– 4 cm

Left ventricular wall thickness—1.3 to 1.5 cm.

Right ventricular wall thickness—0.3 to 0.5 cm.

SA node: Sinoatrial node or pacemaker situated at the atriocaval junction in the upper part of the sulcus terminalis.

AV node: It is situated in the lower and dorsal part of the atrial septum just above the opening of the coronary sinus (triangle of Koch).

How will you measure the valves?
Circumference of the valve is measured by:
a. Graded glass or wooden cones or metal probes 1 to 10 mm.
b. After opening the ring measured by ruler or string.

How to measure thickness of myocardium (ventricular wall)?
Measured 1 cm below the pulmonary valve or mitral valve, only the compact portion of the myocardium is measured and trabecular carneae not included.

Name 3 conditions with right ventricular hypertrophy
1. Tetralogy of Fallot (TOF)
2. Tricuspid regurgitation (TR)
3. Ventricular septal defect (VSD)

Concentric hypertrophy of left ventricle
Hypertension

Asymmetrical hypertrophy of left ventricle
- Aortic stenosis
- Cardiomyopathy
- Aortic regurgitation

Conditions with hypertrophy and dilatations
- Mitral regurgitation
- Aortic regurgitation

Conditions of acute dilatation of right ventricle
- Massive pulmonary embolus
- Wet beriberi

What are fatty streaks and atheromatous plaques stained with?

Fatty streaks and atheromatous plaques are stained with Sudan IV after a few minutes plaques will turn red.

Where is SA node and AV node located?
- *SA node:* At the junction of SVC and RA
- *AV node:* In the triangular space of Koch formed by opening of coronary sinus central fibrous body and tricuspid annulus.

Difference between postmortem clot and antemortem clots.

Table 29.1

Postmortem clot (formed after death)	Antemortem clot (thrombi results from stagnation of blood within the heart or vessels during life)
Moist smooth rubbery slippery homogenous and uniformly darkened	Drier brittle (breaks off sharply, elastic, uneven surface (never smooth and glossy)
Not attached to the endocardium	Attached to the endocardium
No lines of Zahn	Lines of Zahn present

Lines of Zahn

Alternating layer of fibrin and platelets on which more blood is deposited.

What are the different methods of opening the heart?
1. Inflow–outflow method
2. Short axis method
3. Four-chamber method
4. Long axis method
5. Base of heart method
6. Window method
7. Unrolling method
8. Pontition method
9. Injection corrosion method
10. Dissection of the cardiac conduction system.

Some named techniques:
- Schlesinger
- Rodriguez and Rainer

What is perfusion fixation technique?
- Cascade system
- Fixative cascades through stacked plastic containers and flows through nozzles tied into the main bronchus
- An electric pump is mounted to one of the central rails
- Keiserling solution or 10% formalin is used to gravitate perfuse the specimen
- Fixative is circulating
- Distance between each container is maintained (30–33 cm) so that perfusion pressure (30–33 H_2O) is achieved.

What are the organs that are fixed by perfusion fixation method?
- Lungs
- Heart
- Liver
- Kidneys

Vasculature of Heart
1. Arterial supply of heart
2. Right coronary artery supplies
    - Right atrium
    - Major portion of right ventricle except the area adjoining the anterior IV groove
    - A small part of left ventricle adjoining the posterior IV groove

- Posterior part of the IV septum
- Whole of the conducting system of the heart except a part of left branch of AV bundle
- SA node is supplied by left coronary in 40% of cases.

Branches of Right Coronary Artery

Larger branches – Marginal artery
– Posterior interventricular branch

Smaller branches – Nodal arteries in 60% of cases
– Right arterial
– Infundibular
– Terminal

Course of Right Coronary Artery

Arises from the anterior aortic sinus (from ascending aorta)

It passes forward and to the right to emerge on the surface of heart between right auricle and pulmonary trunk.

Runs downwards in the right anterior coronary sulcus to the junction of the right and inferior borders of the heart.

It winds around the inferior border to reach the diaphragmatic surface and runs backwards and to the left in right posterior coronary sulcus to reach the posterior interventricular groove.

Terminates by anastomosing with LCA.

Left Coronary Artery

It is larger than right coronary artery. It arises from the left posterior aortic sinus.

Branches

Large branches: Anterior interventricular branch otherwise called as left anterior descending artery (LAD).

A branch to diaphragmatic surface of left ventricle.

Smaller Branches

- Left atrial
- Pulmonary
- Terminal

Areas of Distribution

- Left atrium
- Left ventricle greater part except a small part adjoining the posterior IV groove
- A small part of right ventricle adjoining the anterior IV groove
- Anterior part of IV septum
- Apart of left branch of AV bundle.

Course of LCA

Arises from the posterior aortic sinus:
- It first runs forward and to the left and emerges between pulmonary trunk and left auricle
- Here it gives of anterior branch (LAD) which runs downwards in the anterior IV groove
- Further continues as left circumflex artery
- It runs towards the left in the left anterior coronary sulcus
- It winds around the left border of the heart and continues in the left posterior coronary sulcus.

Collateral Circulation

a. *Cardiac anastamosis:* The two coronary arteries anastomose with each other in the myocardium.
b. *Extracardiac anastamosis:*
   - Vasa vasorum of aorta and pulmonary arteries
   - Internal thoracic arteries
   - Branchial arteries
   - Phrenic arteries (channels may open up when both coronaries are obstructed)
c. Retrograde flow of blood in the veins may irrigate the myocardium.

Venous Drainage of Heart

1. Greater cardiac vein
2. Middle cardiac vein
3. Small cardiac vein
4. Posterior vein of left ventricle
5. Oblique vein of left atrium (vein of Marshall) develops from the left cardinal vein (duct of Cuvier)
6. Right marginal vein

Lymphatic of Heart

- *Right trunk:* Brachiocephalic nodes
- *Left trunk:* Tracheobronchial nodes

Nerve Supply of Heart

1. Parasympathetic via vagus—cardioinhibitory. On stimulation slows down heart rate.
2. Sympathetic nerve from upper 3–5 thoracic segments, cardioaccelerators. On stimulation increases heart rate.
3. Superficial cardiac plexuses
4. Deep cardiac plexuses.

FAQ

1. What are the methods of autopsy?
2. What are the types of incision?
3. Prerequisites for autopsy.
4. Consent
5. Demonstration of pneumothorax.
6. Difference between antemortem and postmortem clots.
7. Gross examination of all organs (pathological features).
8. Ideal site for blood culture.
9. Branches of aorta.
10. Perfusion fixation, organs fixed by this method.
11. Saddle emboli.
12. Circle of Willis.
13. Signs of cirrhosis.
14. Causes of hepatosplenomegaly.
15. Minimally invasive autopsy.
16. Weight of the organs.
17. Dimension of cardiac valve.
18. Fixation of brain.
19. Portosystemic communications.
20. Should be able to arrive of the cause of death for the given case.

Table 29.2: Portosystemic communications

Site	Portal	Systemic
Umbilicus	Left branch of portal vein	Anterior abdominal wall
Lower end of esophagus	Esophageal tributaries of left gastric vein	Esophageal tributaries of the accessory hemiazygous vein
Anal canal	Superior rectal vein	Middle and inferior rectal vein
Bare area of liver	Hepatic venules	Phrenic and intercostal veins
Posterior abdominal wall	Right colic, left colic, middle colic, splenic with azygous vein	Veins of renal, adrenal
Liver (intrahepatic)	Left branch of portal vein	Inferior vena cava

CHAPTER
30

Important Histochemical Stains

G Barathi, Divya D, Subalakshmi B, GA Vasugi, Archana B, Arthi M, Gokul Kripesh

MASSON'S TRICHROME

Purpose
Used to differentiate between collagen and smooth muscle in tumors, and the increase of collagen in diseases such as cirrhosis. Routine stain for liver and kidney biopsies.

Principle
Three dyes are employed selectively staining muscle, collagen fibers, fibrin, and erythrocytes. The principal rule in trichrome staining is that the less porous tissues are colored by the smallest dye molecule and whenever a dye of large molecular and size is able to penetrate, it will always do so at the expense of the smaller molecule.

The other mechanism is that the tissue is stained first with the acid dye, Biebrich Scarlet, which binds with the acidophilic tissue components. Then when treated with the phosphoacids, the less permeable components retain the red, while the red is pulled out of the collagen. At the same time the collagen is bound to the aniline blue.

Results
Nuclei: Blue black
Cytoplasm, muscle, erythrocytes: Red
Collagen: Blue

APPLICATIONS
- Used to distinguish collagen from muscle and aid in the diagnosis of fibrotic changes, neuromuscular diseases, and tumors of muscle origin.
- Stains type 1 collagen that is normally present in the portal tracts and vessel walls, but also highlights the presence and distribution of reactive fibrosis as a result of liver injury.
- Used for staging of chronic liver diseases, and helps to delineate patterns of injury, such as the perisinusoidal fibrosis associated with steatohepatitis and periductal fibrosis in primary sclerosing cholangitis.
- Used in determining the degree of collagenization in cirrhosis, myelofibrosis, scleroderma and also in diagnosing soft tissue tumors.
- Masson's trichrome highlights the subepithelial deposits (humps) in renal biopsies especially in acute post-streptococcal glomerulonephritis.

STAINS FOR CARBOHYDRATES

Carbohydrates
Main source of energy to the body:
Group 1: Neutral polysaccharides
Group 2: Acid mucopolysaccharides, carboxylated and sulphated.
Group 3: Glycoproteins
Group 4: Glycolipds

Mucin

Clear visicid intracellular secretions and are polysaccharides which are bound to other substances.

PERIODIC ACID-SCHIFF (PAS) STAIN
Principle

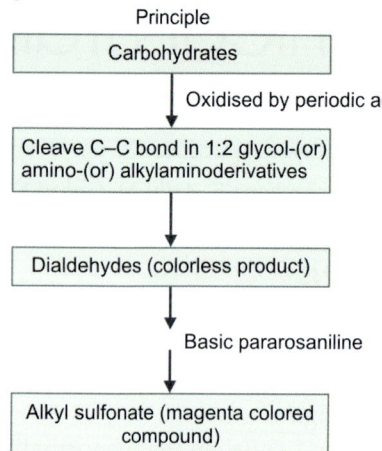

Fig. 30.1

Reagents
- Periodic acid 1% (periodic acid: 1 gm, distilled water: 100 ml)
- Schiff's reagent (basic fuschin: 1 gm, distilled water: 200 ml, Conc. of HCl: 2 ml, activater charcoal: 2 gm)
  Basic fuschin Composition: Rosaniline, pararosaniline, magenta II
  Store at 4°C in a dark container.

Control: Appendix
Results: PAS +ve substances: Magenta
Nuclei: Blue

PAS POSITIVE SUBSTANCES
- A: Alpha 1-antitrypsin, amoebae, amyloid
- B: Basement membrane
- C: Cellulose, collagen, chitin, cerebrosides, corpora amylacea
- E: Elastin
- F: Fibrin, fungus
- G: Gastric mucous neck cells, glycogen, granular cells
- L: Lipofuscin, lymphoblasts
- M: Melanosis coli pigment, megakaryocytes, myelocytes
- N: Neutral mucin, neutrophils
- P: Paneth cell granules, pancreatic zymogen granules, platelets, plasma and serum
- R: Russell bodies, reticulum
- S: Sialomucin, starch
- T: Thyroid (colloid)

Applications
1. Polysaccharides
   - Leukocytes containing glycogen
   - Capsule of bacteria and fungi (neutral polysaccharides)
2. Glycoproteins
   - Mucin and mucoid secretions of the intestinal tract, glands and their ducts.
   - Hormones TSH, thyroglobulin, serum mucoproteins and hyaline proteinaceous renal casts.
   - Russell body (mucoprotein)
   - Bone marrow, collagen, megakaryocytes
   - Sailoglycoproteins of ovarian pseudomucinous cystadenoma
3. Glycolipids
   - Gangliosides (gray matter of the nervous system)
   - Glycolipids of Hurler's syndrome, Whipple's disease
   - Gangliosides of Tay-Sach's disease
   - Epithelioid and globoid cells of Krabbe's neuropathy
4. Noncarbohydrate containing substance
   - Sphingomyelin: Niemann-Pick's disease
5. Pigments and substance
   - Ceroid
   - Pigment in melanosis coli
   - Dubin-Johnson pigment: Lipofuscin
   - Malakoplakia
6. Enzymes
   - Diastase
   - α-amylase
   - β-amylase

7. Others:
- Seminoma
- Ewing's sarcoma
- Alveolar soft part sarcoma
- Endodermal sinus tumors
- Basement membrane of glomeruli
- Metastatic adenocarcinoma and lymphoma
- α_1^- antitrypsin: Liver
- Muscle biopsy to demonstrate increased glycogen.

PAS—Use in Hematology
- AML: Fine positivity
- ALL: Block positivity
- Erythroleukemia (FAB M6): Diffuse cytoplasmic positivity
- Malignant erythroid precursors—PAS positive.

PAS DIASTASE
Principle
The diastase enzyme digests the glycogen and thus on PAS staining shows a negative reaction, thus it confirms the presence of glycogen in the section.
Usually two sections are cut and PAS and PAS D are done simultaneously to confirm the presence of glycogen.

Source of Diastase
1. Malt diastase (commercially available will have both α and β amylase tends to loosen the section)
2. Human saliva (α-amylase)

MUCICARMINE
Principle
Aluminum salts form a chelation complex with carmine, the resulting compound has a net positive charge and attaches to the acid groups of the mucin.

Purpose
To demonstrate neutral or acidic mucin.

Result
- Mucin and capsule of cryptococcus—deep rose or red
- Nuclei—black
- Other tissue elements—blue or yellow

Application
- Metastatic adenocarcinoma
- Mucoepidermoid carcinoma

ALCIAN BLUE
Principle and Purpose
Copper phthalocyanin basic dye:
- Alcian blue when used in 3% acetic acid solution with pH 2
  - Acid mucins
- Alcian blue when used in 0.1 N hydrochloric acid solution and pH 1
  - Strongly sulphated mucins
- Alcian blue pH 1–2.5
  - Weakly sulphated mucins

Results
Acid mucins: Blue
Nuclei: Red

COMBINED ALCIAN BLUE AND PAS
Purpose
Acid and neutral mucin are clearly differentiated.

Rationale
The rationale is that by first staining all acid mucin with alcian blue (nose remaining acidic mucin), which are also PAS positive will not react within the subsequent PAS reaction but only the neutral mucin will.

Application
- Mesothelioma *vs* adenocarcinoma
- Mesothelioma—acid mucin—alcian blue positive
- Adenocarcinoma—neutral mucin—PAS positive.

HALE'S COLLOIDAL IRON FOR ACID MUCOSUBSTANCES
Principle
At low pH, colloidal iron forms a chelate with acid groups which then demonstrated by prussian blue reaction.

If combined with PAS we can differentiate acid and neutral mucins.

Table 30.1

Result	Pas	Hale
Acid	Dark blue	Dark blue
Nuclei	Red	Blue
Neutral mucin	–	Magenta

METACHROMATIC STAIN

Metachromasia

Most of the dye stain the tissue orthochromatically (in the shade of their own dye color). However, certain dye, stains tissue in a color or hue that is quite different from that of the stain itself. For example: Thionine, toluidine blue, new methylene blue, azure B, methyl violet, etc.

Principle

Dye molecules and sulfate groups are stacked closely causing a color shift from blue to purple.

Thus, a metachromatic reaction often indicates the presence of numerous closely packed sulfate groups.

Result

- *Sulphated polysaccharides:* Purple (the metachromatic color)
- *Nucleic acids:* Blue

PERL'S PRUSSIAN BLUE

Aim

- Used for demonstration of ferric iron.

Principle

Loosely bound ferric iron in the tissue combines with potassium ferrocyanide to produce an insoluble blue compound ferric ferrocyanide (prussian blue).

Ferric iron complex (HCl) → ferric iron + protein (potassium ferrocyanide) → ferric ferrocyanide.

Fixative Used

Buffered neutral formalin.

Control

Lung with chronic venous congestion: Heart failure cells.

Preparation of Reagent

- 2% hydrochloric acid
- 2% potassium ferrocyanide
- 0.15% basic fuchsin

Results

- *Ferric iron:* Blue
- *Nuclei:* Red
- *Cytoplasm:* Pink
- *Other structures:* Shades of pink

APPLICATIONS

Pathological Conditions

a. Hemochromatosis
b. Hemosiderosis
c. CVC lung
d. Sclerosing hemangioma

Hematological Conditions

1. To identify iron within nucleated RBCs (sideroblasts) and histiocytes (reticuloendothelial iron)
2. To identify Pappenheimer bodies in erythrocytes
3. Sideroblastic anemia, iron deficiency anemia
4. In MDS to look for ring sideroblasts.

Grading of Perl's Stain

Table 30.2

Grade	Criteria
0	No iron granules observed
1+	Small granules in reticulum cells seen only in oil immersion
2+	A few small granules visible with low power lens
3+	Numerous small granules in all marrow particles
4+	Large granules in small clumps
5+	Dense large clumps of granules
6+	Very large deposits obscuring marrow details

STAIN FOR RETICULIN FIBERS

Introduction
Reticulin fibers are pro-collagen and important constituent of basement membrane. These are fine delicate fibers of type III, which collagen provide supporting framework to organs like lymph nodes, spleen, liver, etc. Metal impregnation technique provides constrast, enabling even the finest fiber to be resolved.

Principle
Reticulin fibers have a little affinity for silver solution. They must be treated with potassium permanganate to produce sensitized site on fiber where silver deposition can be initiated. Silver from silver oxide is deposited on fibers. This appears black after conversion to reduced (metallic) silver by reducing agent (formalin). Gold chloride is used as toner to increase contrast and clarity. Unreduced silver is removed by treatment with sodium thiosulphate.

Methods
- Gomori's method.
- Gordan and Sweet's method.

Applications
- In parenchymal organs such as liver and spleen to outline the architecture.
- In liver biopsies, to show alterations to the normal structure especially early cirrhosis.
- To identify and diagnose myelofibrosis.
- In differentiating carcinomas from sarcomas and certain types of lymphomas. Carcinomas show poor reticulin network patterns, whereas lymphomas show profuse reticulin network.
- Follicular lymphoma (follicles surrounded by retic) *vs* reactive follicular hyperplasia (follicle not surrounded by retic).
- Hemangiopericytoma (reticulin surrounds individual cells) *vs* angioendothelioma (reticulin surrounds groups of cells).
- Glomangioma (cells external to the reticular sheath of blood vessel) and hemangiosarcoma (cells are within the reticular sheath of blood vessel).
- Leiomyosarcoma—reticulin wraps individual cells completely *vs* MPNST—reticulin runs parallel to the spindle tumor cells without surrounding them at the poles.
- Tumors producing abundant reticulin are RMS, angiosarcoma, angiomatous tumor, fibroblastic tumor.
- Absence of reticulin fibers—Ewing's sarcoma of bone.

STAINS FOR MICROORGANISMS

Gram's Stain for Paraffin Sections
1. Crystal violet solution
   - 0.5% crystal violet in 25% alcohol
2. Gram's and Lugol's iodine
   - Iodine: 1 gm, potassium iodide: 2 gm, distilled water: 10 ml
   - 3.1% aqueous neutral red.

Principle
- Differentiates bacteria by the chemical and physical properties of their cell walls
- Gram-positive bacteria—thick cell wall made of peptidoglycan (50–90% of cell envelope), i.e. stained purple by crystal violet.
- Gram-negative bacteria thinner layer—do not retain the purple stain and are counterstained pink by the neutral red.

Result
- *Gram-positive:* Purple-blue
- *Gram-negative:* Red

Quick technique for rapid identification of organism causing a lung abscess, wound infection, septicemic abscesses, or meningitis.

Stains for Mycobacterium
- Ziehl-Neelsen stain
- Fluorescent method
- Wade-Fite (*M. leprae*)

Acid-fast organisms like Mycobacterium—large amounts of lipid substances within their cell walls called mycolic acids. These acids resist staining by ordinary methods such as a

Gram stain. Acid-fast bacteria retain carbol fuchsin so they appear red.

Components

Carbol fuchsin (stain), acid alcohol (destain), methylene blue (counter stain).

Red Color Positivity

- Mycobacteria
- Russell bodies
- Splendore Hoeppli bodies
- Some fungal organisms

Stains for Spirochetes

- Steiner and Steiner method
- Warthin and Starry 1920

Principle

Silver impregnation technique
- Bacteria absorb the silver from the silver solution.
- Reducing agent, the silver is then transformed to a visible metallic state.

Results

- *Spirochetes, Legionella, Campylobacter:* Black
- *Background:* Yellow

Stains for Fungi

- Periodic acid–Schiff (PAS)
- Ziehl-Neelsen
- Gomori methenamine silver

Principle: GMS

Reduction of silver by the aldehyde groups produced after oxidation of fungal wall components with chromic acid.

Stains for *H. pylori*

- Giemsa stain
- Silver stains
- Cresyl violet
- Toluidine blue

Stains for Amoeba

- PAS
- Best carmine
- Iron hematoxylin (Heidenhain)
- PTAH

Stains for Inclusion Bodies

- Phloxine–tartrazine method
- Shikata's orcein method (HBsAg)
- Macchiavello's stain (rickettsia)
- Giemsa stain

Stains for Lipid

Fresh frozen tissue
- Oil red O
- Sudan black B

STAINS FOR PIGMENTS AND MINERALS

1. **Melanin**
   - *Reducing methods:* Masson-Fontana silver technique, Schmorl's ferric ferricyanide reduction test
   - Enzyme method: DOPA reaction
   - Bleaching method
   - Fluorescent methods (formalin induced)

   Melanin bleach
   - Permanganate, chlorate, chromic acid, peracetic acid
   - 0.25% $KMnO_4$, 2% oxalic acid

2. **Lipofuscin**
   - Schmorl's ferric ferricyanide reduction test
   - Long ZN method
   - Sudan black B
   - Aldehyde fuchsin technique

3. **Copper**
   - Rubeanic acid method
   - Modified rhodanine technique

   Useful in:
   - Wilson's disease
   - Primary biliary cirrhosis

4. **Calcium**
   - von Kossa
   - Alizarin red

CYTOCHEMICAL STAINS IN HEMATOLOGY
MYELOPEROXIDASE (MPO)

Stains primary and secondary granules of neutrophils and their precursors, eosinophil granules, azurophilic granules of monocytes.

Principle

In the presence of peroxidase, H_2O_2 is split liberating O_2 that oxidizes benzidine or 4-chlor-1-naphthol

$$H_2O_2 + \text{3-amino-9-ethlyecarbazole or (benzidine dihydrodase)} \xrightarrow{\text{Peroxidase}} \text{Insoluble red brown precipitate}$$

The most primitive myeloblasts are negative granular positivity appearing progressively as they mature toward the promyelocyte stage—positivity may be localized to the Golgi region.

Inference

- Promyelocytes and myelocytes are strongly positive.
- Metamyelocytes and neutrophils—fewer positive (secondary) granules.
- Neutrophils and eosinophils—primary granules.
- Eosinophils—also secondary granules are stained.

Clinical Implications

1. *AML with MDS:* MPO may be aberrant, because patients may develop an acquired MPO deficiency as part of the dysplastic process.
2. *AML-1, 2:* >3% positive
3. *Auer-rods:* MPO +
4. *AML-M3:* MPO is strongly positive with reaction product covering cytoplasm and nucleus
5. *Monoblasts:* MPO negative.
6. *Promonocytes:* Scattered positivity
7. *AML-M7:* Consistently negative for MPO and sudan black B.

SUDAN BLACK

More sensitive than MPO in early precursors. More reliable and stable.

Principle

Sudan black B (SBB) dye is fat soluble, then it stains fat particles (steroles, phospholipids and neutral fats) in the primary and secondary granules of myelocytic and lysosomes in monocytic cells.

Inference

SBB stains the granules of neutrophils (both the primary and the specific granules) and specific granules of eosinophils.

- *Promyelocytes:* A few sudanophilic granules.
- *Neutrophils:* Large numbers of sudanophilic granules.
- *Monoblasts:* Either negative or a few small SBB positive granules.
- *Promonocytes and monocytes:* Variable number of fine positively staining granules.
- *Basophils:* Generally not positive—may show bright red/purple metachromatic staining of the granules.

Clinical Implications

1. Hereditary neutrophil, eosinophil and monocyte peroxidase deficiencies—granules of cells of the deficient lineages are SBB negative.
2. Rare cases (1–2%) of acute lymphoblastic leukemia (ALL) show non-granular smudgy positivity not seen with MPO staining.
3. Acute myeloid leukemia (M1, M2 and M3), Auer rods.
4. *AMML:* Acute myelomonocytic leukemia.
5. *Erythroleukemia:* Postive in myeloblasts, negative in normoblasts.

Esterases

Leucocyte esterases—enzymes that hydrolyse acyl or chloroacyl esters of α-naphthol or naphthol AS. Nine isoenzymes of esterases in leucocytes

- Napthol AS—D chloroacetate (1, 2, 7, 9)
- α-naphthyl acetate
- α-naphthyl butyrate (3, 4, 5, 6)
  Specific myelocyte
  Nonspecific—other cells

SPECIFIC ESTERASE

A specific esterase (capable of liberating naphthol from a naphthol AS-D chloroacetate substrate) is present in the nonspecific granules—granulocytes and mast cells.

Chloroacetate esterase (CAE) has an optimum pH between 7 and 7.6 and is insensitive to fluoride inhibition.

Principle

A naphthol compound is released which combines with a diazonium salt to produce a brightly colored compound at the site of enzyme activity.

Naphthol (AS-D) —Chloroacetate/Esterase→ Naphthol —Fast blue BB→ Blue precipitate

Interpretation

- Myeloid cells (+ve)
- Mast cells
- Monocyte and basophils (–ve) to weak (+ve)
- *Other cells:* Lymphocytes, plasma cells, megakaryocyte, nRBC: Negative.

Clinical Implications

- CAE—more often positive in M2 than in M1 AML.
- Auer rods—usually weak or negative except in M2 AML associated with t(8;21).
- AML-M3 in which Auer rods are often positive for CAE.

NONSPECIFIC ESTERASE (WITH FLUORIDE INHIBITION)

Sodium fluoride, inhibits the activity in monocytes, megakaryocytes, platelets, and plasma cells but not in lymphocytes.

Principle

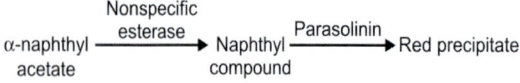

α-naphthyl acetate —Nonspecific esterase→ Naphthyl compound —Parasolinin→ Red precipitate

Interpretation

1. Positive in monocytes and precursor macrophages, megakaryocytes and platelets
2. Mature T cells and T-ALL (cytoplasmic dot)

Clinical Implications

1. AML-M5
2. ALL of T-ALL and in CLL of T-CLL (positive) from B-CLL (negative)

DOUBLE ESTERASE

Sequential combined esterase stain using α-napthyl-acecate esterase (ANAE) and chloracetate esterase (CAE).

Principle

Double esterase combines two substrates: Naphthol AS-D chloroacetate that reacts with primary granules in the neutrophilic series and naphthyl butyrate that stains material in the endoplasmic reticulum of cells in the monocytic lineage.

Inference

- The ANAE—brown reaction product
- CAE—granular bright blue product.
- Staining patterns are identical to those seen with the two stains used separately.

Clinical Implications

1. Identification of monocytic and granulocytic component in AML-M4.
2. In myelomonocytic leukemias—cells staining with both esterases may be present.
3. In MDS and AML with dysplastic granulocytes, double staining of individual cells.
4. Non-clonal dysplastic states such as megaloblastic anemia.

ACID PHOSPHATASE AND ACID PHOSPHATASE WITH TARTRATE RESISTANCE

Enzymes which hyrolyse phosphate esters at acid phosphatase. There are seven isoenzymes (0, 1, 2, 3, 3b, 4 and 5).

Principle

The acid phosphatase hydrolyzes naphthol AS-BI phosphoric acid. The hydrolyzed substrate-dye coloured complex is insoluble which precipitates out at the site of enzyme activity.

Naphthol AS-BI Phosphoric acid $\xrightarrow[\text{Acid pH}]{\text{ACP}}$ Naphthol $\xrightarrow{\text{Parosolinin}}$ Red precipitate

**ACP isoenzymes → (0, 1, 2, 3a, 3b)   Inhibited
(L+)   → (5)   Not inhibited

Tartaric acid when added to the incubation mixture, will not inhibit the enzyme fraction found in hairy cell leukemia.

Clinical Implications

1. Present in all hematopoietic cells. Most intense—macrophages and osteoclasts.
2. Main diagnostic use—diagnosis of T cell ALL and hairy cell leukemia.
3. Lymphocytes from patients with macroglobulinemia.
4. Atypical lymphocytes from infectious mononucleosis (<40 granules).
5. Lymphoblasts from patients with T cell leukemia (Golgi region).

Tartrate resistant acid phosphatase reaction-diffusely prominent in the cytoplasm of neoplastic cells is highly characteristic of hairy cell leukemia.

Not all hairy cells are tartrate resistant and may be positive in other conditions such as:
   a. Infectious mononucleosis has increased acid phosphatase activity with some of the atypical lymphocytes showing tartrate resistance.
   b. Gaucher cells are acid phosphatase positive, tartrate resistantce.
   c. Sezary cells are acid phosphatase positive, tartrate resistant.
   d. Occasionally, some CLL clones are tartrate resistant.

LEUKOCYTE ALKALINE PHOSPHATASE (LAP)

Distinguishing the cells of leukemoid reactions with increase LAP activity from those of (CML) with LAP decreased activity.

Principle

Secondary granules of neutrophils. The substrate naphthol AS-BI phosphate is hydrolyzed by the enzyme at an alkaline pH. This hydrolyzed substrate in combination with a dye such as fast garnet (diamonium dye) produces a colored precipitate at site of the enzyme activity.

*Naphthol AS-M or {naphthol AS-BI} $\xrightarrow[\text{Alkaline pH}]{\text{LAP}}$ Hydrolyzed Substrate $\xrightarrow[\text{RR dye}]{\text{Fast blue}}$ Insoluble precipitate at the site of enzyme activity

Inference

Mature neutrophils, have alkaline phosphatase in specific cytoplasmic organelles which appear as red precipitate of varying intensity.

LAP Score

The cytochemical reaction—within 8 hours of obtaining the blood specimen. Films can be fixed and stored, in the dark, at room temperature.

EDTA—anticoagulated blood is not ideal as enzyme activity is inhibited. Capillary blood or heparinised preferred.

Table 30.3

Score	Intensity of color
0	Colorless
1	Diffuse positivity—occasional granules
2	Diffuse positivity—moderate amount of granules
3	Strong—numerous granules
4	Very strong—dark confluent granules

The reaction is scored from 0 to 4 depending on the number of stained granules and the intensity of the stain. The number of cells is multiplied by the score and added up with a normal range being from 40 to 100.

Clinical Implications

- *Normal:* 20–100
- CML <13
- Leukemoid reaction >100
- *Polycythemia vera:* 100–200
- *Secondary polycythemia:* 10–100

Table 30.4

LAP elevated in	LAP decreased in
Leukemoid reaction	CML
Pregnancy	Paroxysmal nocturnal hemoglobinuria
Polycythemia vera	Sickle cell anemia
Aplastic anemia	Hypophosphatasia
Multiple myeloma	
Obstructive jaundice	
Hodgkin's disease	
Myelofibrosis	
Blast crisis—CML	

CHAPTER 31

Flow Cytometry

N Priyathershini

Flow cytometry is the automated measurement of physical, chemical, and biological properties of individual cells (cytometry) or particles flowing in a single stream (flow) in a fluidic system.

Cyto = cells
Metry = measurement
Flow = in a flow or a stream.

FLOW CYTOMETER

Flow cytometer is an instrument that illuminates cells as they flow in front of a light source and detects and correlates the signals from the illumination.

Unique ability—rapid analysis of thousands of cells, cells flow at a velocity of 5–50 m/s.

Analyze 500–5000 cells/second

Simultaneous illustration of multiple antigens

Major Principles

1. Measurement of physical properties
2. Measurement of antigenic properties

INSTRUMENT COMPONENTS

1. *Fluidics:* Specimen, sheath fluid, flow chamber.
2. *Optics:* Light source(s), mirrors, filters, detectors, spectral separation.
3. *Electronics:* Controls pulse collection, pulse analysis, triggering, time delay, data display, gating, sort control, light and detector control.
4. *Data analysis:* Software—data display and analysis, multivariate/simultaneous solutions, identification of sort populations, quantitation.

Fluidics

A narrow stream of cells flowing in a core within a wider sheath stream.

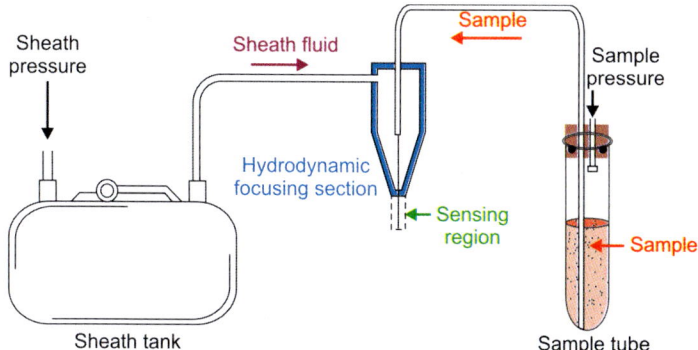

Fig. 31.1

Optics

a. Excitation optics including the LASER (argon) with focusing lenses and prisms
b. Collection optics including dichroic filters and mirrors, photodiode, PMT (photo multiplier tubes).

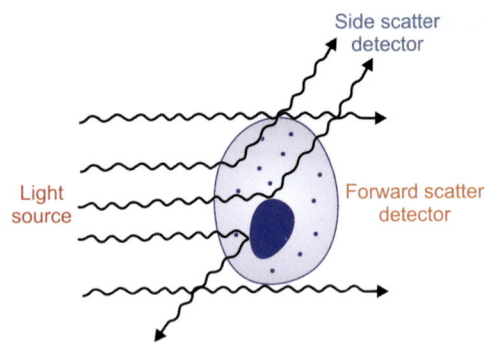

Fig. 31.4

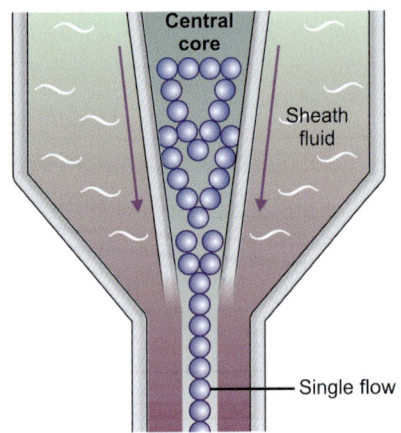

Fig. 31.2

Dichroic Filters

- Can be a long pass or short pass filter or band pass.
- Filter is placed at a 45° angle to the incident light.
- Part of the light is reflected at 90° to the incident light, and part of the light is transmitted and continues on.

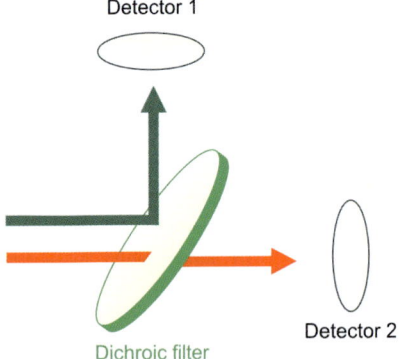

Fig. 31.3

Light Scattering

Light scattering is the result of reflecting and refracting off the cells. Light scattered along the axis of the beam is forward scatter, which is proportional to the size of the cell and the light scattered at greater angles is side scatter which correlates the granularity of the cells.

Fluorescence

Aufluorochrome absorbs laser light (energy) and gets excited. The excited fluorochrome releases that energy in three ways, vibration, heat dissipation, and photon emission. These photons are of a longer wavelength (different color) than the incident laser light.

- The commonly used fluorochromes for conjugation with monoclonal antibodies are fluorescein isothiocyanate (FITC), phycoerythrin (PE), perdin-chlorophyll alpha complex (PerCP), texas red, allophycocyanin.
- The scatter light signals and the fluorescence signals are directed through the filters to the photodiodes and photomultiplier tubes.

Electronics

The photodetectors convert the photons to electric signals.
- Compute pulse height.
- Perform calculations for pulse area and pulse width.
- Convert analog signals to proportional digital signals.
- Interface with the computer for data transfer.

Data Analysis

The electric signals are processed by the computer software and stored in a standard format developed by the society for analytical cytometry. The data are displayed as histogram or dot plot.

Sample Processing

Single cell suspension: all specimens with cells in suspension.
- PB, BMA, CSF, PF, BAL
- Solid tissue
- Fine needle aspirations
- *Tissue suspensions:* Slicing, mincing and teasing = Filtering
- *Sample stabilization:* Anticoagulant—EDTA or Heparin—transport at RT

   Enrichment of cells: For leucocytes
   - RBC lysis—NH_4Cl or
   - Density gradient centrifugation— Ficoll medium

   Antibody staining: Separate cells-wash-incubate with Ab-F in dark
   - *Acquisition:* Acquire the stained cells at earliest or
     Fixed and store in refrigerator
   - *Data Analysis*

Clinical Applications of Flow Cytometry

- Enumeration of lymphocyte subsets (CD4/CD8)
- Immunophenotyping of hematologic malignancies
- Minimal residual disease (MRD)
- Myelodysplatic syndrome (MDS)
- HLA B27 typing
- PNH diagnosis (CD55−/CD59−)
- DNA/RNA analysis and cell cycle studies
- Reticulocyte analysis
- Hemotopoietic stem cell (CD34+)analysis
- Platelet analysis
- Antigen quantitation, e.g. CD20, CD22, CD33, etc.

Less Common Applications

- Microbiology
- Determination of drug resistance to chemotherapy
- Cell function analysis

FCM in Hematolymphoid Neoplasms

The role of flow cytometry in hematolymphoid malignancies includes:
- Accurate diagnosis and classification
- Knowledge of prognostic factors
- Monitoring response
- Diagnosis of early relapse at other sites like CNS

FCM in Diagnosis and Classification of Acute Leukemias

The various steps include:
- Identification of blasts
- Enumeration of blasts
- Assignment of blast lineage

Identification of Blasts

- Low side light scatter
- Weak CD45 expression
- Markers of immaturity such as CD34 and TdT
- Lack markers of maturation
- Myeloblasts—CD11b, CD15, CD16.
- B lymphoblasts—surface light chains kappa/lambda
- T lymphoblasts—surface CD3

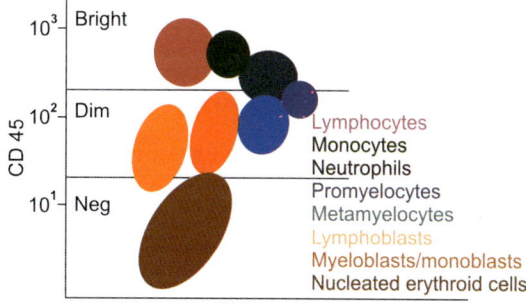

Fig. 31.5

- Abnormal expression of foreign lineage antigens termed aberrant expression.
- Abnormal coexpression of markers of both maturity and immaturity not seen normally. Abnormally increased or decreased expression of an antigen.

Immunophenotypic Markers

- Markers of immaturity—TdT, CD34
- Lineage specific markers
- Myeloid—cMPO
- B cell—cCD22/cCD79a
- T cell— cCD3
- Lineage associated markers
- Myeloid—common—CD13, CD33, CD117
- Other—CD11b, CD15
- Monocytic—CD13, CD33, CD64, CD68, CD117, CD11b, CD14, CD4, cLysozyme
- Erythroid—CD36, CD71, CD105, CD235a (Glycophorin A), Hb
- Megakaryocytic—CD36, CD41, CD42, CD61 and CD62
- B cell—CD19, CD22, CD20, cCD79a, CD10, cIgM, sIg
- T cell—common—CD1a, CD2, CD5, CD7, CD10
- Other—CD4, CD8, CD3,
- NK cell—CD16, CD56, CD57, CD94, KIR
- PDC—CD123, CD4, CD56, CD68, CD33, CD43, BDCA
- Other on PB subset CD2, CD5, CD7

Table 31.1: Immunophenotyping of acute myeloid leukemias

WHO (2008)	FAB	Antigen expression
AML with t(8;21)	AML M2, rarely M1 or M4	CD 34, HLA-DR, MPO, CD 117, CD13, CD33 weak, CD11b, CD 15 and CD65
AML with inv 16	AML M4eo	CD34, HLA-DR, CD117 on primitive blasts, with heterogenous subpopulation of CD13, CD33, CD65, MPO (myeloblasts) and CD4, CD14, CD64 (monoblasts) CD11b pos
APML with t(15;17)	AML M3	High SSC, CD117 (weak), CD13, CD33 and CD64. HLA-Dr, CD 34 Neg CD11b and CD 11c absent. CD 15 and 65 negative
AML with t(9;11)	AML m4 and M5	CD 33, CD15 and HLA DR, monocytic and monoblastic markers CD4, CD11b, CD11c, CD14, CD36 and CD 64
AML t(6;9)	AML M2 or M4	Generic AML phenotype CD13, CD33, HLA-DR usually CD117, CD43, CD15
AML with inv(3)	Any FAB (not M3) M7 common	Generic AML phenotype CD13, CD33, CD34, some CD41 and CD61
AML (megakaryoblastic) with t(1,22)	AML M7	CD13 CD33, CD36, CD41 and CD61
AML with mutated MPM1	Usually M4/M5	CD13, CD33, MPO, most HLA DR.
AML with mutated CEBPA	Mainly AML M1	CD13, CD33, CD34, CD15, CD11b, HLA-DR
AML with MDS related changes	Any FAB (not M3) often AMLM6,	Very variable, non-specific blasts, CD13, CD33, CD34
Therapy related AML		Very variable, non-specific blats, CD13, CD33, CD34
AML with minimal differentiation	AML M0	CD34, HLA-DR, CD 38 usually positive. CD13, CD117 often positive. CD33 positive in 60%
AML without maturation	AML M1	Similar to above with MPO positive in at least some subpopulation

Contd...

Table 31.1: Immunophenotyping of acute myeloid leukemias (Contd.)

WHO (2008)	FAB	Antigen expression
AML with maturation	AML M2	CD13, CD33, HLA-DR, MPO, CD34, CD117, CD11b, CD15, CD65
Acute myelomonocytic leukemia	AML M4	CD34, HLA-DR, CD117 on primitive blasts, CD13, CD33, CD65, MPO (granulocytic) and CD4, CD14 CD64 (monocytic) blasts CD15 is typical of monocytic differentiation
Acute monoblastic and monocytic leukemia	AML M5	CD34, CD117, HLA-DR positive always, CD13, CD33, CD15, CD65, at least two monocytic differentiation
Acute erythroid leukemia	AML M6	Erythroid/myeloid leukemia—similar to M0 or M1 with erythroblasts positive in GPA and CD71 Pure erythroid leukemia—all erythroblasts
Acute megakaryoblastic leukemia	AML M7	CD13, CD33, CD41, CD61 and CD36
Acute basophilic leukemia		CD34, HLA-DR positive always, CD13, CD33, CD9, CD203c, CD123. MPO negative
Myeloid sarcoma		CD13, CD33, CD117 and MPO positive in myeloid differentiation. CD11c, CD14 in monocytic differentiation
Myeloid proliferations related to Down's syndrome, TAM		CD34, CD117, CD13, CD33, CD41 and CD61 positive, HLA-DR positive in 30% MPO negative
Myeloid proliferations related to Down's syndrome, myeloid leukemia		Similar to TAM, CD34 and CD 41 often negative

Table 31.2: Acute lymphoid leukemias

Early or Pro B cell ALL	CD19, CD34, Tdt, CD15 Positive, CD 10 Negative
Common B cell ALL	CD19, CD34, Tdt, CD15, CD 10 positive
Pre B cell ALL	CD10, CD 19 positive, CD34, sIg negative
Mature B ALL	Cd10, CD19, sIg positive, Tdt, HLA-Dr negative
Precursor T lymphoblastic leukemia	cCD3, Tdt, CD7, CD2, CD5

CHAPTER 32

Karyotyping—Basic Essentials

V Pavithra, Divya D

DEFINITIONS

A karyotype is the number and appearance of *chromosomes* in the *nucleus* of an eukaryotic cell. The term is also used for the complete set of chromosomes in an individual organism.

The study of whole sets of chromosomes is sometimes known as karyology.

The chromosomes are depicted (by rearranging a photomicrograph) in a standard format known as a karyogram or idiogram: In pairs, ordered by size and position of centromere for chromosomes of the same size.

HUMAN KARYOTYPE

The normal human karyotypes contain 22 pairs of autosomal chromosomes and one pair of *sex chromosomes*. Normal karyotypes for *females* contain two X *chromosomes* and are denoted 46, XX; *males* have both an X and a Y *chromosome* denoted 46, XY. Any variation from the standard karyotype may lead to developmental abnormalities.

Staining

The study of karyotypes is made possible by *staining*. Usually, a suitable *dye*, such as Giemsa, is applied after cells have been arrested during *cell division* by a solution of *colchicine* usually in *metaphase* or *pro metaphase* when most condensed. In order for the Giemsa stain to adhere correctly, all chromosomal proteins must be digested and removed. For humans, *white blood* cells are used most frequently because they are easily induced to divide and grow in tissue culture. Sometimes observations may be made on non-dividing (*interphase*) cells. The sex of an unborn *fetus* can be determined by observation of interphase cells.

Observations

Six different characteristics of karyotypes are usually observed and compared:
1. Differences in absolute sizes of chromosomes.
2. Chromosomes can vary in absolute size by as much as twenty-fold between genera of the same family.
3. Differences in the position of centromeres.
4. These differences probably came about through translocations.

Differences in relative size of chromosomes
These differences probably arose from segmental interchange of unequal lengths.

Differences in basic number of chromosomes
These differences could have resulted from successive unequal translocations which removed all the essential genetic material from a chromosome, permitting its loss without penalty to the organism (the dislocation hypothesis) or through fusion.

Differences in number and position of satellites

Satellites are small bodies attached to a chromosome by a thin thread.

Differences in degree and distribution of heterochromatic regions.

Note: A full account of a karyotype may therefore include the number, type, shape, and banding of the chromosomes, as well as other cytogenetic information.

CHROMOSOME BANDING

Chromosomes display a banded pattern when treated with some stains. Bands are alternating light and dark stripes that appear along the lengths of chromosomes. Unique banding patterns are used to identify chromosomes and to diagnose chromosomal aberrations, including chromosome breakage, loss, duplication, translocation or inverted segments.

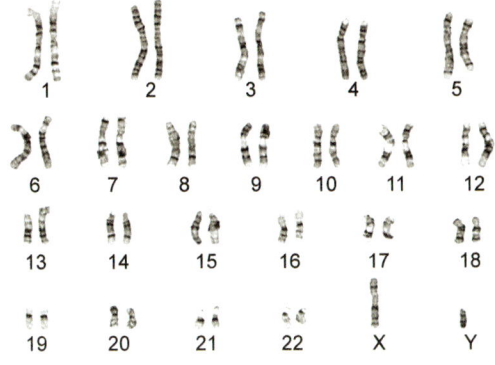

Fig. 32.1: Human male G-bands

R-banding is the reverse of G-banding (the R stands for "reverse"). The dark regions are euchromatic (guanine-cytosine rich regions) and the bright regions are heterochromatic (thymine-adenine rich regions).

C-banding: Giemsa binds to *constitutive heterochromatin*, so it stains centromeres. The name is derived from *centromeric* or constitutive heterochromatin. The preparations undergo alkaline denaturation prior to staining leading to an almost complete depurination of the DNA. Heterochromatin binds a lot of the dye, while the rest of the chromosomes absorb only little of it.

Q-banding is a *fluorescent* pattern obtained using *quinacrine* for staining. The pattern of bands is very similar to that seen in G-banding. They can be recognized by a yellow fluorescence of differing intensity. Most part of the stained DNA is heterochromatin. Quinacrin (atebrin) binds both regions rich in AT and in GC, but only the AT-quinacrin-complex fluorescence. Since regions rich in AT are more common in heterochromatin than in euchromatin, these regions are labelled preferentially. The different intensities of the single bands mirror the different contents of AT.

T-banding: Visualize telomeres.

Silver staining: *Silver nitrate stains the nucleolar organization region-associated protein.* This yields a dark region where the silver is deposited, denoting the activity of rRNA genes within the NOR.

Types of Karyotyping

Classic Karyotype Cytogenetics

- In the "classic" (depicted) karyotype, a dye, often Giemsa (G-banding), less frequently *Quinacrine,* is used to stain bands on the chromosomes.
- Karyotypes are arranged with the short arm of the chromosome on top, and the long arm on the bottom. Some karyotypes call the short and long arms *p* and *q*, respectively.
- In addition, the differently stained regions and sub-regions are given numerical

Types of Banding

Cytogenetics employs several techniques to visualize different aspects of chromosomes

G-banding is obtained with Giemsa stain following digestion of chromosomes with trypsin. It yields a series of lightly and darkly stained bands—the dark regions tend to be heterochromatic, late-replicating and AT rich. The light regions tend to be euchromatic, early-replicating and GC rich. This method will normally produce 300–400 bands in a normal, human genome.

designations from *proximal* to *distal* on the chromosome arms. For example, *Cri du chat* syndrome involves a deletion on the short arm of chromosome 5. It is written as 46, XX, 5p–. The critical region for this syndrome is deletion of p15.2 (the locus on the chromosome), which is written as 46, XX, del(5) (p15.2).

Spectral Karyotype (SKY Technique) (Below Pic)

- Spectral karyotyping is a molecular cytogenetic technique used to simultaneously visualize all the pairs of chromosomes in an organism in different colors.
- Fluorescently labeled probes for each chromosome are made by labeling chromosome-specific DNA with different fluorophores.
- This technique is used to identify structural chromosome aberrations in cancer and leukemic cells and other disease conditions when Giemsa banding or other techniques are not accurate enough.

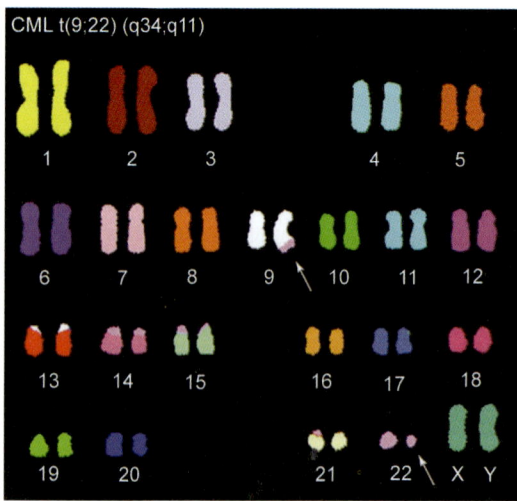

Fig. 32.2

DIGITAL KARYOTYPING

- Digital karyotyping is a technique used to quantify the DNA copy number on a genomic scale.
- Short sequences of DNA from specific loci all over the genome are isolated and enumerated. This method is also known as virtual karyotyping.

Indications

Prenatal Diagnosis

(Amniotic fluid, chorionic villi or fetal blood sampling)

- Late maternal age (35 years old or greater).
- Previous live birth with a chromosome abnormality.
- Previous stillbirth with a potentially viable chromosome abnormality.
- Parental chromosome rearrangement, chromosome mosaicism, or sex chromosome aneuploidy.
- Positive maternal serum screening result indicating an increased risk of a chromosomally abnormal fetus abnormal fetal ultrasound.
- Risk of chromosome breakage syndrome, or other syndrome with specific cytogenetic findings (e.g. Roberts syndrome).
- Resolution of possible fetal mosaicism detected by prior prenatal study.
- Intracytoplasmic sperm injection, or other medical intervention that increases the probability of chromosome abnormalities.

Clinical Indications for Constitutional Karyotyping (Lymphocytes, Bone Marrow, Fibroblasts)

Family history of:
- Chromosome rearrangement
- Mental retardation

Patient with:
- Primary or secondary amenorrhea
- Short stature
- Ambiguous genitalia
- Dymorphism and/or developmental delay
- Multiple congenital abnormalities
- Mental retardation
- Suspected deletion/microdeletion/duplication syndrome

- X-linked recessive condition in a female
- Features of a chromosome breakage syndrome, or other syndrome with specific cytogenetic findings.
- Monitoring after bone marrow transplantation, e.g. other-sex donor in treatment of thalassemia.

Parents with:

- Prenatal diagnosis detection of a chromosome abnormality or unusual variant
- Infertility
- 3 or more pregnancy losses stillbirths with a suspected chromosome abnormality.

Clinical Indications for Cancer Karyotyping (Bone Marrow, Lymph Node, Solid Tumor, Aspirates, Fluids)

- *Acute leukemia:* At diagnosis. If an abnormality is present, follow-up after treatment or at relapse. If an abnormal clone is not detected, reinvestigation at relapse may be indicated.
- *Myelodysplasia (preleukemia):* At diagnosis. Follow-up may be indicated at disease progression.
- *Chronic myeloid leukemia at diagnosis:* Follow-up at disease progression or to monitor therapy.
- *Other chronic myeloproliferative disorders:* At diagnosis and disease progression in selected cases.
- *Malignant lymphoma and chronic lymphoproliferative disorders:* At diagnosis in selected cases.
- *Solid tumors:* For small round cell tumors of childhood, selected sarcomas, lipomatous tumors, and other tumors in consultation with the pathologist.

CHAPTER 33

Fluorescence *in situ* Hybridization (FISH)

Sandhya Sundaram, V Pavithra

DEFINITION

Fluorescence *in situ* hybridization (FISH) refers to the use of labeled nucleic acid sequence probes for the visualization of specific DNA or RNA sequences on mitotic chromosome preparations or in interphase cells.

Steps

Step 1: Denaturation
Conversion of double stranded DNA into single stranded DNA into single stranded form.

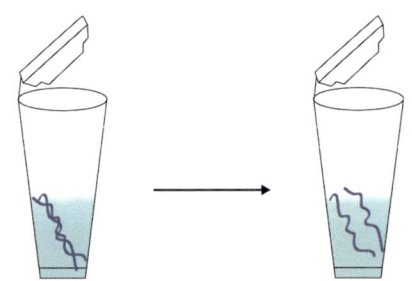

Fig. 33.1: Denaturation of labeled probe DNA

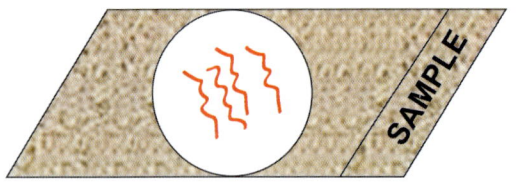

Fig. 33.2: Denaturation of target DNA (interphase nuclei or metaphases on slide)

Step 2: Hybridization
Binding of probe DNA to target DNA

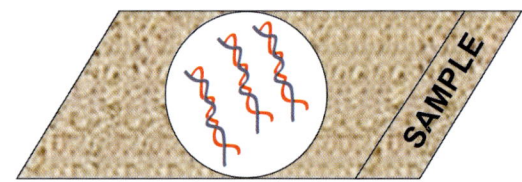

Fig. 33.3

Application of probe DNA to slide and overnight incubation at 37°C

Step 3: Posthybridization washing and detection
Visualization of interphase nuclei/metaphases with bound probe.

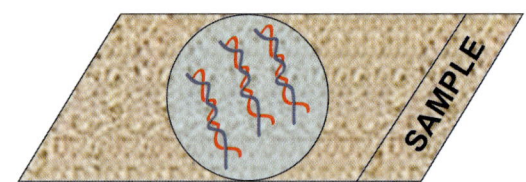

Fig. 33.4

Washing of unbound probe DNA, application of counterstain and visualization using fluorescence microscopy.

PROBES AND SAMPLES USED FOR FISH

Probes can be for the whole chromosome, centromere, or locus specific. FISH probes for the entire genome are also often used.

Interphase nuclei can be obtained from a range of clinical specimens including touch preparations, fine needle aspirates, bone marrow smears, and archival material.

VARIATIONS OF FISH

Interphase FISH

This involves the hybridization of probes to interphase cells and is extremely beneficial when it is not possible to prepare metaphase spreads as in the case of primary tumors. In addition, interphase FISH can be performed on paraffin-embedded, formalin-fixed tissue sections thereby allowing retrospective analysis of samples and correlation of chromosome aberrations with biological and clinical endpoints.

Telomeric FISH (Q-FISH)

Subtelomeric probes are a relatively new addition to the arsenal of cytogenetic tests. A collection of 41 different FISH probes are used to identify rearrangements that cannot be seen by conventional cytogenetic methods. Each of the probes is a different color so that the specific chromosomal segment can be identified. However, it is very expensive and labor-intensive process and can be used when a geneticist suspects a chromosomal abnormality and routine chromosomes are normal or when there is chromosomal material of unknown origin.

RNA *in Situ* Hybridization (RISH)

In many situations, transcription of genes at the cellular level needs to be studied. This application of the FISH technique provides direct visual evidence of gene expression from a particular chromosome.

Primed *in Situ* (PRINS) Labeling

The primed *in situ* (PRINS) labeling method is an alternative to in situ hybridization for chromosomal detection based on the use of chromosome-specific oligonucleotide primers. It has been demonstrated that the PRINS technique is more specific and considerably faster than classical FISH for chromosomal identification.

Fiber FISH (Dynamic Molecular Combing)

The term 'Fiber FISH' refers to the common practice of fluorescence *in situ* hybridization (FISH) conducted on preparations of extended chromatin fibers. FISH on DNA fibers is useful in assessing the length of DNA probes, and to map probes relative to one another, as it can reveal even their degree of overlap. Thus, fiber FISH has superior mapping resolution compared to interphase FISH.

Comparative Genomic Hybridization (CGH)

Comparative genomic hybridization serves as an important global screening test for chromosomal aberrations present within a tumor genome. This technique requires only genomic tumor DNA and metaphase preps from a normal donor, thus circumventing the preparation of high quality tumor metaphase spreads. Once regions of gain or loss have been identified, these regions can be defined further using FISH or molecular genetic techniques. CGH coupled with microarray also known as array CGH has proved to be very informative in many clinical settings.

Combinatorial Binary Ratio Labeling (COBRA) FISH

Combinatorial fluorescence *in situ* hybridization (COBRA FISH) of the DNA of the 24 different human chromosomes with 5 fluorophores in conjunction with spectral or filter-based microscopic imaging has greatly advanced molecular cytogenetic analysis of chromosomes. COBRA FISH allows color discrimination of all of the p and q arms of each chromosome and permits detection and elucidation of intra and interchromosomal rearrangements.

Spectral Karyotyping (SKY) FISH

Spectral karyotyping (SKY) is a molecular cytogenetic technique that allows differential visualization of all human chromosomes in distinct colors with a single hybridization and image exposure.

Multiplex-FISH (M-FISH)

The M-FISH technology has the ability to identify the twenty four different human chromosomes in a metaphase spread by the simultaneous hybridization of chromosome specific DNA probes, each labeled with a different combination of fluorescent dyes. M-FISH differs from SKY only in that it is a filter-based system where separate images are acquired sequentially for each fluorochrome used.

Indications of FISH

Cytogenetics

At present, the entire human genome can be scanned for deletions and duplications at over 30,000 loci simultaneously by array CGH (approximately 100 kb resolution), thus entailing an attractive gene discovery approach for monogenic conditions, in particular those that are associated with reproductive lethality (Fig. 34.5).

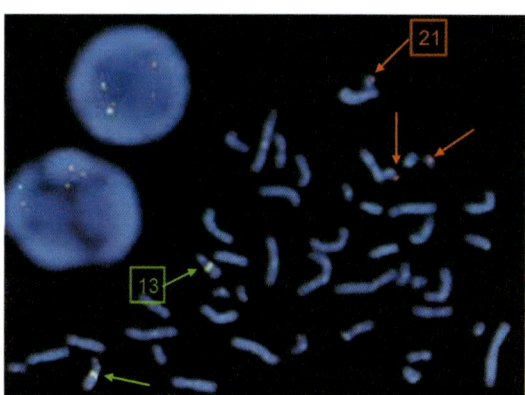

Fig. 33.5: Fluorescence *in situ* hybridization (FISH) chr 21 showed three signals (orange) and two signals for chromosome 13 (green) indicating Trisomy 21—Down's syndrome (image *Courtesy:* Department of Human Genetics, SRMC&RI)

PRENATAL DIAGNOSIS

Prenatal diagnosis employs a variety of techniques to determine the health and condition of an unborn fetus. Numerical chromosome abnormalities are the major cause of inherited diseases. Of these, trisomies for sex chromosomes and chromosomes 13, 16, 18 and 21 account for 50% of chromosomally abnormal abortions.

Preimplantation Genetics

Preimplantation genetic diagnosis (PGD) identifies genetic abnormalities in preimplantation embryos prior to embryo transfer. As mentioned earlier, the correlation between aneuploidy and declining implantation rates with maternal age demands screening of chromosome aneuploidies in human embryos by FISH using 13, 18, 21,X and Y probes should significantly reduce the risk of older patients undergoing *in vitro* fertilization (IVF) delivering trisomic offspring (Fig. 34.6).

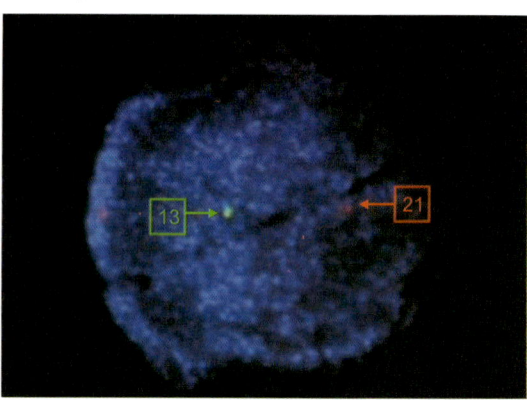

Fig. 33.6: FISH done on a blastomere obtained by embryo biopsy prior to IVF

Fluorescence *in situ* hybridization (FISH) for chromosomes 13 and 21 showed two signals for chromosome 21 (orange) and one signal for chromosome 13 (green) indicating that the blastomere biopsied from the embryo was abnormal.

Cancer Genetics

- Testing ABL/BCR gene fusion in CML: At diagnosis and following therapy.

- Testing APL/RARA gene fusion in acute promyelocytic leukemia: at diagnosis and following therapy.
- Monitoring disease progression following opposite-sex bone marrow transplantation.
- Testing amplication of N-MYC gene in neuroblastoma.

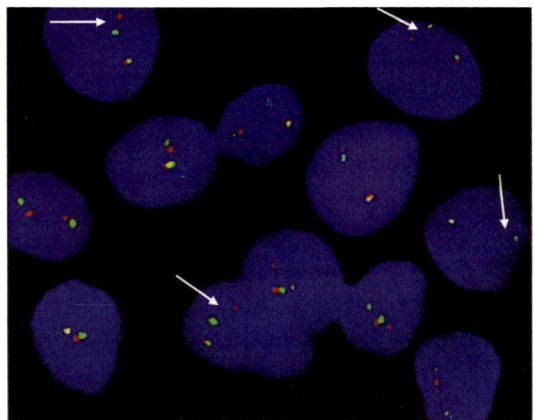

Fig. 33.7: Fusion gene in Ewing's sarcoma

- Follow-up studies for leukemias and other cancers with specific chromosome changes.
- Testing amplification of other oncogenes in consultation with pathologists.

Dual-color FISH with break-apart EWSR1 probes showing nuclei in which one pair of probe signals is split apart due to an EWSR1 region rearrangement.

HER2 Testing by *in Situ* Hybridization

Fluorescence *in situ* hybridization (FISH), chromogenic *in situ* hybridization (CISH), and silver-enhanced in situ hybridization (SISH) studies for HER2 determine the presence or absence of gene amplification. Some assays use a single probe to determine the number of HER2 gene copies present, but most assays include a chromosome enumeration probe (CEP17) to determine the ratio of HER2 signals to copies of chromosome 17.

Failure to obtain results with ISH may be due to the following:
- Prolonged fixation in formalin (>1 week)
- Fixation in non-formalin fixatives
- Procedures or fixation involving acid (e.g. decalcification) may degrade DNA
- Insufficient protease treatment of tissue.

Reporting guidelines: ASCO and CAP have issued recommendations for reporting the results of HER2 testing by ISH.

Dual Probe ISH Group Definitions

Group 1 = HER2/CEP17 ratio ≥2.0; ≥4.0 HER2 signals/cell

Group 2 = HER2/CEP17 ratio ≥2.0; <4.0 HER2 signals/cell

Group 3 = HER2/CEP17 ratio <2.0; ≥6.0 HER2 signals/cell

Group 4 = HER2/CEP17 ratio <2.0; ≥4.0 and <6.0 HER2 signals/cell

Group 5 = HER2/CEP17 ratio <2.0; <4.0 HER2 signals/cell

Reporting Results of HER2 Testing by *in situ* Hybridization (Single-probe Assay)

Result	Criteria (single-probe assay)
Negative	• Average HER2 copy number <4.0 signals/cell • Average HER2 copy number ≥ 4.0 and <6.0 signals/cell and concurrent 1HC 0, 1 + or 2+ • Average HER2 number ≥4.0 and <6.0 signals/cell and concurrent dual probe ISH group 5
Positive	• Average HER2 copy number ≥6.0 signals/cell • Average HER2 copy number ≥4.0 and <6.0 signals/cell and concurrent 1HC 3+ • Average HER2 copy number ≥4.0 and <6.0 signals/cell and concurrent dual probe ISH group I

Reporting Results of HER2 Testing by *in situ* Hybridization (Dual-probe Assay)

Result	Criteria (dual-probe assay)
Negative	• Group 5
Negative* (see comment)	• Group 2 and concurrent IHC 0–1 + or 2+ • Group 3 and concurrent IHC 0–1 + • Group 4 and concurrent IHC 0–1 + or 2+
Positive*	• Group 2 and concurrent IHC 3+ • Group 3 and concurrent IHC 2+ or 3+ • Group 4 and concurrent IHC 3+
Positive	• Group 1

*For groups 2–4 final ISH results are based on concurrent review of IHC, with recounting of the ISH test by second reviewer if IHC is 2+ (per 2018 CAP/ASCO Update recommendations).

Important issues in interpreting ISH are the following:
- **Identification of invasive carcinoma:** A pathologist should identify on the hematoxylin and eosin (H&E) or HER2 IHC slide the area of invasive carcinoma to be evaluated by ISH.
- **Identification of associated DCIS:** In some cases, DCIS will show gene amplification, whereas the associated invasive carcinoma will not. ISH analysis must be performed on the invasive carcinoma.

Some cancers have a low level of HER2 expression as determined by equivocal results by both IHC and ISH analysis. Repeat testing may be helpful to exclude possible technical problems with the assays but often does not result in definitive positive or negative results.

Either the number of HER2 genes or the ratio HER2 to CEP17 can be used to determine the presence of amplification. In the majority of carcinomas both methods give the same result. In unusual cases, the 2 methods give different results, usually due to variation in the number of CEP17 signals. Some studies have shown that chromosome 17 abnormalities can lead to alterations of the HER2/CEP17 ratio, potentially leading to equivocal or incorrect ISH results. In such cases gene copy number may a more accurate reflection of HER2 status. If there is a second contiguous population of cells with increased HER2 signals/cell, and this cell population consists of more than 10% of tumor cells on the slide (defined by image analysis or by visual estimation of the ISH or IHC slide), a separate counting of a least 20 non-overlapping cells must also be done a within this cell population and also reported. An overall random count is not appropriate in this situation.

Radiation Biodosimetry

Biodosimetry involves the identification and scoring of certain biomarkers specific to and induced by radiation. To be useful, a

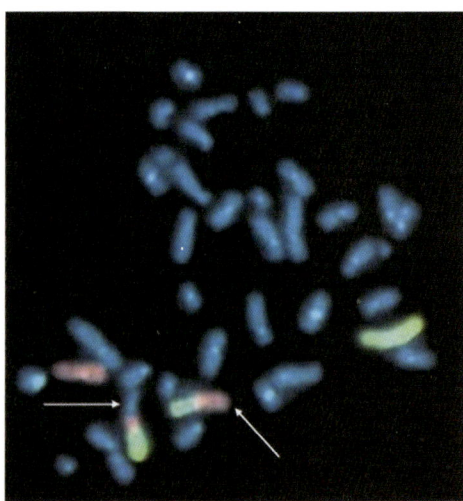

Fig. 33.8: The metaphase shown below shows complex chromosomal aberrations involving chromosome 1 (green) and chromosome 3 (orange), an indication of high doses of radiation exposure. Shows some of the complex aberrations that have been identified by FISH (whole chromosome painting) in peripheral blood lymphocytes exposed to gamma radiation

biomarker for exposure and risk assessment should employ an end point that is highly quantitative, stable over time, and relevant to human risk. Biodosimetry is usually performed by enumerating the number of unstable chromosome aberrations—dicentric chromosomes and centric rings in peripheral blood lymphocytes of exposed individuals. Radiation induced unstable chromosomal exchanges are eliminated from the body within 1–3 years depending on the exposure condition.

CHAPTER 34

Molecular Pathology: Basics

Sandhya Sundaram, C Simon Durai Raj, R Krishnakumar, V Pavithra

Molecular pathology is a discipline of pathology, which focuses on the diagnosis of diseases at the fundamental level in relation to nucleic acid abnormalities. Molecular techniques have revealed diversity among cancers that is now forming the basis for classification of tumors according to their prognostic and, more importantly therapeutic significance.

Genetic information in human cells is encoded in deoxyribonucleic acid (DNA), a double-stranded molecule which is primarily located in the nucleus of each cell. Genes are segments of genomic DNA that encode proteins and other functional products. Ribonucleic acid (RNA) is a single-stranded molecule with a chain of nucleotides on a sugar phosphate backbone. The most abundant type of RNA is ribosomal RNA and tRNA which comprise about 90% of total cellular RNA. They are predominantly located in the cytoplasm and have major function in protein synthesis. Messenger RNA (mRNA) composes only 1–5% of total RNA. Each mRNA molecule is a copy of a specific gene and functions to transfer genetic information from the nucleus to cytoplasm where it serves as a master plan for protein synthesis. After synthesis, the protein undergoes post-translational modifications in order for it to function, to move within the cell, or to fold properly.

SAMPLES USED FOR MOLECULAR DIAGNOSIS

Major Steps Involved in the Molecular Technique

1. The extraction and purification of nucleic acid
2. The amplification of the nucleic acid of interest (target)
3. Nucleic acid analysis.

Several molecular diagnostic methods are used, viz. Polymerase chain reaction and real time PCR, next generation sequencing, DNA microarray, restriction fragment length polymorphism (RFLP), fluorescent *in situ*

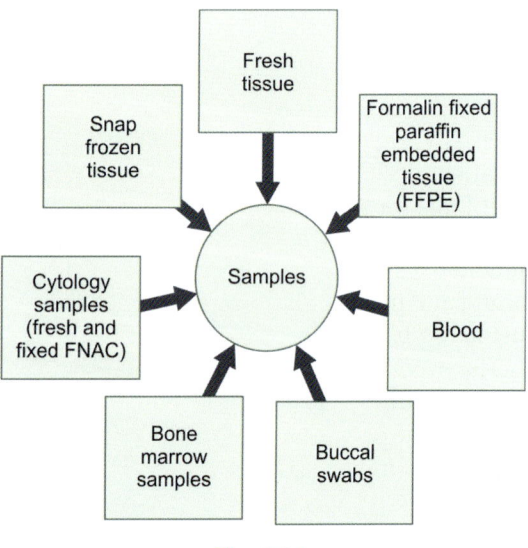

Fig. 34.1

hybridization (FISH), flow cytometry, comparative genomic hybridization and the very sophisticated next generation sequencing.

One of the most commonly performed procedures is the polymerase chain reaction (PCR) which enables the amplification of specific sequences of nucleic acids from an extremely small amount of genetic starting material which can then be subjected to any molecular analysis.

The polymerase chain reaction (PCR) technique was invented in 1985 by Kary B Mullis.

Basic Principle Behind Polymerase Chain Reaction

In PCR, the nucleic acid is selectively amplified up to 1 million-fold, resulting in production of abundant and specific amplicons. It relies on the presence of DNA polymerase to catalyse the reproduction of a specific DNA sequence.

3 Basic Steps in PCR Cycle Denaturing, Annealing, and Extension

During denaturing, the two strands of the helix of the target genetic material are unwound and separated by heating at 90° to 95°C. Annealing, or hybridization, is a process where oligonucleotide primers bind to their complementary bases on the single-stranded DNA at cooler temperature ranging from 55 to 60°C.

Finally, during extension phase at a temperature of 75°C, the polymerase reads the template strand and quickly matches it with the appropriate nucleotides, resulting in two new helixes consisting of part of the original strand and the complementary strand that was just assembled.

The process is repeated 30 to 40 times, each cycle doubling the amount of the targeted genetic material. At the end of the PCR procedure, millions of identical copies of the original specific DNA sequence are generated. This technique offers sensitivity since small amounts of genetic material can be amplified

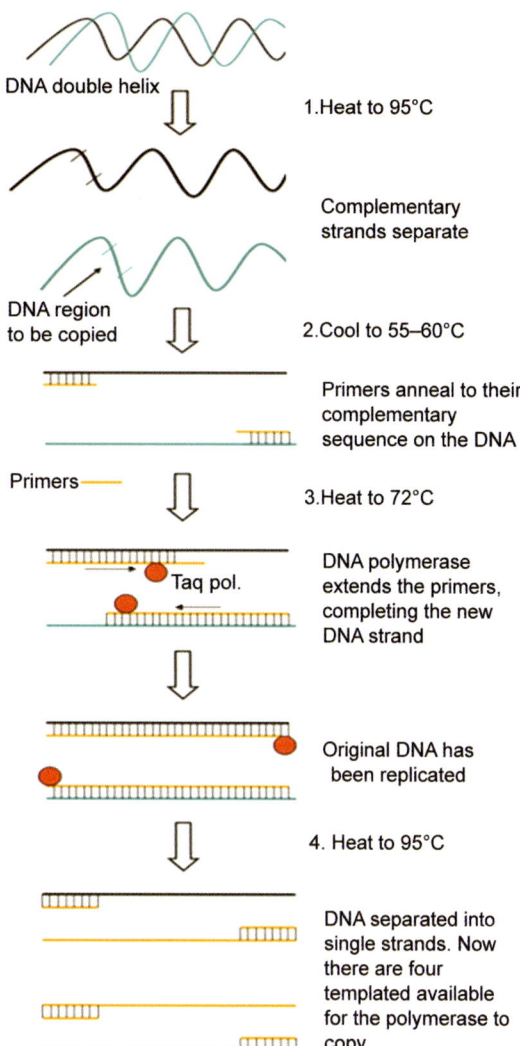

Fig. 34.2

to detect target sequences in a given sample. Also this offers specificity as a specific sequence of DNA is amplified under stringent conditions.

Types of Polymerase Chain Reaction

In recent years, modifications or variants have been developed from the basic PCR method to improve performance and specificity, and to achieve the amplification of other molecules of interest in research such as RNA. A few are mentioned as follow.

Multiplex PCR allows simultaneous amplification of many sequences and is used for diagnosis of multiple diseases in the same sample. Also it can be used to identify exonic and intronic sequences in specific genes.

Nested PCR increases the sensitivity since small amounts of the target are detected by using two sets of primers, involving a double process of amplification. These are specific to an internal amplified sequence in the first PCR. The logic behind this strategy is that if the wrong locus were amplified by mistake, the probability is very low that it would also be amplified a second time by a second pair of primers.

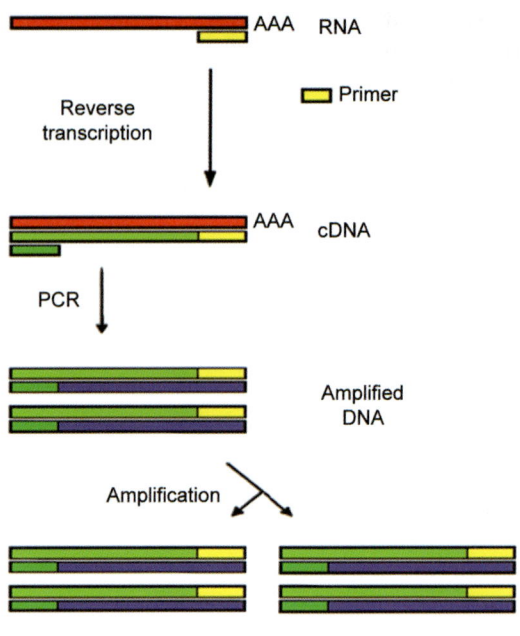

Fig. 34.4

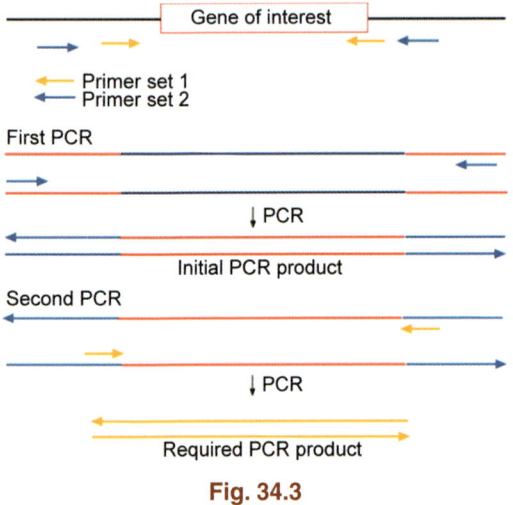

Fig. 34.3

Reverse transcriptase PCR (RT-PCR) is one of many variants of polymerase chain reaction (PCR). In RT-PCR, the RNA template is first converted into a complementary DNA (cDNA) using a reverse transcriptase. The cDNA is then used as a template for exponential amplification using PCR. The use of RT-PCR for the detection of RNA transcript has revolutionalized the study of gene by making it theoretically possible to detect the transcripts of practically any gene, enabled sample amplification and eliminated the need for abundant starting material.

Semiquantitative PCR allows an approximation to the relative amount of nucleic acids present in a sample, then, internal controls (that are used as markers) are amplified. Amplification product is separated by electrophoresis. Agarose gel is photographed after ethidium bromide staining, and optical density is calculated by a densitometer. The disadvantage of the technique is possibility of nonspecific hybridizations, generating unsatisfactory results. Control of specificity is performed using highly specific probes for hybridization.

Real-time PCR

The recent development of "real-time" PCR added great advantages to traditional PCR. Real-time PCR improves upon quantitative endpoint PCR by measuring target amplification early in the reaction when amplification is proceeding during each cycle, using fluorescence-based technology. It can quantify amplicon production at the exponential phase of the PCR reaction in contrast to measuring the amount of product at the end point of the reaction. The amplicon is monitored in "real-time", or as it is being produced, by labeling and detecting the accumulating product with a fluorescently tagged substrate during the amplification procedure. This method has many advantages over conventional PCR including increased speed due to reduced cycle number, lack of post-PCR gel electrophoresis detection of products, and higher sensitivity of the fluorescent dyes used for the detection of the amplicon. It is, moreover, less prone to contamination since the entire process of amplification and quantitation of the original target DNA for each sample is done in a single sealed tube. However, real-time PCR requires sophisticated equipment in comparison to conventional. Nonspecific fluorescent dyes/sequence-specific DNA probes labeled with a fluorescent reporter can quantify messenger RNA by using reverse transcriptase.

Allele-specific polymerase chain reaction is to identify single-nucleotide polymorphism (SNPs). The allele-specific PCR uses primers whose 3' ends cover the SNP. An allele-specific oligonucleotide will only anneal to sequences that match it perfectly, a single mismatch being sufficient to prevent hybridization under appropriate conditions.

Methylation-specific polymerase chain reaction can rapidly assess the methylation status of virtually any group of CpG sites within a CpG island, independent of the use of methylation-sensitive restriction enzymes. Primer pairs are designed to be "methylation-specific" by including sequences complementing only unconverted 5-methylcytosines, or "unmethylation-specific", complementing thymines converted from unmethylated

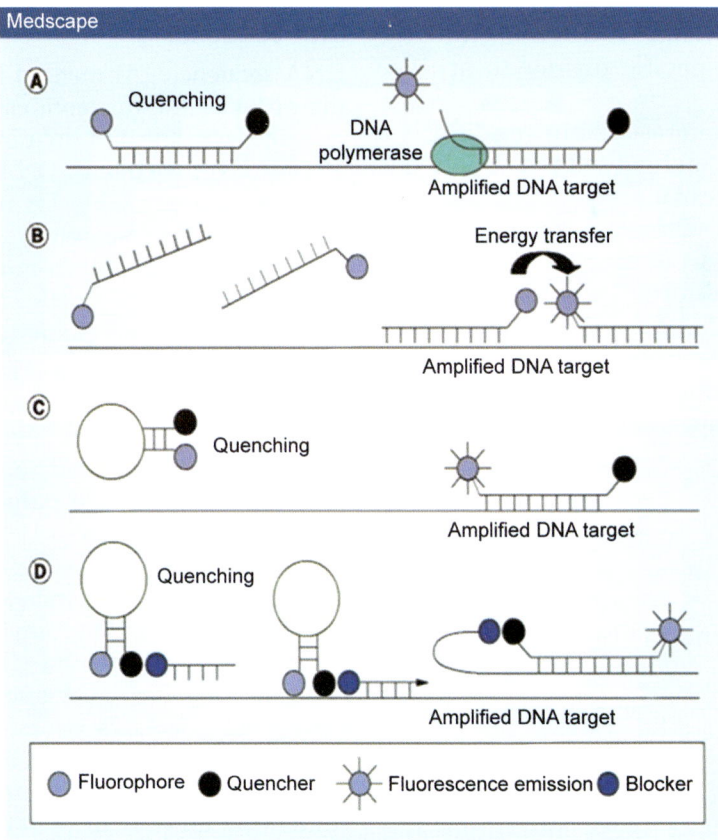

Fig. 34.5

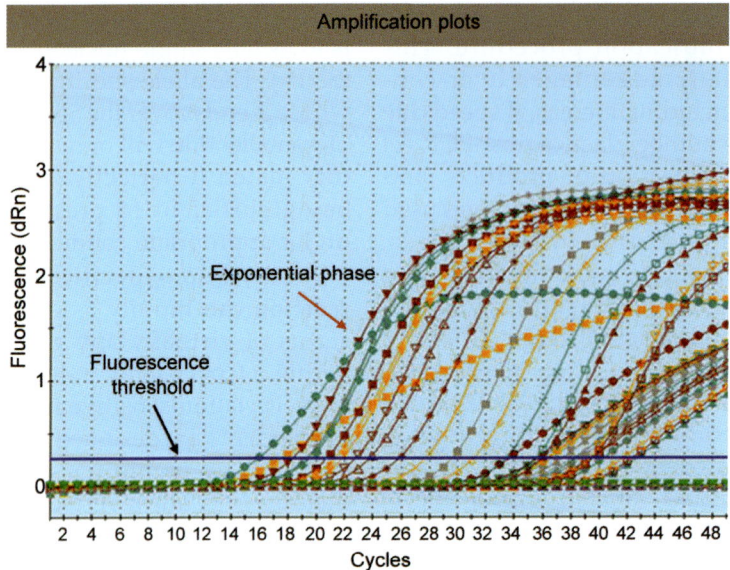

Fig. 34.6

cytosines. Methylation is determined by the ability of the specific primer to achieve amplification.

Inverse polymerase chain reaction is a variant of PCR, and is used when only one internal sequence of the target DNA is known.

Asymmetric polymerase chain reaction is used for synthesis of single-stranded DNA molecules useful for DNA sequencing. Two primers are used in the ratio of 100:1, so that after 20–25 cycles of amplification one primer exhausted and single-stranded DNA will be produce in the successive cycles.

APPLICATIONS OF POLYMERASE CHAIN REACTION

The polymerase chain reaction (PCR) has widespread use in several areas particularly in genetic analysis, medical applications (hematological and solid tumors), infectious diseases, forensic studies, research areas. The final PCR product is analysed using several methods, viz. gel electrophoresis, DNA sequencing, etc. Since cancer involves genetic alterations PCR-based tests assay proves useful in studying these mutations and designing appropriate therapy individually customized to a patient.

DNA Sequencing

DNA sequencing is method for determining the order of the nucleotides bases adenine, guanine, cytosine and thymine in a molecule of DNA. Knowledge of DNA sequences has become indispensable for basic biological research, other research branches utilizing DNA sequencing, and in numerous applied fields such as diagnostic, biotechnology, forensic biology and biological systematics.

The most popular method for doing this is called the chain termination method or Sanger method (named after its inventor, Frederick Sanger). Sanger method requires a single-stranded DNA template, polymerase enzyme, primer, deoxynucleoside triphosphates (dNTPs) and modified nucleotides (ddNTPs) that terminate DNA strand elongation. These ddNTPs lack a 3'-OH group that is required for the formation of a phosphodiester bond between two nucleotides, causing the extension of the DNA strand to stop when a ddNTP is added. The DNA sample is divided into four separate sequencing reactions, containing all four of the standard dNTPs (dATP, dGTP, dCTP, and dTTP), the DNA polymerase, and only one of the four ddNTPs

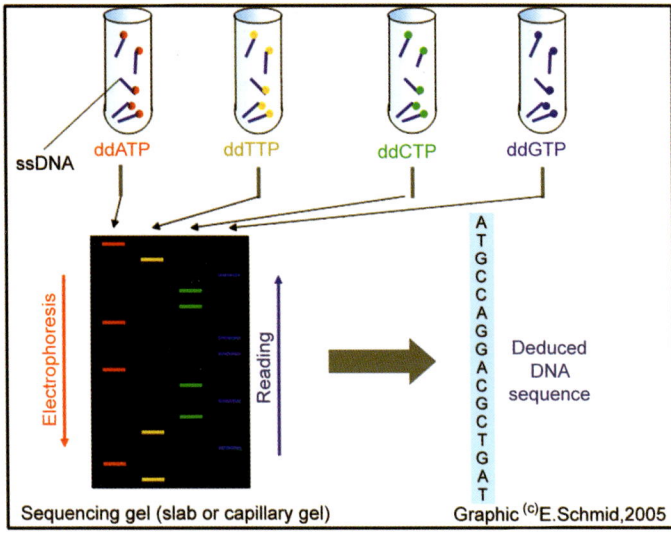

Fig. 34.7

(ddATP, ddGTP, ddCTP, or ddTTP) for each reaction. After rounds of template DNA extension, the DNA fragments that are formed are denatured and separated by size using gel electrophoresis with each of the four reactions in one of four separated lanes. The DNA bands can then be visualized by UV light or autoradiography and the DNA sequence can be directly read off the gel image or the X-ray film. In automated sequencing ddNTPs may be radioactively or fluorescently labeled and the four reactions can be incorporated into one reaction run, and the DNA sequence can be read.

Next Generation Sequencing (NGS)

Next generation sequencing (NGS) and high-throughput sequencing are related terms that describe a DNA sequencing technology. NGS platforms perform sequencing of millions of small fragments of DNA in parallel. Using capillary electrophoresis-based Sanger sequencing, the human genome project took over 10 years and cost nearly $3 billion. Next generation sequencing, in contrast, makes large-scale whole-genome sequencing accessible and practical for the average researcher. Using NGS an entire human genome can be sequenced within a single day.

Illumina (Solexa) sequencing, Roche 454 sequencing, ion torrent: Proton/PGM sequencing and solid sequencing are some of the next generation sequencing platforms.

Illumina Next Generation Sequencing

Illumina next generation sequencing utilizes a fundamentally different approach from the classic Sanger chain-termination method. It leverages sequencing by synthesis (SBS) technology. It has four basic steps: Library preparation, cluster generation, sequencing and data analysis.

Library preparation: DNA or cDNA are randomly fragmented followed by 5′ and 3′ adapter ligation and then PCR amplified.

Cluster generation: Fragments are amplified into distinct, clonal clusters through bridge amplification.

Sequencing: Illumina SBS technology utilizes a proprietary reversible terminator-based method that detects single bases as they are incorporated into DNA template strands.

Data analysis: The newly identified sequence reads are aligned to a reference genome.

Applications of NGS

The information generated by next generation sequencing (NGS)

1. Prepare dinomic DNA sample

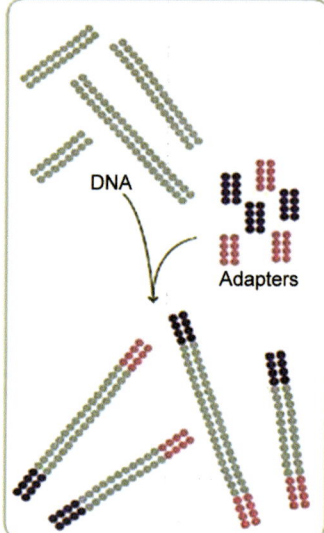

Randomly fragment genomic DNA and ligate adapter to both ends of the fragments.

2. Attach DNA to surface

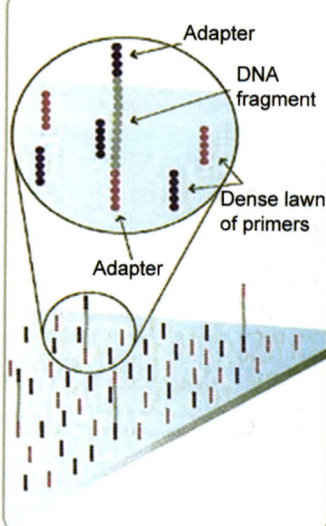

Bind single-stranded fragment randomly to the inside surface of the flow cell channels.

3. Bridge amplification

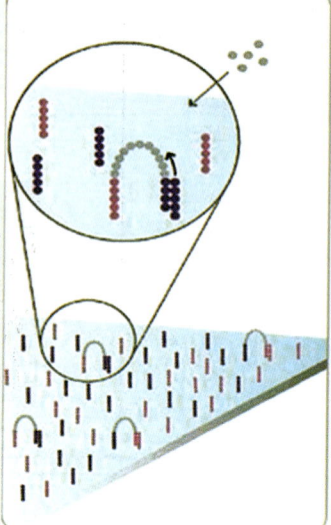

Add unlabeled nucleotides and enzyme to initiate solid-phase bridge amplification.

4. Fragment become double stranded

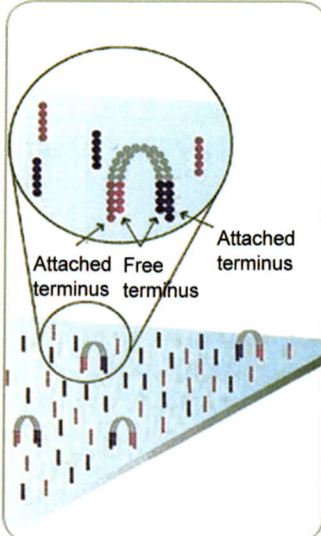

The enzyme incorporates nucleotides to build double-stranded bridge on the solid phase substrate.

5. Denature the double-stranded molecules

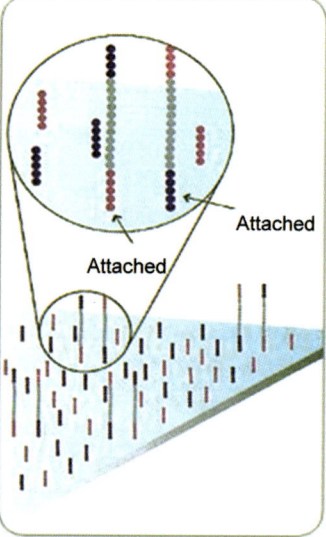

Denaturation leaves single-stranded templates anchored to the substrate.

6. Complete amplification

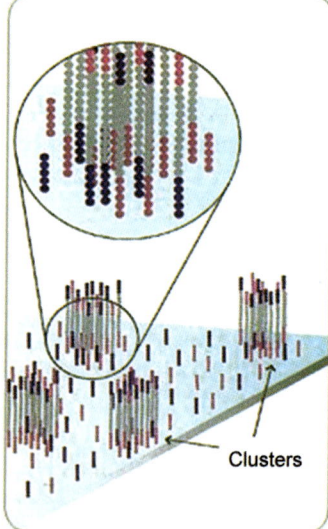

Several millions dense duster of double-stranded DNA is generated in each channel of the flow cell.

Fig. 34.8

technologies enables clinicians to make improved diagnostic and treatment decisions. In genetic screening, several investigators have tested the illumina HiSeq platform in detecting BRCA1, BRCA2, and TP53 from a tumor cell line. In these studies, NGS analysis identified all known variants in the tumor cell line with sensitivity and specificity greater than traditional diagnostic methods, demonstrating the effectiveness of NGS as a diagnostic tool. In diagnostics and assessment, currently, NGS-based gene panels are regularly used for cancer diagnostics. Targeted therapies, a growing group of therapeutic agents with molecular level specificity have greatly changed the treatment and management for many cancers.

Liquid Biopsy

Analyses of circulating nucleic acids are commonly referred to as 'liquid biopsies'. It works on the principle that similar to normal cells the cancer cells undergo necrosis and the small fragments of nucleic acids are released into circulation. The detection of these fragments by ultra-sensitive molecular methods can be used to monitor response to treatment, assess the emergence of drug resistance, and quantify minimal residual disease. In addition to blood, other body fluids such as urine, saliva, pleural effusions, and cerebrospinal fluid, can contain tumor-derived genetic information. The molecular profiles derived from ctDNA (circulating DNA) can be further complemented with those obtained through analysis of circulating tumor cells (CTCs), as well as RNA, proteins, and lipids contained within vesicles, such as exosomes. Liquid biopsies will complement the tissue biopsy allowing more patients to be tested and prove useful in monitoring and in taking therapeutic decision.

To conclude the molecular techniques can be used to confirm, complement and refine the information obtained from routine histological slides. These powerful tools have to be judiciously used and will be an additional adjunct to histomorphology in providing diagnosis, prognosis and theranosis.

Table 34.1: Some of the common applications of molecular testing

S. No	Uses	Gene altered	Description
1.	Lung cancer	EGFR exons 18–21 mutation	Response to EGFR inhibitors
		EGFR T790M mutation exon 20	Resistance to EGFR inhibitors
		KRAS codons 12, 13, 61 mutation	Exclusion of EGFR mutation, poor response to EGFR inhibitors
		ALK	Response to TKI
		ROS1	Response to TKI
		BRAF	Response to anti-BRAF
2.	Colorectal cancer	KRAS codons 12, 13, 61	Lack of response to EGFR monoclonal antibodies
		NRAS codons 12, 13, 61, BRAF	MSI stratification, prognostic factor
		MSI testing following IHC screening	Indicates sporadic MSI tumor
3.	Breast cancer	HER2/neu	Response to HER2 monoclonal antibodies
		BRCA1 and BRCA2	
4.	Gastrointestinal stromal tumor (GIST)	HER2/neu	Response to HER2 monoclonal antibodies
		KIT mutation for exon 9 and 11	Helps to determine prognosis and to predict response to imatinib therapy

Contd...

Table 34.1: Some of the common applications of molecular testing *(Contd...)*

S. No.	Uses	Gene altered	Description
5.	Papillary carcinoma PAX8-PPAR	BRAF mutation, NRAS, HRAS and KRAS, RET-PTC mutation	Preoperative FNA diagnosis and prognosis
	Follicular ca		Preoperative FNA diagnosis
	Medullary ca	RET	Familial in nature
6.	Ewing's sarcoma	EWS-FLI1 translocations	Diagnostic and to differentiate type 1 and type 2 fusions
	Synovial sarcoma	SSX1 and SSX2	Diagnostic, better survival
7.	Cervical and testicular tumors	MYC	Poor prognosis in cervical cancers. Testicular myc-associated protein p62 has better differentiation of the tumors
8.	Bladder and prostate cancer	p53 and p27/Kip1	p53, p27 and kip1 in bladder and prostate carcinoma are found to be biologically more aggressive.
		Glutathione S-transferase P1 (GSTP1) promoter	Methylation specific PCR detects hypermethylation of the GSTP1 promoter in prostate carcinoma
9.	Pancreatic cancers	RAS mutation	Up to 85% of pancreatic cancers have mutations of RAS which can be found in stool samples
10.	Brain tumor	IDH mutation (using IHC surrogates) MGMT, FUS1, MDM2 promoter. p/19q co-deletion in oligodendroglioma BRAF and EGFR	Methylation analysis
11.	Leukemia	t(8;21) mutation	Diagnosis of AML. Indicate a good prognosis, with good response to drugs
		Flt3	Diagnosis of AML. Helps to identify the patients responding to chemotherapy, and who have a high risk of relapse
		t(9;22) (q34;q11) translocation and results in BCR/ABL1 fusion gene	Diagnostic of CML. BCR-ABL1 fusion transcripts are amplified by RT-PCR.
		JAK2 V617F in exon 14	Diagnosis of myeloproliferative neoplasm, polycythemia vera (PV), essential thrombocythemia (ET), primary myelofibrosis (MF), MPN, refractory anemia with sideroblasts and thrombocytosis (RARS-T)
		JAK2 V617F in exon 12	Polycythemia vera

Contd...

Table 34.1: Some of the common applications of molecular testing (Contd...)

S. No.	Uses	Gene altered	Description
12.	Neuroblastoma	N-Myc gene amplification	Correlates with high-risk disease and poor prognosis
13.	Renal cancer	VHL gene mutational analysis SDHx gene mutational analysis	
14.	Malignant Lymphomas	IgH and TCRG clonality analysis	
15.	Thyroid	RET PTC and BRAF for papillary carcinoma thyroid RET mutation in medullary carcinoma	
16.	Hematologic malignancies		Gene rearrangement assays and clonality studies for different categories of lymphomas
17.	Gene testing in established cancers	BRCA1 and BRCA2 p53 MSH2 and MLH1 Rb1	Ovarian cancers Breast carcinoma and childhood sarcomas Colonic carcinoma and polyps retinoblastoma
18.	Single nucleotide Polymorphism (SNP) studies	CYP3A5 (A6986G) and MDR-1 (C3435T)	Allele-specific PCR detected SNP in CYP3A5 (A6986G) and MDR-1 (C3435T) genes in Indian population which has been associated with the toxicity of tacrolimus in case of renal transplant recipients
19.	Microsatellite Instability analysis (MSI) studies		Identification of MSI in several tumors
20.	Identification of micro-metastases		Identification of micro-metastases or minimal residual disease in some cancers particularly in colorectal cancer, neuroblastoma and prostate cancer

CHAPTER 35
Cell Culture and Tissue Banking Techniques

Sandhya Sundaram, Archana B

What is cell culture?

Cell culture refers to the removal of cells from an animal or plant and their subsequent growth in a favorable artificial environment. The cells may be removed from the tissue directly and disaggregated by enzymatic or mechanical means before cultivation, or they may be derived from a cell line or cell strain that has already been established.

Primary Culture

Primary culture refers to the stage of the culture after the cells are isolated from the tissue and proliferated under the appropriate conditions until they occupy all of the available substrate, (i.e. reach confluence). At this stage, the cells have to be subcultured (i.e. passaged) by transferring them to a new vessel with fresh growth medium to provide more room for continued growth.

Cell Lines

After the first subculture, the primary culture becomes known as a cell line or subclone. Cell lines derived from primary cultures have a limited lifespan (i.e. they are finite; see below), and as they are passaged, cells with the highest growth capacity predominate, resulting in a degree of genotypic and phenotypic uniformity in the population.

Cell Strain

If a subpopulation of a cell line is positively selected from the culture by cloning or some other method, this cell line becomes a cell strain. A cell strain often acquires additional genetic changes subsequent to the initiation of the parent line.

Morphology

On the basis of morphology (shape and appearance) or on their functional characteristics. They are divided into three.
- Epithelial like—attached to a substrate and appears flattened and polygonal in shape
- Lymphoblast like—cells do not attach remain in suspension with a spherical shape
- Fibroblast like—cells attached to an substrate appears elongated and bipolar.

Culture Conditions

Culture conditions vary widely for each cell type, but the artificial environment in which the cells are cultured invariably consists of a suitable vessel containing the following:
- A substrate or medium that supplies the essential nutrients (amino acids, carbohydrates, vitamins, minerals)
- Growth factors
- Hormones
- Gases (O_2, CO_2)
- A regulated physicochemical environment (pH, osmotic pressure, temperature)

Most cells are anchorage-dependent and must be cultured while attached to a solid or semi-solid substrate (adherent or monolayer culture), while others can be grown floating in the culture medium (suspension culture).

Cryopreservation

If a surplus of cells are available from sub-culturing, they should be treated with the appropriate protective agent (e.g. DMSO or glycerol) and stored at temperatures below −130°C (cryopreservation) until they are needed. For more information on subculturing and cryopreserving cells, refer to the guidelines for maintaining cultured cells.

Cell Viability

$$\% \text{ of viable cells} = \frac{\text{No. of unstained cells} \times 100}{\text{Total no. of cells}}$$

Basic Equipments Used in Cell Culture

- *Laminar cabinet:* Vertical are preferable
- *Incubation facilities:* Temperature of 25–30°C for insect and 37°C for mammalian cells, CO_2 2–5% and 95% air at 99% relative humidity. To prevent cell death incubators set to cut out at approx. 38.5°C
- *Refrigerators:* Liquid media kept at 4°C, enzymes (e.g. trypsin) and media components, (e.g. glutamine and serum) at −20°C
- *Microscope:* An inverted microscope with 10x to 100x magnification.
- *Tissue culture ware:* Culture plastic ware treated by polystyrene.

Laminar Air Flow

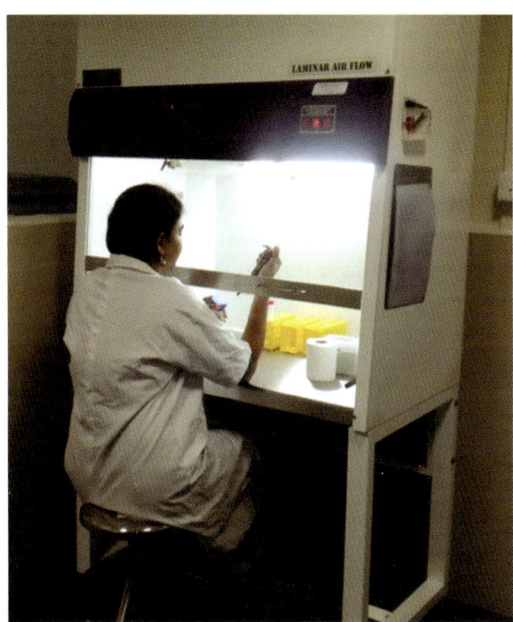

Fig. 35.1

Limitations

- Expertise
- Quantity

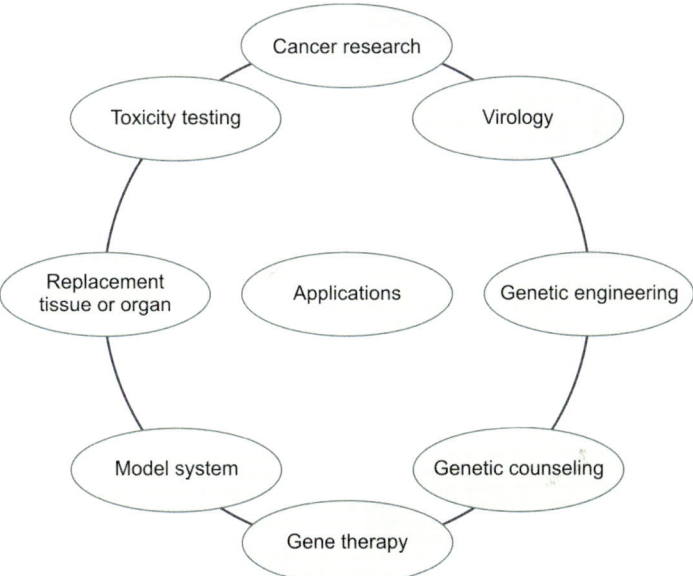

Fig. 35.2

- Dedifferentiation and selection
- Origin of cells
- Instability

Cell Lines Repository

Cell line collections can be procured from by the following organizations:

The National Centre for Cell Science (NCCS), Pune was established as a National Repository of Animal Cell Culture with a mandate of basic research, teaching and training, and as a national repository for cell lines.

http://www.nccs.res.in/

American type culture collection (ATCC) is one of the largest bioresources in the world, and offers a complex array of human, animal, insect, fish and stem cell lines. http://www.atcc.org/

Inverted Microscope

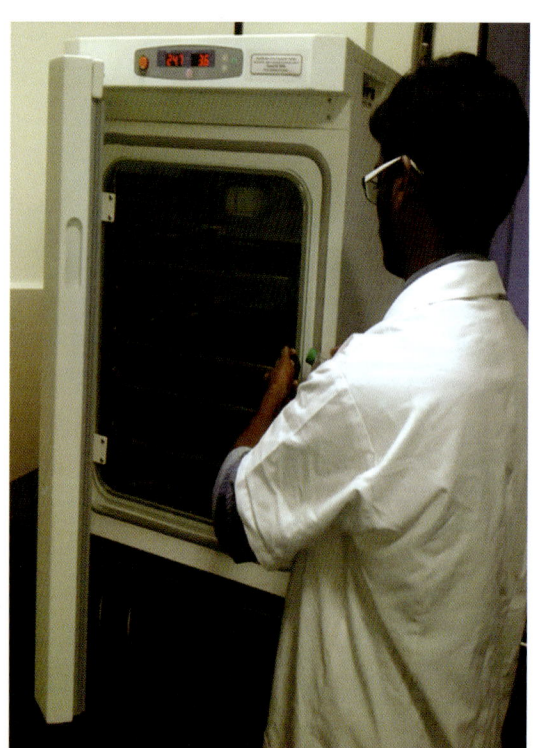

Fig. 35.3

CO_2 Incubator

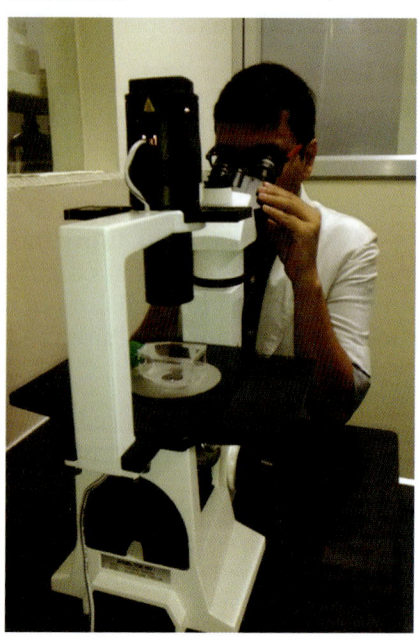

Fig. 35.4

TISSUE BANKING

Synonyms: Biobank, biorepository.

INTRODUCTION

Tissue bank is a collection of biological material, the associated data/information stored in an organised system and made available to investigators to study for clinical and basic research purposes.

NEED FOR TISSUE BANKING

- Finding targets to intervene in cancer treatment.
- Indentifying molecular events in disease progression and heterogeneity.
- Separate patients as likely or not likely to respond to a specific drug (pharmacogenomics).
- Group patients to determine which treatment is appropriate.
- Develop screening tests to diagnose, prognosticate, predict response and detect biomarkers that are associated with specific stages or subtypes of a disease.
- To study disease running in families.

ESTABLISHMENT OF A TISSUE BANK

- Institutional commitment
- Manpower with dedicated staff and resource supervisors
- Infrastructutre and facilities
- Optimum storage conditions
- Safety precautionary measures
- Specimen handling, data collection and recording measures
- Standard operating procedures
- Quality control.

ETHICAL ISSUES AND INFORMED CONSENT

- Tissue bank can be initiated only after permission from a registered ethics committee.
- There are regulatory bodies that monitor the affairs of a tissue bank.
- *Informed consent:*
  1. Mandatory from the patient.
  2. Patient needs to be informed that the tissue which would otherwise be discarded after an appropriate diagnosis would be collected.
  3. The process must be explained clearly.
  4. Strict confidentiality must be ensured regarding the patient's personal and medical information.
  5. The patient has the right to withdraw consent anytime and the donated tissue will be destroyed if they decide to withdraw consent for usage of material for research.
  6. The whole process would be free to the patient and it would not affect treatment in any way.

TISSUES BANKED

- Tissues from any tumors along with normal tissue
- Whole blood, buffy coat and blood cells
- Urine
- Buccal cells and saliva
- Bronchoalveolar lavage, bone marrow aspirates
- CSF
- Semen
- Cervical, urethral swabs
- Hair, nail, etc.

STORING OF BANKED TISSUES

It is stored at –80 in deep freezers for tissues, liquid nitrogen for viable cells, vapor phase of nitrogen for blood, urine and tissues. Dry ice is used for transport and back-up.

The tissue in cryotubes is immersed in freezing medium (isopentane/liquid nitrogen) within 20–30 minutes of surgery.

or

The tissue is placed in RNA later (5 times the volume) which can be stored in 25 degrees for 1 week, 4 degree for 1 month, –20 degrees indefinitely.

or

Paraffin tissue can be stored in a humidity controlled area at 22 degrees for many years.

WORKFLOW

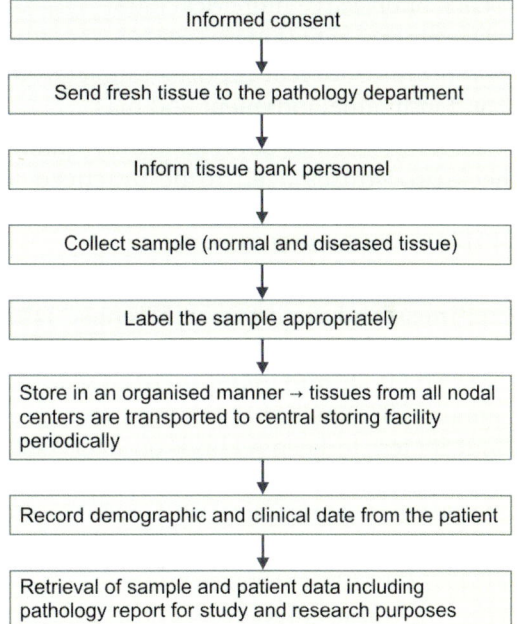

Fig. 35.5

CONCLUSION

Tissue banks are useful as a research tool and pathologists play a key role in this process. Protocols and guidelines need to be followed strictly with appropriate documentation.

Tissue banks are portals of saving more cells and storing more hope for the future.

CHAPTER 36

Quality Control in Histopathology

Lawrence D'Cruze, Shalinee Rao, Sai Shalini, Sandhya Sundaram, S Rajendiran

Assessment and practice of quality control measures in histopathology is a difficult task due to:
- Lack of objective numerical data
- Descriptive nature of reports
- Non-uniformity in reports—subjectivity and individual judgment and bias.

Therefore regular surveillance by quality check procedures need to be practiced to reduce errors and provide more uniform, reliable and consistent reports.

Quality in histopathology aims at accuracy, timeliness and report completeness with easy retrieval and review of reports.

Laboratory should have written quality manual with standard operating procedures about its test to keep a check on every step from specimen collection until delivery of reports. Every paramedical staff, resident and pathologist should be aware of the quality policy of the laboratory.

Quality Assurance (QA)

A set of activities designed to ensure that the development and/or maintenance process is adequate to ensure that a system will meet its objectives. QA activities ensure that the process is defined and appropriate. Methodology and standards development are examples of QA activities.

Quality Control (QC)

A set of activities designed to evaluate a developed work product. QC activities focus on finding defects in specific deliverables, e.g. are the defined requirements the right requirements.

Histopathology laboratory comprises of various subunits and each of these have to be monitored as they have a direct or indirect effect on reporting and final diagnosis. **Histopathology unit is categorized into three phases—pre-analytical, analytical and post-analytical** for monitoring quality of the entire process from receiving the specimen at the lab to delivery of reports.

Table 36.1 is showing the components of histopathology quality control.

Receiving Specimens at Histopathology Laboratory

Confirming unique identification hospital number and name while accepting the specimens. In any case of discordance, immediate communication with clinicians and concerned staff would help resolve the problem of identity. The laboratory should have framed policy regarding specimen handling and every individual should be aware of the policy.

Table 36.1: Components of histopathology quality control

Preanalytical phase	Analytical	Postanalytical
Specimen adequacy	Interpretation of slides with clinical data	Transcription of report
Gross description and sampling of tissue	Reporting	Report delivery
Processing	Critical alerts information	Turnaround time (TAT)
Wax embedding	Correlations: Cytopathology and histopathology when available	Archiving of reported results/slides/blocks/specimen
Sectioning	Frozen routine correlations	Proper disposal of specimen
Staining of slides, mounting, labeling	Intradepartmental consultations	
Slide submission		

Wrong labeling of specimen may result in unwarranted procedures.

"Specimen cannot be rejected in the histopathology laboratory", as all of them are obtained through invasive procedures and at times the entire lesion might have been removed in a particular case.

Check for Fixative and Volume

Fixation is the key step that would not only affect histological section but also antigen retrieval for immunohistochemistry. Poor fixation would result in poor morphology due to autolytic changes limiting the histopathologist for proper interpretation and diagnosis. An inadequate report generated out of poor fixation, in many circumstances would put the clinician in dilemma with regards to further treatment (in case of the lesion that has been completely excised and sent for histopathological examination).

Technician at the reception counter should check each container by taking small amount of fluid in the sent container and by adding 1–2 drops of Schiff's reagent to see the change in color. Change to pink color indicates formalin, while no change in color indicates presence of non-oxidizing fluid such as saline or water.

Unique accession number assigned in histopathology lab to ensure traceability.

Details are entered in nominal records which hold information of all the specimens received in histopathology laboratory.

Requisition forms should include Clinical data with site and laterality Clinical history may influence the accuracy and completeness of reports. Availability of patient's information with respect to age, gender and location would allow the histopathologist to narrow down the differential diagnosis.

Various studies in past have shown that maximum errors occurs in pre-analytical phase

Identification error can be avoided by "Bar coding"

Grossing of specimens forms an important part of pre-analytical phase.

Only if the lesional area has been sampled, one can derive a true picture of pathogenic process. In case of large specimen marking out the bitting area (drawing diagrams) can be a useful step to identify the exact location of the sample tissue studied. Incidence of re-bitting could be an indicator to assess quality of grossing of specimens.

Chemical Processing and Quality Checks

Under-processed tissue and faulty cutting would result in unnecessary re-works. Adhering to strict criteria by the laboratory for chemical change in processing and number of blocks to be cut with each blade would help in bringing out quality sections.

The processing fluids/microtome blades and routine H and E stains are changed as per the following schedule:

Processing fluid: 2000 tissue block/consultant review after daily QC.

Staining (H and E): 1000 slides/weekly or consultant review after daily QC whichever is early. These changes are documented.

When new lots of stains are put into use it is documented verified, and recorded.

Number of blocks cut with a single blade is approximately 25 (soft and medium soft tissue), for bony tissue separate blade –10 tissue blocks/blade, after which the blade is changed.

Temperature Monitoring and Recording

Impregnation and embedding: Paraffin wax-good quality, melting point, paraffin wax – 54–60°C

Water flotation bath: One degree below melting point of wax used.

Slide warming table: 55–60°C

Calibration of instruments should be done at regular intervals

Microtome monitoring
- Good quality
- Serviced regularly
- Proper maintenance of knife
- Use disposable knives
- Sharpening or changing of knives as and when needed based on policy and quality of sections
- Periodic calibration-consistence in thickness of section.

Daily Quality Check in Staining

A well-stained section is one of the hallmarks of a good and proper functioning of histopathology laboratory. Daily running of controls for routine/special stains as a regular procedure is highly recommended quality assessment and improvement step. This as a quality step is practiced to ensure satisfactory sectioning and staining enabling the pathologist in clear identification of morphology.

To assess quality of staining, the first slide from 1st batch is usually taken as the daily internal QC slide. In case of faulty staining in quality check slide, probable cause is identified with rectification and repeat standardization of staining method is done to prevent the subsequent batch from staining errors.

Labeling of stained slides
- Appropriate size
- Identification-legible
- Lab name
- Bar coding system

Participation and performance in external/interlaboratory quality assessment

Tissue sample received in buffered formalin are processed, sectioned and stained along with routine batch of slides. Stained slides are then sent to ILQA-HP (Interlaboratory quality assessment programme for histopathology) lab for preanalytical phase evaluation. Parameters like thickness of section, artefacts and staining quality is scored by external assessing center and an overall score is given.

The laboratory can send minimum of four cases (covering surgical, genitourinary, lymphoreticluar pathology, PAP and FNAC cases) once in 6 months for routine analysis to an approved external laboratory. Any two results can be analysed for major variation and necessary corrective and preventive action may be taken if any. This may be further recorded in the interlaboratory comparasion record.

Recording of Daily Non-conformities

Anything that deviates from normal and has a potential effect on the patient care is defined as non-conformity.

Maintenance of daily non-conformance (NC) register can be a step towards quality improvement and may be helpful in identifying

day-to-day problems. Few of the common non-conformities in this phase includes:
- Floaters
- Improper sectioning
- Poor dehydration and clearing
- Poor staining
- Poor mounting.

Presence of floats can lead to an erroneous diagnosis. Technicians and residents should be aware that it can happen mainly during any of the three steps. One is the pick-up during grossing (contaminated workstation, blades, knifes, forceps), second is at the time of paraffin embedding (contaminated embedding forceps) and the last is floaters from the water bath (poorly cleaned water bath). In cases of 1 and 2, the re-cuts will also show the extraneous material as they are in the paraffin block. However, it will not be seen in the re-cuts if it is has been transferred to the slide (floaters) in the water bath. Continued education regarding this, maybe a useful step to prevent such errors in future.

Policy of thorough washing, cleaning and free flow of running water off the workstation, blade, knife, forceps and other instruments and the embedding forceps at the time of paraffin embedding will avoid the contamination. Immersion of knife, forceps and all the other instruments in a container of water (change regular) can prevent such occurrence.

ANALYTICAL PHASE

This phase is difficult to assess as reporting in histopathology is:
- Subjective
- Descriptive pattern of reporting
- Lack of numerical value
- Lack of uniformity.

Parameters Assessed in Analytical Phase

Assessment based on

Intra-departmental consultation
Comparison with other reports (frozen cytology/histopathology) Random case review. *Intra and inter-departmental conferences (CPC).*

Interlaboratory (external) quality assessment. Interlaboratory quality assessment programme for histopathology (glass slides, pictures, virtual slides). Inter institutional report assessment for complex cases.

Frozen Permanent Correlation

Regular analysis with categorization as concordant, discordant and deferred. Accepted accuracy threshold for major disagreement cases is 3%. An acceptable threshold for deferred cases in intraoperative consultation is 10%. Root cause analysis to be done corrective of preventive action and CAPA to be taken.

Inter-/intraobserver quality assurance performance evaluation

To evaluate consistency in reporting
Precision and accuracy checked.

Tests to be carried out at regular intervals in the department

Histopathology slides comprising of various common systems received in lab should be reviewed with clinical details. Reviewer should be blinded to initial diagnosis. Slides should include cases reported by same pathologist (intraobserver) and different pathologits (interobserver).

High concordance possible with:
- Department policy of specific pattern of reporting.
- Abiding by the formulated guidelines accepted by department
- Well-trained pathologist.

Interlab performance ILQA-HP with a accredited laboratory

H and E stained slide sections from a single block is distributed to participating member

Interpretation and diagnosis to be sent back to assessor. Result is compared by assessing lab with the consensus diagnosis and reported as concordant/discordant. Discordant further classified into not significant (no serious impact on patient management) and significant (serious important on patient management).

Performance in interlaboratory quality assessment is one of the quality indicators of histopathology
- Clinicopathology meets and clinician's feedback
- Regular meets to be conducted and discrepancy should be noted and rectified.

POST-ANALYTICAL PHASE
- Turnaround time
- Report generation without transcription errors
- Report transmission and dispatch to the right person
- Storage of reports and specimens for required time period
- Safe disposal of specimens.

Turnaround Time
Time taken from receiving specimen until dispatch/release of report.

It is one of the quality indicators of histopathology laboratory

Timeliness is one of the main aims in generating quality histopathology reports. Laboratory should make reports available in minimal stipulated time to ensure early treatment. Signing out reports within 48 hrs from receipt of the specimen for small biopsy and 72 hours in large specimens is ideal. Complex cases: Additional time allowed if special procedures are required. TAT for frozen section should also be done. Periodic review of TAT, RCA and CAPA for unsatisfactory TAT should be done.

Guidelines for communication of urgent results ("critical values")

In certain urgent cases, it is necessary to communicate a result directly to the clinician/surgeon. This should be by a telephone call from a staff pathologist or resident, or their designee, to the treating clinician. If the clinician cannot be reached by telephone or page, their office should be called with a request that he or she contact the pathologist.

The communication must occur within six hours of the discovery of the result. All such communication is documented in the pathology report.

Some examples of critical values include:

Unexpected or discrepant findings
- Significant disagreement between frozen section and final diagnosis.
- Significant disagreement between immediate interpretation and final fine needle aspiration (FNA) diagnosis.
- Unexpected malignancy.
- Significant information reported in an addendum not expected by the clinician. Clinicians do not know when an addendum is issued so it is not uncommon for this information to be overlooked unless it is specifically brought to his or her attention.

Cases that have immediate clinical consequences
- Crescents in >50% of glomeruli in a kidney biopsy.
- Leukocytoclastic vasculitis.
- Uterine contents without villi or trophoblast in the setting of suspected pregnancy.
- Fat in an endometrial curettage.
- Mesothelial cells in a heart biopsy.
- Fat in colonic endoscopic polypectomies.
- Transplant rejection.
- Malignancy in superior vena cava syndrome.
- Neoplasm causing paralysis.

Infections
- Bacteria or fungi in cerebrospinal fluid (CSF) cytology in all patients.
- Pneumocystis, fungi, or viral cytopathic changes in bronchoalveolar lavage, bronchial washings, or brushing cytology specimens in all patients.
- Acid-fast bacilli in all patients.
- Fungi in FNA from immunocompromised patients.
- Bacteria in a heart valve or bone marrow.

- Herpes in Pap smears of near-term pregnant patients.
- Candida in placental membranes.
- Any invasive organism in any specimen from immunocompromised patients.

Recommendations for retention times for records and materials are presented in Table 36.2

Ideally, paraffin blocks on patients with cancers would be kept for longer periods of time as these blocks may be of value if the cancer recurs or the patient is taken into an experimental protocol.

In conclusion, though the concept of quality control in histopathology is relatively young and less well-understood, however like in other disciplines of laboratory medicine, quality control is applicable to preanalytical, analytical and postanalytical activities and of late is assuming an important role in histopathology practice.

Table 36.2: Recommended retention time for pathology records and materials

	TJC (the Joint Commission)	Manual CAP (College of American Pathologist)
Gross specimens	7 days after final report	14 days after final report
Paraffin blocks	At least 2 years	10 years
Slides	10 years	10 years
Cytology slides	5 years	5 years
FNAC slides	10 years	10 years
Pathology report	10 years	10 years

CHAPTER 37

Quality Control in Hematology/Clinical Pathology

Febe Renjitha Suman, Rithika Rajendran

Quality is defined by ISO 9000:2000 as the degree to which a set of inherent characteristics fulfils requirements. In the laboratory, quality can be defined as the **accuracy, reliability and timeliness of the reported test results**.

QUALITY MANAGEMENT SYSTEM

Directs and controls an organisation regarding quality. It comprises all the manuals, procedures, reference standards and other documents and records.

QUALITY ASSURANCE

Coordinated effort to organize the various activities in the lab to provide confidence that the best possible service is provided to the patient and physician. It includes controlling and monitoring the competency of staff, specimen collection, quality of methods and materials and reporting of test results to the satisfaction of patients and physicians. Thus it ensures adequate control from the pre-analytical to postanalytical stages.

QUALITY CONTROL (QC)

It involves **operational procedures** used for monitoring and evaluating the characteristics of the testing system.

1. **Calibration:** Calibrator is preserved human/surrogate cell suspension whose laboratory parameters have been determined by multiple reference laboratories and monitored by the distributor. Calibration of the equipment is done by the manufacturer using traceable calibrators. Done at the time of installation, at scheduled intervals and after machine repair.

2. **Internal quality control:**
   i. *Commercial control run:* It involves the analysis of control samples along with patient samples and statistical evaluation of the results to determine the acceptability of the analytical run. The values are plotted in Levey-Jennings chart. QC samples are run depending on the workload of the lab. Minimum 2 level controls to be run. Westgard procedure rules apply and rejection is done accordingly. Automated equipment plot the charts themselves and reject run in case of any deviation. Root cause analysis (RCA) and corrective and preventive action (CAPA) are carried out.

   Shift: Sudden change of values from one level of the mean to another which is due to **constant systematic error** because of abrupt changes to the test system, introduction of new reagents/instruments.

   Trend: Continuous movement of values in one direction over six or more

Major Westgard rules		
Westgard rule	Reason	Action
1^{2s} rule: One control value outside 2SD limit	Possible instrument error or method malfunction	Warning
1^{3s} rule: One control value outside 3SD limit	Random error	Reject run
4^{1s} rule: Four consecutive values on the same side of the 1s range	Systematic error (shift/trend)	Reject run
2^{2s} rule: Two consecutive values are outside the same 2s limits	Systematic error	Reject run

consecutive values due to **deterioration of reagents or problems with pump tubing/light source.**

ii. *Duplicate:* **Two different determinations on the same specimen.** Checks the precision of the routine work. Detects random errors.

iii. *Delta check:* Comparing the result from the analysis of a sample with the result from the **previous sample of the same patient** for the same analyte with the principle that patient values are consistent unless there is a change in treatment/patient condition. The parameters used are MCV, mean platelet volume, RDW. Failure of the delta check indicates analytical error or misidentification. It evaluates precision/accuracy.

iv. *Correlation check:* **Comparing the results of one test method with another relevant test method for the same patient**, e.g. automated DC—manual method, urine automated/manual.

v. *Use of patient data (Bulls algorithm—XB):* Based on the premise that the erythrocyte indices within a patient population are stable. Used to monitor the precision and accuracy of instrument performance. RBC indices on 500 consecutive patient samples are determined and the mean for each index calculated. Acceptable range is ±3%. Automated hematology analyzers employ the unique moving average formula (function).

3. **Inter-lab comparison:** A split sample is send to another accredited laboratory under proper storage conditions. Correlate both the results. Scheduled at regular intervals depending on the workload.

4. **External quality assessment scheme (EQAS):** Reference lab (sends samples and reporting form)→participating labs (analyses and sends report)→reference laboratory (statistical analysis, comparison with reference lab and among participating labs, comments, suggestions)→participating labs (RCA, CAPA).

Analysis of EQA Data

1. **Deviation index—CBC:** Mean, median and SD are calculated by EQA reference lab comparing the participating lab's performance with peer group and with true value. Performance is measured by deviation index DI (Z score) = (Actual result − Mean)/SD. DI score of <0.5%—excellent, 0.5–1% satisfactory, 1–2% acceptable, >2% calibration to be checked, >3% serious defect.

2. **Out with consensus method-coagulation:** Non-Gaussian procedure—blood coagulation median calculated. Participants' results ranked in 5 grades:

   Group A: 25% of all results that are immediately adjacent to and the median

   Group B: The next 10% on each side of A

   Group C: The next 5% on each side of B

   Group D: The next 5% on each side of C

Group E: The final 5% on each side of D and also nonparticipation.

Unsatisfactory performance: Obtained in two consecutive exercises. D-D, E-C, E-D or E-E

QUALITY INDICATORS

Tools used to assess the QC measures of the lab. The important ones are:
  i. *Turn around time:* Time from order receipt to result reporting.
     Various times need to be defined for stat testing, emergency department or intensive care results, routine inpatient testing, and routine outpatient testing.
  ii. *Critical test results:* Results which endanger the life should be telephoned and documented and then released.
  iii. Are the results telephoned to the appropriate defined individuals? Were these individuals available to receive the critical results?
  iv. Computer errors
  v. Patient and physician feedback
  vi. Repeat phlebotomy

ERRORS

Causes of variability in the results of a test procedure.

Sources of Errors

Preanalytical: Specimen collection and handling, quality and cleanliness of the glassware, calibration.

Types of analytical errors	
Systematic errors	*Random errors*
Errors within the test system/method	Errors occurring without prediction/regularity
Caused by incorrect calibration, malfunction of components, failure of some parts of testing process, change in reagents, expired, improper storage	Caused by poor calibration, instrument instability, operator and temperature variability
It affects accuracy	It affects accuracy and precision

Analytical: Instrument errors, reagent stability, room temperature, personnel errors.

Postanalytical: Errors in recording, releasing, computer systems, interpretation (Note: CLSI and ISO quality documents (June 2014) refer to preanalytical, analytical and post-analytical processes as pre-examination, examination and postexamination processes respectively).

Methods to Minimize Errors and Improve Precision

Calibration, preventive maintenance, maintaining room temperature, quality reagents, quality control procedures, assessing quality indicators, qualified and competent staff, and participation in accreditation processes will result in good laboratory practices.

CHAPTER 38

Pearls in Pathology

S Rajendiran

INTRODUCTION

Pathological conditions can be made very interesting by remembering them as valuable points. These may consist of lesions with similar findings (e.g. small blue cells) or specific pattern for any particular conditions (Merkel cell tumor-dot like CK20 positivity). Here we attempt to compile them system wise it is completely... Incomplete... and readers are requested to keep on adding the existing list or to create more... a never ending task ...Happy learning ... to all.

GENERAL

Small Blue Cells

1. Lymphoid cells (LCA)
2. Embryonal rhabdomyosarcoma (desmin, myogenin)
3. PNET/Ewings (CD99, FLI 1)
4. Blastomas (neuro, nephro, hepato, pancreato)
5. Desmoplastic round cell tumor (CK, desmin, neuroendocrine marker)

Large Pink Cells

1. Squamous cell carcinoma
2. Oncocytoma
3. Apocrine carcinoma
4. Acinar cell tumor (salivary gland and pancreas)
5. Hepatocellular carcinoma
6. Adrenal cortical lesions (hyperplasia, adenoma, carcinoma)
7. Leydig cell tumor
8. Granular cell tumor
9. Rhabdomyoma
10. Decidual cells

Plasmacytoid Cells

1. Plasma cell
2. Osteoblast
3. Myoepithelioma
4. Neuroendocrine tumor (e.g. medullary carcinoma of thyroid)
5. Melanoma

Signet Cells

1. Adenocarcinoma
2. Lobular carcinoma of breast
3. Epithelioid hemangioendothelioma
4. Lymphoma
5. Melanoma

Coffee Bean Nuclei

1. Papillary carcinoma of thyroid
2. Chondroblastoma
3. Hemangioblastoma
4. Solid pseudopapillary tumor of pancreas
5. Granulosa cell tumor
6. Brenner tumor

Perineural Tumor Invasion (3Ps)
1. Parotid tumors
2. Pancreatic tumors
3. Prostate tumors

Lesions with Hyaline Globules
1. Hepatocellular tumor
2. Solid pseudopapillary tumor of pancreas
3. Adrenal adenoma (treated with spironolactone)
4. Pheochromocytoma
5. Yolk sac tumor
6. Clear cell tumor of ovary
7. Pregnancy luteoma
8. Juxtaglomerular cell tumor
9. Kaposi's sarcoma

Bag of Worm Appearance
1. Varicocele
2. Mucosal neuroma (MEN 2B)
3. Neurofibromatosis
4. Endometrial low grade stromal tumor

Pagetoid Cells
1. Paget's disease of nipple (CK7 and Her2 neu positive)
2. Extramammary Paget's disease (CK20 positive)
3. Melanoma *in situ* (S100 and HMB45 positive)
4. Toker cells of skin (CK7 positive Her 2 neu negative)

HHV 8 Can Cause
1. Kaposi's sarcoma
2. Primary body cavity lymphoma
3. Smooth muscle tumor in immunocompromised hosts
4. Castleman disease

EBV Virus Causes
1. Infectious mononucleosis
2. Nasopharyngeal carcinoma
3. Burkitt's lymphoma
4. Inflammatory pseudotumor of liver and spleen
5. Post-transplant lymphoproliferative disease (PTLD)

Morphology of HSV Infection (3M)
1. Multinucleation
2. Molding of nuclei
3. Margination

Alk Protein is Positive in
1. Anaplastic large cell lymphoma
2. Inflammatory myofibroblastic tumor
3. Non-small cell carcinoma of lung

HMB 45 Positive Tumors
1. Melanoma
2. Pulmonary lymphangioleiomyoma
3. Pulmonary sugar tumor
4. PECOma (periendothelial cell tumor)
5. Angiomyolipoma
6. Clear cell tumor of tendon sheath (soft tissue melanoma)

CD117 Positive Lesions
1. Myeloid lesions
2. GIST
3. Germ cell tumors
4. Mast cell tumors
5. Melanocytic tumors

HEAD AND NECK

Parathyroid—single gland lesion—adenoma/carcinoma;

- More than one gland enlargement — hyperplasia.
- Weighing the parathyroid is very essential for diagnosis.
- Presence of intra- and intercellular fat (during frozen section with positive lipid stain like Sudan black) is more in favor of hyperplasia.
- Currently intraoperative rapid PTH estimation has replaced the frozen section.

Parotid—refractile tyrosine crystals in FNAC—pleomorphic adenoma

Machine Oil-like Fluid
a. Warthin tumor
b. Craniopharyngioma

Other IgG4 Disease
a. Sclerosing sialadenitis
b. Sclerosing mediastinitis
c. Sclerosing pancreatitis
d. Retroperitoneal fibrosis
   - Microscopic features of IgG4 disease (triad)
     1. Sclerosis
     2. Admixture of lymphocytes, plasma cells and eosinophils
     3. Perivenulitis
e. Thyroid—Riedel thyroiditis—IgG4 disease

Diagnosis of IgG4 disease can be confirmed by serum IgG4 level and increased IHC expression of IgG4.

Thyroid—difference between multinodular goiter and follicular neoplasm.
1. Well-defined capsule in neoplasm with compressed thyroid tissue outside (please remember…thyroid has no capsule…only thyroid neoplasm have capsule). No internal fibrosis in neoplasm …whereas the MNG will have bands of fibrosis inside the lesion (cirrhosis of thyroid…) with secondary degenerative changes.
2. Follicles of same size, shape and distribution in neoplasm. In MNG follicles of varying sizes, shape, and distribution.
3. Background thyroid disease sharply stops at the junction of normal and neoplasm… (e.g. lymphocytic thyroiditis in the background thyroid will not involve the follicular neoplasm but is seen extending into the MNG).

Anaplastic carcinoma of thyroid—large pleomorphic giant tumor cells with neutrophils in the cytoplasm…neutrophils within tumor cells are a clue for anaplastic carcinoma of many organs including lung and pancreas.

Respiratory System
- Adenomatoid malformation of lung—air entry through communication with tracheobronchial tree air is trapped due to lake of cartilage in the lesion.
- Alveolar foamy amorphous material—DD
  1. Alveolar proteinosis
  2. Pnemocystis pneumonia (often associated with CMV infection)
  3. Diffuse alveolar damage

Eosinophilic pneumonia clinically categorized into 4 categories.
1. Loeffler's syndrome
2. Acute eosinophilic pneumonia
3. Chronic eosinophilic pneumonia
4. Tropical eosinophilic pneumonia

Eosinophilic granuloma—common in smokers, interstitial eosinophilic and histiocytic infiltrate—positive for CD1a and Langerin (also remember-Birbeck granule by EM—tennis racquet shaped structures).

Churg-Strauss syndrome—necrotizing granulomatous inflammation of lung with eosinophilic vasculitis.

UIP (usual interstitial pneumonia)—temporal heterogeneity—admixed normal and scarred areas.

Hypersensitivity pneumonitis—interstitial non-necrotizing micro granulomas.

Sarcoidosis—4 inclusions
1. Asteroid bodies
2. Schaumann bodies
3. Calcium oxalate crystals (well seen when polarized)
4. Wesenberg—hamasaki bodies

Silicosis—closely associated with TB and other mycobacterial infection.

Bleomycin—radio recall—Previous irradiation causes damage, unmasked by bleomycin.

Alk positive adenocarcinoma of lung—targeted therapy.

New name for bronchioalveolar carcinoma–Adenocarcinoma with lepidic growth pattern.

Cardiovascular Disease

Arteritis with giant cells
1. Temporal arteritis
2. Buerger disease
3. Polyarteritis nodosa
4. Wegener granulomatosis (new name—granulomatosis with polyangiitis)
5. Vasculitis associated with collagen vascular disease

Polyarteritis nodosa associated with—mnemonic CLASH.
1. Cryoglobulinemia
2. Leukemia
3. Arthritis
4. Sjögren syndrome
5. Hepatitis B

Carcinoid tumor causes endocardial plaque of fibrosis and tricuspid and pulmonary stenosis or regurgitation (right heart is affected and not the left heart—as serotonin, 5-HT (hydroxytryptamine) and other products of the tumor are metabolized by the lungs).

GASTROINTESTINAL SYSTEM—ESOPHAGUS

Esophageal ectopia, atresia and duplication are congenial lesions; diverticula, rings, webs and diaphragmatic hernias are acquired conditions.

Lower esophageal ulcer
1. Candidiasis
2. CMV, HSV infection
3. Reflux esophagitis
4. Pill esophagitis (pill stuck to the esophagus, common in elderly)

Reflux esophagitis: Histology
Triad: Thickened basal layer, elongated papillae, intraepithelial inflammatory cells.
Esophageal pseudoepitheliomatous hyperplasia: Think of submucosal granular cell tumor (it causes overlying epithelial hyperplasia in all the organs including, tongue, trachea and bronchi).

Stomach

Stains for *H. pylori*
1. Giemsa
2. Diff-quik
3. Silver stain
4. IHC

(But the best stain is H&E and careful examination in high power 40X is essential)

In gastric biopsy if the glands appear further apart, please think of:
1. Signet cell carcinoma
2. Xanthoma
3. Lymphoma
4. Infected histiocytes (fungal, mycobacterial)
5. Atrophy

Omphalocele: Failure of formation of abdominal wall.
Gastroschisis: Focal abdominal wall defect.

Intestine

- *Cryptosporidiosis:* Small blue dots on the surface of enterocytes.
- *Microsporidiosis:* Small blue dots in the enterocytes.
- *Diverticulitis:*
  Congenital antimesenteric, all layers present.
  No leading blood vessel.
  Acquired mesenteric, mucosa and submucosa alone leading blood vessel present.

Eosinophilic Gastroenteritis

1. Mucosal involvement—diarrhea
2. Submucosal involvement—intestinal obstruction
3. Mural and serosal involvement—ascites and possible peritonitis.

GVHD: Apoptotic cells in the enterocytes (skin and bile duct also)

Lymphocytic colitis (microscopic colitis)

1. Chronic diarrhea
2. Normal colonoscopy
3. Microscopy—increased number of intraepithelial lymphocytes (25 per 100 epithelial cells)

Collagenous colitis
1. Thickened subepithelial collagen—15 microns (size of 2 RBCs)
2. Atrophy of overlying enterocytes

Radiation colitis: Abnormal stromal fibroblasts and endothelial cells.

Melanosis coli: Lipofuscin laden macrophages in the submucosa.

Brown bowel syndrome: Lipofuscin laden muscularis mucosa and propria.

Adenocarcinoma of small intestine outside the ampullary region: Metastatic tumor.

Hepatobiliary and Pancreas

Focal nodular hyperplasia:
1. Focal nodular lesion with central stellate scar in a noncirrhotic liver (other lesion with classic central stellate scar is renal oncocytoma).
2. Microscopically central fibrous septa with thickened blood vessels with all the components of normal liver.

Adenoma
1. Encapsulated nodule in a noncirrhotic liver.
2. Microscopically bile ducts are absent.

Fibrolamellar HCC—only HCC arising in noncirrhotic liver.

Peliosis hepatis associated with *Bartonella henselae* especially in HIV positive patients.

Epithelioid hemangioendothelioma—grossly multiple well-circumscribed nodules with myxoid center surrounded by hyperemic border.
DD—metastatic carcinoma.

Viral Hepatitis
1. Hep B—ground glass cytoplasm
2. Hep C—triad—portal lymphoid aggregates, biliary epithelial damage, steatosis.

Mallory bodies—Happy World Cup
  H—hepatocellular cancer
  A—alcoholic hepatitis
  Ppy—primary biliary cirrhosis
  W—Wilson's disease
  Cup—chronic cholestasis, childhood cirrhosis (Indian).

Autoimmune hepatitis: Portal plasma cells, lobular rosette formation.

Wilson disease: Cirrhosis, KF rings, CNS dysfunction (hepatolenticular degeneration).

Hemochromatosis: Pigmented cirrhosis, diabetes and cardiac dysfunction.

α_1-*antitrypsin deficiency:* Cirrhosis and pulmonary emphysema.

Serology is very essential in the diagnosis of:
1. Hep B
2. Hep C
3. *Autoimmune hepatitis:*
   Type 1: ANA, SMA
   Type 2: LKM
   Type 3: SLA/LP
4. *Primary biliary cirrhosis:* AMA, elevated IgM.
5. *Primary sclerosing cholangitis:* pANCA.
6. *Autoimmune cholangitis:* ANA, SMA.

Intraductal papillary mucinous tumor (IPMT) of pancreas:
1. Cystic dilatation of pancreatic ducts with mucinous epithelial papillary proliferation.
2. Not associated with ovarian type stroma.

Mucinous cystic tumors:
1. Mucinous cyst adenoma or borderline mucinous tumor or invasive mucinous carcinoma (akin to ovarian tumor) without any communication to pancreatic ductal system.
2. Associated with ovarian type stroma around the cysts.

Solid pseudopapillary tumor—cells with coffee bean nuclei, positive for CD10 and β-catenin (IHC).

Pancreatic islet cell tumors:
1. *Insulinoma:* Whipple triad: Hypoglycemic symptoms, low plasma glucose, relief with glucose.
2. *Glucagonoma:* Dermal migratory necrotizing erythema.
3. *Gastrinoma:* Zollinger-Ellison syndrome (increased gastrin with intractable peptic ulcers).

4. *VIPoma:* Watery diarrhea, hypokalemia and hypochlorhydria.
5. *Somatostatinoma:* Psammoma bodies.

Genitourinary System

- Urothelial carcinoma—muscularis propria invasion has to be evaluated as it need radical cystectomy.
- Rhabdomyosarcoma is the most common mesenchymal tumor of bladder.

Pediatric renal tumors:
1. Wilm's tumor
2. Mesoblastic nephroma
3. Clear cell sarcoma (metastatic to bone)
4. Rhabdoid tumor
5. Xp11 translocation associated tumor.

Renin secreting tumor: Juxtaglomerular cell tumor—rhomboid crystals by EM.

Renal tumor in sickle cell anemia patients: Renal medullary carcinoma.

Female Genital System

Criteria for chronic endometritis
1. Plasma cells
2. Difficult to date
3. Lymphoid aggregates
4. Scattered eosinophils
5. Edematous/fibrotic stroma

Criteria for disordered proliferative endometrium:
1. Proliferative glands of varying size, shape and distribution
2. Stromal balling
3. Fibrin thrombi
4. Absence of apoptosis (apoptosis is seen in menstrual endometrium in non-neoplastic situation).

Atypical polypoid adenomyoma—epithelial and smooth muscle proliferation and squamous metaplasia.

Polypoidal lesion protruding through cervical canal in elderly female—MMMT.

Endometrial Stromal Tumor

1. *Stromal nodule:* Well-circumscribed nodule of endometrial stromal cells (never diagnose this in curettage ... as you cant see the circumscription).
2. *Low-grade stromal sarcoma:* Gross involvement of lymphovascular spaces (bag of worms), infiltrating spindle cells with mild atypia, mitosis <10/10 HPF.
3. *High-grade stromal tumor:* Infiltrative spindle cells with marked cytological atypia and mitosis >10/10 HPF.

All the stromal lesions will have scattered spiral arterioles in between the stromal cells (check it in high power. CD10 positive and SMA negative, to differentiate from smooth muscle tumor).

Symplastic leiomyoma—leiomyoma with focal collection of large atypical cells with bizarre hyperchromatic nuclei. No mitosis (whenever nuclear atypia is not associated with proportionately increased mitosis ... think of degenerative atypia. In schwannoma we call it ancient changes ... also can be seen in endocrine and neuroendocrine tumors and in ischemic fasciitis).

Molar Changes

Complete mole: Villi grape-shaped, no fetal parts, all hydropic rounded villi, diploid, usually 46 XX, both paternal chromosomes. (Father's little daughter)

Partial mole: Club-shaped, fetal parts present normal and hydropic with indentations, triploid, 69 XXX or 69 XXY, one maternal and 2 paternal chromosomes.

Choriocarcinoma: Highly hemorrhagic tumor, with syncytio- and cytotrophoblasts. No villi.

Adenomatoid tumor: Tumor of mesothelial origin showing increased number of tubules/glands (WT1 +).

Can be seen in fallopian tube and in uterine myometrium (also common in paratesticular location).

Polyps of Endometrium

- Endometrial polyp
- Adenomatoid tumor
- Endometrial hyperplasia

- Adenomyoma
- Carcinosarcoma
- Endometrial stromal tumor
- Submucosal fibroid
- Endometrial carcinoma.

Male Genital System

- Prostatic squamous metaplasia—seen in association with infarction related to anti-androgen therapy.
- Spermatocytic seminoma—only germ cell tumor not associated with intratubular germ cell neoplasia.
- Papillary cystadenoma of epididymis—2/3 associated with von Hippel-Lindau syndrome.

Penile squamous cell carcinoma *in situ*.
1. *Bowen disease:* Younger patients, skin of penile shaft.
2. *Erythroplasia of Queyrat:* Older patients, lesion at glans penis or foreskin.

Breast

Diabetic mastopathy—traid:
1. Lymphocytic lobulitis
2. Keloid like stroma
3. Atypical stromal fibroblasts.

Microglandular adenosis: Round ducts with colloid like material. Myoepithelial cells absent (only benign condition without myoepithelial cells).

Complex radial scar: Central scar with cysts of varying sizes, larger cysts in the periphery.

PASH (pseudoangiomatous stromal hyperplasia): Complex, anastamosing, empty slit like spaces.

Tumor commonly associated with BRCA1 gene mutation: Medullary carcinoma of breast.

Male breast carcinoma: Commonly associated with BRCA2 gene mutation.

Ductal epithelial hyperplasia: Proliferation of ductal and myoepithelial cells.

DCIS: Proliferation of epithelial cells alone.

Atypical ductal hyperplasia: DCIS limited to 2 ducts or 2 mm size.

Atypical lobular hyperplasia: Uniform cells involving <50% of lobules, no lobular distension.

LCIS: Uniform cells involving >50% of lobules with lobular distension.

Skin

Painful cutaneous tumors (BANGLES):
B—blue rubber bleb nevus
A—angiolipoma
N—neuroma, traumatic
G—glomus tumor
L—leiomyoma cutis
ES—eccrine spiradenoma

Some people add CO to it—calcinosis cutis and osteoma cutis:

- Munro abscess—neutrophilic abscess in the parakeratotic epidermis: Psoriasis
- Pautrier microabscess—atypical lymphoid cells in the epidermis—mycosis fungoides.
- Lichen planus—civatte body—apototic basal cells; Max-Joseph space—clefts at dermoepidermal junction.
- Bullous lesions of the skin.

Subcorneal/Glandular

- Pemphigus foliaceus and variants
- Staphylococcal scalded skin syndrome
- Bullous impetigo
- IgA pemphigus
- Subcorneal pustular dermatosis.

Suprabasal

- Pemphigus vulgaris and variants
- Paraneoplastic pemphigus
- Darier disease.

Subepidermal

- Epidermolysis bullosa simplex
- Erythema multiforme
- Bullous pemphigoid
- Cicatricial pemphigoid
- Dermatitis herpetiformis
- Bullous systemic lupus erythematosus.

Dermal

- Penicillamine-induced blisters (iatrogenic)
- Immunofluorescence diagnostic of skin lesions:
    Fish net epidermal pattern—pemphigus
    Basal positivity—bullous pemphigoid
    Papillary dermal IgA—dermatitis herpetiformis.

Merkel Cell Carcinoma

1. Very high apoptotic bodies (other tumors with high apoptosis—high grade urothelial carcinoma, high grade lymphoma and small cell carcinoma).
2. Synaptophysin, chromogranin and NSE positive.
3. CK20—dot-like positivity (Golgi apparatus).

SOFT TISSUE LESIONS

- *Nodular fasciitis:* Rapid growth, loose feathery collagenous stroma, extravasated RBCs.
- *Granular cell tumor:* S-100 and inhibin positive (remember the hyperplasia of the overlying epithelium).
- *Malignant triton tumor:* Malignant peripheral nerve sheath tumor with rhabdomyoblastic cells.
- *Bednar tumor:* Melanin pigmented DFSP (dermatofibrosarcoma protuberans).
- *Rhabdomyosarcoma with worst prognosis:* Alveolar RMS.
- *Alveolar soft part sarcoma:* Intracytoplasmic crystals and glycogen—EM—rhamboid crystals.
- *Desmoplastic small round cell tumor:* Immunohistochemically confused tumor, positive for:
  CK and EMA
  NSE
  Desmin

BONE AND JOINT DISEASE

- *Pain in osteoid osteoma:* Due to production of prostaglandin E_2 and prostacyclin.
- *Telangiectatic osteosarcoma:* Associated with long-term Paget disease.
- *Radiological correlation is a must for cartilaginous tumors:* Chondroma and grade 1 chondrosarcoma cannot be differentiated microscopically.
- Myeloma
  1. Solitary myeloma—common in thoracic and lumbar vertebrae
  2. Kappa is the most common light chain produced in myeloma
  3. IgG and IgA are the most common heavy chains produced in myeloma (IgG > IgA).
- *Physaliferous cells:* Diagnostic of chordoma—large cells with central nucleus with bubbly perinuclear vacuoles—Vimentin, CK, EMA and S-100 positive.
- *Gout:* Negatively birefringent needle-shaped uric acid crystals.
- *Pseudogout:* Positively birefringent rhamboid calcium pyrophosphate crystals.
- Giant cell lesions of:
  – Aneurysmal bone cyst
  – Solitary bone cyst
  – Metaphyseal fibrous defect
  – Nonossifying fibroma
  – Langerhans cell histiocytosis
  – Osteitis fibrosa cystica of hyperparathyroidism
  – Giant cell reparative granuloma
  – Osteoid osteoma
  – Malignant fibrous histiocytoma
  – Chondroblastoma
  – Chondromyxoid fibroma
  – Osteoblastoma
  – Osteosarcoma.

LYMPHORETICULAR SYSTEM

Lymph Node

- Toxoplasma lymphadenitis—triad
  1. Follicular hyperplasia
  2. Monocytoid cells
  3. Ill-defined granulomas
- Progressive transformation of germinal centers (PTGC): Large follicles with mantle cells infiltrating the follicular center—seen most commonly in nodular lymphocyte predominant Hodgkin's lymphoma.

- Histiocytic necrotizing lymphadenitis seen in:
  1. SLE
  2. Kikuchi disease
- Stellate neutrophilc abscess in lymph node seen in:
  1. Cat scratch disease—axillary node
  2. Yersinia infection—intra-abdominal LN, especially in the right illiac fossa
  3. Lymphogranuloma venereum—inguinal nodes.
- Folicular hyperplasia varying size, shape and distribution follicular center—present BCL-2 negative *vs*
- Follicular lymphoma follicles—same size
- Follicular center cells absent, BCL-2 negative.

Spleen

- *Small spleen:* Sickle cell anemia, SLE
- *Littoral cell hemangioma:* Vascular channels lined by tall cells with indented nuclei
- *Amyloidosis spleen:*
  1. Sago spleen—involving white pulp
  2. Lardaceous spleen—deposits in the red pulp.

Thymus

- *Normal thymus:* No lymphoid follicles (if you see one ... it indicates autoimmune diseases)
- *Thymoma types and morphology:*
  1. *Type A:* Spindle cells (medullary cells)
  2. *Type B1:* Lymphocyte predominant with a few polygonal cells (predominantly cortical)
  3. *Type B2:* Lymphocytes with many polygonal cells with prominent nucleoli (cortical)
  4. *Type B3:* Polygonal and squamoid cells (well-differentiated thymic carcinoma)
  5. *Type AB:* Mixed spindle and cortical cells
  6. *Type C:* Thymic carcinoam (squamous cell carcinoma, adenocarcinoma).

  Pattern analysis typing of thymoma:
  1. Epithelial predominant—A, B3, C
  2. Lymphocyte predominat—B1, B2
  3. Mixed epithelial and lymphocyte—AB.

CNS

- *Pilocytic astrocytoma:* Loose microcystic areas, Rosenthal fibers, eosinophilic granular bodies.
- *Central neurocytoma:* Morphologically similar to oligodendroglioma but positive for synaptophysin.
- *Meningioma:* EMA and progesterone receptor positive.

Psammoma Bodies (MOST PG)

M—**m**eningioma, **m**esothelioma
O—serous **o**varian carcinoma
S—papillary cancer of **s**alivary gland
T—papillary cancer of **t**hyroid
P—**p**rolactinoma, **p**apillary cancer of RCC
G—**g**lucagonoma

And the list will go on…

CHAPTER 39

Criteria Revisited

Rithika Rajendran, Barathi G, Sandhya Sundaram

This chapter is a quick reference of some of the important criteria that are commonly used. This is not an exhaustive list and is only intended to summarise the key points. The readers are directed to refer to the original papers for the finer details.

Table 39.1: Weiss criteria for malignancy in adrenal cortical lesions

Parameters	Score 1
Architecture	Diffuse architecture (>33% of tumor)
Cellular features	Clear cytoplasm ≤25% of tumor cells Nuclear pleomorphism
Mitosis	>5 mitoses/50 HPF Atypical mitoses
Necrosis	Present
Invasion	Venous invasion Sinusoidal invasion Capsular invasion

Total score >3—Malignancy
Adapted from *Am J Surg Pathol* 1984;8:163.

Table 39.2: Modified Weiss criteria for malignancy in adrenal cortical lesions

Parameters	Score
Mitotic rate >5 per 50 HPF	2
Clear cytoplasm ≤25% of the tumor cells	2
Abnormal mitoses	1
Necrosis	1
Capsular invasion	1

Total score ≥3—Malignancy
Adapted from *Am J Surg Pathol* 2002;26:1612

International Neuroblastoma Pathological Classification System

Modification of Shimada Classification of childhood neuroblastoma and ganglioneuroblastoma. Not graded if metastatic or post-treatment.

Table 39.3: International neuroblastoma pathological classification system

Maturation		Schwannian stroma	Original Shimada	Prognostic group
Neuroblastoma				
<1.5 y	Poorly diff/differentiating + low-intermediate MKI	Stroma poor	Favourable	Favourable
1.5–5 y	Differentiating + low MKI			

Contd...

Table 39.3: International neuroblastoma pathological classification system (Contd.)				
Maturation		Schwannian stroma	Original Shimada	Prognostic group
Neuroblastoma				
<1.5 y	Undifferentiated/high MKI		Unfavourable	Unfavourable
1.5–5 y	Poorly diff/differentiating/ intermediate/high MKI			
>5 y	All			
Ganglioneuroblastoma, intermixed		Stroma rich	Favourable	Favourable
Ganglioneuroma	Maturing Mature	Stroma dominant	Favourable	Favourable
Ganglioneuroblastoma, nodular		Composite (stroma rich/ dom + stroma poor)	Unfavourable	Unfavourable

Adapted from *Cancer 1999;86:364*

Table 39.4: PASS—pheochromocytoma of the adrenal gland scaled score		
Criteria	Score 1	Score 2
Invasion	Vascular Capsular	Periadrenal adipose tissue
Morphology	Profound nuclear pleomorphism Hyperchromasia	Large nests/diffuse growth High cellularity Tumor cell spindling Cellular monotony
Necrosis	—	Focal or confluent necrosis
Mitosis	—	Increased mitosis >3/10 HPF Atypical mitotic figures

PASS <4 Clinically benign; PASS ≥ 4 Clinically aggressive behaviour
Adapted from *Surgery 2008;143:759*.

Table 39.5: Grading of adrenal pheochromocytoma and paraganglioma (GAPP) score			
Parameter	Score 0	Score 1	Score 2
Histological pattern	Zellballen	Large irregular cell nests Pseudorosette	
Cellularity	Low (<150 cells/U *)	Moderate (150–250 cells/U *)	High (>250 cells/U *)
Comedonecrosis	Absent		Present
Vascular/capsular invasion	Absent	Present	
Ki67 index	<1%	1–3%	>3%
Catecholamine type	Adrenaline type (Adr, or Adr + NorAdr) Non-functioning type	Noradrenaline type (NorAdr, or Nor Adr + Dopa)	

U *: Cells in Unit of 10 × 10 mm micrometer under HPF
Score grading 0–2, well differentiated; 3–6 moderately differentiated; 7–10, poorly differentiated
Adapted from *Endocr.-Relat. Cancer 2014;21:405–414*.

Rosen Criteria for Lymphovascular (LV) Invasion

1. Tumor embolus in a LV lumen outside nearby tumor.
2. Definite endothelial lining.
3. Tumor embolus that is different in shape than the surrounding clear LV space.
4. Lymphatics are usually accompanied by blood vessels.

Adapted from *Ann Pathol 1983;18:215–232*.

Table 39.6: Nottingham combined histological grading for invasive breast carcinoma

Criteria	Score 1	Score 2	Score 3
Tubule formation	>75%	10–75%	<10%
Mitosis (/10 HPF)	0–5	6–11	11+
Nuclear pleomorphism	Minimal	Moderate	Marked

Scoring
- 3–5 points, well differentiated (grade I)
- 6–7 points, moderately differentiated (grade II)
- 8–9 points, poorly differentiated (grade III)

Note: Number of mitotic figures for Nikon 40X objective or comparable with field diameter of 0.44 mm; varies with microscope model and field diameter.

Adapted from *Br J Cancer 1957;11:359, Histopathology 1991;19:403, Arch Pathol Lab Med 1983;107:411*.

Table 39.7: Depth of invasion in malignant melanoma

Breslow thickness	2009 AJCC staging
0–0.76 mm	T1 ≤1.00 mm
0.76–1.49 mm	T2 1.01–2.00 mm
1.50–3.99 mm	T3 2.01–4 mm
>4 mm	T4 > 4.00 mm

Note: Measure tumor thickness from top of granular layer of overlying epidermis OR from ulcer base over deepest point of invasion to deepest invasive tumor cells.

Adapted from *Cancer 2000;88:589, Cancer 2001;91:983, AJCC Cancer Staging Manual, 7th ed, 2010*.

Clark levels

I: Within basement membrane (*in situ*)
II: In papillary dermis
III: Interphase between the papillary and reticular dermis
IV: In reticular dermis
V: In subcutaneous tissue

Adapted from *Cancer 2000;88:589*.

WHO/International Society of Urologic Pathology (ISUP) Grading System

Replaces Fuhrman grading system.
Grade 1: Nucleoli absent or inconspicuous and basophilic at 40X.
Grade 2: Nucleoli visible and eosinophilic at 40X; not visible at 10X.
Grade 3: Nucleoli conspicuous and eosinophilic at 10X.
Grade 4: Extreme nuclear pleomorphism, multinucleated cells, rhabdoid or sarcomatoid differentiation.

Adapted from *Am J Surg Pathol 2013; 37:1490*.

French Federation of Cancer Centers Sarcoma Group (FNCLCC) Grading of Soft Tissue Sarcomas

- **Tumor differentiation**
  - 1 point: Resembles normal adult mesenchymal tissue (may be confused with a benign lesion).
  - 2 points: Histologic typing is certain.
  - 3 points: Sarcomas of doubtful tumour type, embryonal and undifferentiated sarcomas.

1 point	2 points	3 points
Leiomyosarcoma—well differentiated	Leiomyosarcoma—conventional	Leiomyosarcoma—epithelioid/poorly differentiated/pleomorphic
Liposarcoma—well differentiated	Liposarcoma—myxoid	Liposarcoma—round cell/pleomorphic
Fibrosarcoma—well differentiated	Fibrosarcoma—conventional	Fibrosarcoma—poorly differentiated
	Myxofibrosarcoma	Angiosarcoma—poorly differentiated/epithelioid
	Angiosarcoma—well differentiated/conventional	MFH-pleomorphic without storiform pattern/giant cell
	MFH-pleomorphic with storiform pattern	Extraskeletal osteosarcoma
		Mesenchymal chondrosarcoma
		Clear cell sarcoma
		Epithelioid sarcoma
		PNET
		Rhabdomyosarcoma—alveolar/embryonal/pleomorphic
		Synovial sarcoma

- **Mitosis (/10 HPF)**
  - 1 point: 0–9 mitoses
  - 2 points: 10–19 mitoses
  - 3 points: 20 or more mitoses
- **Tumor necrosis**
  - 0 points: no necrosis
  - 1 point: < 50% tumour necrosis
  - 2 points: ≥ 50% tumour necrosis
- **Grades:**
  - Grade 1: Total score of 2–3 points
  - Grade 2: Total score of 4–5 points
  - Grade 3: Total score of 6–8 points

Adapted from *Arch Pathol Lab Med* 2006;130:1448.

Table 39.8: Johnsen score for spermatogenesis in testicular biopsy

10	Complete spermatogenesis
9	Disorganised spermatogenesis; many spermatozoa present
8	Few spermatozoa present
7	Many spermatids present
6	Few spermatids present
5	Many spermatocytes present
4	Few spermatocytes present
3	Only spermatogonia present
2	No germ cells present
1	No germ cells or Sertoli cells present

Adapted from *Hormones* 1970;1(1):2–25.

International Myeloma Working Group (IMWG) Updated Criteria for the Diagnosis of Multiple Myeloma

MGUS

IgG/A/M MGUS [All criteria must be met]
Serum monoclonal protein (IgG or IgA or IgM) <3 g/dL
AND
Clonal BM plasma cells <10%
AND
No myeloma defining events (No CRAB or SLiM)

Light chain MGUS (All criteria must be met):
Abnormal sFLC ratio (<0.26 or >1.65)
AND
Increased level of the appropriate involved light chain (increased κ sFLC in patients with ratio >1.65 and increased λ sFLC patients with ratio <0.26)

Contd.

AND
No immunoglobulin heavy chain on immunofixation
AND
Clonal BM plasma cells <10%
AND
Urinary monoclonal protein <500 mg/24h
AND
No myeloma defining events (No CRAB or SLiM)

Smoldering Myeloma

Serum monoclonal protein (IgG or IgA) ≥3 g/dL
OR
Urinary monoclonal protein ≥500 mg/24 h
OR
Clonal BM plasma cells 10–60%
AND
No myeloma defining events or amyloidosis (No CRAB or SLiM)

Multiple Myeloma

Clonal BM plasma cells of ≥10%
OR
Biopsy-proven bony or extramedullary plasmacytoma
AND
1 or more myeloma defining events
≥1 CRAB feature(s) OR
≥1 SLiM feature(s)

Myeloma Defining Events

End organ damage attributable to plasma cell proliferation

CRAB

Calcium elevation (>11 mg/dL or >1 mg/dL higher than ULN);
Renal insufficiency (sr creatinine >2 mg/dL);
Anemia (Hb <10 g/dL or 2 g/dL < normal);
Bone disease (≥1 lytic lesions on X-ray, CT, or PET-CT). If bone marrow has less than 10% clonal plasma cells, more than one bone lesion is required to distinguish from solitary plasmacytoma with minimal marrow involvement.
OR,
In the absence of CRAB; one or more biomarkers of malignancy.

SLiM

S ≥Sixty percent clonal BM plasma cells;
Li serum free light chain ratio involved—uninvolved ≥100;
M >1 focal lesion (≥5 mm each) detected by MRI

Adapted from *Lancet Oncol* 15:e538–e548, 2014.

Table 39.9: Gleason grade groups

Grade group	Gleason score	Histological features
Grade 1	Score 6	Discrete well formed glands
Grade 2	Score 7 (3+4)	Predominantly well formed glands with lesser component of poorly formed/fused/cribriform glands
Grade 3	Score 7 (4+3)	Predominantly poorly formed/fused/cribriform glands with lesser component of well formed glands
Grade 4	Score 8	Only poorly formed/fused/cribriform glands (4+4). Predominantly well formed glands with lesser component of sheets/cribriform glands with comedonecrosis/single cells (3+5)
Grade 5	Score 9/10	Only sheets/cribriform glands with comedonecrosis/single cells

Adapted from *Am J Surg Pathol* 2016;40:244, *Prostate* 2016;76:427.

Table 39.10: Revised Banff 2017 classification of antibody-mediated rejection (ABMR) and T cell-mediated rejection (TCMR) of renal allografts

Category 1	Normal biopsy or Nonspecific changes	Normal/nonspecific biopsy
Category 2	Antibody mediated changes	Active/Chronic active ABMR **Table 39.12**
Category 3	Borderline changes (Borderline for (TCMR)	t > 0 + i0/i1 or t1 + i2/i3
Category 4	TCMR	Acute/chronic active TCMR **Table 39.13**

g, glomerulitis; t, tubulitis; i, interstitial inflammation; v - arteritis

Table 39.11: Antibody Mediated Changes (All 3 criteria must be present for diagnosis. If 1 or 2 criteria are present only suspicious for ABMR can be given)

Parameter	Active ABMR	Chronic active ABMR
Histologic evidence	Any 1 Microvascular inflammation g >0; ptc >0 Intimal or transmural arteritis v >0 Acute thrombotic microangiopathy Acute tubular injury	All 3 Transplant glomerulopathy cg >0 Severe peritubular capillary BM multilayering (EM) New onset arterial intimal fibrosis
Evidence of current/recent antibody interaction with vascular endothelium (1 or more) Serologic evidence of DSA	Liner C4d staining in peritubular capillaries (ptc) (IF/IHC) At least moderate microvascular inflammation in absence of de novo glomerulonephritis. Increased expression of validated gene transcripts/classifiers in biopsy tissue strongly associated with ABMR Thorough DSA testing for HLA and non-HLA antibodies is strongly advised (However C4d staining or expression of validated gene transcripts/classifiers may substitute for DSA)	

Table 39.12: TCMR

Acute TCMR

Grade	i	t	v
IA	i2/i3	t2	
IB	i2/i3	t3	
IIA	+/-	+/-	v1
IIB	+/-	+/-	v2
III	+/-	+/-	v3

Chronic active TCMR

Grade	ti	i-IFTA	t
IA	2/3	2/3	t2
IB	2/3	2/3	t3
II	Chronic allograft arteriopathy		

ti, interstitial inflammation of total cortex; iIFTA, inflammation of sclerotic cortical parenchyma

Table 39.13: Pulmonary neuroendocrine neoplasms, WHO 2015 classification

	Mitosis (/10 HPF)	Necrosis	Ki67 %
Typical carcinoid	<2	Absent	<2
Atypical carcinoid	2–10	Focal	<20
Neuroendocrine carcinoma	>10	Extensive	20–100

Adapted from *Am J Transplant.* 2018;18(2): 293–307.

Table 39.14: Gastroenteropancreatic neuroendocrine neoplasms, WHO 2010 classification

Neuroendocrine tumor	Mitosis (/10 HPF)	Ki67 %
Grade 1	<2	<3
Grade 2	2–20	3–20
Grade 3	>20	>20

Table 39.15: Gastrointestinal stromal tumor (GIST), AFIP risk stratification scheme

Size	Mitotic rate	Stomach	Jejunum/ileum	Duodenum	Rectum
<2	≤ 5/50 HPF	None	None	None	None
2–5		Very low	Low	Low	Low
5–10		Low	Moderate	High	High
>10		Moderate	High	High	High
<2	>5/50 HPF	None	High	Insuff data	High
2–5		Moderate	High	High	High
5–10		High	High	High	High
>10		High	High	High	High

Table 39.16: Smooth muscle neoplasms—uterus, WHO 2016 classification

Smooth muscle neoplasms—uterus	Mitoses (/10 HPF)	Atypia	Coagulative necrosis
Leiomyoma or cellular leiomyoma	<4–10	–	–
Atypical leiomyoma (symplastic, pleomorphic or bizarre)	<10	+	–
Mitotically active leiomyoma	>5	–	–
Leiomyosarcom (2/3)	>10	+	+

Table 39.17: WHO/ISUP consensus classification of non-invasive (*in situ*) papillary urothelial neoplasms

	Thickness	Cellular disorganization	Pleomorphism	Mitosis	Fusion of papilllae
Papilloma	Normal	Absent	Absent	Absent	Absent
PUNLMP	Increased	Absent	Absent	Rare	Rare
LGPUC	Increased	Minimal	Mild	Occasional	Occasional
HGPUC	Increased	Prominent	Mod-severe	Frequent	Frequent

PUNLMP—Papillary urothelial neoplasm of low malignant potential
LGPUC—Low grade papillary urothelial carcinoma
HGPUC—High grade papillary urothelial carcinoma

CHAPTER 40

Pedagogy in Points

G Barathi, Sandhya Sundaram, S Rajendiran, D Prathiba

Pedagogy is a part of the postgraduate pathology examination in many universities and sometimes baffles the student. We list here some of the usual queries asked and important points to present it effectively.

What is it?

Pedagogy is a science or theory of education. In Greek *paidos* means child and *agogos* means lead. (pedagogy to lead a child). Andragogy is the process of teaching the adults.

Types of Communication

- *One-way communication:* Didactic lecture methods in classroom.
- *Two-way communication:* Socratic method.
- Verbal communication
- Nonverbal communication
- Visual communication (charts, graphs, pictogram, tables, maps, poster)

Common Methods of Teaching

Lectures, tutorials, PBL, charts, case review, Internet based teaching, etc.

Advantages and disadvantages of each method are given in Table 40.1 .

Teaching Aids/Media/Technology and Techniques

Chalkboard/Dry Erase Board/White board

Table 40.1

Teaching methods	Advantages	Disadvantages
Lectures	Efficient, cheap way of conveying a topic to a large audience	One-way speaker communication with no active learner participation Difficult to maintain learner's interest
Tutorials	Promotes learning Encourages learners to solve problems, connect and incorporate conceptual knowledge. Promotes social and intellectual experience	Labor intensive
PBL	Promotes independent, active learning Encourages problem solving skills Higher learner satisfaction	Resource intensive Small numbers of learners Facilitator needs to understand group dynamics

Contd...

Table 40.1 (Contd...)

Teaching methods	Advantages	Disadvantages
Charts/case review	Interactive sessions Promotes problem solving, diagnostic, interpretive and management skills Flexible, can be conducted at any time	Time consuming
Internet-based teaching	Accessible, convenient Content can be updated regularly	Needs computing skills

Advantages
Inexpensive, easy to use, widely available.

Disadvantages
Chalk dust, may require practice and prep work to use effectively.

Board Markers
1. *Temporary:* Alcohol-based with special eraser
2. *Permanent:* Cannot be erased.

CHALKBOARD TIPS
Practice drawing diagrams or pictures beforehand so that students can see and understand them. Write legibly—check your writing from the back of the room before class. Highlight important points with a circle, star or underline. Avoid talking with your back to the students. Erase old chalk work completely. Keep your board organized. First-middle panel, second-front panel, third backboard. Follow the 1–10 rule—words and letters should increase in height by 1 inch for each 10 ft increase in viewing distance (e.g. if students are 10 ft way, write letters 1 inch high. If they are 20 ft away your writing should be 2 inches high, and so on). Avoid using all capitals when writing words. Erase the board at the end of the class so that the next instructor has a clean resource with which to work. Erase with up and down strokes rather than side to side.

OVERHEAD PROJECTORS
Advantages
Bright, can be used under regular lighting, use different colors, prepare materials well before class, face students while writing.

Disadvantages
Bulky and difficult to transport, user must stand in one place, may require extra-preparation, transparency film is somewhat expensive.

SLIDE PROJECTOR
Advantages
Vivid colors can be run automatically, inexpensive.

Disadvantages
Can easily be misaligned, trays spill easily must be shown in a dark room, changing the order of the slides difficult.

Overhead Projector Tips
Leave transparencies on the projector for at least 20 seconds. Use a pencil or pen as a pointer by laying it directly on the overhead transparency. Write separate notes so that you know when each transparency should be shown. Use a card or a piece of paper to cover portions of the transparencies and hide information until it is supposed to be discussed.

Designing Transparencies
- Use only 6 to 8 words per line
- Use only 6 to 7 lines per transparency.
- DO NOT USE ALL CAPITAL LETTERS. They are hard to read.

LCD—Liquid crystal display
LED—Light emitting diode

PowerPoint presentation (PPT)
1. Designing presentation.
2. Designing the slides.

Font: Times New Roman, a serif font, Arial—a sans serif font.
- 3 to 4 words per sentence.
- Not more than 20 words per slide.
- JPEG graphics.
- Shadow background better viewed.
- Preferred text color—yellow, white or very light color
- Preferred background dark colour—black, blue, maroon.

Disadvantages
- Time consuming
- Expensive initial set up
- Needs skill
- Continuous power supply (UPS)

The Room
- Is it a comfortable space for students to listen, interact and learn?
- Lights are kept on or off? Most of the lectures are post-lunch session if the lights are switched off they feel sleepy and also eye contact is important for effective teaching.
- Are there enough chairs or spaces at the tables?
- Is the room bright enough?
- How do you operate the lights?
- Will your voice carry to the back of the room easily (so that all students can hear) or will you have to elevate your voice?

Your Voice and Body
You will need to speak loud and clear so that all students in your class can hear you. Ask within the first 10 minutes of class if they can hear you. Students will appreciate your concern. If a student asks a question softly, repeat their question yourself so that the whole class can hear it.

Body
Your body can communicate ideas, emotions and attitudes as easily as your voice. Be cautious about how you appear, act and react to students. Always wear comfortable clothes. Being the teacher does not require that you stay at the front of the room at all times. You can move around while explaining. Keep your discussions interactive and lively.

And of course a smiling expression is always appreciated!

To teach is to learn and learning is lifelong… .

Suggested FAQs
1. Define pedagogy
2. What is androgogy?
3. Type of communication
4. What are the common teaching methods?
5. What are the common teaching media/aids?
6. What is objective?
7. How will you begin your lecture/class?
8. LCD/LED/OHP—all abbreviations?
9. If you forget something during the class. What will you do?
10. If a student is talking/coming late/playing with mobile?
11. PPT:
    i. How many slide?
    ii. How many lines in a slide?
    iii. How many words in a line?
12. If there is a power failure during your class what will you do?
13. Duration of class—attention span-related questions?
14. Best method of teaching?
15. Vertical/horizontal integration?
16. Advantages and disadvantages of all teaching methods?
17. What is self directed learning—SDL?
18. Episcope/microprojector/virtual teaching/digital, etc.?
19. Ambience related question?
20. How will you assess your class is effective or not?

CHAPTER 41

Current Updates in Pathology

Sandhya Sundaram, V Pavithra, Divya D, Archana B, Gokul Kripesh

GENITOURINARY SYSTEM UPDATES
- Eighth edition of the American Joint Committee on Cancer (AJCC) cancer staging manual and corresponding College of American Pathologists (CAP) cancer protocols should be followed.
- Testicle and penis have undergone substantial changes to the pT categorization.
- Pheochromocytoma/paraganglioma has a newly created pTNM staging system.

Testis
Major changes to the pT categorization for testicular tumors:
- Germ cell tumor subtype now impacts pT categorization in the orchiectomy. Tumor subtype continues to be critical in the subsequent retroperitoneal lymph node dissection and other metastatic locations.
- If there is non-teratomatous tumor in these specimens, additional chemotherapy is given.
- Pure seminoma is subcategorized based on a size threshold of 3 cm-pT1a if <3 cm and pT1b if ≥3 cm, therefore, an accurate gross measurement is relevant.
- Epididymal and hilar soft tissue invasion is now pT2. Rete testis stromal invasion is associated with more aggressive tumors but not impact pT category.
- Discontinuous invasion of the spermatic cord is now pM1b, lymphovascular invasion in the spermatic cord is pT2 (not pT3).
- Node pN category is based on the size of the involved lymph node stage.

Impact on Clinical Management in Seminoma
If node negative, usually surveillance is recommended with adjuvant single agent carboplatin or radiation considered. If node positive, adjuvant chemotherapy or radiation is given.

Impact to Clinical Management of Mixed Germ Cell Tumor
If pT2, the patient undergoes a retroperitoneal lymph node dissection or receives chemotherapy. If pN2-3, chemotherapy is utilized.

Penis
Categorization of Penile Squamous Cell Carcinoma
- Tumor with perineural invasion is now categorized as pT1b.
- Invasion of the corpus vernosum is now pT3 rather than pT2.
- Invasion of the urethra, which had been pT3, is no longer included in pT categorization.

Impact to Clinical Management
Patients that are pT1b-4, an inguinal lymph node dissection is commended. If pN2-3, a pelvic lymph node dissection, chemotherapy and radiation are considered.

Prostate
- pT2 is no longer subcategorized so laterality of the tumor need not be mentioned.
- Grade group has been added to the CAP cancer protocol as a required element. This does not replace Gleason score.

Impact to Clinical Management
If the tumor is pT3a or higher, has positive surgical margins or is pN1, adjuvant androgen deprivation or external beam radiation therapy can be considered.

Urethra
No substantive changes.

Impact to Clinical Management
If pT3-4, pN1-2 or a positive margin, adjuvant chemotherapy, chemoradiation or additional surgery are considered.

Bladder, Ureter, Renal Pelvis
No substantive changes.

Impact to Clinical Management
If the bladder tumor is pT3-4 or pN1-3 and no neoadjuvant chemotherapy was given, adjuvant chemotherapy may be utilized. In uretor and renal pelvis, if pT2-4 or pN1-2, adjuvant chemotherapy is considered.

Kidney
- To note coagulative necrosis and rhabdoid morphology, in addition to sarcomatoid differentiation. Do not impact standard clinical management currently.
- Microscopic identification of tumor in the renal vein or its branches is now sufficient for the T3a category.
- Muscle no longer needs to be visualized for a vessel to be classified as a renal vein segmental branch.
- Pelvicaliceal invasion is now a part of pT3a.

Impact to Clinical Management
If a renal cell carcinoma is clear cell histologic type and pT2-4 or N1, the patient has the option of adjuvant sunitinib or placement in clinical trial.

Adrenal Cortex
- To note the histologic types of adrenal cortical carcinoma as per the CAP cancer protocol
- To grade the tumor as high or low grade based on number of mitotic figures with a threshold of 20 mitoses per 50 high powered fields—high grade, if >20 mitoses and low grade if ≤20 mitoses.

Impact to Clinical Management
If the tumor is high grade, has positive margins, is a large sized or has a ruptured capsule, adjuvant external beam radiation therapy and mitotane are considerations.

Pheochromocytoma/Paraganglioma
- New AJCC pTNM staging system but currently no CAP cancer protocol.
- Size is used in pT categorization based on a threshold of 5 cm—pT1, if <5 cm and pT2, if ≥5 cm.
- Invasion into surrounding tissue is pT3.

Impact to Clinical Management
None. Patients undergo surveillance.

Since the various findings impact clinical management, they have to be meticulously documented.

BREAST PATHOLOGY UPDATES
- To follow 8th edition of the American Joint Committee on Cancer (AJCC) cancer staging manual and corresponding College of American Pathologists (CAP) cancer protocols
- Most of the updates were on HER2 guidelines from ASCO/CAP, PDL1 staining, recommendations and reporting for handling neoadjuvant therapy specimens and DCIS active surveillance clinical trials.

Breast Cancer Staging, AJCC, 8TH Edition
- Lobular carcinoma *in situ* (LCIS) has been removed from pTis because it has been considered as a benign risk lesion.
- Histological grade and biomarker status (including ER, PR and HER2) has been incorporated into clinical prognostic staging.

College of American Pathologists (CAP) Cancer Protocols
- The data element modified for **resection specimens from patients with ductal carcinoma *in situ* (DCIS) of the breast** is specification of the closest uninvolved DCIS margin(s) is now conditionally required, if <2 mm and in non-core reporting sections the distance to other margins, if margins are involved.
- The following data elements were modified in the **resection specimens from patients with invasive carcinoma of the breast:**
  - To specify the closest uninvolved margin—is now a non-core (optional) element.
  - Specifying the closest uninvolved DCIS margin(s)—is now conditionally required, if <2 mm.
  - Size of largest metastatic deposit—is now a core (required) element.
- The following data elements were added in the resection specimens from patients with invasive carcinoma of the breast:
  - Distance to other margins, if margins are involved.
  - Distance to other margins, if margins are involved by DCIS.
  - Added Ki-67 to ancillary studies.

2018 Update to the ASCO/CAP HER2 Guidelines
- A 2+, equivocal HER2 result by IHC is now defined as weak to moderate complete membrane staining in >10% of invasive tumor cells.
- HER2 negative result on core biopsies does not necessitate repeat testing on the excision in all case. It may be repeated on excision, if the tumor is grade 3 and the amount of invasion in the core biopsy is small or there is a high grade region in the excision that is morphologically distinct from that in the core.
- HER2 should not be repeated on excision, if the initial core biopsy is HER2 negative and is either hormone receptor positive or tubular, mucinous or adenoid cystic carcinoma.
- The FISH testing algorithm was updated. IHC is needed for equivocal FISH results (see below), and if still equivocal (2+), additional cells for FISH are counted. If the ratio and average HER2 remain the same, the final result is interpreted as HER2 negative with a comment **(Arch Pathol Lab Med 2018;142.1364.**

Formerly equivocal FISH results:
a. Ratio ≥2.0 and HER2 copy number <4.0 signals per cell.
b. Ratio <2.0, average HER2 copy number ≥6.0 per cell.
c. Ratio <2.0, average HER2 copy number >4.0 and <6.0.

PD-L1 Testing
- PD-L1 positivity in the IMpassion 130 trial was defined as PD-L1 expression (using ventana SP142 antibody) in >1% tumor infiltrating immune cells and has demonstrated prolonged progression free survival in patients with metastatic triple negative breast cancer (ER/PR/HER2 negative) and PD-L1 positive immune cells, treated with the PD-L1 inhibitor, atezolizumab.
- In March 2019, the FDA approved the SP142 assay as a companion diagnostic to identify patients of breast cancer eligible for treatment with atezolizumab plus chemotherapy.

Recommendation of Standardized Evaluation and Reporting Response to Neoadjuvant Therapy in Breast Cancer Surgical Specimens

- Neoadjuvant chemotherapy is routinely used for triple negative and HER2 positive tumors.
- Multiple systems exist for assessing post-neoadjuvant therapy specimens to quantify the response to therapy (i.e. Miller-Payne, Sataloff, Chevallier methods) but the new recommendations were recently made based on **standardization of pathologic evaluation and reporting of postneo-adjuvant specimens in clinical trials of breast cancer: Recommendations from an international working group** (Modern Pathology, **volume 28**, pages 1185–1201 (2015).
- An image (drawing, photo or radiograph) of the sliced specimen should be maintained with a map of submitted tissue sections.
  - In small specimens with no gross tumor, submit the entire specimen.
  - Attempt to quantify residual tumor in large specimens, sample any grossly visible tumor or location of biopsy clips; in the absence of gross tumor, sample the largest cross-sectional area of the pretreatment tumor area (submit 5 blocks per 1–2 cm pretreatment size, up to 25 total blocks).
- Complete pathologic response (pCR) means no residual invasive tumor, lymphatic or lymph node involvement.
- Residual DCIS only is considered pCR (AJCC 8th agrees).

DCIS Active Surveillance Clinical Trials

- Overdiagnosis and overtreatment of ductal carcinoma *in situ* (DCIS) is an ongoing debate and there has been recent clinical trials exploring the active surveillance as a substitute to surgical management.
- Since DCIS grade and comedonecrosis are specific inclusion/exclusion criteria for these trials, it is important to report these features in core biopsies too.

THYROID UPDATES

There were updates in the **WHO** classification, in the **AJCC** system of reporting and minor updates in the **Bethesda** system of reporting thyroid neoplasms.

Who Classification of tumours of Endocrine Organs, 4th Edition (2017)

- A group of borderline thyroid tumors was introduced: **NIFTP** (noninvasive follicular thyroid neoplasm with papillary-like nuclear features), **FTUMP** (follicular tumor of uncertain malignant potential) and **WDT-UMP** (well-differentiated tumor of uncertain malignant potential).
- These borderline tumors are now considered to be similar to carcinoma *in situ* in other organs.
- **Hobnail variant** of papillary carcinoma is the latest addition to the list of variants of papillary carcinoma. It is considered to be very aggressive.
- Follicular thyroid carcinomas are divided into **minimally invasive** (capsular invasion only), **angioinvasive** (grossly encapsulated with vascular invasion) and **widely/grossly invasive**.
- **Hurthle cell tumors** are reintroduced as a separate entity and not merely as variants.
- **Turin criteria** for the diagnosis of poorly differentiated thyroid carcinoma:
  a. Presence of a **solid/trabecular/insular** growth pattern,
  b. **Absence** of the conventional nuclear features of papillary carcinoma, and
  c. Presence of at least one of the following: convoluted nuclei, ≥3 mitoses per 10 high powered fields, tumor necrosis.
- **Micromedullary carcinoma vs. nodular C cell hyperplasia:** Suspect invasion, if C cell proliferation plus stromal desmoplasia is seen confirmed by collagen IV stains.

Noninvasive Follicular Thyroid Neoplasm with Papillary-like Nuclear Features (NIFTP)

- Additional exclusion criteria are: **No true papillae** (no more 1% cutoff), no BRAFV 600E or TERT promoter mutations, no distant metastasis.
- NIFTP **is not staged by AJCC;** only size, location and margin status should be reported.

Thyroid Cancer Staging, AJCC, 8th Eeition (2017)

- Differentiated thyroid cancer:
  - Age cut off for staging was increased from 45 to 55 years.
  - Minimal extra-thyroidal extension detected only on histologic examination was removed from the definition of pT3.
  - **pT3a**—tumors >4 cm confined to the thyroid gland; and **pT3b**—tumors of any size demonstrating gross extrathyroidal extension into strap muscles.
  - <55 years at diagnosis, N1 disease is stage I.
  - 55 years, N1 disease is stage II.
  - Presence of psammoma bodies on the cervical node is considered N1 irrespective of malignant cells present or not.
  - Microscopically positive margins (R1) have no prognostic significance
- **Anaplastic thyroid cancer:** pT definition same as differentiated thyroid cancer.
- **Medullary thyroid cancer:** Most staging parameters are the same as differentiated/anaplastic thyroid carcinoma and is age independent.

Bethesda System for Reporting Thyroid Cytopathology, 2nd Edition (2018)

- Only minor updates: 6 diagnostic categories remain the same.
- Risk of malignancy based on when NIFTP is not considered a malignancy and when NIFTP is still considered a carcinoma.
- Atypia of undetermined significance (AUS/FLUS) and follicular nodules/suspicious for follicular nodules (FN/SFN) now has the option of **molecular testing.**
- **Diagnostic criteria for category** IV (FN/SFN) are revised in light of NIFTP.
- **Diagnostic criteria for PTC**—only classic PTC.
- Optional notes may be used to acknowledge NIFTP for subsets of categories IV-VI with cytological features suggestive of follicular variant of PTC/NIFTP.

HEMATOLOGY UPDATES—PART 1

Changes to lymphoid malignancies include the revised WHO classification of tumors of hematopoietic and lymphoid tissues, 4th edition, 2017 as well as molecular data for prognosis and treatment.

Large B Cell Lymphoma

- **High grade B cell lymphoma (HGBL)** with rearrangements of MYC and BCL2 or BCL6: New categories for "double hit" or "triple hit" lymphomas are included; Excludes cases that fulfill criteria for follicular or lymphoblastic lymphoma.
- **HGBL, not otherwise specified (NOS):** Blastoid or intermediate between diffuse large B cell lymphoma (DLBCL) and Burkitt morphology but lack MYC and BCL2 or BCL6 rearrangement
- **Double expressor phenotype:** Expression of MYC (> 40%) with BCL2 (> 50%), often without MYC/BCL2 translocation; may be more aggressive than DLBCL, NOS but generally less so than HGBL.
- **Burkitt-like lymphoma with 11q aberration:** Lacks characteristic MYC rearrangements; has chromosome 11q alterations and more cytologic pleomorphism than Burkitt; frequently nodal.
- **DLBCL, NOS:** Cell of origin subclassification is required: Either germinal center B cell-like (GCB) or activated B cell-like (ABC)/non-GCB; associated with different chromosomal alterations, signaling pathways and clinical outcome (ABC typically worse), immunohistochemical algorithms acceptable (e.g. Hans algorithm).

- **Genetic landscape of DLBCL:** Large scale sequencing suggests revision to DLBCL subsets, risk stratification and potential treatment strategies.
- **EBV+ DLBCL, NOS:** Elderly term now dropped but typically affects immunocompetent patients >50 years old; generally worse prognosis than EBV cases; excludes specific EBV+ subtypes (e.g. lymphomatoid granulomatosis).

Mantle Cell Lymphoma (MCL)

Classically aggressive but now two clinically indolent variants recognized:
- **Leukemic non-nodal MCL:** Has IGHV mutated SOX11-B cells; usually involves blood, bone marrow, often spleen; indolent but secondary abnormalities (e.g. TP53 mutation) may result in aggressive disease.
- *In situ* **mantle cell neoplasia:** Replaces "*in situ* MCL"; often incidental; cyclin D1+ cells in the inner mantle zones of follicles but lacks other features to suggest MCL.

Revised Follicular Lymphoma (FL) Variants

- *In situ* **follicular neoplasia:** Replaces *in situ* FL; has low rate of progression, often associated with prior or synchronous overt lymphomas; distinguish from partial involvement by FL.
- **Duodenal type FL:** Now recognized as distinct from other GI tract FL; features overlap with *in situ* follicular neoplasia and MALT lymphoma; has excellent outcome, often with a watch and wait strategy.
- **Pediatric type FL:** Now a definite entity affecting children and young adults; is a localized nodal disease with low malignant potential; has expansile, highly proliferative follicles but no BCL2, BLC6 or MYC rearrangements.
- **Large B cell lymphoma with IRF4 rearrangement:** New provisional entity of children and young adults affecting Waldeyer ring or cervical lymph nodes; typically low stage; has strong IRF4/MUM1, BCL6 expression and high proliferation rate.
- **CD10–, IRF4/MUM1+ FL:** Often associated with high grade morphology; older individuals.

Other Low Grade B Cell Lymphomas

- **Hairy cell leukemia:** BRAF V600E mutations in almost all cases
- **Hairy cell leukemia variant:** MAP2K1 mutations, preferential IGHV4—34 gene family usage.
- **Splenic diffuse red pulp small B cell lymphoma:** Provisional entity; uncommon; diffuse involvement of splenic red pulp and bone marrow sinusoids by small, monomorphic lymphocytes and circulating villous lymphocytes.
- **Lymphoplasmacytic lymphoma:** MYD88 L265P in 90% of cases but not specific (also in DLBCL ABC type); concurrent CXCR4 mutations (30%) associated with higher bone marrow involvement.
- **Monoclonal B cell lymphocytosis:** Has up to 5×10^9/L circulating monoclonal B cells, often with a CLL phenotype, but no other lymphomatous features; "low count" (up to 0.5×10^9/L) only rarely progresses.

Immunosuppression Related

- **DLBCL associated with chronic inflammation:** Long-standing chronic inflammation, EBV+, includes pyothorax-associated lymphoma and fibrin-associated DLBCL.
- **EBV+ mucocutaneous ulcer:** Provisional entity with Hodgkin-like features, age related or iatrogenic immunosuppression, typically indolent with spontaneous regression.
- **EBV+ marginal zone lymphoma:** Now considered a post-transplant lymphoproliferative disorder.

T Cell Lymphomas (TCL)

Peripheral T cell lymphoma (PTCL), NOS: Very heterogeneous group actively studied to better subclassify:

Nodal lymphomas of T follicular helper (TFH) cell origin:
- *Angioimmunoblastic T cell lymphoma (AITL)* remains a distinct entity with characteristic morphologic findings and systemic disease.
- *Follicular TCL:* Morphology resembles follicular lymphoma or progressive transformation of germinal centers; lacks the vascular proliferation and expanded dendritic meshworks of AITL.
- *Nodal PTCL with TFH phenotype:* No longer part of PTCL, NOS; shares recurrent genetic alterations with AITL.
- *Node-based EBV+ PTCL:* Associated with immunodeficiency; most neoplastic cells are EBV+; no angioinvasion or necrosis as seen in extranodal NK / TCL.

- **ALK-anaplastic large cell lymphoma (ALCL):** No longer provisional, improved criteria to distinguish from CD30+ PTCL, NOS; rearrangements at DUSP22 and IRF4 locus (6p25) provide superior prognosis; TP63 rearrangements (small subset) are very aggressive.
- **Breast implant associated ALCL:** Usually confined to seroma/fibrous capsule enabling conservative management.
- **Enteropathy associated TCL:** Formerly EATL type I; closely linked to celiac disease; cells are typically polymorphic.
- **Monomorphic epitheliotropic intestinal TCL:** Formerly EATL type II; not associated with celiac disease; cells are monomorphic, usually CD8+, CD56+ and CD5- with gains in chromosome 8q24 (MYC).
- **Primary cutaneous CD4+ small/medium T cell lymphoproliferative disease:** Indolent, localized, TFH phenotype which lacks the genetic profile of nodal TFH lymphomas.
- **New provisional entities are indolent T cell lymphoproliferative disorder of the GI tract and primary cutaneous acral CD8+ TCL (first identified on ear);** both are clonal, usually CD8+ and indolent.

- **Systemic EBV+ TCL of childhood:** No longer "lymphoproliferative disorder" due to fulminant clinical course usually associated with a hemophagocytic syndrome.

Lymphoblastic Lymphoma
- **Early T precursor acute lymphoblastic leukemia (ALL):** Retains some myeloid and stem cell features by immunophenotype and gene expression profile; CD7+, CD1a-, CD8-; positive for at least one myeloid/stem cell marker.
- **B lymphoblastic leukemia/lymphoma BCR-ABL1-like:** New provisional category with similar gene expression as ALL with BCR-ABL; often has translocations of other tyrosine kinases such as ETV6-JAK2 or BCR-JAK2 or involving CRLF2; has poor prognosis.

HAEMATOLOGY UPDATES—PART 2

It includes highlights from the revised WHO classification of tumours of haematopoietic and lymphoid tissues, 4th Edition, 2017, European Leukemia Network and American Society for Hematology (ASH) and College of American Pathologists (CAP) guidelines for diagnosis of acute leukemias.

Myeloid Neoplasms with Germline Predisposition
- Three categories are distinguished:
  - Without pre-existing disorder/organ dysfunction (e.g. DDX41*, AML with germline CEBPA)
  - With pre-existing platelet disorder (e.g. ANKRD26*, ETV6*, RUNX1*)
  - With other organ dysfunction (e.g. GATA2, bone marrow failure syndromes, Down syndrome*).

  *Lymphoid neoplasms also reported.
- Specific underlying genetic defect or predisposition syndrome should be noted as part of the diagnosis.

Acute Myeloid Leukemia (AML)
- Conventional cytogenetics remain the standard of care.
- Molecular testing:
  - Actionable targets: FLT3-ITD and TKD (recommended for all AML), IDH1/2.
  - Consider testing TET2, WT1, DNMT3A, TP53 (European Leukemia Network guidelines); test for KIT mutations in core binding factor AML (worse prognosis).
  - Diagnostic of AML even with <20% blasts if t(8;21), inv(16), t(16;16) or PML-RARA present.
- Eight categories of AML with three defined by molecular characteristics.
  - **AML with biallelic mutated CEBPA:** Better prognosis; single mutations do not count.
  - **AML with mutated NPM1:** High NPM1 mutant allele burden at diagnosis may correlate with minimal residual disease at first remission and a worse prognosis.
  - **AML with mutated RUNX1 (provisional):** Worse prognosis; MDS related cytogenetics or prior therapy takes precedence for diagnosis.
  - **AML with myelodysplasia-related changes:** Prior MDS, specific cytogenetic abnormalities (del(9q) and monosomy 5 removed) or multilineage dysplasia.
  - **Therapy related AML:** Should designate along with any specific genetic abnormality.
  - **AML with BCR-ABL1 (provisional):** A type of de novo AML (must exclude CML), most are p210 fusions, additional cytogenetic abnormalities common; may benefit from tyrosine kinase inhibitor (TKI) therapy.
  - **Acute erythroid leukemia, erythroid/myeloid type:** Removed as subcategory of AML, NOS; myeloblasts should always be counted as a percentage of total marrow cells.
  - **Minimal residual disease in AML:** Independent prognostic indicator for risk stratification and treatment; can be performed through flow cytometric or molecular techniques

Myelodysplastic Syndrome (MDS)
- Diagnostic categories no longer refer to the specific type of cytopenia; complete karyotype critical for determining prognosis.
- **MDS del(5q):** The only cytogenetic or molecular abnormality that defines an MDS subtype, can have 1 other chromosomal abnormality—except monosomy 7 or del (7q); TP53 mutation identifies adverse prognostic subgroup.
- **MDS with ring sideroblasts (MDS-RS):** If SF3B1 mutation, ≥5% ring sideroblasts sufficient for diagnosis.
- **NPM1 mutated myeloid neoplasms** with < 20% blasts are rare but appear biologically distinct; patients may demonstrate an aggressive course and benefit from more intensive therapeutic regimens.

Myeloproliferative Neoplasms (MPN)
- **Chronic myeloid leukemia (CML), BCR-ABL1+:** Chronic phase can largely be diagnosed on peripheral blood with detection of BCR-ABL1 but bone marrow essential for complete karyotype and morphologic confirmation of disease phase.

  Accelerated phase: Criteria include additional clonal chromosomal abnormalities at diagnosis in Ph(+) cells and provisional criteria related to TKI response.
- **BCR-ABL negative MPNs:** CALR mutations provide proof of clonality and have prognostic significance in addition to JAK2 and MPL; JAK2 V617F is not specific for any MPN type and can rarely be seen in de novo AML and MDS.
- Semiquantitative grading for bone marrow fibrosis now includes collagen and osteosclerosis in addition to reticulin.
- **Chronic neutrophilic leukemia:** Rare, strongly associated with CSF3R mutation, often together with SETBP1 or ASXL1; JAK2 V617F reported in a subset.

- **Polycythemia vera (PV):** Revised hemoglobin criteria to avoid under diagnosis (>16.5 g/dL men, >16.0 g/dL women); bone marrow morphology is a reproducible criterion for diagnosis.
- **Primary myelofibrosis (PMF):** Prefibrotic PMF now includes minor clinical criteria (anemia, leukocytosis, palpable splenomegaly, elevated LDH) to help differentiate from essential thrombocythemia.
- **PMF with absolute monocytosis** (15% of cases) associated with worse outcome.
- **Chronic eosinophilic leukemia, NOS (CEL):** Must have clonal abnormality; increased blasts (≥ 5% bone marrow or ≥2% peripheral blood); excludes rearrangements of PDGFRA/PDGFRB, FGFR1, PCM1-JAK2, ETV6-JAK2, BCR-JAK2.

Myeloid/Lymphoid Neoplasms with Eosinophilia

- **Myeloid/lymphoid neoplasms associated with eosinophilia and rearrangement of PDGFRA, PDGFRB or FGFR1 or with PCM1-JAK2:** Diagnosis does not require eosinophilia and may be absent in a subset.
- **Myeloid neoplasm with t(8;9)(p22;p24.1); PCM1-JAK2 (provisional):** Rarely presents as B or T lymphoblastic leukemia; responds to JAK2 inhibitors.
- **ETV6-JAK2 and BCR-JAK2** neoplasms more frequently present as B lymphoblastic leukemia and best included in the new category BCR-ABL1-like B-ALL.
- **STAT5B:** Recurrent activating STAT5B N642H mutations now described in myeloid neoplasia with eosinophilia.

MDS/MPN

- **MDS/MPN with ring sideroblasts and thrombocytosis:** Formerly RARS-T, now accepted as a full entity, ≥15% ring sideroblasts required even if SF3B1 mutation in contrast to MDS-RS.
- **Chronic myelomonocytic leukemia (CMML):** Blast percentage of prognostic import, now stratify as CMML –0, –1 or –2; molecular and clinical differences between proliferative type (WBC count ≥ 13 × 10^9/L) and dysplastic type (WBC <13 × 10^9/L); TET2, SRSF2, ASXL1 mutations common; ASXL1 mutations associated with worse prognosis.
- **MDS/MPN unclassifiable:** Features of an overlap syndrome but do not meet criteria for defined WHO entities; NOT for evolution of dysplasia in a previously defined MPN.
- **MDS/MPN unclassifiable with isolated isochromosome 17q:** <20% blasts and not meeting criteria for CMML or other well-defined category, may have distinct clinicopathologic features and poor prognosis.
- **Atypical CML:** SETBP1 or ETNK1 mutations; generally lack CSF3R mutations.
- **Juvenile myelomonocytic leukemia:** Mutually exclusive genetic aberrations that alter RAS/MAPK pathway (PTPN11, KRAS, NRAS, CBL or NF1).

Mastocytosis

- New category, separate from MPN.
- Revised nomenclature for combined disorders: Systemic mastocytosis with an associated hematological neoplasm (SM-AHN).
- Revised nomenclature for combined disorders: Systemic mastocytosis with an associated hematological neoplasm (SM-AHN).

GASTROINTESTINAL UPDATES

Type	Subject	Change in 2019 classification
Esophageal adenocarcinoma	Etiology and epidemiology	7% of these cancers are thought to be familial. The role of gastroesophageal reflux in the inflammation–metaplasia–dysplasia adenocarcinoma model has been proposed.
Esophageal adenocarcinoma	Prognosis and prediction	The use of antibodies targeting ERBB2 (HER2) in patients overexpressing this molecule is included, and the need for testing.
Esophageal squamous carcinoma and esophageal squamous dysplasia	Etiology and pathogenesis	Other environmental factors, including the importance of TP53 mutation is now clear, and studies have identified alterations in genes that regulate cell cycle, cell differention (especially NOTCH pathway), and EGFR (HER1).
Gastric adenocarcinoma	Etiology and pathogenesis	Most sporadic gastric cancers are now considered to be inflammation-driven, usually related to *Helicobacter pylori* infection.
Gastric adenocarcinoma	Classification	Heterogeneity of poorly cohesive carcinoma (PCC) is discussed, including signet-ring cell carcinoma and PCC-NOS. Rare subtypes are described, such as gastric adenocarcinoma of fundic gland type.
Gastric adenocarcinoma	Prognosis and prediction	ERBB2 testing is used to predict potential response to anti-ERBB2 therapy. MSI-H and EBV positivity are markers of good prognosis with potential therapeutic importance, namely for immunotherapy targeting the PD1/PDL1 axis (under investigation in clinical trials). A large number of other reported markers are described, but not yet in practice.
Small intestinal and ampullary carcinomas	Pathogenesis	These are split into ampullary and non-ampullary types, on the basis of anatomy. Pathogenesis seems similar to colorectal carcinoma, though more information is required.
Goblet cell adenocarcinoma of the appendix	Classification	This is a change from goblet cell carcinoid/carcinoma as it is now recognised to have a minor neuroendocrine component.
Serrated lesions of the colon, rectum and appendix	Classification and pathogenesis	The preferred name is serrated lesion, as these may be flat rather than polypoid, and the association with BRAF or KRAS mutation delineates two separate neoplastic pathways.
Anal squamous dysplasia	Diagnostic molecular pathology	P16 and HPV testing is recommended.
Neuroendocrine neoplasms (NEN)	Classification and molecular pathology	Dividing NEN (neuroendocrine neoplasm) into neuroendocrine tumours (NET) and neuroendocrine carcinomas (NEC) based on their molecular differences. Mutations in MEN1, DAXX, and ATRX are entity-defining for well-differentiated NETs, while NECs usually have TP53 or RB1 mutations.

Contd.

Type	Subject	Change in 2019 classification
Precursor lesions	Classification	The term "dysplasia" is preferred for lesions in the tubal gut, whereas "intraepithelial neoplasia" is preferred for those in the pancreas, gallbladder, and biliary tree. Use of the term, 'carcinoma in situ' is not recommended.
Hepatocellular tumors	Classification	Revision based on molecular profiling studies. Fibrolamellar carcinoma defined by DNAJB1-PRKACA translocation.
Intrahepatic cholangiocarcinoma	Classification	Two specific main subtypes: A large duct type, which resembles extrahepatic cholangiocarcinoma, and a small duct type, which shares etiological, pathogenetic, and imaging characteristics with hepatocellular carcinoma.
Pancreatic intraductal neoplasms	Classification	Intraductal oncocytic papillary and intraductal tubulopapillary neoplasms are distinguished from intraductal papillary mucinous neoplasms and ductal adenocarcinoma by the absence of KRAS in these lesions.
Acinar cystic transformation of the pancreas	Classification	Previously called acinar cell cystadenoma, but now demonstrated to be non-neoplastic by molecular clonality analysis.
Hematolymphoid tumors and mesenchymal tumors	Classification	Grouped together in separate chapters, to ensure consistency and avoid duplication.
EBV positive inflammatory follicular dendritic cell sarcoma of the digestive tract	Classification	This name change is necessary due to new information on the EBV relationship of this tumor type, previously known as 'inflammatory pseudotumor-like fibroblastic/follicular dendritic cell tumor'.
Genetic tumor syndromes of the digestive system	Classification, pathogenesis and diagnostic molecular pathology	Common syndromes are updated. A new section on GAPPS (gastric adenocarcinoma and proximal polyposis of the stomach) syndrome is presented. Tumor predisposition syndromes that confer a raised risk of various gastrointestinal tumors are described.

CHAPTER 42

FAQs in Histotechniques

Barathi G, Priyathersini

1. Define fixation.

Fixation is the process by which the constituents of the cells are fixed in a physical and partly chemical state so that they will withstand subsequent treatment with various reagents with minimal loss of significant distortion or decomposition and keep the tissue in as life-like manner as possible.

2. Write the criteria for an ideal fixative.
- Penetrate the tissue quickly
- Rapid in action
- Isotonic
- Cheap
- Stable
- Non-toxic
- Safe to use
- Causes minimal alteration of tissue components

3. What is the amount of fixing fluid to be used?

The volume of fluid should be 10 to 20 times the volume (size) of sample.

4. What is the routine fixative used in your lab? How do you prepare it?

10% Neutral buffered formalin

Preparation
- 37% formaldehyde stock solution—100 ml
- NaH_2PO_4—4 g/L
- Na_2HPO_4—6.5 g/L
- Distilled water—900 mL

5. What is buffered formalin? What is its advantage over unbuffered formalin?
- Buffered formalin is used to maintain optimum pH.
- At the acidic pH of unbuffered formaldehyde, hemoglobin metabolic products is chemically modified to form a brown-black, insoluble, crystalline, birefringent pigment. Acidic pH also disrupts the tertiary structure of protein.
- To avoid the formation of formalin pigment, neutral buffered formalin is used as the preferred formaldehyde-based fixative.

Unbuffered formalin
- 100 mL 37% formalin + 900 mL of distilled water
- Commonly used buffers—phosphate, bicarbonate and acetate

6. What are the advantages and disadvantages of formalin?

Advantages
- Rapid in action, even and uniform in penetration.
- Does not shrink the tissue because of its low osmolality.
- Easy availability and cheap.
- Easy to prepare and relatively stable.
- Does not over harden the tissue, it fixes the tissue moderately and hence permits use for various special stains.

- Fixes lipids for frozen sections.
- Ideal for mailing.
- Best fixative for CNS tissue.

Disadvantages
- Irritant to the nose, the eyes and mucous membrane.
- Formation of precipitate of paraformaldehyde.
- Formation of black formalin pigment, acid formaldehyde hematin.

7. What is the fixative used for electron microscopy?

Fixative for EM is 3% glutaraldehyde

8. What are the advantages and disadvantages of glutaraldehyde?

Advantages
- Better preservation of ultrastructure
- Relatively inexpensive
- Easily available

Disadvantages
- Lipids and most phospholipids are not fixed and will be extracted during subsequent processing without secondary fixation.
- Has a pungent odour
- Respiratory irritant

9. Classify fixatives.

Simple fixatives	Compound fixatives
Formalin	Micro-anatomical:
Ethyl alcohol	– Formal saline
Mercuric chloride	– Neutral buffer formalin
Acetone	– Zenker fluid
Osmium tetroxide	– Bouin fluid
Picric acid	Cytological
	Nuclear: Carnoy
	Cytoplasmic: Champy
	Histochemical:
	– Cold acetone
	– Ethanol

10. Mercury-containing fixatives: Zenker's, Helly's and Heidenhain's susa.

Mercuric chloride is favored for its qualities of enhancing the staining properties of tissues, particularly for trichrome stains. Hence, it is the fixative of choice for photography.

Mercury-based fixatives are toxic and should be handled with care. They should not be allowed to come into contact with metal and should be dissolved in distilled water to prevent precipitation of mercury salts. These fixatives penetrate slowly, so specimens must be thin. Mercury and acid formaldehyde haematin pigments may deposit in tissues after fixation. Mercury fixatives are no longer used routinely in laboratories except for fixing hematopoietic tissues. A major disadvantage of mercuric chloride fixation is the inevitable formation of deposits of intensely black precipitates of mercuric pigment in tissues.

11. Chromate-containing fixatives: Orth's fluid, Regaud's fluid.

Chromium trioxide dissolves in water to produce an acidic solution of chromic acid, with a pH of 0.85. Chromic acid is a powerful oxidizing agent which produces aldehyde from 1,2 diglycol residues of polysaccharides. The fixation and hardening reactions are not understood completely but probably involve the oxidation of proteins, which varies in strength depending upon the pH of the fixative, plus interaction of the reduced chromate ions directly in cross-linking proteins. Chromium ions specifically interact with disulfide bridges and attacks lipophilic residues such as tyrosine and methionine. Chromate is reported to make unsaturated but not saturated lipids insoluble upon prolonged (>48 hours) fixation and hence mitochondria are well preserved by dichromate fixatives. Dichromate containing fixatives have primarily been used to prepare neuroendocrine tissues for staining, especially normal adrenal medulla and related tumours (pheochromocytomas).

12. Picric acid containing fixatives: Bouin's, Rossman's, Gendre's.

Acidic coagulants, such as picric acid, change the charges on the ionizable side chains of proteins and disrupt electrostatic and hydrogen bonding. These acids may also insert a lipophilic anion into a hydrophilic region and hence disrupt the tertiary structures of proteins. Picric acid slightly dissolves in water to form a week acid solution. In reactions, it forms salts with basic groups of proteins, causing the proteins to coagulate. If the solution is neutralized, precipitated protein may re-dissolve. Picric acid fixation produces brighter staining, but the low pH solutions of picric acid may cause hydrolysis and loss of nucleic acids.

13. Composition of Bouin's fixative.
- Saturated aqueous picric acid—750 ml
- Formalin—250 ml
- Glacial acetic acid—50 ml

14. Uses of Bouin's fixative.
- It is an effective rapid cytological preservative specifically used for trichrome staining.
- Glycogen is preserved with this fixative, hence can be demonstrated by it.
- It hardens the tissue hence very useful for gastrointestinal tract, embryo and endocrine gland preservation.
- Small fragments of tissue like renal biopsies are better demonstrated, since they pick up the yellow colour.
- It is an excellent fixative for testicular biopsies as it gives good nuclear details.

15. Alcohol-based fixatives.
1. Clark's solution:
   - Absolute ethanol—60 mL
   - Glacial acetic acid—20 mL
2. Carnoy's fixative:
   - Ethanol—60 mL
   - Chloroform—30 mL
   - Glacial acetic acid—10 mL
3. Methacarn:
   - Methanol—60 mL
   - Chloroforrm—30 mL
   - Glacial acetic acid—10 mL
4. Gendre's solution:
   - 95% ethanol saturated picric acid—80 mL
   - Formalin—15 mL
   - Glacial acetic acid—5 mL
5. Rossman's solution
   - Tap water—10 mL
   - Formaldehyde—10 mL
   - Absolute ethanol—80 mL
   - Lead nitrate—8 g
6. Alcohol formalin
   - 95% ethanol—895 mL
   - Formalin—10 mL
   - Glacial acetic acid—5 mL

16. What are the advantages of Carnoy's fluid?
- Carnoy's fixative composition: Absolute ethanol—60 mL, chloroform—30 mL, glacial acetic acid—10 mL.
- It preserves tissue glycogen, carbohydrates, RNA and Nissel substances.
- It penetrates very rapidly and is an excellent nuclear fixative.

17. How do you fix brain specimen?
- After removal and macroscopic examination of the whole brain in the autopsy room, it should be thoroughly washed with saline solution to remove the blood.
- Whole brain specimens should be fixed by injection of fixative into the basilar artery.
- After injection of the fixative, a linen thread is passed under the basilar artery, or by hooking the basilar artery to the thread with a curtain hook or safety pin (avoid safety pin because it tends to rust). Tie the basilar artery with long length of linen thread.
- Brain suspension by the basilar artery: The thread is then tied to a glass or wooden rod laid over the top of the 10-liter bucket containing formalin fixative. Suspend/immerse the brain by the thread so that the brain (which floats) remains suspended in the center of the fixative fluid.
- Duration of fixation: The brain should then be left to fix in formalin for 3 or more weeks.
- If molecular techniques are likely to be required, portions of brain may be snap frozen in liquid nitrogen.

18. **How to orient and fix a muscle biopsy tissue?**
    - Orientation of fibers is of utmost importance since most of the information is provided by transverse sections. The biopsy should be oriented under a dissecting microscope and sample is divided as follows: For electron microscopy, 2–3 mm fragments are kept in cacodylate buffered glutaraldehyde and preserved at 4°C.
    - For cryosections, biopsy piece is fresh frozen in isopentane cooled in liquid nitrogen (–170 to –180°C) and then sections are cut in cryostat at –18 to –20°C. These sections are stained with H and E, MT, modified Gomori's trichrome (MGT). The various enzyme histochemical stains done include myosine adenosine triphosphate (ATPase) pre-incubated at pH 9.4, 4.6 and 4.3, succinate dehydrogenase and nicotinamide adenine dinucleotide- tetrazolium reductase.
    - A part of the biopsy is used for routine processing after fixing in buffered formalin.
    - For molecular biology, biochemical and genetic analysis, a small tissue is preserved in 80°C.

19. **How to soften hard tissue?**
    - Softening of hard tissue, like finger nails, hyperkeratotic skin lesions, fibroid, is done by Lendrum's method.
    - Method: First wash the tissue in running water overnight, followed by placing the tissue in 4% aqueous phenol for 1–3 days.

20. **What is secondary fixation?**
    - Secondary fixation, also known as post-fixation, is the term used for the practice of initially fixing with 10% formalin, then re-fixing with another fixative. The second fixative re-fixes the tissue so that some of its characteristics can be obtained. In this way, it is possible to obtain fixation with different characteristics on different blocks from the same bulk tissue. One advantage of this procedure is that it can be applied to tissues that have been fixed with a formalin variant and stored in the fixative for some time.
    - The most popular secondary fixatives are often those that contain mercuric chloride, such as formal sublimate or Helly's solution.
    - Advantages of secondary fixation are:
      – Sections are more easily cut and flatten better than using only formaldehyde.
      – Stain more brilliantly hence better for photography.

21. **What is formalin pigment? How to remove it?**
    Formalin pigment is a brown, granular, doubly refractile deposit seen both intracellularly and extracellularly in tissues which have been fixed with a simple formalin solution, such as formal saline. It is also known as acid formaldehyde hematin, as it is formed from hemoglobin by the action of formaldehyde at acid pH. The hematin being referred to in this context is the derivative of hemoglobin and not the oxidation product of hematoxylin, called hematin.

22. **Removing formalin pigment.**
    Bring sections to water via xylene and ethanol. Place into saturated picric acid in absolute ethanol for 1 hour. Optionally, treat with saturated aqueous lithium carbonate to remove picric acid discoloration. Wash well with water and continue with the staining method.

    Note: Most formalin pigment will be removed fairly rapidly, and the time given should be adequate. Heavy deposits may take longer. Sections may be left overnight, if necessary. Treatment with lithium carbonate is only required, if picric acid discoloration interferes with staining.

23. **Schedule of automated tissue processing in your lab.**
    8–13 hours minimum.

24. **Thickness of a routine H and E tissue section.**
    4–6 microns, 9 microns minimum, if staining for amyloid.

25. Steps in tissue processing.
1. *Fixation:* Stabilization and hardening of tissue with fixative.
2. *Dehydration:* Removal of water by using hydrophilic solution before embedding it in paraffin wax.
3. *Clearing:* Using alcohol as an intermediary between the dehydration and infiltration solution.
4. *Impregnation and embedding:* Permeation of tissue with a support medium with wax most commonly.

26. Mention the names of clearing agents.
1. Most common clearing agent in the laboratory is xylene.
2. Toluene
3. Chloroform

Other clearing agents: Esters, Cedar wood oil, Limonene

27. Advantages and disadvantages of xylene.

Advantages:
a. Rapid action
b. Cost-effective
c. Better quality of tissue sections
d. Maintains good staining quality
e. Possible to determine end point with some accuracy.

Disadvantages:
a. Long-term immersion of tissue in xylene results in tissue distortions, therefore, tissues should not be left in it for more than 3 hours.
b. Inflammable
c. Vapour is an irritant, may cause skin erythema.
d. Acute neurotoxicity

28. What is impregnation and embedding?

Impregnation
- Impregnation is the process in which the clearing agent is replaced by paraffin or its substitute that completely fills all the tissue spaces and gives a firm consistency to the specimen. This allows easier handling and cutting of thin sections without any damage to the tissue or its cellular constituents.
- Impregnation is done at the melting point temperature of wax in use, i.e. 54–64°C, in case of paraffin wax.
- The volume of the wax should be 25–30 times the volume of the tissue.

Embedding: Embedding is the process by which processed tissues are surrounded by a support medium such as agar, gelatin or wax, which on solidification will provide sufficient support during sectioning.

29. Criteria for ideal embedding medium.
- Soluble in processing fluids
- Suitable for sectioning and ribboning
- Capable of flattening after ribbon cutting
- Molten between 30 and 60°C
- Translucent or transparent; colorless at its melting point
- Stable
- Nontoxic
- Odorless
- Easy to handle
- Inexpensive.

Paraffin wax is routinely used as an impregnating and embedding media.

Paraffin wax forms a matrix that gives hardness and support to the tissues, thus preventing tissue sectioning distortion and provides easy ribbon during microtomy.

30. Various methods of embedding (4 types of molds).

a. *Leuckart/Dimmock embedding irons (L molds):* Leuckart method is the conventional method of blocking. These consist of two L-shaped pieces of heavy brass. Glycerin is applied to the L pieces and also to the metal plate. The tissue is then embedded within the molten wax. After cooling, the molds are removed and wax cakes formed.

b. *Paper blocks/boats:* Waxed paper blocks are suitable for embedding. The block is convenient to release from the paper mold. Blocked tissue may be stored with an identifying number for a long time.

c. ***Peel-a-way system using disposable plastic molds:*** Peel-a-way systems are present in different sizes. The plastic walls are peeled off, once the wax gets solidified. The block requires no trimming and may be placed directly on the microtome.

d. ***Tissue-tek system:*** Plastic embedding system of this type has replaced all other types of embedding. The plastic molds support the block during sectioning and also eliminate the step of mounting the block to the holder.

31. When is cellodin embedding used?
Cellodin is used in the embedding of neuropathological specimens.

32. Write the advantages and disadvantages of cellodin.
Advantages:
a. Causes less distortion and shrinkage.
b. Suitable for embedding eye and brain tissue.

Disadvantages:
a. Longer process
b. Rarely used because of special requirements to house the processing reagents.

33. What is the use of gelatin embedding?
Used in small friable tissues and frozen section for necrotic tissue.

34. What is the volume of gelatin embedding?
Volume—0.5 ml

35. What is double embedding?
If Agar and paraffin wax is used, it is called double embedding.

36. What is the embedding medium used in EM?
Epoxy resins are the embedding medium of choice in EM. Epoxy resins usually comprise four ingredients: The monomeric resin, a hardener, an accelerator and a plasticizer.

37. What is the melting point of wax?
Paraffin wax has a melting point ranging from 56 to 64°C.

38. What is vacuum embedding?
- Tissues are loaded into a retort chamber where they remain throughout the process. Reagents and melted paraffin wax are moved sequentially into and out of the retort chamber using vacuum and pressure. Each step could be customized by controlling time, temperature, or pressure/vacuum.
- The advantages of this system are that vacuum and heat can be used at any stage, customized schedules for tissue processing are possible, and there is fluid spillage containment and elimination of fumes.

39. What are hard wax and soft wax?
The hardness of the wax depends upon the melting point of wax. The wax with a higher melting point is used for embedding hard tissue like bone so that it is easy to get thin sections but can cause difficulty in ribboning. The wax with a low melting point is soft and is not suitable for hard tissues. Ribboning is easier with soft wax but it is difficult to obtain thinner sections.

40. How do you order for wax?
Wax is ordered in the form of wax pellets in packets of 2 or 2.5 kg depending upon the case load in a laboratory.

41. How do you order for cover slip?
They are available in cartons of 10 g each, containing cover slip of 22 × 40 mm. A large carton contains 10 packs of cover slips, 10 g each. Suitable number of cartons are ordered depending upon the case load of a laboratory.

42. What are the additives used in wax?
An additive is a chemical substance which is added to paraffin wax to adjust the hardness of the wax, so that it is compatible with the tissue to be embedded. Commonly used additives now are plasticisers and resin. Previously beeswax, rubber, ceresin and diethylene glycol distearate were used as additives.

43. What are the types of microtome?
- Rotatory microtome
- Base sledge microtome
- Rotary rocking microtome
- Sliding microtome
- Ultra-microtome

44. What are the types of microtome knives?
- Disposable blades
- Glass and diamond knives

45. What are the parts of a knife?
- Handle
- Heel
- Blade
- Toe

46. How do you assess the sharpness of the cutting edge?

Done by manual or automatic methods:
- Honing
- Stropping

47. What is honing? What are the types of hone used?

Honing is done to restore the straight cutting edge and to correct bevel.

Types of hone: Belgian black vein, Arkansas, aloxite, Tam O' Shanter Scotch hone, carborundum plate glass.

48. What are the lubricants used?
- Paraffin oil
- Vegetable oil
- Soap water

49. Define stropping? What are the types of strop?

It is a process of polishing an already fairly sharp edge. Blunt knife cannot be sharpened on a strop.

Types: Flexible/hanging, and rigid.

50. Rake angle.

It is the angle between the upper bevel of the knife and the perpendicular line drawn from the surface of the block. Increased rake angle makes the section cutting easier.

51. Angle of clearance.

It is the angle between the lower bevel of the knife and the surface of the block. It is usually around 5°. The angle of clearance is related with the friction between the block and knife. Lower the angle of clearance, the less will be the compression on the block.

52. Temperature of water bath used in microtomy.

The constant temperature (usually 40–50°C) is maintained in the water bath. This is usually 5–10°C lower than the melting point of the paraffin.

53. H&E staining procedure.

Most widely used technique in histopathology.

Principle: Acidic component of cells have the affinity to basic dye and basic components of cells have affinity to acidic dye. Hematoxylin stains the acidic part of cell (nucleus), thus it is a nuclear stain. While eosin stains the basic part of cell (cytoplasm).

Procedure:
1. Slide fixed in isopropyl alcohol or ethanol for 5 min.
2. Nuclear staining—stain in hematoxylin for 3–5 min.
3. Wash in running tap water.
4. Differentiation—dip in 1% acid alcohol. (Selective removal of excess dye from the section.)
5. Blueing—wash in tap water and blueing for 3 min.
6. Counterstaining—stain in 1% eosin for 2 min. Wash in tap water for 1–2 min.
7. Dehydrate and mount.

Interpretation:
- Nuclei—blue/purple
- Cytoplasm—pink

54. Hematoxylin.
- It is extracted from heartwood of tree *Haematoxylin campechianum.*
- Hematoxylin itself is not a stain, but hematin the major oxidization product is a natural dye responsible for color properties.
- Hematin can be produced from hematoxylin in two ways:
  1. *Natural oxidation or ripening:* This is a slow process. Ehrlich's and Dalafield's hematoxylin solutions are examples of naturally ripened hematoxylins.

2. **Chemical oxidation:** Ready for use immediately after preparation. Shorter useful life than naturally oxidized hematoxylins.
- Hematin is anionic with poor affinity for tissue and is inadequate as nuclear stain without the presence of mordant. The metal cation in mordant confers net positive charge.
- Type of mordant used influences the type of tissue components stained and their final color.
- Hematoxylin solutions are classified according to mordant used:
  - Alum hematoxylin
  - Iron hematoxylin
  - Tungsten hematoxylin
  - Molybdenum hematoxylin
  - Lead hematoxylin
  - Hematoxylins without mordant.

55. What is blueing?
It is the process by which soluble red-colored hemalum is converted into the insoluble blue colored substance in alkaline pH. Bluing solution has alkaline pH which causes the mordant dye-lake to form a permanent blue color product.

56. Name bluing solutions.
Scotts tap water and lithium carbonate

57. Eosin.
- It is a fluorescent, xanthene dye which binds to salts with eosinophilic compounds containing positive charges. It is the most suitable stain to combine with an alum hematoxylin to demonstrate the general histological architecture of tissues.
- Eosin has the ability, with correct differentiation, to distinguish between the cytoplasm of different types of cell, connective tissue fibers and matrices, by staining these differing shades of red and pink
Types of eosin: Eosin Y, Eosin R, Eosin B

58. Decalcification.
- It is softening of bones due to the removal of calcium ions, and to make the tissue suitable for sectioning as a histological technique to study bones and preserve DNA for molecular studies.
- Surface decalcification can be performed by placing paraffin block face down in 10% formic acid 15–60 min or 5% HCl for 10 min.
- Best decalcifying fluid is—3% nitric acid.

59. Methods of decalcification.
- Acid decalcification
- Ion-exchange resin
- Electrical ionization
- Chelating solution
- Surface decalcification

60. Methods to detect end-point of decalcification.
- Radiographic examination—X-ray
- Chemical test—checking decalcifying agent for the presence of calcium
- Physical test—bending the tissue or inserting a pin into the tissue

61. Special stain for calcium.
- Von kossa
- Alizarin red S
- Azan stain

62. Characters of good decalcifying agent.
- Complete removal of calcium
- Absence of damage to tissue cells or fiber
- Non-impairment of subsequent staining technique
- Reasonable speed of decalcification

63. Frozen section.
Frozen sections have important clinical and research applications. Clinically use of frozen sections for intraoperative consultations, Moh's procedure for surgical margins and sentinel node evaluation has great significance in patient care and maintenance.

Uses:
- Rapid production of sections for intra-operative diagnosis
- Diagnostic and research enzyme histo-chemistry for labile enzymes.
- Immunofluorescent methodology

- IHC techniques when heat and fixation may inactivate or destroy the antigens
- Diagnostic and research non-enzyme histochemistry, e.g. lipids and some carbs
- Silver demonstration methods

Techniques for suitable freezing include—liquefied nitrogen (–190c), isopentane cooled by liquid nitrogen (–150c), dry ice (–70c), CO_2 (–70c).

Best frozen tissue sections obtained when tissue is frozen very quickly without artefact.

64. Cryostat.

To produce thin, high quality, frozen sections, tissue must be properly frozen and embedded correctly, conditions of cryostat must be optimal, block temperature must be correct for tissue being cut, and blade must be clean and properly secured. It is a refrigerated cabinet in which a speciality microtome is present. All controls for microtome are operated outside cabinet. Most unfixed material will section well between –15°C and –23°C. Tissues with more water will section best at warmer temperature, harder tissues and tissues that contain fat require colder temperature. If there is cutting problem, microtome is to be defrosted or oiled. Cryoembedding media is based on temperature, freezing mode and type of tissue to be frozen.

Potpourri of Cases

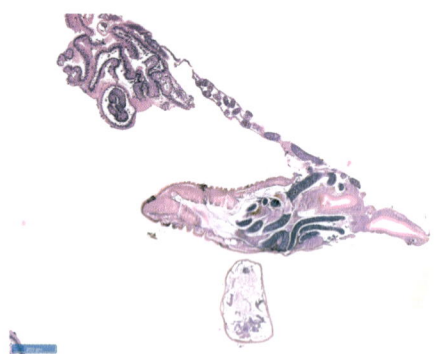

Fig. 1: Intestinal hookworm—duodenal biopsy

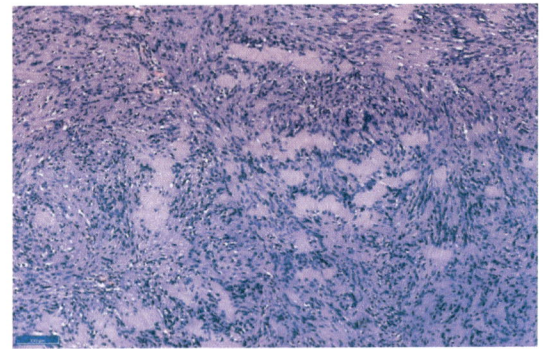

Fig. 3: Verocay bodies—Schwanomma

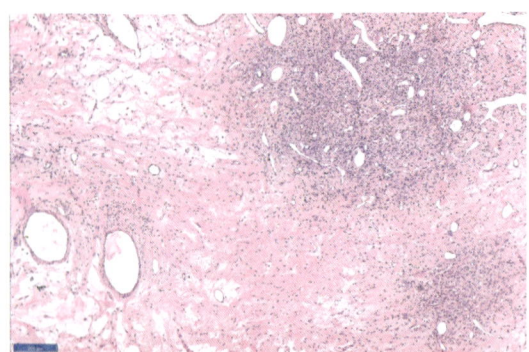

Fig. 2: Sclerosing stromal tumor of the ovary

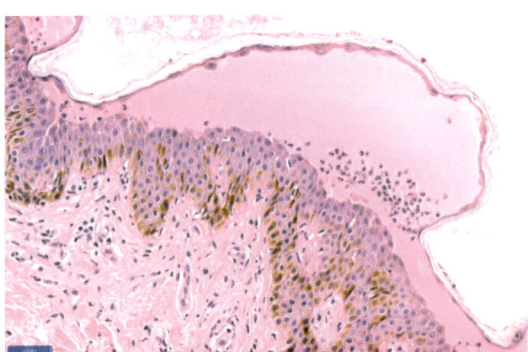

Fig. 4: Subcorneal bullae—pemphigus foliaceous

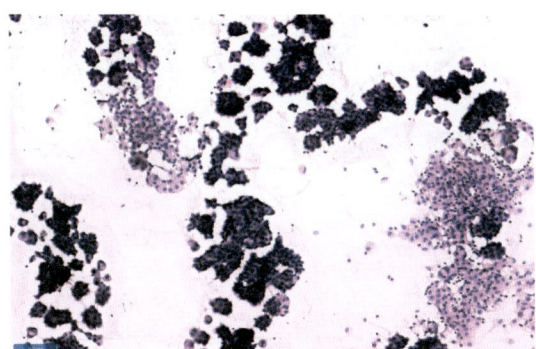

Fig. 5: Serous papillary carcinomatous deposit in ascitic fluid

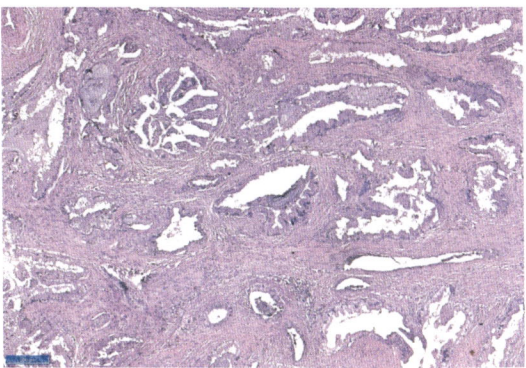

Fig. 8: Minimal deviation adenocarcinoma of the cervix

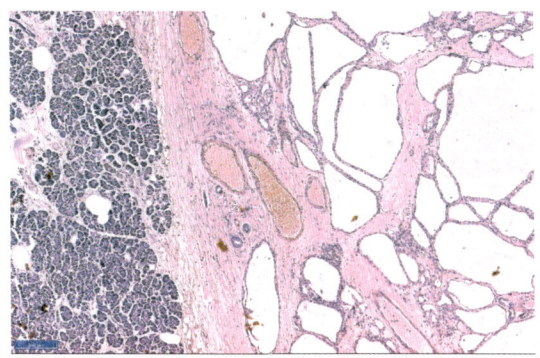

Fig. 6: Pancreatic serous cystadenoma

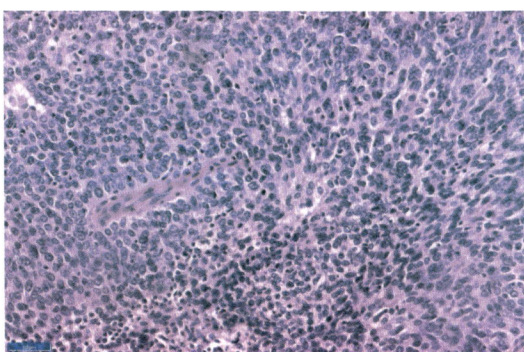

Fig. 9: Lymphoepithelial carcinoma

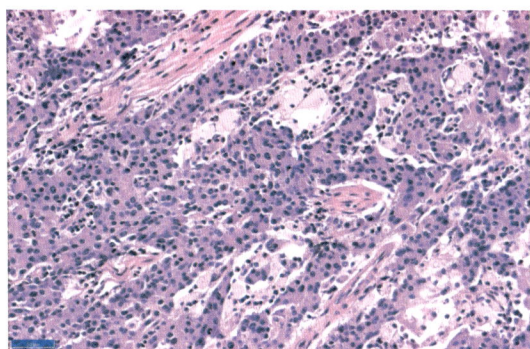

Fig. 7: Pancreatic acinar variant—gastric adenocarcinoma

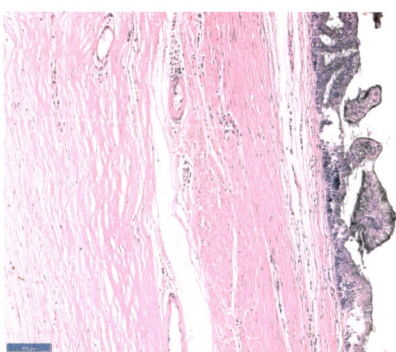

Fig. 10: Low grade appendiceal mucinous neoplasm

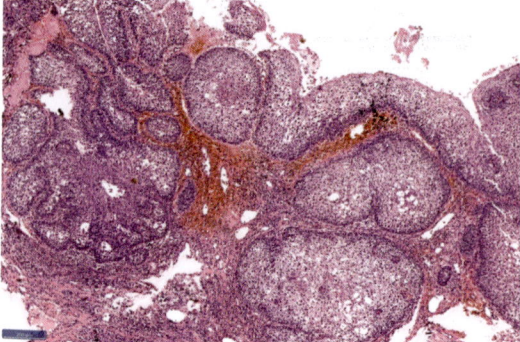
Fig. 11: Inverted papillary urothelial carcinoma

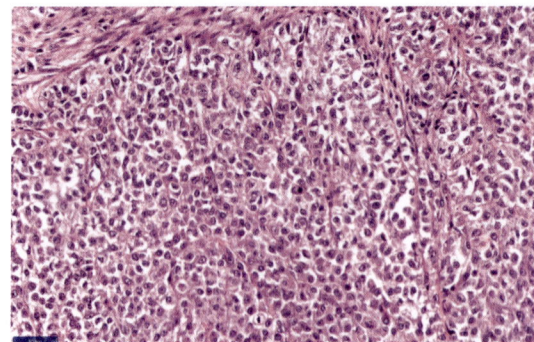
Fig. 14: Gastrointestinal neuroectodermal tumor

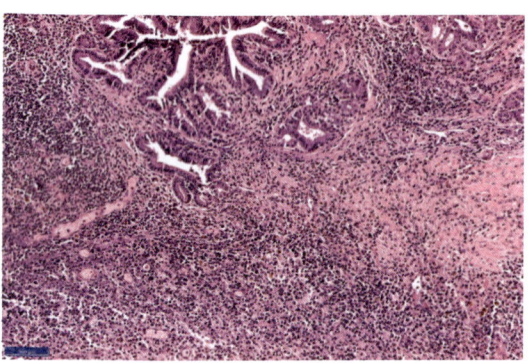
Fig. 12: IgG4 disease of the pancreas

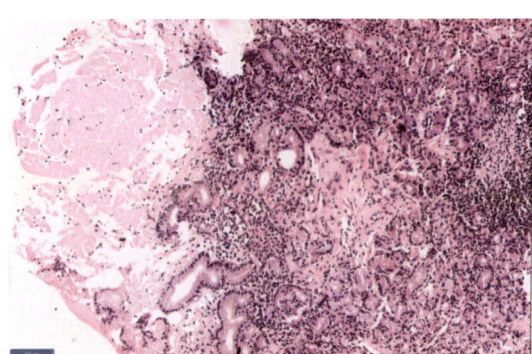
Fig. 15: Gastric amyloidosis

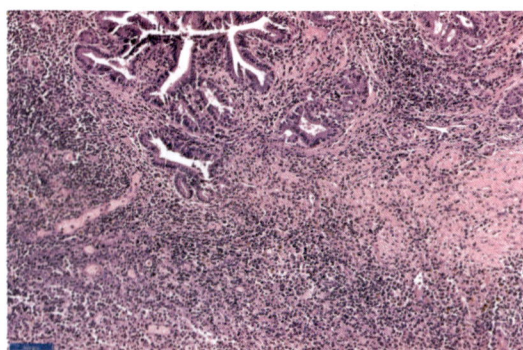
Fig. 13: Hamartomatous polyp

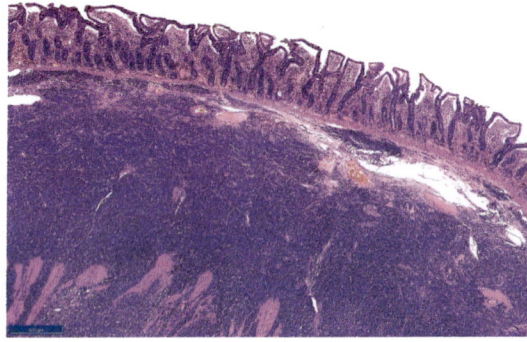
Fig. 16: Diffuse large B cell lymphoma of small intestine

Potpourri of Cases

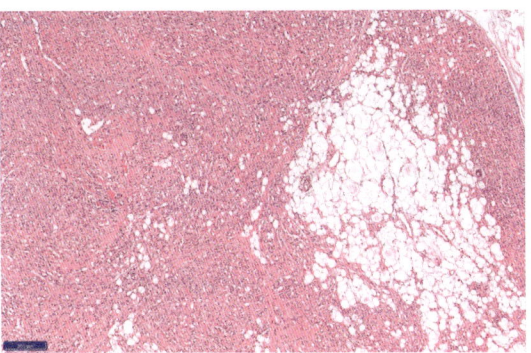

Fig. 17: Angiolipoma

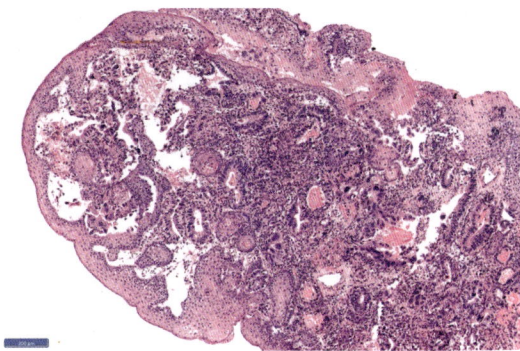

Fig. 19: Adenosquamous carcinoma of the gastroesophageal junction

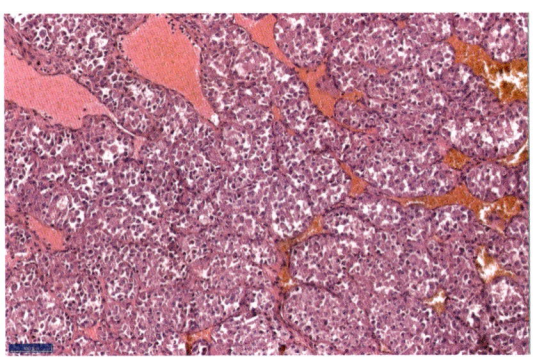

Fig. 18: Alveolar soft part sarcoma

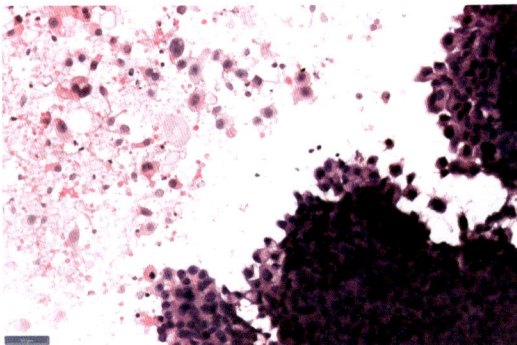

Fig. 20: Urine cytology—high grade urothelial carcinoma

General Tips for the Examination Going Postgraduates

Sandhya Sundaram, S Rajendiran, Febe Renjitha Suman, J Thanka, Leena Joseph, D Prathiba

Below we give a general outline of MD pathology examination as conducted in our university. There may be minimal variations among different universities; however, the general trend remains the same.

THEORY

For written examination, usually there are 4 papers encompassing the topics:

Paper 1: General pathology and immunology,

Paper 2: Systemic pathology,

Paper 3: Clinical pathology, hematology, cytology, and blood bank

Paper 4: Recent advances. In our university, each paper has 2 parts composed of 1 essay (20 marks) and 3 short notes (10 marks) for each part (in total 2 essays and 6 short notes per paper). A few universities also have very short objective type questions. Knowing this will help you in appropriate preparation.

Method of Presentation is Very Important

Please write your answers with subheadings and small paragraphs. Please highlight or underline the headings and major points. Use simple diagrams and tables (have mercy on the examiner…..!!). Schematic diagrams and flowcharts will be an added advantage. Also, a neat and legible handwriting (to the extent possible) will keep the examiner happy.

Please attempt all the questions

Essays should be of 6 pages in length (each page—20 lines)… and short notes up to 3 pages.

Reading the following is a must for the theory examination (Minimal)

a. Past 10 years' examination question papers of your university
b. Recent advances in histopathology –5 recent issues
c. Robbin's Pathologic Basis of Diseases—latest edition—page to page, word by word
d. Review articles from the following journals (past 2 years) recommended (list is by no means complete)
   i. Histopathology
   ii. Archives of Pathology and Laboratory Medicine
   iii. American Journal of Surgical Pathology
   iv. Diagnostic Cytopathology
   v. Journal of Clinical Pathology
   vi. British Journal of Hematology, Blood
   vii. American Journal of Hematology

PRACTICAL

It is usually conducted for 2 days. As in theory, be acquainted with all the components of the practical examination. The standard schedule as follows:

a. Day 1
   i. Autopsy
   ii. Gross specimen examination
   iii. CP cases
   iv. Hematology and cytology slides
b. Day 2
   i. Pedagogy
   ii. Histopathology slides
   iii. Histotechniques, cytotechniques, and charts

iv. Blood bank and special procedures
v. Grand viva

Some Highlights of the Major Exercises

1. *Autopsy:* This exercise tests the candidate's ability to clinicopathologically correlate the given history in addition to autopsy techniques, to arrive at the cause of death. So the clinical corelation consequences of the particular lesion, it's effect on the other systems, possible complications should be known.
   For example, hemodynamic alterations in valvular heart disease, pathogenesis and complications of cirrhosis liver. It is advised to read a standard General Medicine textbook to understand these aspects better. The candidate should be able to give an anatomical diagnosis and then discuss the specific cause of death in the particular cause.

2. *Gross specimens:* Try to see if you can recognize the organ. Generally it is possible. Descriptive terminology should be standard one, as used in textbooks. If there are specific terms like "cut cabbage appearance", etc... please mention it.

3. *Clinical pathology exercise:* Analyze the case given and derive as much information as possible from the history to arrive at a probable diagnosis. List out investigation in a order.... CBC, ESR, PS, Urine/motion any other CP, biochem, micro, others—radiology, genetics, etc. Justify your requests.
   Peripheral smear staining—Monitor the procedure till you dilute and take care to prevent deposits. Do not pour off, wash over the slides. Present a neat labeled slide. Urine—be through with manual/dip stick method. PT/APTT/INR-calculation and interpretation. Be conversant with 2nd line investigations, if required. Of course all normal values with units should be at your fingertips!!

4. *Slide diagnosis session:* A good performance in each component is essential but the most vital exercise is slide evaluation (histopathology, hematology, and cytology). Slides are brought by the external examiner and generally this exercise carries more marks.

   a. Timing is very essential. Make sure you are done with ... at least 50% of slides by half way of the allotted time (e.g. 5 out of 10 slides should have been reviewed by 30 minutes of 1 hr allotted time).
   b. 75% of the slides will be very straight forward and simple thinking is very essential. They will be generally
      i. Common lesions in uncommon sites
      ii Uncommon lesions in common sites.
   c. First… read the history and see the slide grossly. Sometimes it gives a clue (tubular structures, solid or cystic tumors). Clinical history like age and specific symptoms, e.g. headache, projectile vomiting in CNS lesions will be useful clues. For bone lesions it is a must to correlate with age, X-ray and bone involved.
   d. Ask the following questions for each slide:
      i. Normal organ seen or not?
      ii. What is the pattern of the lesion? For example, glandular, papillary, nesting, cribriform storiform…
      iii. Is the lesion neoplastic or non-neoplastic?
      iv. If neoplastic…benign or malignant?
      v. Primary or secondary?
      vi. What is the origin of the tumor? (Epithelial, stromal, hematolymphoid, melanocytic, germ cell…)
      vii. Write a good description… always start with low power findings… followed by mid and high power features (a good description will bring you additional points…)

viii. If not able to settle on a single diagnosis… list reasonable differential diagnosis (from most likely to least likely)… followed by special stains request…. (start from deeper, histochemisty, immunohistochemistry, and other special tests like… EM, flowcytometry, molecular work-up…. do not start with high end like molecular work-up first).

5. The grand viva: Gives you a chance to rectify things to your favor and hence before appearing…

   a. Please read the theory questions … especially the ones that you have not answered well.
   b. Find out the answers for the questions that you did not answer during the practical examination (it gives you a chance to show that you have an attitude to learn immediately).
   c. Have an attitude to accept healthy criticisms and as mentioned before… be ready to learn as the real examination starts after getting the degree … and each patient will be your external examiner.
   d. Be ready to list the journals that you read regularly.
   e. Dissertation topics are always discussed. So be prepared. Please train yourself to summarize the results of your thesis in an interesting and effective way.

Always Remember

Your performance will be suboptimal if you are tense or serious
So, don't stress, do your best, forget the rest
All the Very Best

NOTEWORTHY BODIES

Pathological body	Conditions
Asteroid-Schaumann bodies	Sarcoidosis, tuberculosis, leprosy, fungal infections, and foreign body reactions
Call-Exner bodies	Granulosa cell tumor
Civatte bodies	Lichen planus
Councilman bodies	Virus infections, yellow fever and hepatitis
Donovan bodies	Granuloma inguinale
Embryoid bodies	Polyembryoma
Gamna-Gandy bodies	Cirrhosis
Guarnieri bodies	Smallpox
Hematoxylin bodies	Systemic lupus erythematosus (SLE) (Renal glomeruli)
Hamazaki-Wesenberg bodies	Sarcoidosis
Heinz bodies	Glucose-6-phosphate dehydrogenase deficiencies but also found in congenital hemolytic anemias and in premature infants.
Hirano bodies	Alzheimer's and Creutzfeldt-Jacob disease
Kamino bodies	Spindle cell naevi
Lamellar bodies	Pulmonary mucosa-associated lymphoid tissue (MALT) Lymphomas and sclerosing hemangiomas of the lung
Leishman-Donovan bodies	Leishmaniasis and kala-azar
Lewy bodies	Parkinson's and Alzheimer's disease.
Lipschütz bodies	Primary infection with herpes simplex virus.
MacCallum bodies	Rheumatic heart disease
Mallory bodies	Cirrhosis and alcohol related diseases
Mallory-Denk bodies	Chronic hepatitis C
Masson bodies	Cryptogenic organising pneumonia (COP) and Bronchiolitis obliterans organising pneumonia (BOOP)
Melon seed bodies	Tuberculous tenosynovitis
Michaelis-Gutmann bodies	Malakoplakia
Molluscum bodies (Henderson-Patterson bodies)	Molluscum contagiosum
Negri bodies	Rabies
Nemaline bodies	Nemaline myopathy
Owl's eye bodies	CMV infection
Pale bodies	Parkinson's disease
Papillary mesenchymal bodies	Trichoepithelioma
Psammoma bodies	Papillary cancer of the ovary but may also be found in papillary carcinomas of the thyroid and meningiomas
Pustulo-ovoid bodies	Granular cell tumors
Reinke bodies	Leydig cell tumor
Rice bodies	Rheumatoid arthritis
Rokitansky bodies	Benign cystic teratomas
Schiller-Duval bodies	Yolk sac tumor
Verocay bodies	Schwannoma
Warthin-Finkeldey bodies	Measles

Glossary

Head and Neck
Nasopharyngeal angiofibroma
Epithelial myoepithelial carcinoma
Mucormycosis
High grade mucoepidermoid carcinoma
Adenoid cystic carcinoma
Warthin's tumour
Salivary duct carcinoma
Olfactory neuroblastoma
Basal cell adenoma
Clear cell carcinoma
Acinic cell carcinoma
Branchial cleft cyst
Sinonasal papilloma
Carcinoma ex-pleomorphic adenoma
Nasopharyngeal carcinoma

Oral Lesions
Odontogenic keratocyst
Unicystic ameloblastoma
Ameloblastoma
Ameloblastic carcinoma
Giant cell granuloma
Adenomatoid odontogenic tumor
Calcifying odontogenic cyst
Odontome

CNS Lesions
Diffuse astrocytoma grade-II
Rhabdoid meningioma grade-II
Ependymoma grade-II
Glioblastoma multiforme grade-IV
Craniopharyngioma
Meningothelial meningioma grade-I
Pilocytic astrocytoma grade-I
Myxopapillary ependymoma grade-I
Oligodendroglioma-II
Anaplastic oligodendroglioma-III
Medulloblastoma grade-IV
Central neurocytoma grade-II
Choroid plexus papilloma
Metastatic carcinoma
Hemangioblastoma grade-I
Phaeohyphomycosis
Melanotic progonoma of infancy
Chordoid meningioma
DNET grade-I
Papillary glioneuronal tumor

Ophthalmic Lesions
Malignant melanoma of choroid
Cancerous acquired melanosis
Retinoblastoma
Sebaceous hyperplasia
Sebaceous gland carcinoma
Myoepithelioma of lacrimal gland
Syringocystadenoma papilliferum
Conjunctival amyloidosis
Fibrosarcoma of the orbit
Apocrine carcinoma
Orbital teratoma
Filarial lesion
Pleomorphic adenoma of lacrimal gland

Spectrum of Breast Lesions
Granulomatous mastitis with abscess
Tubular adenoma
Intraductal papilloma
Papillary DCIS or indraductal papillary carcinoma
Adenomyoepithelioma
Sclerosing adenosis
Mucocele like lesion
Pseudoangiomatous stromal hyperplasia (PASH)
Benign phyllodes
High grade malignant phyllodes tumor
Ductal carcinoma *in situ*
Paget's disease of nipple
Squamous cell carcinoma—breast
Metaplastic carcinoma with heterogenous elements
Metastatic carcinoma with apocrine differentiation—lymph node
Carcinoma with medullary features—breast
Invasive lobular carcinoma

Invasive micropapillary carcinoma
Invasive mammary carcinoma with lobular features
Tubular carcinoma
Mucinous carcinoma—breast
Rosai-Dorfman disease of breast
Adenosquamous—breast
Angiosarcoma—breast
Pleomorphic sarcoma—breast
Granular cell tumour—breast
Lactating adenoma
   (a) Encapsulated papillary carcinoma
   (b) Invasive papillary carcinoma

Lesions of the Lung

ARDS with hyaline membrane
Metastatic lymphangitic carcinomatosis
Bronchiectasis
Metastatic chordoma to the lung
Metastatic endometrial stromal sarcoma
Neuroendocrine tumor—classical carcinoid
Aspergillus with pneumocystis pneumonia
Pulmonary hamartoma/chondroma
Aspergillus with poorly differentiated squamous cell carcinoma
Pulmonary-hydatid cyst
Adenocarcinoma—acinar and papillary types
Cryptococcal mucoid pneumonia
Cryptococcal granulomatous nodule
Carcinosarcoma lung
Aspiration pneumonia
Blastomycosis—necrotizing granuloma
Coccidioidomycosis—necrotizing granuloma
Eosinophilic granuloma
Malignant mesothelioma
Solitary fibrous tumor of the pleura
Small cell carcinoma lung
Extranodal marginal zone B-cell lymphoma of mucosaassociated lymphoid tissue (MALT lymphoma)
Adenocarcinoma—bronchoalveolar type, non-mucinous variety with clara cell differentiation
Alveolar septal pulmonary amyloidosis
Nodular pulmonary amyloidosis
Adenocarcinoma—BAC, mucinous type
CMV pneumonitis
Busulphan pneumonitis

Upper Gastrointestinal Lesions

Candidiasis esophagitis
CMV esophagitis
HSV esophagitis
Barrett esophagus
Mod. Diff. sq. cell ca.
Adenocarcinoma with focal papillary pattern
Barrett esophagus
Poorly differentiated ca.
Basaloid sq. cell ca.
H. pylori with chronic gastritis with moderate activity
Gastric fundic gland polyp
Peutz-Jegher polyp
Hyperplastic polyp with xanthoma
Poorly diff. ca. with focal signet cells
Signet cell ca stomach
Mucinous ca. of stomach with focal signet ring cells
Mod. diff. adenoca—intestinal type
Lymphangiectasia
GIST-LMP

Lower Gastrointestinal Lesions

S. stercoralis with focal pyloric metaplasia
Whipple disease
Diverticulosis
High grade dysplasia, lymphangitis carcinomatosa
Eosinophilic appendicitis
E. vermicularis
Neuroendocrine ca. grade I (carcinoid)
Hirschsprung disease
CMV colitis
C/W Ulcerative colitis
Ischemic colitis sigmoid volvulus
Radiation colitis
Tubular adenoma
Mod. Diff. adenoca. and tubular adenomas
Mucinous adenoca. with focal signet ring cells
NHL-diffuse large B-cell type—rectal
NHL-diffuse large B-cell type—ileocaecal
Malignant GIST
Fibroepithelial polyp—anal canal
Benign granular cell tumor
Malignant melanoma—anal canal

Histological Approach to Hepatobilliary and Pancreatic Lesions

Chronic active hepatitis
Chronic active hepatitis with cirrhotic changes
NASH
Neonatal hepatitis
Cirrhosis
Haemophagocytic syndrome
Extramedullary hematopoiesis
Hydatid cyst
Overlap syndrome

Mesenchymal hamartoma
Intraductal papillary biliary neoplasm
HCC
Fibrolamellar HCC
Hepatoblastoma
Mets: Leiomyosarcoma
Mets: NE carcinoma
Mets: Mucin secreting AdenoCa

Pancreaticobiliary Lesions

Adenoma gallbladder
Adenocarcinoma gallbladder
CMV cholangitis
Granular cell tumour—CBD
Mucinous neoplasm pancreas
Intraductal papillary neoplasm with high grade dysplasia
Pancreatic microcystic adenoma
Solid pseudopapillary pancreatic tumour
Adenocarcinoma pancreas with its variants (mucinous)
Adenocarcinoma pancreas with its variants (ductal)
Adenocarcinoma pancreas with its variants (adenosquamous)
Neuroendocrine tumour pancreas
Nesidioblastosis

Medical Renal Disease

Cast nephropathy
Primary membranous nephropathy
Crescentic glomerulonephritis: Antiglomerular basement membrane disease
Infection related glomerulonephritis
Diabetic nephropathy
Amyloidosis
Acute tubular injury
Hypertensive arterionephrosclerosis
Granulomatous tubulointerstitial nephritis
Diffuse lupus nephritis
Focal segmental glomerulosclerosis (FSGS)
Minimal change disease (MCD)
Acute tubulointerstitial nephritis (Tin)
IgA Nephropathy
Atheroembolic renal disease (AERD)

Kidney and Urinary Bladder

Wilms tumour, favorable histology
Neuroblastoma, Ganglioneuroblastoma, Ganglioneuroma
Papillary variant of RCC
Chromophobe variant of RCC
Clear cell RCC, Sarcomatoid RCC, Rhabdoid, Sarcomatoid clear cell RCC with cystic change
Multicystic renal dysplasia
Angiomyolipoma
Clear cell sarcoma kidney
Xanthogranulomatous pyelonephritis
Low grade urothelial ca
High grade urothelial ca
Urothelial carcinoma (UC)
UC with squamous differentiation
UC—microcystic variant
UC—lymphoepithelial variant
NHL B-cell type—Unirary bladder
Collecting duct carcinoma
Renal oncocytoma
Multicystic nephrom, Multicystic clear cell renal cell carcinoma
Malakoplakia
Cystitis cystica, cystitis cystica glandularis
Urachal villous adenoma with adjacent mucinous adenocarcinoma
Tubulovillous adenoma with HG dysplasia and focal signet ring cell
Chronic pyelonephritis with actinomycosis
Micropapillary ca of bladder
Urothelial ca of ureter and renal pelvis
Renal lymphoma

Male Genital Tract and Prostate

Seminoma
Mixed germ cell tumor (embryonal + yolk sac tumor + teratoma)
DLBCL
Leydig cell tumor
Sertoli cell only syndrome
TB epididymo orchitis
Prostatic adenocarcinoma
Rhabdomyosarcoma
Urothelial carcinoma of prostate
SCC
Verrucous carcinoma
High grade dysplasia and carcinoma *in situ*
Granulomatous prostatitis
Adenomatoid tumor

Female Genital Tract

Borderline papillary serous cystadenofibroma
Micropapillary serous carcinoma
Borderline mucinous neoplasm with Brenner component
Clear cell carcinoma
Fibrothecoma
Adult granulosa cell tumour

Adult granulosa cell tumour with sertoli cell component
Juvenile granulosa cell tumour
Sex cord tumour with annular tubules
Steroid cell tumour (NOS)
Dysgerminoma
Mature cystic teratoma with gliomatosis peritoni
Immature teratoma
Yolk sac tumour
Signet ring cell carcinoma
Carcinoid
Tubular Kruckenberg tumour
Actinomycosis
Partial mole
Chorangioma
Endometrioid adenocarcinoma
Endometrial stromal sarcoma
Leiomyosarcoma
MMMT predominantly epithelial with heterologous component
Choriocarcinoma
Glassy cell carcinoma
Diffuse mesonephric hyperplasia of cervix
Angiomyxoma
Uterine stromal sarcoma with sex cord stromal differentiation.
Solid and cystic APBT with APMT
High grade serous carcinoma with chemotherapy induced changes
Ovarian fibroma with minor sex cord elements
Osseous metaplasia of endometrium

Soft Tissue Tumors and Tumor Like Lesions

Synovial sarcoma
Glomus tumour
Scar endometriosis
Dermatofibrosarcoma protuberance (DFSP)
Myxoid liposarcoma
Malignant triton tumor
Rhabdomyosarcoma—embryonal
Granular cell tumour
Solitary fibrous tumour
Malignant fibrous histiocytoma—storiform pleomorphic
Alveolar soft part sarcoma
Fibromatosis
Nodular fasciitis
Inflammatory myofibroblastic tumour
Angiosarcoma
Paraganglioma
Plexiform neurofibroma
Aggressive angiomyxoma
Cysticercosis
Fibrosarcoma
Perineurioma
Angiomatoid fibrous histiocytoma
Epithelioid sarcoma

Lesions of Bone and Joints

Tumoral calcinosis
Aneurysmal bone cyst
Osteoid osteoma
Osteochondroma
Chondromyxoid fibroma
Chondrosarcoma
Giant cell tumour/osteoclastoma
Giant cell tumour of tendon sheath
Myositis ossificans
Ewings' sarcoma
Synovial chondromatosis
Enchondroma
Langerhans cell histiocytosis
Chondroblastoma
Rheumatoid arthritis
Follicular carcinoma—metastasis to bone
Neuroendocrine carcinoma metastasis to bone
Fibrous dysplasia
Gout
Coventional osteosarcoma
Paget's disease
Small cell osteosarcoma
Parosteal osteosarcoma
Extraskeletal mesenchymal chondrosarcoma
Telengiectatic osteosarcoma

Skin Lesions

Leucocytoclastic vasculitis
Seborrheic keratosis
Verruca vulgaris
Nodular melanoma
Hidradenoma papilliferum
Lupus vulgaris
Lepromatous leprosy
Scleroderma
Intradermal nevus
Trichoepithelioma
Sebaceous gland carcinoma
Chondroid syringoma
Basal cell carcinoma
Pilomatricoma
Psoriasis
Lichen planus

Nodular hidradenoma
Eccrine spiradenoma
Cryptococcus
Bullous pemphigoid
Pemphigus vulgaris
Bowens disease
Cutaneous lymphoma
Lichen nitidus
Amyloidosis

Non-Neoplastic Lesions of the Lymph Node

Kikuchi lymphadenopathy
Castleman lymphadenopathy
Reactive lymphoid hyperplasia—follicular
Sinus histiocytes with multiple lymphadenopathy (Rosai Dorfman disease)
Sinus histiocytosis
Tuberculous lymphadenitis
Cryptococcus lymphadenitis
Measles lymphadenitis
Kimura disease
Progressive transformation of germinal centre
Intranodal palisading myofibroblastoma

Neoplastic Lesions of the Lymph Node

CLL/SLL
Follicular lymphoma
NHL mantle cell
Burkitt's lymphoma
T-lymphoblastic lymphoma
Diffuse large B cell lymphoma
Classic Hodgkin lymphoma and nodular sclerosis
Nodular lymphocyte predominant Hodgkin lymphoma
Hairy cell leukemia
ALK+ Anaplastic large cell lymphoma

Endocrine Pathology

Pituitary adenoma (null cell)
Papillary carcinoma, (cystic) arising in a background of Hashimoto's thyroiditis
Papillary carcinoma thyroid—classical type
Papillary carcinoma—follicular variant
Papillary carcinoma multifocal arising in the background of a follicular adenoma, microfollicular pattern dominant
Papillary carcinoma—diffuse sclerosing variant
Follicular adenoma—oncocytic variant (hurthle cell adenoma)
Follicular carcinoma—minimally invasive with capsular invasion
Follicular carcinoma—widely invasive with capsular and vascular invasion
Poorly differentiated thyroid carcinoma
Medullary carcinoma thyroid
Papillary carcinoma—thyroid involving parathyroid
Thymoma (lymphocytic predominant)
Thymoma predominantly epithelial type
Malignant thymoma (invasive)
Metastatic hepatocellular carcinoma in the adrenal gland
Adrenal myelolipoma with adrenal carcinoma
Adrenocortical carcinoma
Phaeochromocytoma
Parathyroid adenoma
Parathyroid carcinoma
Pancreatic neuroendocrine tumor, well differentiated
Pancreatic neuroendocrine tumor—Insulinoma
Colonic metastases to the adrenal
Craniopharyngioma—papillary variant
Craniopharyngioma—adamantinomatous type

Cytology Slide Case Discussion Part I

Diagnosis	Sample
Metastatic adenocarcinoma deposits	Pleural fluid
Lymphocytic effusion of pleural fluid—possibly primary effusion lymphoma	Pleural fluid
Mucinous adenocarcinoma deposit	Peritoneal fluid
Squamous cell carcinoma	Bronchial brush
Adenocarcinoma	Lung-FNA
Lobular ca	Breast-FNA
Intraductal papilloma	Breast nipple discharge
Phyllodes tumour	Breast-FNA
Hashimoto's thyroiditis	Thyroid-FNA
Dequervians thyroiditis	Thyroid-FNA
Anaplastic ca	Thyroid-FNA
Metastatic papillary ca	Lung-FNA
Hodgkin's lymphoma	Node-FNA
Metastatic melanoma deposits	Node-FNA
Thymoma	Mediastinum-FNA
Mucoepidermoid ca	Salivary gland-FNA
Pleomorphic adenoma	Salivary gland-FNA
Adenoid cystic ca	Salivary gland-FNA
Malignant myoepithelioma	Salivary gland-FNA
Hepatocellular ca	Liver-FNA
Hepatoblastoma	Liver-FNA
Mixed germ cell tumour	Testis-FNA

Papillary cystadenocarcinoma	Ovary-POD aspirate
Pancreatic endocrine tumour	Pancreas-FNA
Neuroendocrine tumour	Git-FNA
Plasmacytoma	Bone-FNA
Oncocytoma	Kidney-FNA
Spindle cell sarcoma	Soft tissue-FNA
Calcinosis cutis	Soft tissue-FNA
Chordoma	Soft tissue-FNA
Squamous cell ca	Squash cytology
Granulomatous inflammation	Infection
Extramedullary hematopoiesis	Liver nodule
Small cell carcinoma—lung	Pleural fluid
Colloid carcinoma of breast	Breast-FNA
Myelolipoma	Retroperitoneal mass-FNA
Warthin's tumour	Parotid-FNA
Chondroid syringoma	Forearm-FNA
Organizing abscess parotid with non-tyrosine crystalloids	Parotid-FNA

Cytology Slide Case Discussion Part II

Diagnosis	Sample
Cysticercosis	Eyelid-FNA
Cystic pleomorphic adenoma with extensive squamous metaplasia	Parotid-FNA
Adenoid cystic carcinoma	Mandible-FNA
Non-Hodgkin lymphoma/ Hodgkin lymphoma	Neck swelling-FNA
Ewing sarcoma/PNET	Supraclavicular region—swelling
Malignant endothelial neoplasm	Liver-FNA
Wilm's tumour	Abdominal mass-FNA
Synovial sarcoma	Inguinal region-FNA
Langerhans cell histiocytosis	Scalp lesion
Hepatocellular carcinoma	Liver-FNA
Gouty arthritis	Synovial fluid
Low grade papillary urothelial carcinoma	Urine
Tuberculous pleural effusion	Pleural fluid
Metastasis from carcinoma breast	Cutaneous nodule
Pilar cyst/pilomatrixoma	Scalp swelling
LE cell	Pericardial fluid

Haematology

Peripheral Smear

Microcytic hypochromic anemia
Hereditary spherocytosis
Microangiopathic hemolytic anemia
Plasmodium vivax and *Plasmodium falciparum*
Hemolytic anemia due to hemoglobinopathy probably HBS/beta-thalassemia
Thalassemia major
Chronic lymphocytic leukemia
Chronic myeloid leukemia—chronic phase
Acute leukemia, probably myeloid in origin—AML M2 (FAB)
Acute lymphoblastic leukemia
Acute leukemia: Probably lymphoid in origin—T cell origin
Megaloblastic anemia

Bone Marrow Aspirate

Lymphoproliferative disorder probably chronic lymphocytic leukemia
Lymphoproliferative disorder—Burkitt's lymphoma
Myelodysplastic syndrome (MDS/MPN)
Acute leukemia probably of myeloid origin—AML-M4 (FAB)
Acute leukemia—probably lymphoid in origin (ALL)
Myeloma

Bone Marrow Biopsy

Aplastic anemia
Burkitt's lymphoma
Plasma cells myeloma
Myelofibrosis—fibrotic phase
Myelofibrosis—prefibrotic phase
Chronic lymphocytic leukemia
Acute myeloid leukemia—probably M4–EO
Acute leukemia, probably acute lymphoblastic leukemia
Chronic granulomatous inflammation of tuberculous origin
Metastatic deposit—small round cell tumor, probably neuroblastoma
Metastatic carcinoma
Pure red cell aplasia
Storage disorder—Gaucher's disease
Lymphoproliferative disorder—Hairy cell leukemia

Bibliography

- John R. Goldblum MD FCAP FASCP FACG, Laura W Lamps MD, Jesse K McKenney and Jeffrey L Myers MD (2017) *Rosai and Ackerman's Surgical Pathology* (11th Edition), Elsevier
- Victor E, MD Reuter Joel K, MD. Greenson Stacey, E Mills Stacey E Mills and Hornick Jason L, MD (2015) *Sternberg's Diagnostic Surgical Pathology* (6th Edition), Wolters Kluwer
- Digestive System Tumours, WHO Classification of Tumours, 5th Edition, 2019
- WHO Classification of Skin Tumours, WHO Classification of Tumours, 4th Edition, 2018
- WHO Classification of Tumours of Endocrine Organs, WHO Classification of Tumours, 4th Edition, 2017
- WHO Classification of Tumours of Haematopoietic and Lymphoid Tissues
- WHO Classification of Tumours, Revised 4th Edition, 2017
- WHO Classification of Tumours of the Urinary System and Male Genital Organs, WHO Classification of Tumours, 4th Edition, 2016
- WHO Classification of Tumours of the Central Nervous System, WHO Classification of Tumours, Revised 4th Edition, 2016
- WHO Classification of Tumours of the Lung, Pleura, Thymus and Heart, WHO Classification of Tumours, 4th Edition, 2015
- WHO Classification of Tumours of Female Reproductive Organs, WHO Classification of Tumours, 4th Edition, 2014
- WHO Classification of Tumours of Soft Tissue and Bone, WHO Classification of Tumours, 4th Edition, 2013
- WHO Classification of Tumours of the Breast, WHO Classification of Tumours, 4th Edition, 2012
- Dr Christopher Fletcher (2013) *Diagnostic Histopathology of Tumors* (4th Edition)

Lesions of the Head and Neck

- Vijaya B. Reddy MD MBA, Paolo Gattuso MD, et al (2014) *Differential Diagnosis in Surgical Pathology*, (3rd Edition), Elsevier
- Lester DR. Thompson MD (2018) *Head and Neck Pathology: A Volume in the Series: Foundations in Diagnostic Pathology* (2nd Edition), Elsevier

Oral Lesions

- Brad W. Neville DDS, Douglas D. Damm DDS, Carl M. Allen DDS MSD, Angela C. Chi DMD (2015) *Oral and Maxillofacial Pathology*, (1st South Asia Edition), Elsevier
- B Sivapathasundharam (2016), *Shafer's Textbook of Oral Pathology*, (8th edition). Elsevier

CNS Lesions

- Matthew J. Schniederjan, Daniel J. Brat (2011), *Biopsy Interpretation of the Central Nervous System (Biopsy Interpretation Series)*, Wolters Kluwer
- Seth Love, Arie Perry, James Ironside, Herbert Budka, (2015), Greenfield's *Neuropathology*, (9th Edition)

Ophthalmic Lesions

- Gottfried OH Naumann, L Holbach, FE Kruse (2010), *Applied Pathology for Ophthalmic Microsurgeons*, (1st Edition), Springer

Spectrum of Breast Lesions

- Stuart J. Schnitt, Laura C. Collins (2012), *Biopsy Interpretation of the Breast (Biopsy Interpretation Series*, (2nd Edition), Wolters Kluwer
- Syed A. Hoda, Edi Brogi, Frederick C. Koerner, Paul Peter Rosen, (2014), *Rosen's Breast Pathology*, (4th Edition), Wolters Kluwer

Lesions of the Lung

- Saul Suster, Cesar A. Moran (2012), *Biopsy Interpretation of the Lung (Biopsy Interpretation Series)*, (1st Edition) Wolters Kluwer
- Bryan Corrin, Andrew G. Nicholson MA, (2011), *Pathology of the Lungs*, (3rd Edition), Churchill Livingston, Elsevier

Approach to Gastrointestinal Biopsies and Case Files of GIT Lesions

- Elizabeth A. Montgomery, Lysandra Voltaggio (Vol 1 2017 and Vol 2 2012), *Biopsy Interpretation of the Gastrointestinal Tract Mucosa*, (Vol 1 3rd Edition and Vol 2 2nd Edition), Wolters Kluwer
- Robert D. Odze, John R. Goldblum (2014), *Surgical Pathology of the GI Tract, Liver, Biliary Tract and Pancreas*, (3rd Edition), Elsevier

Histological Approach to Hepatobiliary Lesions

- Robert D. Odze, John R. Goldblum (2014), *Surgical Pathology of the GI Tract, Liver, Biliary Tract and Pancreas*, (3rd Edition), Elsevier
- Stephen A. Geller, Lydia M. Petrovic (2009), *Biopsy Interpretation of the Liver (Biopsy Interpretation Series)*, (2nd Edition), Wolters Kluwer

Patterns in Pancreatic and Gallbladder Lesions

- Robert D. Odze, John R. Goldblum (2014), *Surgical Pathology of the GI Tract, Liver, Biliary Tract and Pancreas*, (3rd Edition), Elsevier
- Ralph H. Hruban Martha Bishop Pitman, David S. Klimstra (2007), *Tumors of the Pancreas (AFIP Atlas of Tumor Pathology, Series 4,)*

Medical Renal Disease

- J. Charles Jennette, Vivette D. D'Agati, Jean L. Olson, Fred G. Silva, (2014), *Heptinstall's Pathology of the Kidney*, (7th Edition), Wolters Kluwer
- Xin J. Zhou, Zoltan Laszik, Tibor Nadasdy, Vivette D'Agati, Fred G. Silva, (2009), *Silva's Diagnostic Renal Pathology*, (2nd Edition), Cambridge

Pathologic Lesions of Kidneys, Urethra and Urinary Bladder

- Victor Reuter Jonathan I. Epstein Victor E. Reuter Mahul B, Amin Mahul B. Amin (2016), *Biopsy Interpretation of the Bladder (Biopsy Interpretation Series)*, (3rd Edition), Wolters Kluwer
- Ximing Yang, (2014) *Atlas of Practical Genitourinary Pathology*, Mc Graw Hill

Male Genital Tract Lesions including Prostate

- EPSTEIN, (2015), *Biopsy Interpretation of the Prostate (Biopsy Interpretation Series)*, (5th Edition), Wolters Kluwer
- Jae Y. Ro, David J. Grignon, Alberto G. Ayala (1996), *Atlas of Surgical Pathology of the Male Reproductive Tract: A Volume in the Atlases in Diagnostic Surgical Pathology Series*, (1st Edition), Saunders

Diseases of the Female Genital Tract

- Robert J. Kurman, Lora Hedrick Ellenson, Brigitte M. Ronnett (2019), *Blaustein's Pathology of the Female Genital Tract*, (7th Edition), Springer
- Malpica A, (2015), *Biopsy Interpretation of the Uterine Cervix and Corpus*, (2nd Edition), Wolters Kluwer

Soft Tissue Tumors and Tumor-like Lesions

- John R. Goldblum, Sharon W. Weiss, Andrew L. Folpe, (2013), *Enzinger and Weiss's Soft Tissue Tumors*, (6th Edition), Elsevier
- Markku Miettinen, *Modern Soft Tissue Pathology: Tumors and Non-Neoplastic Conditions*, (1st Edition), Cambridge

Lesions of the Bone and Joint

- G. Petur Nielsen, Andrew E Rosenberg, (2017), *Diagnostic Pathology: Bone*, (2nd Edition), Elsevier
- Bullough (2009), *Orthopaedic Pathology*, (5th Edition), Elsevier

Skin Lesions

- Elder, (2019), *Lever's Histopathology of the Skin*, (11th Edition), Wolters Kluwer
- Calonje (2011), *McKee's Pathology of the Skin*, (4th Edition), Elsevier

Non-Neoplastic Lesions of the Lymph Node and Diagnostic Approach to Lymphoma

- Harry L. Ioachim, L. Jeffrey Medeiros (2008), *Ioachim's Lymph Node Pathology*, (4th Edition), Wolters Kluwer
- L. Jeffrey Medeiros Roberto N. Miranda, (2017), *Diagnostic Pathology: Lymph Nodes and Extranodal Lymphomas*, (2nd Edition), Elsevier

Endocrine Pathology

- Boerner, (2012) *Biopsy Interpretation of the Thyroid*, (2nd Edition), Wolters Kluwer
- Vania Nosé, (2018), *Diagnostic Pathology: Endocrine*, (2nd Edition), Elsevier

Pap Smear—Gynecological Cytology

- Ritu Nayar, David C. Wilbur (2015), *The Bethesda System for Reporting Cervical Cytology*, (3rd Edition), Springer
- Pranab Dey, (2017) *Handbook of Cervical Cytology Special Emphasis on Liquid-Based Cytology*, (1st Edition), Jaypee

Cytology Slide Case Discussion Part I and Part II

- Svante R. Orell AM ML, Gregory F. Sterrett MB, (2011), *Orell and Sterrett's Fine Needle Aspiration Cytology*, 5th Edition, Churchill Livingston
- Koss L.G., (2018), *Koss Diagnostic Cytology and its Histopathologic Bases*, 5th Edition, Wolters Kluwer

Haematology

- John P. Greer, Daniel A. Arber, Bertil E. Glader, Alan F. List, Robert T. Means, Frixos Paraskevas, George M. Rodgers, John Foerster (2013), *Wintrobe's Clinical Hematology*, 13th Edition, Wolters Kluwer
- Barbara J. Bain, David M. Clark, Bridget S. Wilkins (2019), *Bone Marrow Pathology*, 5th Edition, Wiley-Blackwell
- Barbara J Bain (2017), *Dacie and Louis Practical Hematology*, 11th Edition, Elsevier Health - UK

Approach to Bleeding Disorders

- Barbara J Bain (2017), *Dacie and Louis Practical Hematology*, 11th Edition, Elsevier Health - UK
- Nigel S. Key, Michael Makris. David Lillicrap (2017) *Practical Hemostasis and Thrombosis*, 3rd Edition, Wiley-Blackwel

Automation in Haematology and Clinical Pathology

- Barbara J Bain (2017), *Dacie and Louis Practical Hematology*, 11th Edition, Elsevier Health - UK
- Godkar PB (2005), *Text book of Medical Laboratory Technology* 3rd Edition, Bhalani Publishing House

Component Preparation and Therapy/Blood Bank—Laboratory Procedures

- Transfusion Medicine Technical Manual, Directorate General of Health Services, Government of India
- Technical Manual, AABB, sixteenth edition

Immunohistochemistry

- David J Dabbs MD (2018) *Diagnostic Immunohistochemistry: Theranostic and Genomic Applications*, 5th Edition, , Elsevier

Autopsy Highlights

- Dhaneshwar Lanjewar, Pradeep Vaideeswar (2017), *Autopsy Practices*, 1st Edition, Jaypee Brothers Medical Publishers

Histotechniques/Important Histochemical Stains

- Kim S Suvarna MBBS BSc FRCP FRCPath , Christopher Layton PhD, John D. *Bancroft (2018), Bancroft's Theory and Practice of Histological Techniques*, 8th Edition , Elsevier

Flow Cytometry

- Doyen T. Nguyen ,Lawrence W. Diamond ,Raul C. Braylan (2007), *Flow Cytometry in Hematopathology: A Visual Approach to Data Analysis and Interpretation*, 2nd Edition, Humana
- Tsieh Sun (2012), *Flow Cytometry, Immunohistochemistry, and Molecular Genetics for Hematologic Neoplasms*, 2nd Edition, Lippincott Williams and Wilkins

Karyotyping—Basic Essentials

- Linda R. Adkison PhD (2011), *Elsevier's Integrated Review Genetics: With Student Consult Online Access*, 2nd Edition, Saunders

Fluorescence *in situ* Hybridization (FISH)

- Thomas S.K. Wan (2016), *Cancer Cytogenetics: Methods and Protocols (Methods in Molecular Biology)*, 1st Edition. Humana
- Thomas Liehr (2018), *Fluorescence in Situ Hybridization (FISH): Application Guide (Springer Protocols Handbooks)*, 2nd Edition , Springer

Molecular Pathology : Basics

- Mohammad A. Vasef MD , Aaron Auerbach MD MPH (2015), Diagnostic Pathology: Molecular Oncology,1st Edition, Elsevier
- William B. Coleman, Gregory J. Tsongalis (2010), Essential Concepts in Molecular Pathology ,1st Edition, Academic Press

Cell Culture and Tissue Banking Techniques

- George Galea (2014), *Essentials of Tissue Banking, 1st Edition*, Springer
- Dusko Ilic (2016), Stem Cell Banking (Stem Cell Biology and Regenerative Medicine), 1st Edition, Springer

Quality Control in Histopathology

- Iyengar JN. Quality control in the histopathology laboratory: An overview with stress on the need for a structured national external quality assessment scheme. Indian J Pathol Microbiol 2009; 52: 1–5

Quality Control in Hematology/Clinical Pathology

- Barbara J Bain (2017), Dacie and Louis Practical Hematology, 11th Edition, Elsevier Health - UK
- Godkar P.B (2005), Text book of Medical Laboratory Technology,3rd Edition, Bhalani Publishing House.